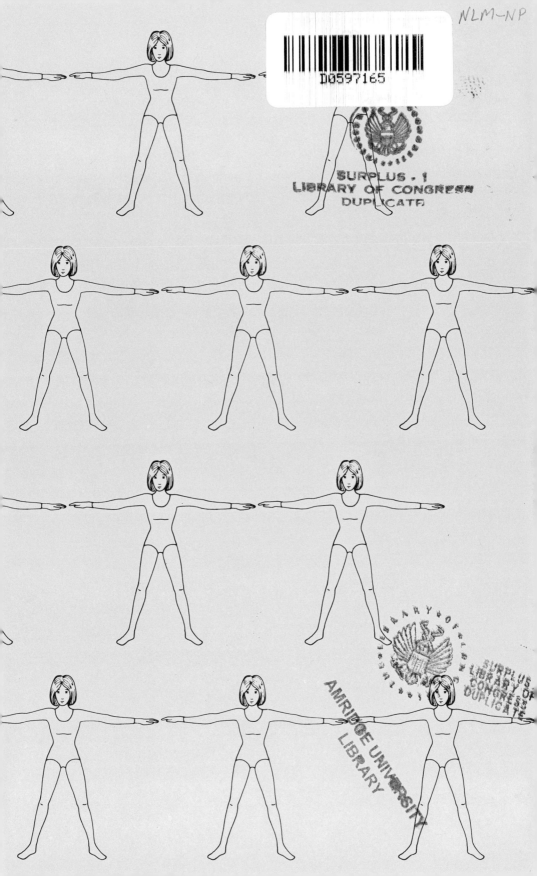

EVERYWOMAN'S HEALTH

The Complete Guide to Body and Mind

EVERYWOMAN'S HEALTH

The Complete Guide to Body and Mind

Revised Edition

By 17 Women Doctors

June Jackson Christmas, M.D. • Elizabeth B. Connell, M.D.

Frances Drew, M.D. • Barbara Gastel, M.D. and Maureen Mylander

Toby Graham, M.D. • Mary Jane Gray, M.D. • Christine E. Haycock, M.D.

Dorothy Hicks, M.D. • Adele Hofmann, M.D. • Lonny Myers, M.D.

Carol Nadelson, M.D. • Margaret A. Nelsen, M.D. • Malkah Notman, M.D.

Kathryn Schrotenboer, M.D. • Kathryn Stephenson, M.D.

Louise Tyrer, M.D. • Joan J. Zilbach, M.D.

DOUGLASS S. THOMPSON, M.D., CONSULTING EDITOR

ILLUSTRATED BY LEONARD D. DANK

R A
778
.E93
1980

Doubleday & Company, Inc.
Garden City, New York

Library of Congress Cataloging in Publication Data
Main entry under title:

Everywoman's health.

    Includes bibliographies and index.
    1. Women—Health and hygiene. 2. Medicine, Popular—Dictionaries. I. Christ-
mas, June Jackson. II. Thompson, Douglass S. [DNLM: 1. Gynecology—Popular
works. WP120 E94]
RA778.E93   613'.04244

ISBN: 0-385-15567-0

Library of Congress Catalog Card Number 79-6095

Contributors

Consulting Editor DOUGLASS S. THOMPSON, M.D.
Clinical Professor of Obstetrics and Gynecology and Clinical Associate Professor of Community Medicine, University of Pittsburgh School of Medicine; Clinical Professor, Department of Health Services Administration, University of Pittsburgh Graduate School of Public Health; Medical Director, Ob-Gyn Medical Care Center, Magee-Womens Hospital, Pittsburgh, Pennsylvania

Illustrator LEONARD D. DANK
Consultant Medical Illustrator, St. Luke's–Roosevelt Hospital Center and Woman's Hospital, New York City

Authors

JUNE JACKSON CHRISTMAS, M.D., Past President, American Public Health Association

ELIZABETH B. CONNELL, M.D., Associate Professor of Obstetrics and Gynecology, Northwestern University School of Medicine, Chicago, Illinois

FRANCES DREW, M.D., M.P.H., Professor of Community Medicine and Associate Dean for Student Affairs, University of Pittsburgh School of Medicine, Pittsburgh, Pennsylvania

BARBARA GASTEL, M.D., M.P.H., National Institute on Aging, National Institutes of Health, Bethesda, Maryland

TOBY GRAHAM, M.D., Assistant Professor of Medicine, University of Pittsburgh School of Medicine, Pittsburgh, Pennsylvania

MARY JANE GRAY, M.D., Professor of Obstetrics and Gynecology, University of North Carolina Medical School, Chapel Hill, North Carolina

CHRISTINE E. HAYCOCK, M.D., Associate Professor of Surgery, New Jersey Colleges of Medicine and Dentistry, New Jersey Medical School, Newark, New Jersey

DOROTHY HICKS, M.D., Professor of Obstetrics and Gynecology, University of Miami School of Medicine; Director, Rape Treatment Center, Jackson Memorial Hospital, Miami, Florida

ADELE HOFMANN, M.D., Associate Professor of Pediatrics and Director, Adolescent Medical Unit, New York University Medical Center–Bellevue Hospital, New York City

HELENE MACLEAN, medical writer

LONNY MYERS, M.D., Director of Sexual Health Services, Midwest Population Center, Chicago, Illinois

MAUREEN MYLANDER, National Institute on Aging, National Institutes of Health, Bethesda, Maryland

CAROL NADELSON, M.D., Professor of Psychiatry, Tufts University School of Medicine; Vice Chairman, Department of Psychiatry, Tufts–New England Medical Center, Boston, Massachusetts

MARGARET A. NELSEN, M.D., Associate Director for Utilization Control, Surveillance Utilization Review and Education, EDS Federal, Raleigh, North Carolina; Assistant Professor of Surgery, 1975–1979, University of North Carolina School of Medicine, Chapel Hill, North Carolina

MALKAH NOTMAN, M.D., Associate Clinical Professor of Psychiatry, Harvard Medical School; Psychiatrist, Beth Israel Hospital, Boston, Massachusetts

KATHRYN SCHROTENBOER, M.D., Assistant Attending Physician, Obstetrics and Gynecology, New York Hospital–Cornell Medical Center; Clinical Instructor, Cornell Medical School, New York City

KATHRYN STEPHENSON, M.D., Plastic Surgeon, Santa Barbara Cottage Hospital, Santa Barbara, California

LOUISE TYRER, M.D., Vice-President for Medical Affairs, Planned Parenthood–World Population

JOAN J. ZILBACH, M.D., Associate Clinical Professor of Psychiatry, Tufts University School of Medicine, Boston, Massachusetts; Co-Director, Family Therapy and Research Program, Judge Baker Guidance Center, Harvard Medical School, Boston, Massachusetts

Contents

PART ONE   GUIDE TO TOTAL HEALTH

3   The Healthy Woman   JUNE JACKSON CHRISTMAS, M.D.

KNOW HOW YOUR BODY FUNCTIONS · The Skeletal Muscular System: The Framework · The Circulatory System: Movement of Blood · The Respiratory System: Supply of Oxygen · The Digestive System: Nourishment · The Urinary System: Removal of Waste · The Nervous System: Communication and Control · The Endocrine System: Internal Control and Balance · The Reproductive System: Perpetuation of the Species · The Menstrual Cycle · The Relationship Between Physical and Mental Health · TAKE RESPONSIBILITY FOR YOUR OWN HEALTH · Primary Prevention: Prevention of Illness · Secondary Prevention: Early Diagnosis and Treatment · Tertiary Prevention: Rehabilitation · Economic Benefits of Prevention · BE AN ACTIVE, EQUAL PARTNER IN HEALTH CARE · Holistic Health · Self-Care · Improving Health Services

36   Nutrition and Weight   TOBY GRAHAM, M.D.

THE NUTRIENT CONTENT OF FOOD · Protein · Carbohydrates · Fat · Vitamins · Minerals · Water and Fiber · Balanced Nutrition · SELECTION OF FOODS FOR BALANCED NUTRITION · Food Groups · Food Labeling · Food Additives · Fast Foods · WEIGHT · Determining Ideal Body Weight · Calorie Requirements to Maintain IBW · NUTRITIONAL NEEDS AT SPECIAL AGES AND STAGES · Nutrition in Pregnancy · Nutrition When Breast-Feeding · Nutrition for the Older Woman · OBESITY · Diet · Exercise · Diet Pills · Group Therapy and Behavior Modification · ANOREXIA NERVOSA

66   Fitness   CHRISTINE E. HAYCOCK, M.D.

BENEFITS OF PHYSICAL FITNESS · YOUR BODY'S ENERGY · THE FIRST STEP—A PHYSICAL EXAMINATION · SUITABLE CLOTHES AND PROPER EQUIPMENT · IN-

JURIES · DEVELOPING A FITNESS PROGRAM TO CONDITION YOUR BODY · THE EXERCISE ROUTINE · Routines Suitable for Various Age Groups · Exercises on the Job

102   Sexual Health   LONNY MYERS, M.D.

SEXUAL STAGES · Born Free—Infancy and Childhood · Adolescence · Adulthood · SEX AND HEALTH CARE · LOVE · SELF-RESPECT · FEMALE SEXUAL RESPONSE · Physiological Response · Questions Often Asked About Orgasm · SEXUAL ENRICHMENT FOR COUPLES · SEXUAL THERAPY · Sexual Dysfunction—Physical Conditions · Sexual Dysfunction—Psychological Causes · SEX AND NONSEX FOR SINGLE WOMEN · EXTRAMARITAL SEX · ALTERNATIVES IN SEXUAL EXPRESSION · Masturbation · Sexual Fantasies · Lesbianism and Bisexuality · SEX AND EDUCATION FOR PARENTHOOD BY CHOICE

133   Contraception and Abortion   ELIZABETH B. CONNELL, M.D.

RISK-BENEFIT RATIO · SELECTION OF METHODS · HORMONAL METHODS—FEMALE · Major Severe Side Effects · Contraindications · Minor Adverse Side Effects · Beneficial Side Effects · Injectables · "Morning After" Pill · HORMONAL METHODS—MALE · INTRAUTERINE CONTRACEPTIVES · Currently Marketed IUDs · Side Effects · Contraindications · BARRIER CONTRACEPTIVES · Diaphragm · Condom · Cervical Cap · Methods in Combination · NATURAL FAMILY PLANNING · COITUS INTERRUPTUS · LACTATION · STERILIZATION · Female Sterilization · Male Sterilization · Current Issues · INDUCED ABORTION · Techniques · Counseling · AVAILABILITY AND FURTHER DEVELOPMENT OF EFFECTIVE CONTRACEPTION

165   Pregnancy and Childbirth   KATHRYN SCHROTENBOER, M.D.

DECIDING TO HAVE A BABY · CONCEPTION AND EARLY DEVELOPMENT · DIAGNOSIS OF PREGNANCY · Signs and Symptoms · Pregnancy Tests · WHO WILL DELIVER YOUR BABY? · Obstetrician-Gynecologist · Family Practitioner · Nurse-Midwife · Lay Midwife · WHERE WILL YOU HAVE YOUR BABY? · Hospital Delivery · Home Delivery · Maternity Center Delivery · HEALTH CARE DURING NORMAL PREGNANCY · Emotional Changes · Diet · Smoking, Alcohol, and Drugs · Activity · COMPLICATIONS OF PREGNANCY · Bleeding and Spontaneous Abortion · Ectopic Pregnancy · Pre-eclampsia and Eclampsia · Chronic and Genetic Diseases · Infections · Rh Disease · Intrauterine Fetal Death · Hydatidiform Mole · EVALUATING FETAL HEALTH · Amniocentesis · Sonography · Fetal Monitors · Chemical and Hormone Studies · LABOR AND DELIVERY · Natural Childbirth · First Stage of Labor—Dilatation of the Cervix · Anesthesia · Second Stage of Labor—Delivery · Third Stage of Labor—Afterbirth · CESAREAN SECTION · AFTER THE DELIVERY · Rooming-in · The "Baby Blues" · Physical Recovery · Breast-Feeding

206   **Infertility**   KATHRYN SCHROTENBOER, M.D.

CAUSES OF MALE INFERTILITY · TESTS FOR MALE INFERTILITY · TREATMENT
FOR MALE INFERTILITY · CAUSES OF FEMALE INFERTILITY · TESTS FOR FEMALE
INFERTILITY · Basal Body Temperatures · Endometrial Biopsy · Hormone
Tests · Hysterosalpingogram · Rubin Test · Postcoital Test · Laparoscopy ·
TREATMENT FOR FEMALE INFERTILITY · ARTIFICIAL INSEMINATION

221   **Gynecologic Diseases and Treatment**   MARY JANE GRAY, M.D.

FINDING CAUSES OF COMMON PROBLEMS · History · Pelvic Examination · Pap
Smear · X-ray, Sonography, Laparoscopy, and Colposcopy · Biopsy · PROB-
LEMS AND DISEASES · Menstrual Problems · Other Vaginal Bleeding · Lower
Abdominal Pain · Vaginal Discharge · Prolapse of the Uterus · Infections ·
Tumors · Endocrine Problems · TYPES OF GYNECOLOGIC TREATMENT · Treat-
ment of Infection · Hormone Therapy · Cautery · Surgery · Radiation Ther-
apy · Chemotherapy · Counseling

245   **Sexually Transmissible Diseases**   LOUISE TYRER, M.D.

WHAT WOMEN NEED TO KNOW ABOUT STD · DESCRIPTION OF SPECIFIC STDS ·
Chancroid · Chlamydial Infections · Cytomegalovirus (CMV) · Fungal In-
fections (Tinea Cruris) · Gonorrhea · Granuloma Inguinale · Hemophilus
Vaginalis (HV); Corynebacterium Vaginale · Herpes Simplex Virus Infec-
tion · Molluscum Contagiosum · Pelvic Inflammatory Disease (PID) · Pubic
Lice · Scabies · Syphilis · Trichomoniasis · Vaginitis (Nonspecific) · Vene-
real Warts (Condyloma Acuminata) · Yeast Infections (Monilia) · OTHER
STDS AND SEXUAL PRACTICES · Amebiasis · Shigellosis · Viral Hepatitis

265   **Breast Care**   MARGARET A. NELSEN, M.D.

GROWTH AND DEVELOPMENT OF THE BREAST · BREAST SELF-EXAMINATION ·
EVERYDAY BREAST CARE · BREAST DISORDERS · Anatomical Abnormalities and
Endocrine Dysfunction · Normal Physiologic Changes · Benign Cysts and
Tumors · Infections · Malignant Disease · DIAGNOSIS · TREATMENT · Non-
malignant Disorders · Breast Cancer

293   **Cosmetic Surgery**   KATHRYN STEPHENSON, M.D.

DECIDING TO UNDERGO COSMETIC SURGERY · CONSULTATION WITH THE COSMETIC
SURGEON · SURGICAL PROCEDURES · Rhinoplasty · Rhytidoplasty · Abrasion,
Chemosurgery, and Collagen Injection · Maxilloplasty, Mandibuloplasty, Mentoplasty, and Malarplasty · Blepharoplasty · Eyebrow Lift · Otoplasty · Mammaplasty · Lipectomy · Spider Hemangioma and Capillary Varicosities

318   Drugs, Alcohol, and Tobacco—Their Use and Abuse
ADELE HOFMANN, M.D.

DEFINITIONS · THE UNIVERSALITY OF DRUG USE · KNOW YOUR FACTS · WOMEN AND DRUGS TODAY · WHAT YOU SHOULD KNOW ABOUT DRUGS IN GENERAL · How Drugs Are Taken · Frequency, Strength, and Purity of Contents · Experience and Environment · Individual Vulnerability to Drug Abuse · Effect of Availability, Popularity, and Acceptance of Drug Use · DRUGS IN COMMON USE TODAY · Depressants · Stimulants · Hallucinogens · Narcotics · Tobacco · Miscellaneous Drugs · DRUGS AND PREGNANCY · Sedatives and Tranquilizers · Alcohol · Stimulants · Hallucinogens · Narcotics · Tobacco · SIGNS OF TROUBLE · Motivation for Help · Treatment · Sources of Information · DRUG ABUSE EMERGENCIES · PERSONAL DECISIONS ABOUT DRUGS

362   Rape and Spouse Abuse—Two Crimes of Violence
DOROTHY HICKS, M.D.

SEXUAL ASSAULT: FORCIBLE RAPE · History · The Startling Facts: Current Statistics · Myths About Rape · Protecting Yourself · What You Should Do If Attacked · Treatment · Sexual Abuse of Children · SPOUSE ABUSE

383   Your Mind and Feelings—Mental and Emotional Health
JOAN J. ZILBACH, M.D.

DEFINITION OF MENTAL HEALTH · Normal Tension and Anxiety · Universal Stresses—Individual and Family Life Cycles · MECHANISMS TO MAINTAIN EQUILIBRIUM · IMPAIRED MENTAL HEALTH · Stress Overload · Effects of Overload—Signs of Imbalance · Neurosis · Severe Mental Illness and Psychosis · The Need for Help · TYPES OF HELP · Psychotherapy · Drug Therapy · Hospitalization for Mental Illness · Self-Help and Support Groups

403   Changing Roles—Women from 18 to 40   CAROL NADELSON, M.D.

RIGIDITY OF ROLE EXPECTATIONS · CHANGING ATTITUDES, VALUES, AND BEHAVIORS · THE SINGLE WOMAN · THE MARRIED WOMAN · THE DECISION TO HAVE CHILDREN · THE CAREER-FAMILY DILEMMA · DIVORCE · NONTRADITIONAL LIFE STYLES · THE FUTURE

421   Midlife Transitions   MALKAH NOTMAN, M.D.

WHAT IS MIDDLE AGE? · WOMEN, MIDDLE AGE, AND CHILDREN · MENOPAUSE · Estrogen Replacement Therapy · MIDLIFE FAMILY ISSUES · Departure of Children · Elderly Parents · Years Alone · Returning to Work and School

442   Aging Healthfully—Your Body   BARBARA GASTEL, M.D., M.P.H.

AGE-RELATED CHANGES IN PARTS OF THE BODY · Skin · Eyes · Ears · Teeth and Gums · Nervous System · Heart and Blood Vessels · Lungs · Digestive System · Urinary and Reproductive Systems · Sexual Response · Bones and Joints · Feet · Diabetes · Infection · GOOD MEDICAL CARE · MEDICATION · EXERCISE · SAFETY

466   Aging Healthfully—Your Mind and Spirit   MAUREEN MYLANDER

ECONOMIC, SOCIAL, AND PSYCHOLOGICAL PROBLEMS RELATED TO OLD AGE · Income · Housing and Transportation · Crime · Widowhood · Social Supports · Sex and Sensuality · Self-image · Depression · Sleep Problems · Drugs and Alcohol · Suicide · Psychotherapy and Personal Growth · ADAPTATION · Earning Power · Learning Power · Networks · Loving · Group Living · Exercise · Life Work · Leverage · Looking Ahead

488   You, Your Doctors, and the Health Care System
FRANCES DREW, M.D., M.P.H.

CHOOSING YOUR DOCTORS · Choosing a Primary Physician · Payment Plans · Hospital Outpatient Departments · Choosing a Specialist · BEING A WOMAN AND A PATIENT · EMERGENCY CARE · HOSPITALS · WHAT YOU HAVE A RIGHT TO EXPECT FROM YOUR PHYSICIAN · WHAT YOU SHOULD NOT EXPECT FROM YOUR PHYSICIAN · WHAT YOUR PHYSICIAN HAS A RIGHT TO EXPECT FROM YOU · THE COMMUNITY OF HEALTH CARE

511   PART TWO ENCYCLOPEDIA OF HEALTH AND MEDICAL TERMS

737   Appendixes

Suggested Health Examinations for Well Women · Immunization Guide · Common Medical Terms · How to Read a Prescription · Commonly Prescribed Brand Name Drugs and Generic Equivalents · Directory of Health Services

752   Index

List of Illustrations

PART ONE

Skeletal System 6–7

Voluntary Muscular System 8

Circulatory System 9

Respiratory System 11

Digestive System 12–13

Urinary System 16

Nervous System 18

Endocrine System 20

Female Reproductive System 22–23

Male Reproductive System 24

Menstrual Cycle 27

Fitness Exercises 78–96

Common Contraceptive
  Methods 135

Intrauterine Contraceptive
  Devices 145

Barrier Contraceptives 151

Permanent Contraceptives:
  Tubal Sterilization and
  Vasectomy 157

Dilatation and Evacuation 160

Female Genital Tract:
  Ovulation, Fertilization,
  and Implantation 168

Uterine–Fetal Relationship 170

Weight Gain During Pregnancy 178

Amniocentesis 190

Stages of Labor 197

Positions of the Fetus 200

Causes of Male Infertility 208

Causes of Female Infertility 210–11

Tests for Infertility 214–15

Vaginal Examination 223

Bimanual Examination of
  Uterus 224

Abdominal and Vaginal Hysterectomy 240

Pelvis after Hysterectomy 241

Development of the Breast 268

Cross-Section of the Breast 269

How to Examine Your Breasts 272–73

Cystic Disease 278

Signs of Breast Cancer 282

Growth of Breast Cancer 283

Cosmetic Surgery of the Nose 300

Cosmetic Surgery of the Face 303

Cosmetic Surgery of the Breast 311

Emotions and the Body 392

A Woman's Body: Structure and Functions
A 16-page full-color portfolio

Part two

Anemia   524
Angina Pectoris   527
Antibodies   529
Appendicitis   532
Arthritis   533
Atherosclerosis   537
Biopsy   541
Cystitis   542
Blood Composition   543
Bursitis   551
Chest Pains   558
Heredity   561
Colitis   563
Colostomy   564
Diabetes   577
Slipped Disc   583
Ear   589
Ectopic Pregnancy   591
Endometriosis   594
Episiotomy   596
Eye   599
Gallbladder   607
Glaucoma   610
Goiter   612
Gonorrhea Pathway   613

Headache   617
Heart   621
Heart Attack   622
Heimlich Maneuver   624
Hemorrhoids   626
Hernias   628
Hymen   632
Immunology   635
Kidney   642
Knee Disorders   643
External Eye   644
Mouth and Larynx   645
Liver   648
Lymph Nodes   651
Medic Alert   653
Pap Smear   673
Prolapse of Uterus   684
Rh Factor   691
Sex-Linked Abnormalities   699
Sickle Cell Trait   701
Skin   703
Stroke   710
Ulcer   722
Uterine Fibroids   725
Vocal Cords   731

Acknowledgments

Many people gave generously of their time during the development of this book. While the facts and opinions offered in *Everywoman's Health* reflect the individual authors' viewpoints, both they and the editors are grateful to the following people for their advice, information, and encouragement:

Tenley Albright, M.D., New England Baptist Hospital, Boston, Massachusetts; Ann W. Burgess, Ph.D., Boston College School of Nursing; Ronald A. Chez, M.D., Professor and Chairman, Department of Obstetrics and Gynecology, Pennsylvania State University; Bill Cohen, Editor, Haworth Press; Theodore Cooper, M.D., Ph.D., Dean, Cornell University Medical College; Harriet P. Dustan, M.D., Past President, American Heart Association; Penelope S. Easton, Ph.D., R.D., Miami, Florida; Andrea R. Fox and Kenneth S. Thompson II, students, Boston University School of Medicine; Michael J. Halberstam, M.D., Washington, D.C.; Pauline H. Hord, R.N., American Public Health Association; Mary C. Howell, M.D., Boston, Massachusetts; Detective Ellen King, Rape Crisis Program, Beth Israel Hospital, New York City; Dorothy C. Kolodner, R.D., M.S., Pittsburgh, Pennsylvania; Maggie Kuhn, National Convenor, Gray Panthers; Jim Lichtenberg and Laura Spechler, Council on Family Health, New York City; Richard Lincoln, Director of Publications, Alan Guttmacher Institute; Helene MacLean, medical writer; Frederick Martens, M.D., New York

Hospital–Cornell Medical Center; Edward T. Mazilauskas, Clayton & Edward Inc., New York City; Andra Medea, author; Sgt. Gladys Pollikoff, New York City Police Sex Crimes Unit; Betty Rollin, author; Jane Shure, Information Officer, National Institute on Aging; members of the Departments of Obstetrics–Gynecology and Community Medicine, University of Pittsburgh School of Medicine; Estelle Vappas, American Board of Plastic Surgery; and Carol Winograd, M.D., Stanford University Medical Center.

For hours of professional help and good humor during the preparation of manuscript and illustrations, we extend thanks to: Cathy Bakos, Cindy Godek, Carol Hill, and Regina Muraca, typists; Judith Kahn, copyeditor; Robin Markovits, assistant medical illustrator; Fran Gazze Nimeck, designer; and for their special contributions and support, thanks to Diana Klemin, Nancy Tuckerman, Jean Anne Vincent, Marjorie Goldstein, and the staff of Nelson Doubleday Books.

DOUGLASS S. THOMPSON, M.D., Consulting Editor

BARBARA S. GREENMAN, Project Editor

Part One

GUIDE TO TOTAL HEALTH

The Healthy Woman

JUNE JACKSON CHRISTMAS, M.D.

Past President, American Public Health Association

Health is a positive state—not merely the absence of disease. Yet, we often describe health in a negative way. We may consider ourselves healthy because, at the moment, we have no aches or pains and are not under the care of a doctor. But health is a condition of wellness, a state of physical, mental, and emotional well-being. Although this definition expresses an ideal, it suggests that our health is our most precious asset. It is too valuable to be described by what it is not. It is too important to be left entirely in the hands of others, whether they are doctors, advertisers, druggists, neighbors, or friends.

You are responsible for your health. It is up to you to develop the knowledge and attitudes that enable you to recognize and promote this state of well-being, to maintain your health and when necessary, to help regain it.

There are three things you can do for your health.

- Know how your body functions, what factors influence health, and how to deal with them.
- Take responsibility for your health and make wise decisions to promote health.
- Be an active, equal partner in health care.

KNOW HOW YOUR BODY FUNCTIONS

Many people have described the body as a machine, yet this is too simple a comparison. The body is a living, dynamic organism, one that is constantly replacing or repairing its old or damaged parts. It consists of many systems which are interrelated and dependent upon each other for effective functioning. A weakness in one system frequently leads to malfunction in others. The function of the brain and nervous system affects all parts of the body. The pituitary gland influences growth, reproduction, metabolism, and a number of other activities, including uterine contractions at childbirth. These interrelationships are certainly too complex to be compared to a machine!

The brief descriptions and illustrations that follow summarize how the systems of your body work. The Encyclopedia (pages 513–736) provides more detailed information about the organs or parts that comprise each system.

The Skeletal Muscular System: The Framework

Your skeletal muscular system forms the framework of your body. It consists of bones, muscles, tendons, ligaments, and joints. The skin can also be considered part of this system in that it constitutes part of the framework. These elements give the body its shape, enable the body to move, and protect the vital organs such as the heart and brain.

Muscles are attached to bones by tendons. The bones are held together by ligaments of connective tissue which allows movement between the bones when the muscles contract. Joints are the points at which two bones meet and are classified as hinge, pivot, or ball-and-socket, according to the kind of motion their structure allows. Joints of the skull are fixed, or nonmovable.

Muscles are composed of bundles of fibers that have the ability to contract in response to a complex system of electrochemical signals transmitted from the brain through the nervous system. All muscle fibers store fuel for activity in the form of glycogen, a sugar created by the body's metabolic process.

The approximately 600 muscles of the human body make up about half its total weight. They are divided into three types. The voluntary muscles normally are controlled by the conscious mind. The involuntary muscles control the functions of internal organs, such as the caliber of the arteries and the size of the pupils, via impulses arising automatically in the brain. The cardiac, or heart muscle (myocardium), is a third, distinct type.

The voluntary muscles move the skeletal and other parts of the body and maintain posture. When seen under a microscope these muscle fibers appear to be striped; thus they are referred to as striated muscles. These are the muscles we use to walk, to speak, to gesture. The state of partial contraction in which the voluntary muscles are held is called muscle tone. Exercise and proper nutrition are necessary to maintain tone and condition. If these muscles are not used regularly, they may become slack and atrophy. They are also subject to fatigue if extended use both depletes their supply of stored glycogen and causes a build-up of lactic acid.

The involuntary muscles function continually during respiration, digestion, and circulation. These muscles are not striated and are called smooth muscles. They do not atrophy when not used regularly. For example, the uterine muscle maintains the capacity to contract even if it is never used or is used only once or twice in a lifetime.

The cardiac muscle is unique in its composition. It is made up of partially striated fibers which contract and relax continuously through a lifetime. This muscle has its own "built in" nerve conduction system.

The skin, the largest organ of the body, completes the body framework. It contains the sense of touch, keeps fluids in and foreign bodies out, and helps to regulate temperature. Changes in the condition of the body and in emotional states are reflected in skin color, temperature, and moisture, for example, the flush of fever or embarrassment.

The Circulatory System: Movement of Blood

The circulatory system consists of the heart and a network of blood vessels throughout the body. As the pumping action of the heart moves the blood through the network, oxygen, nutrients, and other substances are distributed to all parts of the body. Perhaps the most surprising thing about the heart is not that it fails, but that it works as hard and as long as it does. It weighs only about a pound. If the pathways through which the blood circulates were laid out end to end, they would cover a distance of about 75,000 miles. In order to keep approximately 5 quarts of blood circulating through these pathways, the heart pumps about 8,000 quarts of blood every 24 hours and continues to do so over a life span—27,000 days or 75 years.

The heart, essentially a muscular pump, consists of four chambers, the left and right atria and left and right ventricles. Blood from each atrium flows into its corresponding ventricle. There is a valve between each atrium and ventricle (the tricuspid valve on the right and the mitral valve on the left) which prevents blood from flowing from the ventricle back to the atrium. The right atrium receives blood from the entire body except the lungs and contracts to pump it into the right ventricle. The right ventricle pumps blood into the pulmonary artery and then to the lungs. The left atrium receives blood from the lungs and pumps it into the left ventricle. The left ventricle pumps blood into the aorta and then to the rest of the body. There is a heart valve (pulmonic) at the junction of the right ventricle and the pulmonary artery and another (aortic) at the junction of the left ventricle and the aorta. These valves prevent the blood from flowing backward. Automatic nervous system impulses from the brain to a part of the heart called the sinoauricular node (the heart's pacemaker) control the

SKELETAL SYSTEM

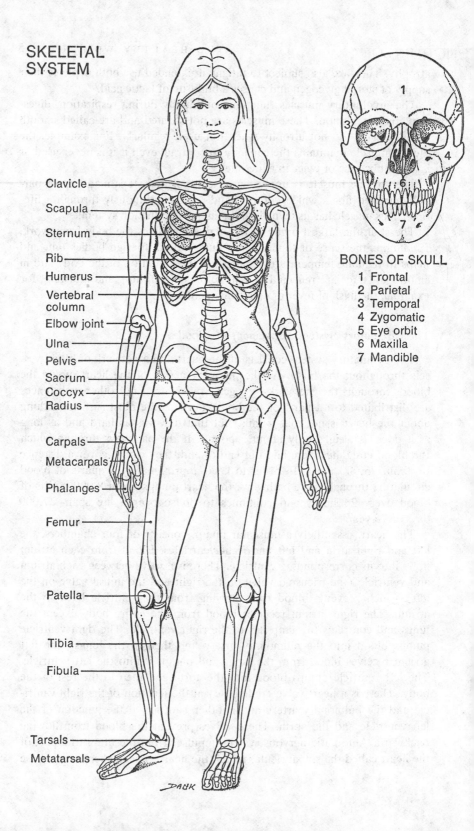

Clavicle

Scapula

Sternum

Rib

Humerus

Vertebral column

Elbow joint

Ulna

Pelvis

Sacrum

Coccyx

Radius

Carpals

Metacarpals

Phalanges

Femur

Patella

Tibia

Fibula

Tarsals

Metatarsals

BONES OF SKULL

1 Frontal
2 Parietal
3 Temporal
4 Zygomatic
5 Eye orbit
6 Maxilla
7 Mandible

DANK

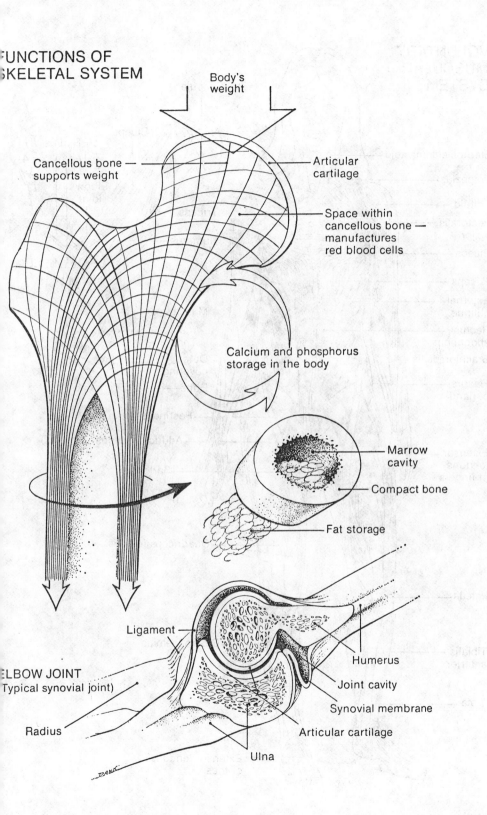

FUNCTIONS OF SKELETAL SYSTEM

Body's weight

Cancellous bone supports weight

Articular cartilage

Space within cancellous bone — manufactures red blood cells

Calcium and phosphorus storage in the body

Marrow cavity

Compact bone

Fat storage

Ligament

Humerus

ELBOW JOINT
(Typical synovial joint)

Joint cavity

Synovial membrane

Radius

Articular cartilage

Ulna

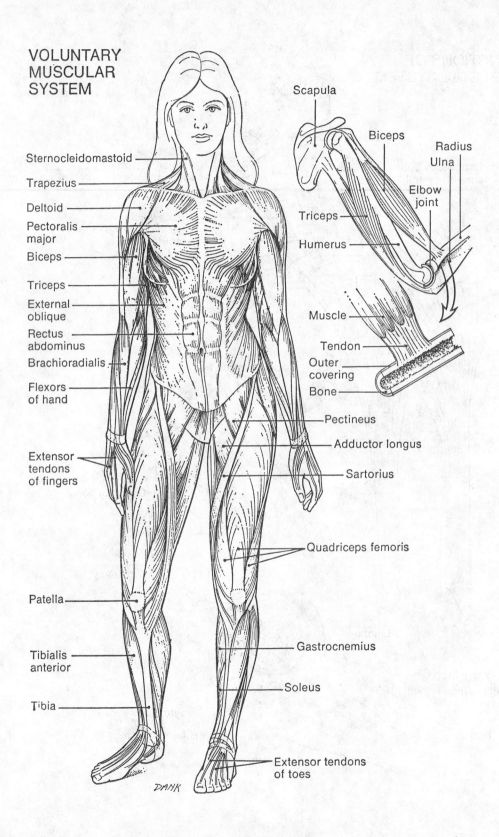

VOLUNTARY MUSCULAR SYSTEM

Scapula

Biceps

Radius
Ulna

Sternocleidomastoid

Trapezius

Deltoid

Triceps

Pectoralis major

Elbow joint

Biceps

Humerus

Triceps

External oblique

Rectus abdominus

Brachioradialis

Muscle

Tendon

Flexors of hand

Outer covering

Bone

Pectineus

Adductor longus

Sartorius

Extensor tendons of fingers

Quadriceps femoris

Patella

Gastrocnemius

Tibialis anterior

Soleus

Tibia

Extensor tendons of toes

DANK

CIRCULATORY SYSTEM

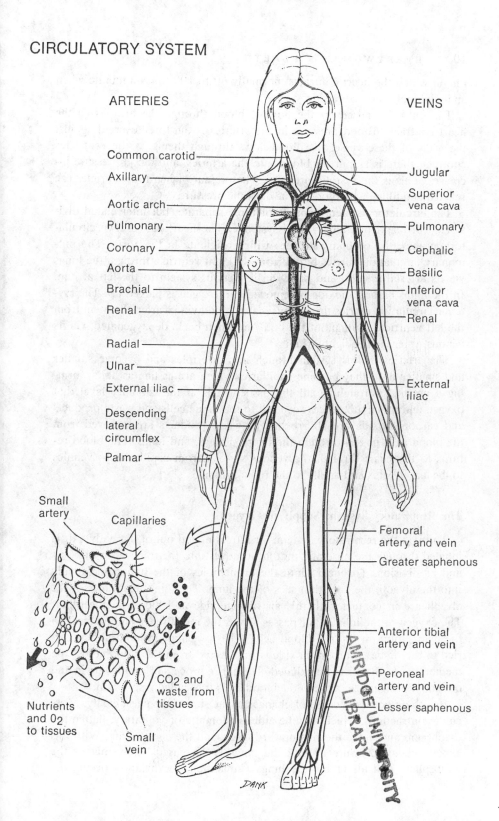

ARTERIES

VEINS

Common carotid

Axillary

Aortic arch

Pulmonary

Coronary

Aorta

Brachial

Renal

Radial

Ulnar

External iliac

Descending lateral circumflex

Palmar

Jugular

Superior vena cava

Pulmonary

Cephalic

Basilic

Inferior vena cava

Renal

External iliac

Small artery

Capillaries

Nutrients and O$_2$ to tissues

CO$_2$ and waste from tissues

Small vein

Femoral artery and vein

Greater saphenous

Anterior tibial artery and vein

Peroneal artery and vein

Lesser saphenous

DANK

rate at which the heart contracts, normally 60 to 100 times a minute when an individual is not exercising.

The pulse is caused by the flow of blood through the arteries as the heart contracts. Blood pressure in the arteries is the force exerted against the walls of these vessels as blood flows through them. As the ventricles contract, there is a spurt of blood into the arteries, and blood pressure increases. This is the systolic pressure. The pressure when the ventricles are relaxed and filling with blood is the diastolic pressure.

The circulatory system consists of three separate, but interrelated divisions: coronary, pulmonary, and systemic. The heart has its own circulatory system, the coronary arteries which originate in the aorta. The pulmonary circulation carries blood from the right ventricle through the lungs via its arterial system, and back via its venous system to the left atrium. In the lungs carbon dioxide is removed and oxygen is picked up. The systemic circulation carries this reoxygenated blood via its arterial system from the left ventricle throughout the body and then back, deoxygenated, via its venous system to the right atrium.

The arteries in this system branch into arterioles and become smaller and smaller until they become capillaries which are as fine as hairs, forming a network throughout all the tissues. It is at the capillary level that oxygen and other substances seep out to the tissue cells and waste products and carbon dioxide are absorbed. The waste products are removed from the blood as it passes through the liver, kidneys, and lungs. The blood returns to the heart through the venous system, from capillaries to venules to the larger veins and finally to the right atrium.

The Respiratory System: Supply of Oxygen

Through the respiratory system, air moves in and out of the body. Air is inhaled through the nose and mouth; it moves into the trachea (windpipe) and its divisions (bronchi) into the bronchioles of the lungs, and finally into the alveoli, the very thin sacs of the lung. The thin membranes of the alveoli are in contact with this air on one side and blood on the other. The oxygen in the inhaled air passes across the membranes and unites with the hemoglobin in the red blood cells. The oxygenated blood is then carried to the tissues. Carbon dioxide is transferred from the blood across the membranes to the air to be exhaled. The entire process of air moving in and out and the exchange between the blood and air is called respiration.

Breathing occurs because of changes in the size of the chest cavity. Muscular contractions, which may be either automatic or voluntary, flatten the diaphragm and move the ribs upward to expand the chest cavity. With this expansion, air pressure around the lungs is decreased below that of the atmosphere and air enters the lungs (inhalation). Exhalation occurs be-

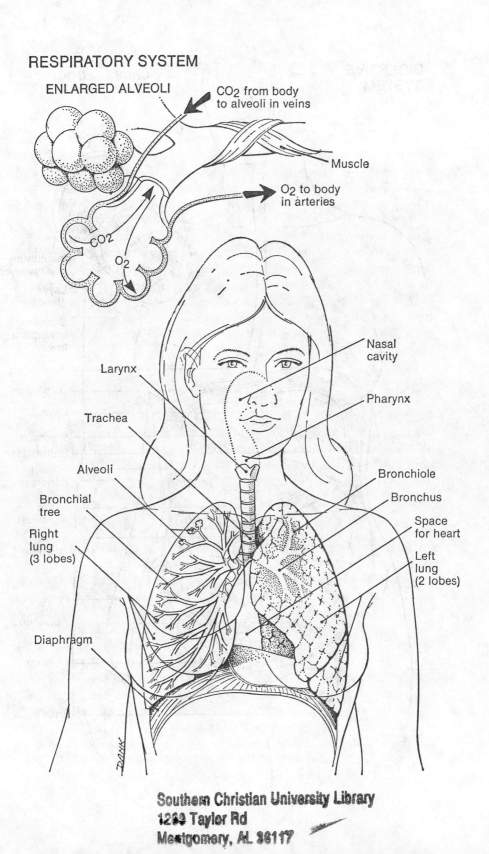

RESPIRATORY SYSTEM

ENLARGED ALVEOLI

CO₂ from body
to alveoli in veins

Muscle

O₂ to body
in arteries

CO2

O2

Larynx

Trachea

Alveoli

Bronchial
tree

Right
lung
(3 lobes)

Diaphragm

Nasal
cavity

Pharynx

Bronchiole

Bronchus

Space
for heart

Left
lung
(2 lobes)

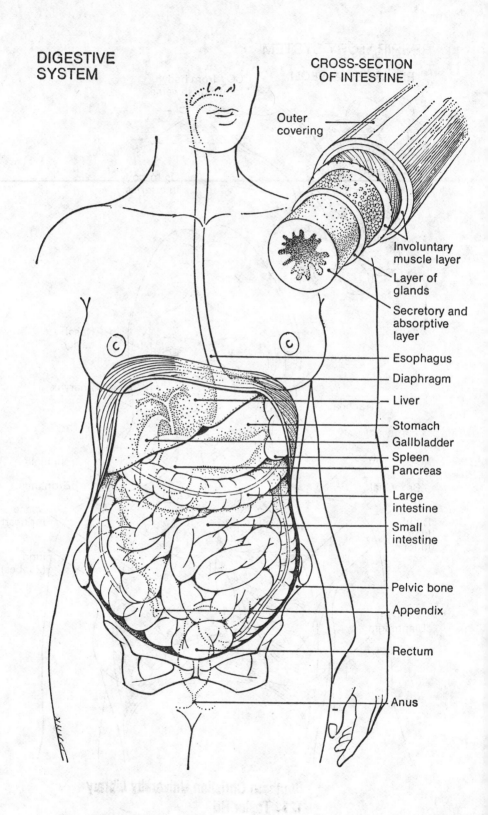

DIGESTIVE
SYSTEM

CROSS-SECTION
OF INTESTINE

Outer
covering

Involuntary
muscle layer

Layer of
glands

Secretory and
absorptive
layer

Esophagus

Diaphragm

Liver

Stomach

Gallbladder

Spleen

Pancreas

Large
intestine

Small
intestine

Pelvic bone

Appendix

Rectum

Anus

FUNCTIONS OF DIGESTIVE SYSTEM

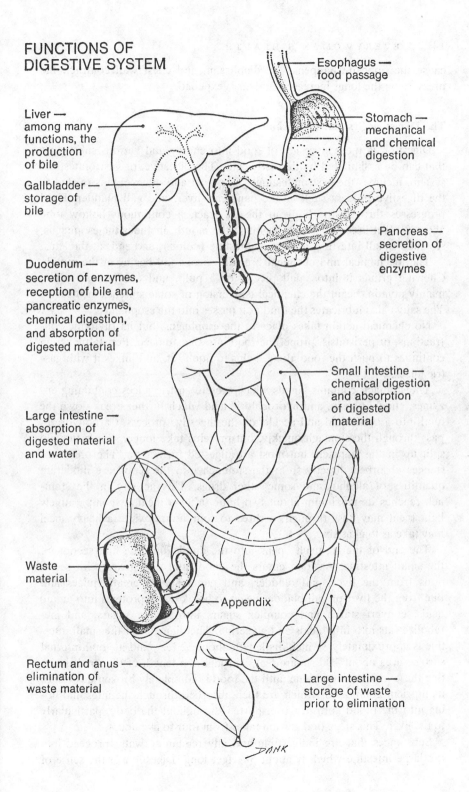

Esophagus — food passage

Stomach — mechanical and chemical digestion

Liver — among many functions, the production of bile

Gallbladder — storage of bile

Pancreas — secretion of digestive enzymes

Duodenum — secretion of enzymes, reception of bile and pancreatic enzymes, chemical digestion, and absorption of digested material

Small intestine — chemical digestion and absorption of digested material

Large intestine — absorption of digested material and water

Waste material

Appendix

Rectum and anus — elimination of waste material

Large intestine — storage of waste prior to elimination

DANK

cause the opposite happens; the diaphragm and chest wall contract, the pressure on the lungs increases, and air is expelled.

The Digestive System: Nourishment

Digestion is the conversion of food into energy and various substances that can be assimilated by the body cells. The digestive, or gastrointestinal system, includes the gastrointestinal (GI) tract and other organs related to the digestive process such as the pancreas, liver, and gall bladder. Food progresses through the body in the GI tract, a continuous hollow tube about 30 feet in length which begins at the mouth, includes the esophagus, stomach, small intestine, and large intestine (colon), and ends at the anus.

The mechanical and chemical breakdown of food begins in the mouth. Chewing grinds it into small pieces, or a pulp, and enzymes in saliva, mainly ptyalin, begin the chemical conversion of some starches into sugar. The saliva also lubricates the food as it passes into the esophagus.

No chemical action takes place in the esophagus, but its rhythmic contractions, or peristalsis, propel the food into the stomach. Peristaltic action continues to push the food along, helps to liquify it, and mixes it with gastric juices.

The stomach contains glands which secrete gastric juices containing enzymes, chiefly pepsin, and hydrochloric acid which further break down the food into a semiliquid and accelerate the digestive process. Carbohydrates pass through the stomach quickly, but proteins take longer. Some fats are split up in the stomach, but most are digested further on. The only substances absorbed directly from the stomach into the blood are moderate quantities of alcohol and some other drugs. This activity in the stomach reaches its maximum about two hours after a meal. A comparatively light meal may pass through in three to four hours, while a heavy meal may take as long as six.

The end of the stomach opens into the duodenum, the first section of the small intestine. As food enters the duodenum it is mixed with secretions from the liver, gall bladder, and pancreas. Pancreatic juices and bile from the liver or gall bladder begin to break down proteins into amino acids, convert starch and complex sugars into simple sugars, and metabolize fats into fatty acids and glycerine. The diameter of the small intestine is approximately ½ inch, its length about 22 feet, and its total internal surface area about 100 square feet. Through the length of the small intestine these processes continue until the food is completely broken down into its nutrient compounds which are then absorbed through the intestinal lining into the blood and then transported throughout the body, particularly to the liver. This stage of digestion takes from four to five hours.

Substances that are indigestible and any remaining water proceed into the large intestine which is about 5½ feet long. Digestion in the sense of conversion of food into nutrient compounds is completed in the small intestine, but the first part of the large intestine absorbs some remaining nutrients. Liquid waste is absorbed through the lining of the large intestine into the blood. The remaining solids, or feces, reach the final segment of the large intestine, the rectum, and are evacuated through the anus. This final aspect of digestion may take from five to twenty-four hours.

The Urinary System: Removal of Waste

Your body must not only build up the substance of its tissues and gain energy from the food you eat, but it must also get rid of the end products of body metabolism. These waste products continuously reach the blood and are carried to various places for excretion. Carbon dioxide and water (in the form of water vapor) are exhaled from the lungs; salts and other water pour out through sweat; others such as urea, uric acid, and creatinine are removed by the kidneys and excreted in urine.

The kidneys are the main filtering organ of the body. They also help to maintain the balance between salts and fluid in the body and to keep body minerals in balance. The kidneys filter blood plasma and thus form urine. While the amount of urine produced from hour to hour can vary considerably, the daily total is 2 to 3 pints. Many factors account for the varying rate of urine formation. The ingestion of alcohol, tea, and coffee, all of which are diuretics, increases the amount as does cold weather. Conversely, stress, perspiration due to hot weather or strenuous exercise, and limited intake of fluid decrease the amount.

The ureter leads from each kidney to the urinary bladder. The urethra leads from the bladder to the external opening, called the meatus, through which you urinate.

The Nervous System: Communication and Control

The nervous system is a complex organization of integrated structures which control an individual's reaction and adjustment to both internal and external environments. These reactions and adjustments include the rapid actions of the body such as muscular contractions, various visceral activities such as peristalsis, and the secretory activity of some endocrine glands.

The nervous system is composed of special cells called neurons, each of which contains fibers that reach out toward, but do not touch, other neurons. There is an electrochemical contact between them, called a synapse, which transmits the impulse. The nervous system functions primarily through a vast number of reflexes and reflex arcs. This reflex system starts with the stimulation of a receptor organ, such as the skin. This stimulation initiates an impulse which is transmitted by a conduction system to an ef-

URINARY SYSTEM

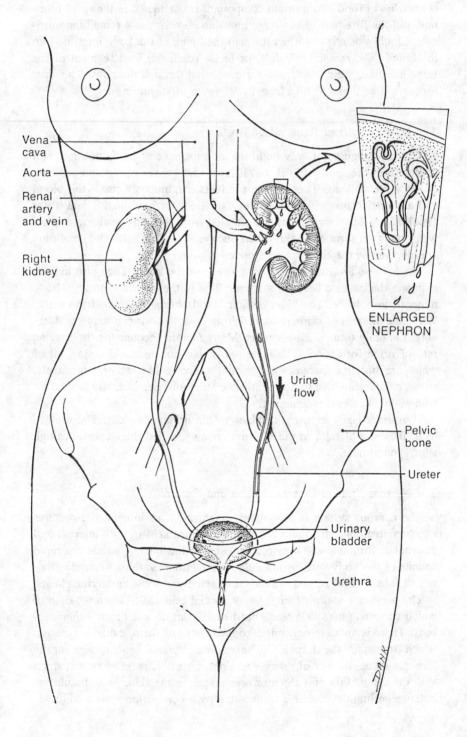

Vena cava

Aorta

Renal artery and vein

Right kidney

ENLARGED NEPHRON

Urine flow

Pelvic bone

Ureter

Urinary bladder

Urethra

fector organ such as a skeletal or a smooth muscle that responds to the initial stimulus. This conduction system is composed solely of nerves or of nerves plus hormones secreted by endocrine glands.

The nervous system is separated for descriptive purposes into two large segments, the central and the peripheral nervous systems. The former is made up of the brain and the spinal cord. The brain is in the cranium and has many parts, the major one being the right and left occipital lobes or hemispheres which are linked together on their lower surfaces, thus forming several structures including the medulla oblongata (bulb) which is also the beginning of the spinal cord. Another major part of the brain is the cerebellum which also has two hemispheres that are linked together. Memory, intellectual processes, perceptions of emotion, sensory perception, and both voluntary and involuntary motor functions are controlled and integrated with each other by the brain. The major parts of the brain make up what is called the cerebrum; hence such words as "cerebral" and "cerebration" are used to describe the brain and its function.

The spinal cord extends from the base of the brain downward through the vertebral canal. In an adult it is about 18 inches in length and ½ inch in diameter. It contains both motor and sensory nerve tracts which traverse its entire length. The spinal cord and the brain are covered by three layers of protective membranes (meninges) between two of which the cerebrospinal fluid circulates.

The peripheral nervous system consists of many paired nerves which conduct impulses to and from the brain and spinal cord. Twelve of them originate in the brain and are referred to as the cranial nerves. They control the muscles of the face, eyes, tongue, etc. They serve also as the nerves for the special senses of sight, hearing, smell, and taste. There are 31 pairs of spinal nerves along the entire length of the spinal cord, which course through the bony spinal column, and reach the muscles, blood vessels, organs, and skin surface of the entire body except the face. These nerves group together at several points and form plexi such as the sacral plexus.

A special group of peripheral nerves make up the autonomic (involuntary) nervous system which has two divisions, the sympathetic and parasympathetic. The former arise from the middle portions of the spinal cord, the latter from the brain and lowest portion of the spinal cord. In general both divisions innervate the same organs such as the pupils, heart, lungs, blood vessels, gastrointestinal tract, adrenal and other glands, and liver. Each division is physiologically antagonistic to the other. Thus the sympathetic system serves to mobilize energy for sudden activity—dilates the pupils, increases the heart rate, etc.—while the parasympathetic system acts to slow such activities to conserve energy. Ordinarily, however, they balance each other to maintain all the body's vital functions in a state of equilibrium or homeostasis.

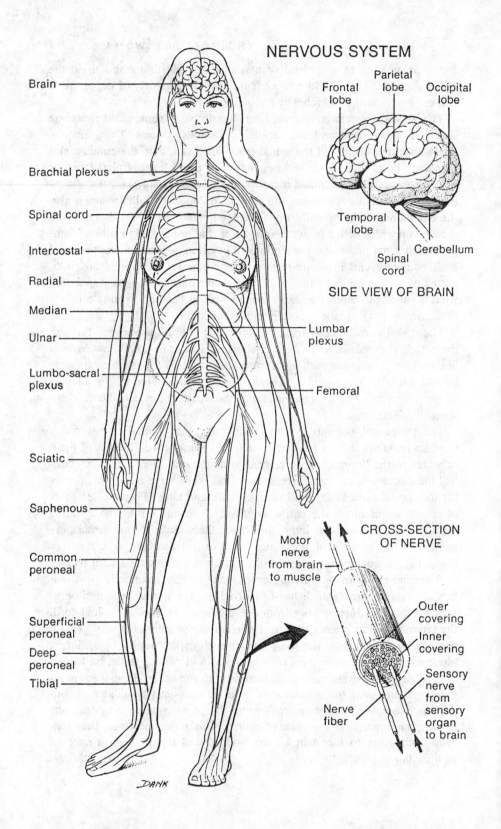

NERVOUS SYSTEM

Brain

Brachial plexus

Spinal cord

Intercostal

Radial

Median

Ulnar

Lumbo-sacral plexus

Sciatic

Saphenous

Common peroneal

Superficial peroneal

Deep peroneal

Tibial

Lumbar plexus

Femoral

Frontal lobe

Parietal lobe

Occipital lobe

Temporal lobe

Cerebellum

Spinal cord

SIDE VIEW OF BRAIN

CROSS-SECTION OF NERVE

Motor nerve from brain to muscle

Outer covering

Inner covering

Sensory nerve from sensory organ to brain

Nerve fiber

DANK

The Endocrine System: Internal Control and Balance

The endocrine system is often referred to as a master control system. It consists of nine glands. These glands are ductless; they secrete chemicals (hormones) directly into the bloodstream and they form an interconnected system. Their function affects and is affected by the entire nervous system, and they are the major regulators of growth, sexual development, secretion of other glands, metabolism of sugar and protein, and emotional states.

The hypothalamus is the master gland of endocrine activity. Located in the base of the brain it secretes at least ten substances that trigger or block the release of specific hormones by the pituitary gland which is attached to it by a stalk. It is the center in which the activities of the central nervous and endocrine systems are integrated.

The pituitary gland has an anterior portion and a posterior portion. The anterior pituitary secretes hormones called tropic hormones and stimulating hormones which stimulate hormone secretions in several other endocrine, or target glands. These are detailed in the illustration of the endocrine system. The hormones produced by these target glands in turn regulate the secretion of their tropic hormones. The anterior pituitary also secretes prolactin which, among other things, initiates and maintains lactation after pregnancy, and growth hormone (GH), which is essential for cell growth and proliferation. Overproduction of GH prior to full growth causes gigantism and after full growth, acromegaly. Underproduction prior to full growth results in pituitary dwarfism. The posterior pituitary secretes vasopressin which conserves body water. Another of its secretions (oxytocin) stimulates smooth muscles, including those of the uterus at the time of childbirth, and contributes to the ejection of breast milk.

The thyroid gland regulates the rate at which the body utilizes oxygen and food through the production of thyroxin. Underproduction of this hormone (hypothyroidism) produces cretinism in infants and the listlessness and drowsiness of myxedema in adults. Overproduction causes hyperthyroidism.

The paired parathyroid glands secrete parathyroid hormone (PTH) which controls the blood levels of calcium and phosphate in the body. Underproduction results in low levels of calcium and can cause muscle cramps, even convulsions; overproduction drains the bones of calcium and can produce kidney stones.

The islets of Langerhans, thousands of cell clusters scattered throughout the pancreas, regulate the body's use of carbohydrates through the production of insulin and glucagon. An underproduction of insulin is associated with diabetes mellitus; an overproduction causes hypoglycemia (low blood sugar). Glucagon acts in the opposite way.

The paired adrenal glands have a cortex or outer portion and a medulla

ENDOCRINE SYSTEM

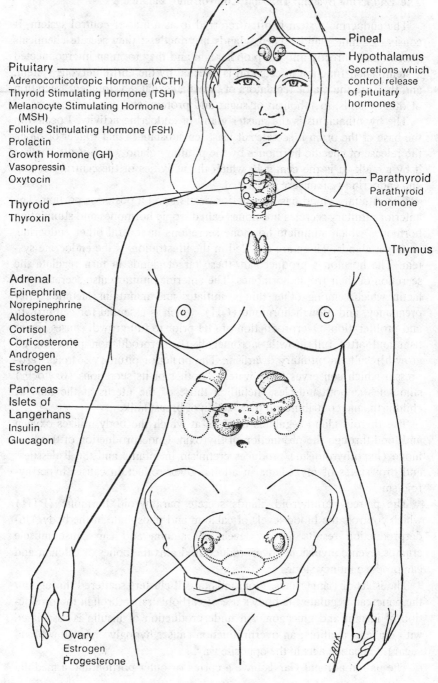

Pituitary
Adrenocorticotropic Hormone (ACTH)
Thyroid Stimulating Hormone (TSH)
Melanocyte Stimulating Hormone (MSH)
Follicle Stimulating Hormone (FSH)
Prolactin
Growth Hormone (GH)
Vasopressin
Oxytocin

Thyroid
Thyroxin

Adrenal
Epinephrine
Norepinephrine
Aldosterone
Cortisol
Corticosterone
Androgen
Estrogen

Pancreas
Islets of
Langerhans
Insulin
Glucagon

Ovary
Estrogen
Progesterone

Pineal

Hypothalamus
Secretions which
control release
of pituitary
hormones

Parathyroid
Parathyroid
hormone

Thymus

or inner portion. The cortex produces steroid hormones—glucocorticoids (cortisone and several others), which control the metabolism of protein and sugar; mineralocorticoids (aldosterone), which control the balance of mineral substances and fluids; and sex hormones (androgen, mainly testosterone, and estrogen). Underproduction of both groups of corticoids produces a rare condition called Addison's disease. Overproduction causes Cushing's syndrome. Excess androgen production can induce the development of masculine secondary sex characteristics in females and young boys. Excess estrogen production has little effect on mature women. In young girls it can lead to enlargement of the breasts and early maturation of the uterus and vagina. In males it can lead to breast enlargement (gynecomastia). The medulla produces catecholamines (epinephrine, or adrenalin, and norepinephrine). These are produced also in the endings of the sympathetic nerves. They normally contribute to the maintenance of homeostasis, but they also enable the body to respond to danger, fright, anger, or sudden physical stress with an increased heart rate and faster breathing.

The male sex glands, the testes, produce sperm and the male sex hormone testosterone which is responsible for the development of male secondary sex characteristics such as voice change and facial hair. Overproduction of testosterone produces virilism; insufficiency, eunuchism. The female sex glands, the ovaries, produce ova or eggs; they also secrete estrogen and progesterone, hormones needed for menstruation, reproduction, feminine secondary sex characteristics, and skeletal development, plus androgens. Excessive production of these hormones occurs very rarely and then only with certain ovarian tumors. Absence of them early in life causes female eunuchism. Underproduction of them later in life causes menstrual irregularities and, ultimately, menopause. (The relationship of the pituitary to the female gonads is discussed further in the next section.)

The functions of the thymus gland and the pineal gland are not well understood. The thymus gland appears to play a role in the body's resistance to disease, metabolism of calcium, and development of the skeleton and sex glands. The pineal gland's functions appear to be related to preventing excessive growth and overactivity of sex glands in early life.

The Reproductive System: Perpetuation of the Species

The female reproductive system consists of internal and external sex organs. The external sex organs are called the vulva. The mons pubis (mons veneris) is a pad of fatty tissue in front of the pubic bone which from puberty on is covered with pubic hair. Two folds of fatty tissue covered with skin, the labia majora (outer lips) and the labia minora (inner lips), protect the vaginal and urethral openings which lie between them. The labia minora are sensitive to touch and sexual arousal. Just below the mons the labia minora join to form a hood over the clitoris. The clitoris, the most

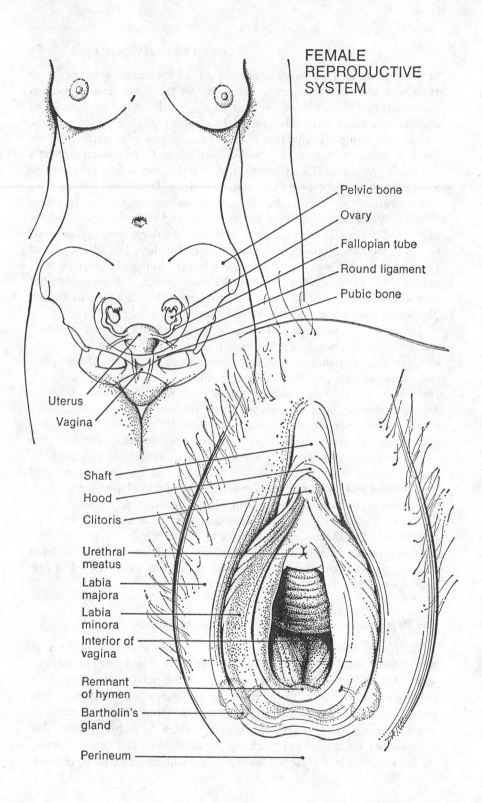

FEMALE
REPRODUCTIVE
SYSTEM

Pelvic bone

Ovary

Fallopian tube

Round ligament

Pubic bone

Uterus

Vagina

Shaft

Hood

Clitoris

Urethral
meatus

Labia
majora

Labia
minora

Interior of
vagina

Remnant
of hymen

Bartholin's
gland

Perineum

SIDE VIEW OF EXTERNAL AND INTERNAL GENITALIA

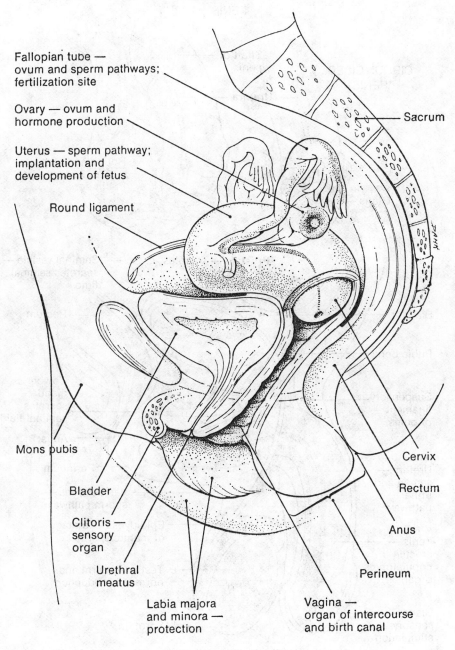

Fallopian tube — ovum and sperm pathways; fertilization site

Ovary — ovum and hormone production

Uterus — sperm pathway; implantation and development of fetus

Round ligament

Sacrum

Mons pubis

Bladder

Clitoris — sensory organ

Urethral meatus

Labia majora and minora — protection

Vagina — organ of intercourse and birth canal

Perineum

Anus

Rectum

Cervix

MALE REPRODUCTIVE SYSTEM

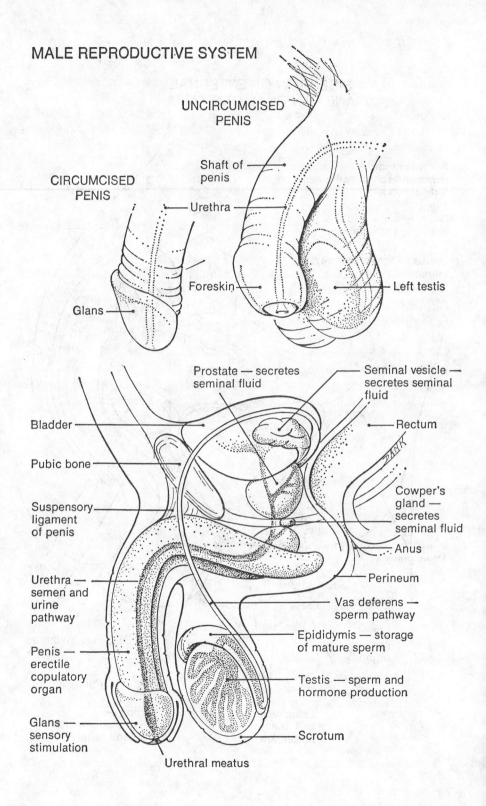

UNCIRCUMCISED
PENIS

CIRCUMCISED
PENIS

Shaft of
penis

Urethra

Foreskin

Glans

Left testis

Prostate — secretes
seminal fluid

Seminal vesicle —
secretes seminal
fluid

Bladder

Rectum

Pubic bone

Suspensory
ligament
of penis

Cowper's
gland —
secretes
seminal fluid

Anus

Urethra —
semen and
urine
pathway

Perineum

Vas deferens —
sperm pathway

Epididymis — storage
of mature sperm

Penis —
erectile
copulatory
organ

Testis — sperm and
hormone production

Glans —
sensory
stimulation

Scrotum

Urethral meatus

sexually responsive female organ, is composed of erectile tissue which becomes engorged with blood during sexual activity. It is homologous to the penis.

Below the clitoris is the urethral meatus, the external opening of the urethra. Below that is the vaginal opening or introitus. The hymen is a thin fold of mucous membrane across the introitus, partially blocking it. After being stretched by ordinary physical activity, insertion of tampons, or intercourse, only a ridge of tissue usually remains around the introitus. Beyond the hymen on each side of the vaginal opening is a mucus-secreting gland (Bartholin's gland). The perineum is the area between the external genitals and the anus.

The internal sex organs include the vagina, the uterus, the fallopian tubes, and the ovaries. The vagina is a tubular, muscular structure covered with skin which extends from the vulva upward and backward to the uterus. The vaginal walls stretch and contract during intercourse; during childbirth, they expand greatly. Continuous secretions from the vaginal wall keep the vagina clean, maintain acidity to prevent infection, and provide lubrication for intercourse.

The uterus (womb) is a hollow, pear-shaped organ, about the size of a lemon. In a nonpregnant state, its walls (myometrium) are one of the strongest muscles in the body. The cervix, the base or neck of the uterus, projects into the vagina and has a small opening (cervical os) in its center up through which sperm can travel and down through which menstrual blood flows.

The fallopian tubes (oviducts) are paired muscular narrow canals which extend from each side of the top of the uterus to the ovaries and in an adult are about 5 inches long. The end near the ovary is open and enlarged so that an ovum, when released from the ovary, can be "trapped" by, enter, and travel along the tube.

The ovaries, organs about the size of an almond, are located on either side of the uterus. The breasts (discussed in detail in the chapter on "Breast Care") produce milk following the birth of a baby.

The male reproductive system consists of the penis, urethra, scrotum, testes, and some glands. The penis contains erectile tissue, a collection of veins; on sexual arousal it is engorged with blood and becomes erect, thus facilitating sexual intercourse. The urethra is the tube in the center of the penis through which urine and semen leave the body. The prostate gland and Cowper's glands, located at the junction of the bladder and urethra, produce the seminal fluid in which sperm cells are mixed, thereby forming semen.

The Menstrual Cycle
The menstrual cycle is a dramatic example of the delicate balance and

interactions maintained by your body. A series of complex feedback interactions among several organs and glands stimulate ovulation (production of the reproductive cell, the egg), prepare the uterus for pregnancy, and, if conception does not occur, make adjustments so that the process can begin again. Menstruation is the process by which tissue, built up in the uterus in readiness for the implantation of a fertilized ovum, is discharged through the vagina if conception does not occur.

The cycle is repeated throughout the reproductive years of a woman's life from menarche, the onset of menstruation, to menopause, the cessation of menstruation. Menarche occurs between the ages of 10 and 16, when certain secretions from the hypothalamus begin and thus stimulate the pituitary. Menopause occurs between the ages of 45 and 55 when ovarian follicular function ceases. Its onset is gradual.

The complete menstrual cycle takes approximately a month, that is, the time from the beginning of one menstrual period to the beginning of the next ranges from 25 to 35 days. The menstrual flow or period lasts from 2 to 7 days. The length of the cycle and of the menstrual period varies from woman to woman and in any one woman from time to time.

There are three phases in each menstrual cycle and the primary organs involved are the hypothalamus/pituitary, ovary, and uterus.

Menstrual phase. We consider the first day of the menstrual cycle to be the day menstruation begins. As the estrogen and progesterone levels fall (see postovulatory phase below) the functional layers of the endometrium (the lining of the uterus) begin to shed and appear as menstrual flow. As menstruation continues, estrogen and progesterone levels drop further and follicle-stimulating hormone (FSH) from the pituitary increases. FSH stimulates the proliferation, usually only in one ovary, of masses of cells called follicles which secrete estrogen. FSH also stimulates the enlargement of the ovum in a follicle. The estrogen stimulates further development of the ovum; a drop, via negative feedback system, in FSH; and, via a positive feedback system, an increase in LH which stimulates further follicle development and with it an increase in estrogen secretion. This additional estrogen stimulates the start of the "rebuilding" of the endometrium which, of course, causes menstruation to end and marks the beginning of the preovulatory phase.

Preovulatory (proliferative or follicular) phase. Estrogen levels continue to increase, FSH to decrease, and LH to increase slightly. The endometrium further thickens and its glands and blood vessels increase. One of the follicles (the dominant follicle) and its ovum continue to mature while the others shrink. Finally there is a surge of LH from the pituitary which triggers the dominant follicle to rupture.

Ovulation. This is not a phase of the menstrual cycle but is an event that more or less marks the change from one phase to another. After the follicle ruptures, the ovum is expelled from it (ovulation), and the follicle

MENSTRUAL CYCLE

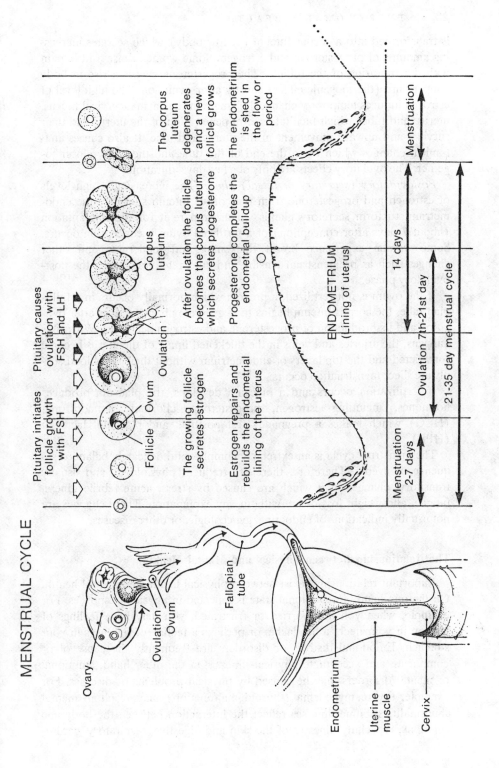

Pituitary initiates follicle growth with FSH

Pituitary causes ovulation with FSH and LH

Follicle   Ovum   Ovulation

Corpus luteum

The corpus luteum degenerates and a new follicle grows

The growing follicle secretes estrogen

After ovulation the follicle becomes the corpus luteum which secretes progesterone

The endometrium is shed in the flow or period

Estrogen repairs and rebuilds the endometrial lining of the uterus

Progesterone completes the endometrial buildup

ENDOMETRIUM (Lining of uterus)

Menstruation 2-7 days

Ovulation 7th-21st day

14 days

Menstruation

21-35 day menstrual cycle

Ovary

Ovulation   Ovum

Fallopian tube

Endometrium

Uterine muscle

Cervix

is transformed into a corpus luteum (yellow body) which secretes increasing amounts of progesterone and estrogen. Some women sense a little pain with the rupturing of the follicle. The progesterone causes a rise in body temperature (thermogenic effect) shortly after ovulation. The high level of estrogen induces temporary chemical changes in the vagina, cervical mucus, uterus, and tubes which facilitate sperm penetration of the uterus and their survival and upward movement in the uterus and tube. It also causes anatomical changes which bring the end of the tube and the ovary closer together. The ovulatory effects are only of a few days' duration.

Postovulatory (secretory or luteal) phase. The increasingly high levels of estrogen and progesterone from the corpus luteum stimulate the endometrium to form secretory glands which prepare it for the implantation (about 7 days after conception) of a fertilized ovum if conception occurs. Some women experience breast thickening and tenderness and other changes such as premenstrual tension and fluid retention during the postovulatory phase.

If the ovum is not fertilized, a process which normally occurs in a fallopian tube, the corpus luteum begins to degenerate about 14 days after ovulation and its production of progesterone and estrogen decreases. When this happens, the arteries and veins in the thickened lining of the uterus become constricted and the top layers of endometrium without their rich blood supply are shed; menstruation occurs.

If fertilization occurs and a placenta develops, the placenta produces hormones, including estrogen, progesterone, chorionic gonadotropin (HCG) which makes a pregnancy test positive, and placental lactogen (HPL).

The menstrual cycle is an extremely complex and delicately balanced sequence of events. Therefore, there are frequent physiologic, and usually transitory, changes in it which are caused by stress, acute febrile illness, fatigue, and weight loss or are without any explanation. These changes are not usually indications of endocrine, gynecologic, or other diseases.

The Relationship Between Physical and Mental Health

Important relationships exist between physical health and mental health. On the one hand, an emotional state is reflected in physical responses. For example, when you are worried or frustrated, you may have feelings of tension in your neck, a headache, or perhaps a feeling of tightness in your stomach. Emotional distress or disorders are frequently the cause of or complicate and accentuate physical illness. On the other hand, emotional or mental disorders may be caused by physical problems or diseases. For example, severe myxedema (thyroid malfunction) may result in mental abnormalities. Some illnesses reflect the interaction between the body and emotions, especially illnesses of the skin and digestive, respiratory, cardiovascular, and urinary systems. These parts of the body are under the control of the involuntary nervous system. Thus, emotional factors can contribute to such disorders as certain types of skin allergies, dermatitis, colitis, ulcers, asthma, changes in heart rate and rhythm, hypertension, and urinary frequency. Emotional factors may possibly contribute to arthritis and rheumatism as well.

Emotional states such as anxiety, restlessness, loss of appetite, or overeating should not be ignored. They are as real as any physical disorder and should be dealt with appropriately. An attempt should be made to find their underlying cause and to treat the cause, whether it be organic or emotional.

TAKE RESPONSIBILITY FOR YOUR OWN HEALTH

Our definition of health as a condition of wellness does not mean that you should ignore the possibility of disorders and disease. Quite the contrary, an important part of maintaining health is being aware of the sources of potential illness. Promoting your own well-being involves prevention of illness, early treatment of illness, and minimizing disability.

Primary Prevention: Prevention of Illness

There are three levels of prevention. Primary prevention is directed toward keeping a disorder from occurring. Immunization is the classic example of primary prevention. Today, primary prevention includes the vaccinations which children receive against whooping cough, diphtheria, tetanus, German measles, measles, and poliomyelitis. As an adult, you may have been immunized against influenza or, when you were planning to travel, against hepatitis, yellow fever, or other infectious diseases. Environmental health controls are another form of primary prevention. They include fluoridation of water to prevent dental cavities, proper sewage disposal, purification of water, and air pollution control. These all have a profound effect on your personal health.

The term primary prevention, however, also refers to choices you make in behavior and activities that may affect your health. Because of the effectiveness of sewage control, immunization, and antibiotics, devastating infectious diseases are no longer serious health problems. They have been replaced in this country as the major cause of death by cardiovascular disease, lung disease, cancer, alcoholism, automobile accidents, homicide, and suicide. Now, the interesting thing about all of these is that each reflects, to a degree, an element of choice. In regard to at least some of the factors that contribute to the likelihood that you will become ill or die from any of these causes, the way you live your life is particularly relevant. The choices you make are not related to public health measures, shots or services a doctor provides, but they are critical to the level of well-being you can maintain.

Some of the choices are commonplace but still important. Do you practice regular oral hygiene? Do you use seat belts? Some involve activities that are so habitual that you may rarely give them any thought. For example, how much sleep do you usually get? What kind of food do you eat? Do you eat breakfast regularly? Perhaps because of current interest in food additives and jogging you have given some thought to the quality of your food and to physical fitness, but many people pay little attention to them.

Clearly, eating a well-balanced diet, not smoking, and drinking in moderation if at all are activities which have a major effect on your health and are within your power to control. Also, although you may not be able to eliminate sources of stress in your life, you can take a good look at how you handle it. If you are a businesswoman and/or homemaker, the difficulty of adapting to the critical stages in your life can reinforce the tendency to use a crutch for help in dealing with everyday stresses. Perhaps your life consists of busy, tension-producing days during your working years or when your children are young, and a frantic search for activities after your retirement or "when the nest is empty." At such times of change in your life, you may find yourself uncertain as to how to make an adjustment to the next stage of life. Then, the need to avoid stress, tension at work, or pressures at home may encourage you to respond to the media appeals to turn to a variety of drugs, from nicotine to alcohol, for relief.

Are you quick to take aspirin at the first sign of a headache, to rely on sleeping pills in order to get a good night's sleep, to seek (and to receive) tranquilizers because some of the problems of everyday living seem to be too difficult? We are constantly exposed to, and many of us come to rely on, a variety of drugs, from aspirin and other over-the-counter pills to prescription medications. Some women become dependent on alcohol, the most serious drug abuse problem in our country. For others, it is those drugs which everyone more readily labels addictive or dependency-producing. You may find yourself smoking or eating too much. All these activities are not conducive to promoting your health. If any of these habits continues, you may be placing yourself at a greater risk of hypertension; of heart, liver, or lung disease; or cancer.

Secondary Prevention: Early Diagnosis and Treatment

Secondary prevention refers to early diagnosis, detection, and treatment of a disease in order to reduce its consequences, duration, and severity. Screening programs to detect cancer of the cervix or hypertension fall into this category. Breast self-examination for early detection of cancer is a similar example. Early care for pregnancies is an example of efforts to prevent congenital defects or other abnormalities in the health of the child or mother.

Tertiary Prevention: Rehabilitation

Finally, there is a third level of prevention—rehabilitation following a serious disorder. Rehabilitation is directed toward minimizing disability, chronic conditions, or the limitations that might result. You may feel that this kind of prevention comes very late. Yet, if help is given early in the course of a chronic illness, rehabilitation can prevent further deterioration and improve the chances for social, psychological, and physical adjustment.

Economic Benefits of Prevention

Beside preventing pain, discomfort, and anxiety, prevention has another important advantage—it usually saves you money. Health promotion and maintenance cost less than providing medical care once disease has occurred. This is particularly important since hospital care in particular and health care generally have become increasingly expensive. Prevention programs, particularly primary prevention, reduce the demand on the medical care system and give it more opportunity to prevent, treat, or rehabilitate other diseases.

An example may illustrate the importance of this issue. The difference in cost for caring for one breast cancer patient whose disease is diagnosed early and one who is diagnosed late has been estimated at $5,000. It is estimated that nearly 20,000 cases of breast cancer would be discovered each year in the United States by more early screening programs (secondary prevention). Taking into account the costs of screening, this could result in savings of nearly $100,000,000 annually; the human value of this preventive activity is beyond measure.

BE AN ACTIVE, EQUAL PARTNER IN HEALTH CARE

To be an active and equal partner means that you recognize your right to be informed about your own health, to receive the kind of information which will help you to play your part as a consumer of health care services. Being an active, equal partner also means taking responsibility for follow-through, for questioning, and for expressing both satisfaction and dissatisfaction, not just being a compliant, passive recipient. As an informed consumer, you can take much better care of yourself because you understand how your body functions, what the relationship between you and your health care provider should be, and how to improve your health. You will then be less likely to be in awe of the health care practitioner and more able to contribute to your own health maintenance. Most important, as an active participant with knowledge, with a sense of responsibility, following a health-promoting life style, you will be more likely to maintain a healthy body, to recover from illness, and to function in spite of whatever disability you may have.

Sometimes it may seem that there are many forces and pressures working against a positive state of health. Medical care is organized in such a way that people have to seek out the "correct" doctor. "Sickness care" is a better name than health care for the kinds of services most people have available. Your insurance company is unlikely to reimburse you for most preventive services or for many of the outpatient visits you make, while reimbursement for costly inpatient hospitalization is extensive. And many physicians seem more interested in your ailments than in your well-being, in your individual parts than in you as a whole person, and in your presenting symptoms than in your whole life.

Holistic Health

There is an increasing interest in looking at people as whole human beings living in their family, community, and social environments, rather than as isolated organs or systems. New attention to holistic health reflects this orientation.

The concern with the whole person is the essential element of the holistic approach. It does not compartmentalize you into the various parts of your body or even according to kinds of specialists that you might see. Because there is an overemphasis on specialization in medical care, interest has recently been expressed in a return to the family physician, to the primary care physician, to that person who can deal with the individual on many levels. There is certainly a need for this.

Women, especially, seem to be penalized in the way our health care is organized in this country. If we choose, for example, to go to an internist or a family physician for our general health care, in many instances this physician does not care for our reproductive health, for our breast care, or for our concerns related to the genitourinary system. It may be a while before you as a woman have all of your basic health care needs met by someone who has the experience to deal with you as a whole person as well as the understanding and sensitivity to your emotional and physical needs.

Self-Care

In the search for better health care, while holistic medicine attempts to reduce overreliance on specialists, self-care is directed toward reducing overreliance on medical services in general. Self-care as a concept can be considered to be enlightened self-interest. For example, this means that you as a woman do a regular monthly breast examination, so that you are able to detect any suspicious findings and bring them to the attention of your health care provider. It also means an emphasis on a more health-promoting life style. For some people it also means turning from total reliance on medical care.

To take full advantage of the benefits of self-care you should approach it with the same sense of responsibility you apply to medical services. At its most extreme the self-care movement is characterized by those who would avoid all doctors and actively reject any kind of medical intervention. Although the body has wonderful curative abilities and many ailments and disorders will respond to home remedies, rest, and tender loving care, there also are many that will not. Your knowledge of when to turn to the doctor, rather than slavish reliance as a passive patient or an equally extreme rejection of any outside help, is part of health promotion.

You should also be aware that self-care, like so many aspects of life in the United States, has been used by those who take advantage of people's interest and worry to sell a product. Manuals of self-knowledge, self-understanding, and health care flood the market. This presents a challenge to you as a reader to know when you are enriching your knowledge to complement health care and when you are being given panaceas and simplistic solutions for problems that may be more complex and that require the skills of health workers.

One of the innovative approaches that is related to the increasing interest in self-care has been the development of self-help groups. You are probably aware of Weight Watchers, Overeaters Anonymous, and Alcoholics Anonymous. Now there are self-help groups for almost any disorder you could think of, from diabetes to hypertension, from muscular dystrophy to allergies. Self-help groups have been organized to provide information, to clarify the role of medical care in dealing with problems, and to help people through serious physical and emotional problems or through life crises such as bereavement and loneliness.

The benefit of self-help groups comes from the fact that when you are with someone who is your peer, who has some of the same problems you have, you tend to share positive experiences as well as burdens, and to generalize or universalize your experiences. In doing this you gain some insight and understanding. Self-help groups provide both the knowledge and the emotional support that membership in any group gives.

Some of these self-help groups have led to the establishment of clinical services for women, including medical services provided by women health practitioners, counseling programs, and educational and consciousness-raising discussion groups. These are consistent with the increased participation of consumers in making decisions.

With increased awareness of health care, it is hoped that changes and reform may come in how all services are organized and provided. The consumer movement has caused consternation among many people in medicine whose attitudes and approaches had never been questioned by the people who use their services. This is particularly true of physicians who have occupied a sacrosanct position. The desire for change, especially by women whose emotional and intellectual needs have not been met, is very much related to your becoming an equal participant in the health care partnership.

Improving Health Services

Citizen participation in health service has gone beyond hospital lay advisory boards and voter control of funding. It now extends to the establishment of alternative health care services, particularly those in which potential patients carry on health care activities themselves. In some instances women's groups have banded together for education—to understand how their bodies function, to learn what to expect during an examination by a gynecologist, during childbirth, during sexual intercourse, to become informed about all aspects of sexuality and reproduction of which women as patients have been kept ignorant. Other groups seek to ensure less sexist behavior on the part of physicians, generally males, or to demand their rights as patients to accept or not to accept a doctor's recommendation for sterilization, hysterectomy, or mastectomy. Still others are concerned with abortion rights and reproductive freedom.

Even if you feel that the medical care you personally receive is adequate, you might consider that active participation in a women's health group (to whatever degree seems best for you) can have an effect in the long run on the health care system. Your participation will help to influence those within the medical community to be more attuned to the needs of the individual patient. Your participation can help to demonstrate that the patient can be an equal in a process which depends on persons on both sides of the relationship. The progress of treatment and rehabilitation can be influenced by your attitude, knowledge, and involvement in the health care partnership. Already, there have been many influential forces. The patients' rights movement, the women's movement, the public's increased concern with elitism in medical practice, and demands for more citizen participation in the affairs of hospitals, clinics, and health centers have already affected the attitudes of health care providers.

This exchange of information gives those in the field of health care a better sense of what helps you accept their guidance and follow their recommendations. This issue has sometimes been referred to as "patient compliance," a misnomer. Ideally it should be a more active process, in which a knowledgeable person (1) understands her role in the process of becoming or staying well; (2) asks pertinent questions; and (3) knows to whom to turn for further information or help. Unfortunately, when knowledge and understanding are lacking, you may often find yourself misunderstanding directions, confused as to what the problem is, and reluctant to follow instructions.

Alternative health services may be effective in dealing with such issues, but there is a need for real reform in the way health care is organized and provided. Health care should emphasize health rather than sickness, partnership rather than hierarchy, and quality health care as the right of all women—and of all people.

FURTHER READING

Boston Women's Health Book Collective. *Our Bodies, Ourselves.* New York: Simon & Schuster, 1976.

British Museum. *Human Biology: An Exhibition of Ourselves.* London: Cambridge University Press, 1977.

Cooke, Cynthia W., M.D. and S. Dworkin. *Ms. Guide to a Woman's Health.* New York: Doubleday, 1979.

Diagram Group. *Woman's Body: An Owner's Manual.* New York: Bantam, 1977.

Miller, Benjamin F. and Lawrence Galton. *The Family Book of Preventive Medicine.* New York: Simon & Schuster, 1971.

Nutrition and Weight

TOBY GRAHAM, M.D.
Assistant Professor of Medicine,
University of Pittsburgh School of Medicine,
Pittsburgh, Pennsylvania

We are what we eat! Our food choices affect our health, energy, appearance, and disposition. Eating the right amounts and kinds of foods supplies us with energy and stamina for work and play, provides for our growth, maintains our bodies in good health, and helps to keep us mentally alert. That's what nutrition is all about. It is unfortunate, but too often true, that many women become interested in nutrition only when they are pregnant or breast-feeding, they are overweight and want to diet, they have children with a weight problem, or they develop symptoms stemming from inadequate nutrition, such as fatigue resulting from iron-deficiency anemia. Hopefully, this chapter will encourage increased attention to good nutrition, not as treatment for a problem but as the basis for good health and well-being.

THE NUTRIENT CONTENT OF FOOD

Nutrition is the process whereby our bodies use food to supply us with energy; build, maintain, and repair body tissues; and regulate body processes. Nutrients, those chemical substances obtained from food during digestion, can be grouped into five classes—protein, carbohydrate, fat, vitamins, and minerals. Two other substances, water and fiber, although not technically considered nutrients, are also essential in the diet. The amount of energy a nutrient can supply is measured in calories.

Protein

Protein is the basic substance of all living cells and is therefore vital in the diet for cellular growth, replacement, and repair. Protein is composed of combinations of amino acids, organic compounds containing nitrogen and hydrogen. The material needed for different types of body cells, such as enzymes, hormones, red blood cells, and antibodies, is provided by different combinations of the amino acids. The protein derived from animal foods, such as meat, fish, eggs, and dairy products, contains all of the amino acids we need to construct proteins in our body (essential amino acids), and is therefore known as complete protein. The protein derived from plant food, such as nuts, legumes, and grains, usually lacks some essential amino acids in the amounts needed and is therefore incomplete. However, complete protein can be obtained by eating plant foods if they are combined to complement one another, that is, to supply in combination all the required amino acids. Examples of such complementary foods are dried beans and corn, peanuts and wheat, and fried beans and rice. One third of one's daily protein requirement should be eaten at the first meal of the day to assure maximum energy during the day.

Carbohydrates

Carbohydrates, the sugars and starches, supply most of the body's energy needs. They are also necessary for protein digestion and certain brain functions. Some forms are rapidly absorbed into the bloodstream unchanged to provide immediately available energy. Others are converted by digestion into a form which can be stored for later use. Their presence in adequate amounts allows the body to preserve protein, which also supplies energy, primarily for body building and maintaining functions. Carbohydrates are obtained from fruits, vegetables, and grains.

Fat

Fats and oils (fats which are liquid at room temperature) are composed mainly of fatty acids. Fats are an excellent source of energy, providing more calories per gram than do protein or carbohydrates. Fatty acids contain or are involved in the digestion of the fat soluble vitamins—A, D, E, and K. Stored body fat helps to maintain body temperature by providing insulation and also protects body structures and organs. Fats are found in abundance in animal and plant products, including meats, dairy products, nuts, and some vegetables.

Both the quantity and quality of fat in the diet should be considered. Obviously, eating more than the body needs usually leads to excess body fat, but the type of fat consumed may be equally important. Fatty acids differ in their chemical structure. If one additional hydrogen atom can be incorporated into the carbon chain, the fatty acid is called an unsaturated fat. If the hydrogen cannot be incorporated, it is a saturated fat. If two or more hydrogen ions can be added, it is known as a polyunsaturated fat. The polyunsaturates are almost exclusively vegetable in origin: corn oil, safflower oil, soybean oil, and the like. Practically all animal fats are saturated. The fats found in milk and cream substitutes as well as those that are in solid white shortenings derived from palm oil or cocoanut oil are also saturated. Excess consumption of saturated fats is thought to raise the amount of cholesterol, a lipid, in the bloodstream. In the blood plasma, cholesterol and other lipids are combined with proteins and circulate as lipoproteins. There is some not yet totally clear relationship between the amount and ratio of saturated and unsaturated fats one eats, the level and density of lipoprotein (particularly cholesterol) in the blood plasma, and disease of the arteries (atherosclerosis).

Vitamins

Vitamins, sometimes referred to as micronutrients, are organic substances which are present in foods and are needed in very small amounts (a few micrograms or milligrams) to enable specific metabolic reactions to occur. They generally serve as coenzyme catalysts for intracellular enzyme system reactions. Each vitamin has a specific function. Since only small amounts of vitamins are needed to trigger and control these reactions and since they are used again and again, only small amounts are needed daily for replenishment. Although some vitamins can be synthesized by humans, we consider that all vitamins are needed in our daily diets.

A woman in normal health who is eating properly prepared and adequately balanced meals does not need supplemental vitamins. However, women over 55 or 60 years of age may need them because their diets are inadequate or because, as some clinicians believe, their gastrointestinal absorption mechanisms are impaired. Women on special or restricted diets should discuss the advisability of vitamin supplements with their doctor. When a situation exists which increases tissue requirements for vitamins, such as hyperthyroidism, pregnancy, or postoperative convalescence, or when there is disturbance in vitamin absorption as occurs in hypothyroidism, the doctor usually prescribes any necessary vitamin supplements. In addition, some women who regularly take certain medications such as Dilantin, isoniazid, and possibly oral contraceptives may need supplemental vitamins.

The possible adverse effects on the body of excessive intake of vitamins either in foods or in pills are not thoroughly understood. It does not appear that overdoses of most vitamins have toxic or adverse effects, except for vitamins A and D. A disorder, known as hypervitaminosis, can result from taking A or D in amounts far in excess of the standard recommended daily requirements.

The beneficial effects, if any, of taking more than the recommended amounts of vitamins in the absence of a physiological deficiency are even less clear. This is referred to as pharmacologic or megadose vitamin use. Some have suggested that such doses of vitamin C can prevent upper respiratory infections and that such doses of multivitamins can be used to treat chronic fatigue, depression, and certain mental illnesses.

Terminology in vitamin science is confusing because over the years some vitamins have been assigned letters, some have been given names, and some are referred to by both a letter and a name. Names are used on food packages. Vitamins can be divided into two main groups—fat soluble and water soluble.

FAT-SOLUBLE VITAMINS

The fat-soluble vitamins are A, D, E, and K. Because dietary excesses can be stored in the body, they are not absolutely necessary in the diet every day and evidence of deficiencies is slow to develop.

Vitamin A is essential to keep healthy the skin and the mucous membranes which line the eyes and respiratory, gastrointestinal, and urinary tracts. Also it keeps our tear ducts functioning, makes night vision possible by combining with a protein to form visual purple, seems to be involved in reducing susceptibility to general infection, and contributes to bone growth. Carotene, a substance which the body converts to vitamin A, is present in fruits and vegetables, particularly those which are yellow, green, or orange. Vitamin A itself is present only in animal products, particularly liver, and to a lesser extent in milk, eggs, butter, and margarine.

Intake of vitamin A far in excess of the recommended daily amounts can cause liver damage, interfere with growth, destroy bone, and cause mental malfunction. Deficiencies can lead to night blindness, diarrhea, eye and respiratory infections, and loss of tooth enamel.

Vitamin D helps to regulate the absorption and utilization of calcium and phosphorus which are needed to form strong bones and teeth. It is found naturally in a few foods of animal origin, primarily eggs, milk, and butter, but only in small amounts. Generally, therefore, these foods, and particularly milk, are enriched with vitamin D. In the presence of sunlight on the skin the skin synthesizes vitamin D.

Doses far in excess of the recommended amounts may produce abnormally high levels of blood calcium which can cause kidney damage, high blood pressure, and depression of brain function. Deficiencies cause rickets in children and bone softening in adults.

Vitamin E (*tocopherol*) is an antioxidant and thus serves as a food pre-

TABLE 1.

A Guide to the Vitamins

Vitamin	Best Sources
A	liver; eggs, cheese, butter, fortified margarine and milk; yellow, orange, and dark green vegetables (e.g., carrots, broccoli, squash, spinach)
B_1 (thiamin)	pork (especially ham), liver, oysters; whole grain and enriched cereals, pasta and bread, wheat germ; brewers yeast; green peas
B_2 (riboflavin)	liver, meat; milk; dark green vegetables; whole grain and enriched cereals, pasta and bread; mushrooms
B_3 (niacin)	liver, poultry, meat, tuna; whole grain and enriched cereals, pasta and bread; nuts, dried beans, and peas; made in body from amino acid tryptophan
B_6 (pyridoxine)	whole grain (but not enriched) cereals and bread; liver; avocados, spinach, green beans; bananas
B_{12} (cobalamin)	liver, kidneys, meat, fish, oysters; eggs; milk
Folic acid (folacin)	liver, kidneys; dark green leafy vegetables; wheat germ; brewers yeast
Pantothenic acid	liver, kidneys; whole grain bread and cereal; nuts; eggs; dark green vegetables; yeast
Biotin	egg yolk; liver, kidneys; dark green vegetables, green beans; made in intestinal tract
C (ascorbic acid)	many fruits and vegetables, including citrus, tomato, strawberries, melon, green pepper, potato, dark green vegetables
D	milk; egg yolk; liver, tuna, salmon; made on skin in sunlight
E	vegetable oils; margarine; whole grain cereal and bread, wheat germ; liver; dried beans; green leafy vegetables
K	green leafy vegetables; vegetables in cabbage family; milk; made in intestinal tract

Main Roles	Deficiency Symptoms
formation and maintenance of skin and mucous membranes, bone growth, vision, reproduction, teeth	night blindness, rough skin and mucous membranes, no bone growth, cracked or decayed teeth, drying of eyes
release of energy from carbohydrates, synthesis of nerve-regulating substance	beriberi, mental confusion, muscular weakness, swelling of heart, leg cramps
release of energy to cells from carbohydrates, proteins, and fats; maintenance of mucous membranes	skin disorders, especially around nose and lips; cracks at mouth corners; eyes very sensitive to light
works with thiamin and riboflavin in energy-producing reactions in cells	pellagra: skin disorders, especially parts exposed to sun; smooth tongue; diarrhea; mental confusion; irritability
absorption and metabolism of proteins, use of fats, formation of red blood cells	skin disorders, cracks at mouth corners, smooth tongue, convulsions, dizziness, nausea, anemia, kidney stones
building of genetic material, formation of red blood cells, functioning of nervous system	pernicious anemia, anemia, degeneration of peripheral nerves
assists in forming body proteins and genetic material, formation of hemoglobin	anemia with large red blood cells, smooth tongue, diarrhea
metabolism of carbohydrates, proteins and fats; formation of hormones and nerve-regulating substances	not known except experimentally in man: vomiting, abdominal pain, fatigue, sleep problems
formation of fatty acids, release of energy from carbohydrates	not known except experimentally in man: fatigue, depression, nausea, pains, loss of appetite
maintenance of health of bones, teeth, blood vessels; formation of collagen, which supports body structure; antioxidant	scurvy; gums bleed; muscles degenerate; wounds don't heal; skin rough, brown, and dry; teeth loosen
essential for normal bone growth and maintenance of strong bones	rickets (in children): retarded growth, bowed legs, malformed teeth, protruding abdomen; osteomalacia (in adults): bones soften, deform, and fracture easily, muscular twitching and spasms
formation of red blood cells, muscle, and other tissues; prevents oxidation of vitamin A and fats	breakdown of red blood cells; symptoms in animals (reproductive failure, liver degeneration, muscular dystrophy, etc.) not seen in man
essential for normal blood clotting	hemorrhage (especially in newborns)

SOURCE: © 1979 by The New York Times Company. Reprinted by permission.

servative. In the body it is involved in cellular respiration and in muscle and red blood cell formation. It is found in a wide variety of foods including green leafy vegetables, whole grains, liver, and dried beans. Deficiencies are almost never seen in humans, but can reduce the stability of red blood cells. Claims that vitamin E will ward off the effects of aging, enhance fertility, and restore or improve libido (sexual drive) and potency have not been substantiated.

Vitamin K is needed to form the prothrombin factor that must be present for blood to coagulate (clot). It was named from the Danish word *Koagulation*. It is present in green leafy vegetables and cabbage and is synthesized by bacteria in the digestive tract. Deficiencies characterized by diffuse internal bleeding are sometimes seen in adults with liver disease that impairs absorption capacities because of insufficient bile, persons on antibiotic therapy that causes changes in intestinal bacteria, and in newborn infants. They are treated by giving injections of vitamin K.

WATER-SOLUBLE VITAMINS

The water-soluble vitamins are the so-called B complex vitamins and vitamin C. Two additional substances, choline and inositol, are sometimes considered to be B vitamins, but they are actually not vitamins. Each B vitamin is unique and there is now no functional justification for continuing to refer to them as a group. Dietary excesses of water-soluble vitamins can be stored only in limited amounts. Ascorbic acid can be stored for longer periods. Therefore, they must be supplied every day and deficiencies often develop rapidly.

Thiamin (B_1) is necessary as an oxidizing agent in the release of energy from carbohydrates and in the synthesis of certain nerve regulating substances. Since no one food is exceptionally high in thiamin, we must eat a selection of foods to get our daily supply. Good sources are whole grains, dried beans, leafy vegetables, milk, and liver and other meats, especially pork. It is important to note that some thiamin is lost when foods are cooked in water or at high temperatures. Severe thiamin deficiency causes beriberi, one of the first deficiency diseases to be recognized. Its major signs and symptoms are those of peripheral neuritis with weakness, aching, and burning, especially in the legs; central nervous system manifestations such as irritability and confusion; cardiovascular problems such as rapid heart beat and enlarged heart; and gastrointestinal symptoms such as loss of appetite and constipation.

Riboflavin (B_2) is essential in hydrogenation processes which release energy from carbohydrates, proteins, and fats. It also is essential for healthy skin and mucous membranes and for good vision in bright light. Milk and cheese are the best sources, and liver, eggs, and yeast are also rich in riboflavin. Although not affected by heat in cooking, riboflavin is soluble in water, and some of it can be lost when foods are cooked in water. Riboflavin deficiency causes cracks around the corners of the mouth (cheilosis), inflammation of the lips, and tongue changes (glossitis).

Niacin (*nicotinic acid, nicotinamide, B_3*) works with thiamin and riboflavin to produce energy in cells. It is needed to change glucose to glycogen, our only storage form of carbohydrate, and has a role in the synthesis of fat and cholesterol. Liver and yeast are the most concentrated sources of niacin, but the best commonly eaten food sources are meats, poultry, fish, and legumes. It also is synthesized in the body from tryptophan, an amino acid. A lack of it causes pellagra with skin eruptions, sore and swollen tongue, diarrhea, and impaired brain function.

Pyridoxine (*B_6*) facilitates reactions in which amino acids (the building blocks for protein) are absorbed and metabolized, and it plays a role in the formation of red blood cells. The list of chemical reactions which require pyridoxine is enlarging continually as research efforts progress. The best sources are those containing the other B vitamins—liver, whole grain cereals and bread, green beans, spinach, and bananas. When wheat is made into white flour, most of this vitamin is lost, and food processing also has a destructive effect on it. Requirements for pyridoxine increase when the protein of the diet is increased, as in pregnancy. Old age and medications such as birth control pills and hormones may also increase requirements. The main signs of pyridoxine deficiency are secretory and weepy lesions of the skin around the nose and mouth and sore mouth and tongue.

Pantothenic acid, another of the B vitamins, is essential for the metabolism of carbohydrates, proteins, and fats. It is involved in hormone formation also. Its physiologically active form is known as coenzyme A. A deficiency of pantothenic acid has almost never been seen in man, possibly because it is present in ordinary foods, particularly liver, eggs, and wheat germ.

Folacin (*folic acid, folate, pteroylglutamic acid or PGA*) is essential for the formation of new cells, the production of red blood cells, and protein synthesis. Liver, yeast, and fresh green vegetables are rich sources, but it is present in nearly all foods. However, because 50 to 90 percent of folacin may be destroyed by prolonged cooking or by canning, some people have a deficiency, particularly those on very marginal diets, many of whom are alcoholics. Pregnant and nursing women generally are thought to need extra folacin. Deficiency leads to megoblastic (large red blood cells) anemia, inflammation of the tongue, and diarrhea. Antifolic acid preparations are used to treat some types of cancer since folacin is essential for cells to divide and multiply.

Cobalamin (*cyanocobalamin, B_{12}*) is essential for the normal functioning of all cells in the body, particularly the blood-producing cells in the bone marrow and the cells of the nervous system and digestive tract. It is found only in foods of animal origin. Plants, including yeast, which are good sources of other B vitamins provide no cobalamin. Beef, liver, lamb, cheese, and oysters are exceptionally good sources. A lack of cobalamin generally results from malabsorption rather than from a dietary inadequacy. Deficiency causes pernicious anemia, a rare but once fatal disease, which now is "cured" by periodic injections of this vitamin.

Biotin, another B vitamin, is involved in the metabolism of carbon dioxide. It is present in egg yolk, dark green vegetables, liver, and green beans. It is synthesized in the gastrointestinal tract. Deficiency of it is unknown except experimentally.

Ascorbic acid (vitamin C) is needed to form collagen, the protein which binds our cells together. It promotes wound and bone healing and normal blood clotting. By maintaining the elasticity and strength of blood vessels, vitamin C prevents easy bruising. It is also needed for the absorption of iron. The best sources are fruits including strawberries, oranges, and grapefruit. Vegetable sources include broccoli, tomatoes, cauliflower, and green pepper.

Scurvy, which results from ascorbic acid deficiency, has been known since early Egyptian times. It is the subject of much of the fiction and nonfiction written about the British Navy where in 1753 a Scottish doctor discovered that sailors who got lemon juice during long voyages at sea remained healthy. Those who did not developed extreme lassitude, bleeding gums, and skin bruises.

While there is some indication that stress and infection (including colds) increase our need for ascorbic acid, there is no proven reason to take excessively large amounts of it. In fact, to do so may be harmful.

Minerals

Calcium circulating in the bloodstream helps blood to clot, is required for muscle contraction and relaxation, and helps to regulate nerve activity. The most important muscle of all, the heart, contracts and relaxes in large measure because of an adequate and controlled level of calcium. Combined with phosphorus as calcium phosphate, it forms the hard material of bones and teeth. Calcium in bone is absorbed and replaced continually to maintain the proper level in the blood. Calcium absorbed from the teeth, however, cannot be replaced. Therefore, broken bones heal, but teeth cannot repair themselves.

Vitamin D is essential in the diet for the proper metabolism of calcium from food sources. Important sources are milk, milk products, and egg yolk.

Iron is the constituent of hemoglobin that enables the red blood cells to transport oxygen to all parts of the body. Only 15 milligrams of dietary iron are needed each day to replace the red blood cells that are destroyed in the body's processes. During menstruation a woman needs an additional 3 milligrams to compensate for the blood loss. These daily requirements are easily obtained in a diet containing such foods as eggs, lean meat, liver, peanut butter, molasses, kidney beans, raisins, and green leafy vegetables.

Other minerals required by the body are phosphorus (milk and meat), iodine (fish and any plants grown near the sea), potassium (fish, milk, vegetables), magnesium (grains and vegetables), and sodium (salt).

Water and Fiber

Two substances which are technically not nutrients, but are essential to healthy function and structure are water and fiber. Water, the most abundant substance in our bodies, is needed for all of the nutrients and wastes carried to and from our cells and regulates body temperature. Fiber (cellulose in plant food) speeds and stimulates the digestive process and the elimination of unused and indigestible foods.

Balanced Nutrition

Nutrients work together. Each nutrient has specific functions, several may be necessary for a particular function, and one may affect how another operates in the body. For example, vitamin A cannot be absorbed unless the right amount of vitamin D is present. A sudden increase in the amount of phosphorus without a proportionate increase in calcium, makes the unchanged amount of calcium inadequate for the body's needs. An extra supply of one nutrient cannot make up for the deficiency of another. Therefore, good nutrition means balanced nutrition, with all the necessary nutrients supplied in the right proportions.

SELECTION OF FOODS FOR BALANCED NUTRITION

Food Groups

All the required nutrients cannot be obtained from any single food. In order to be sure of balanced nutrition we must select our nourishment from a variety of food products. For convenience in making that selection foods with similar nutrient content are grouped together.

Foods in the milk group supply us with calcium, protein, and riboflavin (B_2). The group includes all types of milk and milk products, such as cheese and yogurt.

Foods in the meat group supply protein, niacin, iron, and thiamine

(B$_1$). It includes meats (pork, veal, lamb, beef), fish and shellfish, poultry, eggs, and certain plant foods which supply large amounts of protein, such as legumes and nuts.

The fruit-vegetable group supplies vitamin A, vitamin C, some minerals, carbohydrates, and cellulose.

Foods in the grain group supply carbohydrates, B vitamins, iron, and cellulose. The group includes all grains and cereals, such as barley, buckwheat, corn, oats, rice, rye, and wheat.

Table 2 lists the four basic food groups and gives specific examples of foods for each, the amount in each serving, and the recommended number of servings per day based on age and whether women are pregnant or breast-feeding. Note that Table 2 refers specifically to nutrients and not to calories.

TABLE 2.

Recommended Servings of Basic Food Groups to Supply Essential Nutrients

Number of Servings Per Day		*Food Group/Serving Size*
Child	3	MILK
Adolescent	4	1 cup (8 oz) or yogurt; 1½ slices (1½ oz)
Adult	2	cheddar cheese; 1 cup pudding; 1¾ cups ice
Pregnant Woman	4	cream; 2 cups cottage cheese
Breast-feeding Woman	4	
Child	2	MEAT
Adolescent	2	2 oz cooked, lean meat, fish, poultry; 2 eggs;
Adult	2	2 slices (2 oz) cheddar cheese; ½ cup cottage
Pregnant Woman	3	cheese; 1 cup dried beans, peas; 4 tbsp peanut
Breast-feeding Woman	2	butter
Child	4	FRUIT-VEGETABLE
Adolescent	4	1 cup raw fruit or vegetable; ½ cup cooked
Adult	4	fruit or vegetable; 1 medium fruit, e.g., apple,
Pregnant Woman	4	banana; ½ cup juice
Breast-feeding Woman	4	
Child	4	GRAIN (Whole grain, fortified, or enriched)
Adolescent	4	1 slice bread; 1 cup ready-to-eat cereal; ½ cup
Adult	4	cooked cereal, pasta, cornmeal, rice, or grits;
Pregnant Woman	4	1 small muffin or biscuit; 5 saltines; 2 graham
Breast-feeding Woman	4	crackers

SOURCE: Adapted from recommendations of National Dairy Council, Rosemont, Ill., 1978.

Food Labeling

Thanks to the consumer advocacy movements, food shoppers are increasingly aware of and interested in the nutrition information on package labels. The Recommended Daily Dietary Allowances (RDAs) are the levels of intake of essential nutrients that are considered by the Food and Nutrition Board of the National Research Council to meet the known needs of "practically all healthy people." The United States Recommended Daily Allowances (U.S. RDA) are a simplified form of the RDA devised for use in nutrition labeling. On most canned or packaged foods, the ingredients must be listed on the label. Any additives used in the products also must be listed, but colors and flavors need not be listed by name. Under a Food and Drug Administration (FDA) regulation, the word "imitation" must be used on the label when a product varies in content from an established standard for the product it resembles and for which it is a substitute.

Nutrition labeling is required only if a manufacturer adds nutrients or makes a nutritional claim on the label or in advertising. The nutrition label gives the size of a serving; the number of servings in the container; the number of calories in one serving; the grams of protein, carbohydrate, and fat in one serving; and the percentage of the U.S. RDA in one serving for protein, vitamins A, B_1, B_2, niacin, and C, calcium, and iron.

Some foods carry a grade on the label, such as "U.S. Grade A." Grades are set by the U.S. Department of Agriculture and are based on the inherent quality of a product—its taste, texture, and appearance. Milk and milk products in most states carry a Grade A Label which is based on FDA recommended sanitary standards for production and processing. The grade is not based on nutritional value.

Food Additives

Food additives have received much publicity in the recent scientific and lay press. The FDA defines food additives as "substances added directly to food, or substances which may reasonably be expected to become components of food through surface contact with equipment or packaging materials, or even substances that may otherwise affect food without becoming part of it."

Food additives are divided into two groups. One consists of newly developed additives regulated by the FDA and the other includes substances in use for a long time and called the Generally Recognized as Safe List (GRAS).

Most intentional additives, such as spices, herbs, flavorings, and oil extracts, are added for flavor. Some, such as monosodium glutamate, are flavor enhancers. Foods lose quality or become unsafe to eat because of chemical changes within the food or because bacteria or molds develop. Antioxidants, such as butylated-hydroxy anisole (BHA), prevent fats from becoming rancid and are added to oils, salad dressings, fried foods, potato chips, margarines, and baked goods or cake mixes which contain shortening. Ascorbic acid (vitamin C) is added to keep peeled and cut fruits from turning brown. Sugar, the oldest additive, is used to prevent molds from growing in bread, baked goods, cheese, syrup, candy, and jams, and jellies. Additives such as salt, sodium nitrate, and sodium nitrite are used to cure meat, thus preventing harmful bacteria from developing.

Mineral and vitamin additives are used to enrich the nutritive value of foods, most commonly bread and flour. Milk is enriched with vitamin D while margarine, skim milk and nonfat dry milk are enriched with vitamin A. Potassium iodide is added to table salt to prevent thyroid goiter, and fluoride is added to water because of its preventive action against tooth decay.

Additives which are used to give or maintain texture include emulsifiers, stabilizers, and thickeners which give body or greater consistency. Emulsifiers keep chocolate candy from changing color if it becomes warm and keep ice cream smooth and creamy by helping fats and other liquids to mix and stay mixed. Stabilizers keep solids and liquids from separating, as in chocolate milk, and prevent flavor loss from cake and pudding mixes.

Chemical substances such as citric acid (lemon juice) and acetic acid (vinegar) are used to give flavor and texture to foods such as jellies and jams, pickles, and salad dressings. Sodium hydroxide provides the glaze on pretzels.

While food colors were once derived from plants, 90 percent of all colors now in use are synthetic and are obvious in such foods as ice cream, soft drinks, pudding mixes, and gelatin desserts. Many of the synthetic dyes used to color foods, especially dyes prepared from aromatic compounds, were banned several years ago as a result of toxicity tests. Recent tests indicate that excessively high levels of colors violet 1, red 2, and red 4 produce tumors in rats and mice. As a result of a Federal law's "Delaney clause," which bars from use any food additive which induces cancer in man or animals, the number of permitted food colorings has decreased.

There are additives to keep foods moist called humectants and others to keep salt and powdered sugar free-flowing. Firming agents help canned tomatoes hold their shape, and sequestrants keep soft drinks clear by removing trace metals which cloud the water. Sodium nitrite, sodium nitrate which is converted to nitrite in the body, and sodium chloride (table salt) have been used for centuries to keep meat from spoiling. Before the advent of refrigeration and freezing, salting was the only way to keep meat. The formation of botulism toxin, the most deadly of all food poisons, can be prevented by the sodium nitrite in the salting mixture used to cure meats. In addition, sodium nitrite prevents fat from becoming rancid, produces the popular cured flavor, and gives the meat a pleasant pink color. These substances are added to all cured and smoked meats (bacon, bologna, ham, frankfurter, corned beef, and so forth).

During the last decade there has been a great deal of research on factors in food and the environment which might cause cancer. Among the compounds found to produce cancer in rats were nitrite and its precursor, nitrate. Though cancers occurred only when the intake of either was high, the results cast suspicion on the safety of cured meats. Harmful compounds are more easily formed at a high temperature. For instance, nitrosamines, which are derivatives of nitrate and nitrite, are carcinogenic agents, formed when bacon which has been cured with nitrate or nitrite is cooked. The nitrosamines then are present in the bacon and also are released into the air. As a result neither nitrate nor nitrite is used now in many cured meats such as bacon, and when they are used, the amount has been reduced to the minimum needed to preserve the product.

The leading food additive used in the United States is sugar. The prejudice against sugar is conspicuous in the supermarket where an increasing number of foods are labeled "natural," "no sugar added," or "in natural juice." The concern about sugar stems from a preoccupation with obesity and tooth decay. But a calorie is a calorie, whether it comes from sugar, starch, or fat; obesity or excessive calorie intake is no more a consequence of sugar intake than of starch or fat intake. And tooth decay results from food deposits left on the teeth, not just the presence of sugar in the diet.

The concern about excess sugar in food has prompted the development of artificial, non-nutritive sweeteners, such as saccharin, which taste sweet because they stimulate taste receptors in the same way but which cannot be oxidized by the body to yield energy. Links between saccharin and bladder cancer in rats have been an important factor in efforts by the FDA to restrict its use. While new studies do not prove that saccharin is entirely harmless, they show *no* evidence that it has played a significant role in cancer of the urinary tract, including the bladder. The risk for children, especially those exposed in utero, and for older people with lifelong heavy use, has yet to be determined.

Salt (sodium chloride), probably the oldest and most widely used food additive, can be harmful, even under common conditions of use. Sodium and chloride, along with potassium, are the regulators for the passage of nutrients in and out of the cells. Though the process is complicated, the most important factor is balance. Too much or too little salt upsets this balance. While the average daily intake of salt is between 7 and 13 grams, the amount needed to stay healthy is only about 200 milligrams a day. It's the sodium which concerns us most; it can cause fluid retention and is a vital factor in controlling high blood pressure. Salt is restricted in the diets of people with high blood pressure to 1 or 2 grams daily. For most people, such restriction makes meal planning difficult and often requires the assistance of a dietitian.

While most natural unprocessed food is relatively low in sodium, processed and factory-made food is overdosed with sodium in the form of salt and other additives. Peas from your garden contain 1 milligram of sodium per 3 ounces, while the same quantity of canned peas contains 240 milligrams of sodium. Since the amount of salt essential to our health is more than adequately provided in the foods we buy, salt shakers on our table are superfluous and should be removed. Labels on processed foods should be reviewed carefully regarding sodium content.

Fast Foods

Many of us eat more than half our meals away from home. As a result fast-food chains have thrived and the industry continues to grow. We are attracted to them because they are fast, filling, easy, inexpensive, attractive to our children, and sometimes taste quite good. While not synonymous with "junk," which provides little or no nutrients other than sugar and calories, fast foods are not nutritionally balanced. For the number of calories they provide, fast-food meals tend to oversupply us with fats and salt, while undersupplying us with vitamins. While the meals at fast-food chains may be low in sugar, the beverages (soft drinks and shakes) and desserts are not. In terms of food groups, these meals are severely deficient in vegetables (except potatoes) and fruit. Therefore, we should be certain to eat salad, vegetables, and fruit at our other meals on those days when we eat fast food in order to assure that our daily nutrition is properly balanced.

The french fries especially are a nutritional pitfall. Potatoes are nutritional and in proportion to their calories they provide relatively large amounts of protein, vitamins, and minerals. But when fried in deep fat, they become a high-fat, high-calorie food, and when doused with salt and ketchup, their sodium content is high.

As shown on Table 3, the calories in our favorite burger-with-everything-on-it are high. For example, a Burger King Whopper has 606 calories and a McDonald's Big Mac 541. Sodium content is excessive with levels of 909 milligrams and 962 milligrams in each of the burgers cited. Pizza is one of the better balanced fast foods with plenty of protein and less fat than many other fast-food meals. But again, the high level of sodium is a major nutritional drawback.

TABLE 3.

Nutritional Content of Popular Fast Foods

Item	Calories	Protein (grams)	Carbo-hydrates (grams)	Fat (grams)	Sodium (milligrams)
HAMBURGERS					
Burger King Whopper	606	29	51	32	909
McDonald's Big Mac	541	26	39	31	962
Burger Chef hamburger	258	11	24	13	393
FISH					
Arthur Treacher's fish sandwich	440	16	39	24	836
Burger King Whaler	486	18	84	46	735
McDonald's Filet-O-Fish	402	15	34	23	709
Long John Silver's fish (2)	318	19	19	19	N.A.*
CHICKEN					
Kentucky Fried original dinner	830	52	56	46	2285
Kentucky Fried crispy dinner	950	52	63	54	1915
OTHER ENTREES					
Pizza Hut Thin 'N Crispy cheese pizza (half of 10-inch pie)	450	25	54	15	N.A.
Pizza Hut Thick 'N Chewy pepperoni pizza (half of 10-inch pie)	560	31	68	18	N.A.
McDonald's Egg McMuffin	352	18	26	20	914
Taco Bell taco	186	15	14	8	79
Dairy Queen brazier dog	273	11	23	15	868
SIDE DISHES					
Burger King french fries	214	3	28	10	5
Arthur Treacher's cole slaw	123	1	11	8	266
Dairy Queen onion rings	300	8	33	17	N.A.
Burger King vanilla shake	332	11	50	11	159
McDonald's chocolate shake	384	11	60	9	329
McDonald's apple pie	300	2	31	19	414

* N.A. = Not available.

SOURCE: © 1979 by The New York Times Company. Reprinted by permission. Data supplied by companies.

WEIGHT

Determining Ideal Body Weight

There is a weight that is physiologically best for each of us. It depends on age, physical activity, height, and body build. Your best or ideal body weight (IBW) for height and body build can be determined from standard actuarial tables as in Table 4. Note that these weights apply to women age 25 and over.

TABLE 4.

Ideal Body Weights for Women Ages 25 and Over, According to Body Build (in Pounds)

Height		Small Build	Medium Build	Large Build
4 ft	8 in	89– 90	93–104	101–116
4	9	91– 98	95–107	103–119
4	10	93–101	98–110	106–122
4	11	96–104	101–113	109–125
5	0	99–107	104–116	112–128
5	1	102–110	107–119	115–131
5	2	105–113	110–123	118–135
5	3	108–116	113–127	122–139
5	4	111–120	117–132	126–143
5	5	115–124	121–136	130–147
5	6	119–128	125–140	134–151
5	7	123–132	129–144	138–155
5	8	127–137	133–148	142–160
5	9	131–141	137–152	146–165
5	10	135–145	141–156	150–170

SOURCE: Adapted from table prepared by Metropolitan Life Insurance Company. Derived primarily from data of the Build and Blood Pressure Study, 1959, Society of Actuaries.

When a woman at age 25 has reached her best or ideal weight, continued weight gain after that age is not normal or necessary for basic biologic function.

IBW can also be calculated easily without a table. Allow 100 pounds for the first 5 feet of height, add 5 pounds for each additional inch of height, and adjust for body build by adding 10 percent of the total for a large build or subtracting 10 percent for a small build. As an example, for a large-framed woman, 5 feet 5 inches tall:

first 5 feet	100
each additional inch	+ 25
	125
10 percent of total	+ 12½
IBW	137½ pounds

Calorie Requirements to Maintain IBW

Calories do count! There is never a time or an age when calories don't count. Food supplies energy to your body and energy is measured in calories just as body weight is measured in pounds. When the total amount of food we eat in one day provides our bodies with more calories than are needed for the day's activities, the extra calories are stored as fat and weight is gained. When fewer calories are consumed than the body needs, weight is lost.

In 1980 the Food and Nutrition Board of the National Academy of Sciences of the United States published revised guidelines of energy requirements for all age groups; these appear in Table 5. The recommended number of calories represents an average needed daily to maintain an average IBW at the ages listed, based on a moderate level of activity. Activities such as swimming, tennis, running, bicycling, and disco dancing are classified as strenuous; making beds, polishing a car, light gardening, and a brisk walk are moderate; reading, eating, typing, and office work are sedentary. Without access to such a table, we can calculate our total daily calorie needs by adding the calories needed for basal metabolic function to calories required for activity.

Calories needed for basal metabolic function: IBW (in lb) × 10
Calories needed for activity:

Sedentary	IBW	× 3
Moderate	IBW	× 5
Strenuous	IBW	× 10

For example, let us calculate the calorie needs for a 35-year-old woman, 5 feet 5 inches tall and of medium build, who works 8 hours a day as a draftsperson and then returns home where she prepares the evening meal and machine launders clothes for her family of four before relaxing with her evening paper.

Basal calorie needs	125 lb (IBW) × 10	1,250
Activity	125 lb × 4 (av. of 3 + 5)	500
Total		1,750 calories

TABLE 5.

Recommended Energy Requirements for Basal Metabolic Function with Moderate Activity

Category	Age years	Weight kg	Weight lb	Height cm	Height in	Energy Needs (with range) kcal
Infants	0.0–0.5	6	13	60	24	kg × 115 (95–145)
	0.5–1.0	9	20	71	28	kg × 105 (80–135)
Children	1–3	13	29	90	35	1300 (900–1800)
	4–6	20	44	112	44	1700 (1300–2300)
	7–10	28	62	132	52	2400 (1650–3300)
Males	11–14	45	99	157	62	2700 (2000–3700)
	15–18	66	145	176	69	2800 (2100–3900)
	19–22	70	154	177	70	2900 (2500–3300)
	23–50	70	154	178	70	2700 (2300–3100)
	51–75	70	154	178	70	2400 (2000–2800)
	76+	70	154	178	70	2050 (1650–2450)
Females	11–14	46	101	157	62	2200 (1500–3000)
	15–18	55	120	163	64	2100 (1200–3000)
	19–22	55	120	163	64	2100 (1700–2500)
	23–50	55	120	163	64	2000 (1600–2400)
	51–75	55	120	163	64	1800 (1400–2200)
	76+	55	120	163	64	1600 (1200–2000)
Pregnancy						+300
Lactation						+500

SOURCE: *Recommended Dietary Allowances, Revised 1980,* Food and Nutrition Board, National Academy of Sciences-National Research Council, Washington, D.C.

TABLE 6.

Calorie Estimates of Daily Required Servings of Basic Food Groups

Food Group	Estimated Calories per Serving	Minimum Servings (Adult)	Approximate Calories
Milk	150	2	300
Meat	125	2	250
Fruit-vegetable	50	4	200
Grain	75	4	300
		Total	1050

Listed in Table 6 are calorie estimates per serving for each of the food groups reviewed in Table 2. Though only rough approximations, the calorie estimates can be used to measure total daily calorie intake which can then be compared with the total daily calorie needs just calculated. A woman who eats the minimum number of servings in each basic food group, that is, two servings each from the milk and meat groups and four servings each from the fruit-vegetable and grain groups, will consume an estimated 1,050 calories per day. This is a low calorie intake for most women and should not be reduced further except on the advice of a physician. Our draftsperson, whose daily calorie requirement is 1,750 calories, can add to these minimum servings another 600 calories. For example, based on the calorie estimates per serving, she might add 1¾ cups of ice cream as an evening snack (150 calories), an extra meat serving with her dinner meal (125 calories), an apple for a mid-afternoon snack (50 calories), an extra slice of buttered toast for breakfast (75 calories for toast, 72 calories for 2 teaspoons of butter), and an extra glass of milk or cup of yogurt (150 calories).

NUTRITIONAL NEEDS AT SPECIAL AGES AND STAGES

The general information we have presented on ideal body weight, calorie requirements, and balanced nutrition applies to the healthy woman age 23 through 50 who is not pregnant and not lactating. Older women and those who are pregnant or lactating have special nutritional needs.

Nutrition in Pregnancy

Pregnancy is a unique and special time in the life of a woman. All women want their babies to be healthy. The main reason some babies die or are not healthy is that they weigh 2,500 grams (5.5 pounds) or less at birth. While there are many causes of this low birth weight problem, the major one involves inadequate maternal nutrition during the pregnancy and even before conception.

Adequate nutrition is needed to provide the caloric energy, essential nutrients such as proteins, vitamins, and minerals required by the growing fetus, and the many physiologic and metabolic changes that occur in the mother. Nutritional needs for a healthy, well-nourished woman who is not underweight during pregnancy require about 300 extra calories each day over the nonpregnant diet of approximately 2,100 calories (see tables 2 and 5). These ideally should be provided from food in the following ratios: 40 to 50 percent from carbohydrates (preferably starch); 15 to 20 percent from protein (animal and vegetable); and 30 to 35 percent from fat. Such a 2,400 calorie daily diet will provide all her energy needs.

Of the essential nutrients, protein is most important because it is vital to the formation and growth of the fetal brain which is more fully developed at birth than the rest of the body. The healthy woman described above needs approximately 76 grams of protein each day, particularly in the last three months of pregnancy. This is 30 grams more than an acceptable nonpregnant daily protein diet of 46 grams. A quart of milk contains 32 grams of protein. One third of the protein should be animal in origin. Vegetarian diets are often deficient in certain types of amino acids and special care must be taken to eat the complementary foods to get complete proteins.

Another essential nutrient is iron, used by the body to make the needed additional maternal hemoglobin which carries oxygen to all the tissues, including the fetus. Since many women have insufficient stored iron and no diet can supply the increased amounts necessary, ferrous sulfate is often prescribed—one 5-grain tablet a day is sufficient—starting as early in pregnancy as possible and continuing for about a month after birth. Daily folic acid is often prescribed, too, to prevent both folate deficiency and a rare kind of anemia called megaloblastic anemia. Accumulating evidence suggests that a supplement of other vitamins also is important during pregnancy.

Since individual eating habits vary so much and since only 20 to 30 percent of women in the United States begin pregnancy in a good nutritional state, it is crucial for every pregnant woman to discuss her nutritional needs with her health care provider early in her pregnancy or even before pregnancy, if possible. Women with poor or marginal diets, adolescents, women underweight, and women carrying twins, for example, need more calories and protein than the amounts noted above.

As your pregnancy continues the most convenient way to assess your nutritional status is by observing your weight changes from week to week. This should be about 2–4 pounds of tissue, not fluid (edema), during the first trimester, and then a little less than 1 pound a week thereafter for a total gain of around 27 pounds. Such a gain suggests good nutritional intake. Lesser gains usually indicate inadequate nutrition and the possibility of a resultant low birth weight baby. Most obese women also should gain this amount. Slightly greater gains ordinarily are not a problem for the baby or mother.

In the past salt restriction was invariably suggested, if not demanded. We now know that salt restriction is unnecessary and unwise except when pregnant women have certain chronic diseases, like congestive heart failure, which are often treated by restricting salt. One problem with excessive salt is that it tends to be associated with empty calorie foods, like potato chips, which may replace foods containing other essential nutrients.

Nutrition When Breast-Feeding

Proper nutrition is essential for successful breast-feeding. The energy and nutritional costs to the nursing mother are high. Compared to her pre-pregnancy needs, she needs as much as an extra 1000 calories per day for the first three months and more from the fourth month on if breast-feeding continues. She needs an extra 20 grams of protein daily. Needs for vitamins A and C are modestly increased. The high calcium content of breast milk requires an extra 400 milligrams per day in the diet. The extra calcium, vitamin A, and protein can be supplied by drinking an extra 1¼ pints of milk each day; the extra vitamin C can be supplied by two additional servings of citrus fruit or tomatoes.

During a normal full term pregnancy, about 3 kilograms of nutrients (fat and protein) are stored in the body. These provide 200 to 300 calories of energy a day for three months. Women who breast-feed their babies lose most of this extra tissue by six months unless they maintain a very high intake of food. Women who do not breast-feed but wish to lose weight must restrict their caloric intake or increase their activity to get rid of the additional fat gained during pregnancy. Regular eating and drinking habits and responding to thirst usually assure an appropriate amount of fluid.

Nutrition for the Older Woman

As we grow older, we need the same essential nutrients we have always needed, but we need fewer calories. Our calorie requirement at age 30 slowly decreases as we age as a result of decreases in rate of basal metabolism and physical activity.

To get the essential nutrients every day, eat recommended servings from the four basic food groups listed in Table 2. To avoid exceeding your energy requirements, use the recommended daily calorie intake in Table 5 as a guide in selecting additional foods. According to the table, the average woman in the 51–75 age group requires 1,800 calories a day, a drop of 200 calories from what was needed between ages 23–50. For women 76 years of age and over, the need is 1600 calories.

If mealtime is a chore rather than a pleasure, alter your mealtime habits. Instead of the standard three "squares" a day, have two meals—a late breakfast or brunch and an early dinner when you are most hungry. Take a brisk walk and sip a glass of wine before dinner to stimulate your appetite. Make meals which are appetizing; include colorful vegetables and garnish with a parsley sprig. With age the sense of taste becomes less acute, and food may seem bland and unappealing. Avoid adding large and potentially harmful amounts of salt and sugar to your meals. Herbs and spices can be good substitutes to enhance flavor. Be realistic about your chewing ability. If your teeth are not up to the rigors of chewing a steak or if you wear dentures, you will find cubed or chopped foods easier to chew. A different atmosphere does wonders to improve mealtime. A few fresh flowers on the table or candlelight can make mealtime different and fun, even when you eat alone. Books about "cooking for one" can give you new ideas for attractive meals. When possible, invite a friend or relative for dinner and use this as an occasion to try out a new recipe.

Foods high in fiber are especially important to help counter several common problems among the elderly, especially constipation and diverticular disease. There is some research to suggest that increased bulk in the diet may prevent colon cancer.

Excess phosphorus tends to enhance the loss of bone as we get older, yet the typical American diet contains proportionately more phosphorus than calcium in foods such as meats, soft drinks, snacks such as potato chips and crackers, and cheeses, especially processed cheeses which contain phosphorus in the form of phosphates used as additives.

Since the ability of our bodies to process sugar may decline with age, restricting sweets and starches as we get older may avoid or forestall problems in metabolizing carbohydrates.

Many older women require special diets for their health. For example, if you have heart disease or high blood pressure you may need to restrict your intake of salt. Diet is the main way to control many cases of diabetes that begin in the later years of life. Women taking blood pressure medication often require foods rich in potassium. Women on special diets should obtain written instructions from doctors or qualified nutrition specialists. Cookbooks containing a wide variety of appetizing dishes for those on restricted diets are available.

When illness and disability occur, shopping for and preparing nutritious foods can become difficult. Check around your community for agencies that deliver meals, group meal programs, homemaker services, and stores that deliver groceries. And sharing of food by relatives and neighbors has been a gesture of aid throughout the ages.

OBESITY

Having reviewed the general principles of balanced nutrition and the more specific nutritional needs of women at various stages and ages of life, I want to discuss now a disorder of nutrition which is all too common, especially among women—obesity. Defined in most studies as a weight 20 percent or more above IBW, obesity affects more than 30 percent of the adult women in the United States. This prevalence increases with age from 12 percent for women in their twenties to 46 percent for women in their fifties.

Obesity results from an imbalance between calories consumed and calories used as energy. When calories consumed are greater than those needed and burned for energy, the excess is stored primarily as fat. The factors known to be involved in keeping body weight normal include learned behaviors associated with eating, physiologic factors implicated in the regulation of food intake, change in hormonal status, effects of early nutritional status, genetic endowment, level of activity, and differences in fat cell number and size. The limitations of space preclude reviewing all of these, but we should review factors involved in the early onset of obesity, nutrition and eating patterns during infancy and adolescence and the impact of fat cell number and size.

There is some evidence that fat infants may become fat children who then become fat adults. While it is possible that heredity has some influence on why a child becomes fat, most physicians and students of nutrition are convinced that the most important factor in childhood obesity is how a child is fed during his early years. Children become fat because they are overfed and stay fat because (1) eating patterns and attitudes formed in early life continue and (2) fat infants develop more fat cells than do those of normal weight. Once excess fat cells are acquired, they are not lost through dieting. When an excess number of fat cells is present, the obese child, and later the obese adult, can become thinner only by reducing the fat cell size to smaller than normal. Prospective studies have shown that 60 to 80 percent of infants who are overweight during the first year of life will be of normal weight by 4 to 7 years of age, but a significant proportion, up to 20 percent, will remain overweight and probably be obese. The chance of becoming an obese child and an obese adult is definitely greater for an obese infant than for one of normal weight. Consequently, prevention of obesity in infancy by educating parents in sound nutritional principles and closely monitoring weight during infancy is important.

The initial onset of obesity is not as common during adolescence as it is during the preadolescent period. Many obese teenagers were obese children. The typical obese teenager has exogenous obesity, that is, the excess weight results simply from an excessive caloric intake in relation to body energy needs and expenditure. Primary glandular or endocrinologic abnormalities, such as thyroid or adrenal malfunction, are rare.

In general, controlling obesity is difficult and frustrating. The statistics on treatment leave no doubt that treatment rarely produces a permanent and sustained weight reduction. While any method of weight reduction (and there are more than 17,000 such methods published to date) will produce some degree of weight loss in almost all motivated obese women, maintenance of the reduced body weight occurs in something less than 10 percent. After reviewing the studies on obesity and treatment programs, one must conclude that the only sure-fire way to reduce the prevalence of obesity is to prevent its occurrence!

The goals of treatment are basically to decrease calorie intake and to increase calorie expenditure (negative calorie balance). Although the biologic and physiologic mechanisms leading to a positive calorie balance are often unclear, the fact remains that for a woman to add fat to her body stores, she must eat more calories than she is using in her daily activities. This can occur because her food intake is excessive, her calorie expenditure (physical activity) or basal metabolic needs are lower than normal, or because her absorption of food from her gastrointestinal tract is greater than normal.

Motivation is the fundamental factor for the success of any weight reduction program. The obese woman must want to lose weight. An impending marriage is a most potent factor motivating weight loss. Short-term, but significant weight loss often accompanies the desire to fit into that formal dress for a special event. In most instances weight loss is a matter of personal pride and vanity augmented by the present fashion. Pregnancy, as noted before, is an inappropriate time to diet since the nutritional needs of pregnancy are high.

Basically, there are four major areas of treatment; diet, exercise, drugs, and group therapy including behavior modification.

Diet

Diets are popular, but as is the case with fashion, the popularity of any one diet is short-lived. Dr. Herman Taller in the 1960s tried to convince us that "calories don't count" when he proposed a low-carbohydrate diet which emphasized the "right" amount of polyunsaturated fat in the form of safflower capsules and margarine. He claimed that by stimulating the pituitary gland, safflower gets body fat burned at a higher rate. In truth, the only proven effect of safflower oil is to add calories, approximately 125 per tablespoon!

The "magic" in the Magic Mayo Diet was grapefruit, which was recommended with every meal and was supposed to act as a catalyst to burn body fat. Meat, fish, and eggs were unlimited and sugars and starches were taboo. While grapefruit is an excellent source of vitamin C there is no evidence to support its "magic" as a fat-burning catalyst. Then, too, this diet is high in saturated fats and cholesterol which may promote atherosclerosis or hardening of the arteries.

Dr. Atkin's Revolutionary Diet and Dr. Tarnower's Scarsdale Diet are other popular versions of the low-carbohydrate, high-protein diet which proposes an unlimited consumption of proteins and fats while severely limiting carbohydrates. Women on such a diet often lose up to 8 pounds in the first week, but since carbohydrate restriction has a diuretic effect, the weight lost is mostly water. The severe restriction on carbohydrates, below 60 grams a day, can also result in ketosis as fat is used as an alternative fuel. When the breakdown products of fat, called ketone bodies, build up in the blood, the breath smells fruity and women may complain of an unpleasant taste and nausea. The end result is usually a loss of appetite, so food intake is curbed. If this type of diet is maintained for only a short time, say, one or two weeks, the ketosis is short-term and probably not harmful. However, any episode of ketosis may have harmful effects on an unborn child, so none of the low-carbohydrate, high-protein diets is recommended for pregnant women. Also, the high protein consumed in such diets can be harmful to patients with kidney disease.

Dr. Stillman captured the interest of many diet-conscious readers with his Quick Inches-Off Diet which proposed high-carbohydrate, low-protein meals, specifically forbidding meat, seafood, poultry, milk, and cheese. His magic formula was supposed to allow women to lose inches wherever wanted or needed. It is true that if a woman has abnormal fat deposits and loses weight, these deposits, like all of her body fat, will get smaller. However, disproportionately large thighs will remain disproportionately large!

Dr. Stillman's version of low-carbohydrate, high-protein diet is his Quick Weight-Loss Diet in which eggs, meat, poultry, fish, and seafood are unlimited; dairy foods, with the exception of cottage cheese, are forbidden; 8 glasses of water are to be consumed daily; and the dieter is advised against counting calories.

I will mention the simple "starvation" diet to decry its use, except under the careful direction and supervision of a physician. Its principles are simple—do not drink or eat anything but water and lose 1 pound a day. The hazards of starvation or fasting are many including ketosis, dehydration, nausea, fatigue, and loss of minerals, such as potassium, calcium, and magnesium. The weight loss is due to loss of muscle mass and water, the latter quickly regained when the period of starvation, short-term for obvious reasons, is over.

The large variety of diets as well as the transcience of their popularity indicates that none can guarantee long-term success. Of course, any diet which results in a negative calorie balance, meaning that fewer calories are consumed than are burned for energy, will allow the obese woman to lose weight. However, no single diet is good for everyone, and there is no real evidence that any particular dietary mixture accelerates the rate of weight loss. The main reasons for the failure of these fashionable diets are that they do little to educate the woman with a serious and chronic weight problem in the basic and sound nutritional principles necessary to achieve and maintain the weight which is best for her, nor do they address either the underlying emotional issues or behavior patterns which cause overeating.

The Weight-Watcher's Diet Plan is a step in the right direction. While not the diet or weight reduction program for everyone, this plan counts calories for its members and at the same time makes sure they get all the required nutrients in the proper balance while losing weight.

In my concept of a weight reduction program *calories do count*. A calorie is a calorie whether supplied as carbohydrate, fat, or protein. A diet which has hope for long-term success is one that has a negative calorie balance, is nutritionally balanced, and is suited to the individual's economic constraints, life style, and personal tastes. I recommend, therefore, that whether you are moderately overweight or obese, you design your own diet plan using the guidelines presented herein. Use Table 4 and the formulas provided to determine your IBW and the calories needed for basal metabolic function at that weight. To basal needs add 200 to 300 calories for activity (whatever your IBW or level of activity). As an example, we'll return to the 35-year-old, 5 feet 5 inch draftswoman. Let's say she weighs 160 pounds and wants to reduce to the 125 pounds established as her IBW. We can calculate the calorie intake which will allow her to lose weight.

IBW	125 lb
Basal needs (125 × 10)	1,250
Activity	200
Total	1,450 calories

From Table 2 and Table 6 we know that the minimum servings recommended for adults from each of the four basic food groups will provide approximately 1,050 calories and be nutritionally balanced. Her remaining 400 calories can be added as she chooses, either as larger portions, as additional servings at or between meals, or as a frivolous ice cream sundae.

Exercise

Physical activity is an important factor in determining caloric needs and, clearly, inactivity promotes obesity. Obese adults, by and large, are less active than normal weight individuals. Not only do they spend less time in physical activity, but even when they participate, their time is spent less vigorously.

While exercise can be an important factor in any weight reduction program, the use of exercise in the treatment of obesity is surrounded by faddism. Despite the advertisements of reducing salons, there is no evidence to support the claims that by mechanical means you can selectively mobilize fat from one part of the body. In studies done with tennis players, the greater amount of exercise in the playing arm was not accompanied by any decrease in fat deposits in that arm.

Without a reduction in calorie consumption, exercise is not an effective way to reduce weight since it takes far too much activity to burn up a significant number of calories. Would you walk 3 to 4 miles for a piece of cake? That's the distance it takes to burn up the energy in the cake's calories.

It is important to point out, however, that exercise is accompanied by a reduction in excessive food intake, apparently by reducing appetite. Not only can exercise decrease food intake, but it can also decrease body fat. Studies involving college students have shown that a program of mild to moderate jogging or walking on a treadmill reduced body fat, increased lean body mass, and decreased body weight without other dietary control.

With grossly obese patients, though it is harder to achieve effective levels of exercise, more weight is lost through exercise than in patients of normal weight. In a study of 12 massively obese patients all maintained on the same liquid formula diet, 6 had an exercise program and 6 did not. In the 6 who exercised, the rate of fat loss and weight loss was clearly increased.

In summary, exercise in combination with diet produces greater weight loss than diet alone. If you are trying to lose weight, drive less and walk more. On public transportation signal for a stop before you reach home and walk the rest of the way. Climb stairs instead of pushing the elevator button, especially when you must negotiate three or fewer flights. Walking daily is the easiest form of exercise and 1 mile a day costs your body more than 500 calories a week. In a year that's 8 pounds walked away. By reducing food intake by 100 calories each day, you will take off another 10 pounds.

Diet Pills

Drugs are not effective treatment of obesity and may in fact be harmful. Used not only to suppress appetite, but supposedly to break down fat, their effectiveness, if any, is short-term. And, there are inherent side effects and potential dangers associated with the use of thyroid hormone, amphetamines, and diuretics.

Group Therapy and Behavior Modification

A number of successful weight reduction organizations administer their programs in a group setting. Weight-Watchers, TOPS (Take Off Pounds Safely), and Overeaters Anonymous are the best known self-help organizations for the obese. In general, the cost to the individual is modest and less than that of standard medical therapies. Studies evaluating the effectiveness of group treatment compared to standard medical treatment in achieving weight loss suggest that patients in group programs stay in treatment longer and are more successful in losing weight. Presumably, this is because people with a similar problem reinforce and encourage one another.

Behavior modification in a group setting appears to be the most effective method to date for treating obesity. The basic principle of this approach is the assumption that eating is a learned behavior. If a woman is obese, then her eating behavior is maladapted and should be unlearned. Appropriate behavior conducive to achieving and maintaining a normal body weight can be substituted. The following are some simple suggestions for changing eating patterns. Eat only while seated at a proper eating place and using proper utensils. Eliminate eating in front of the television or snacking by the kitchen sink. Concentrate solely on eating, not on the television, a magazine article, or the conversation around you. Be aware of every bite.

Eat slowly, chew slowly, and pause between bites. Overeaters are frequently fast eaters who are unaware of how much they eat.

Plan menus for the week in advance and count calories *every* time you eat. Compulsive women may find that careful records of meals and snacks prevent splurging and spontaneous eating. Shop for groceries after you have planned your menu and after you have eaten a meal. Never grocery shop when you are hungry!

Eat because you are hungry and stop when you are no longer hungry; don't eat because you are depressed, it is a holiday, you need a reward, or you are anxious to please your hostess.

These changes in eating habits can aid you in losing weight, and when such learned behaviors become automatic, they will help you maintain the weight which is best for you.

I remind you that what I have offered here is no "magic," no mysterious combination of special foods assuring instant, painless weight reduction. Instead, I have presented basic information about nutrition so you can plan meals which are well-balanced and provide calories which are appropriate for your metabolic needs and activity level. Dieting becomes necessary only when these basic guidelines are not followed and overweight results.

ANOREXIA NERVOSA

Anorexia nervosa, fortunately a rare disorder of nutrition, afflicts adolescent and young women with sufficient frequency that we should discuss it before concluding our review of nutrition and weight. It is the relentless pursuit of thinness through self-starvation. Basically, anorexia nervosa is a psychiatric disorder with the main issue a struggle for control and a sense of identity. Many young women affected with this disorder have struggled for years to make themselves over and to be "perfect" in the eyes of others. Their concept of their own body image becomes distorted and even when they are less than ideal body weight for their age, height, and body frame, they see themselves as fat when looking in a mirror.

The outstanding characteristic of this disorder is reduced calorie intake. Not only is the amount of food rigidly restricted, but the whole pattern of eating becomes disorganized in bizarre ways. The absence or denial of hunger alternates with an uncontrollable impulse to gorge oneself. After gorging, the anorectic may induce vomiting or take laxatives to purge herself. Paradoxically, anorexia nervosa is often preceded by obesity and usually begins or becomes overt with dieting. However, in contrast to the ordinary dieter, who makes the supreme sacrifice each time she rejects an ice cream sundae or suffers every time she declines her hostess' offer of chocolate cake, the anorectic adolescent will insist that she is not hungry, does not need to eat and that not wanting to eat is "normal." In contrast to her emaciated appearance, she is overly active, often exercising religiously for many hours each day or increasing her participation in sports. She is an overachiever and her parents will describe her as "a real perfectionist." Secondary amenorrhea, the cessation of menstrual periods, though a characteristic feature of anorexia nervosa, is not an essential part of the disorder. Because the menstrual cycle is so easily affected by emotional disturbances, loss of periods is commonly observed in women under severe stress and the psychological as well as nutritional stresses on the anorectic are indeed severe. In advanced stages of emaciation which these young women often reach, true loss of appetite may result from severe nutritional deficiency, similar to the complete lack of interest in food which occurs in the late stages of starvation during a famine.

It must be apparent from these brief comments that anorexia nervosa is a serious, even grave, condition which manifests as a nutritional dysfunction but is really a psychiatric illness. As such it must be approached psychotherapeutically by a psychiatrist, psychologist, or family therapist with expertise in handling such patients.

FURTHER READING

Diets '79. Consumer Guide Publication. Sold at magazine and news counters; reviews the pros and cons of various weight control programs.

Jordan, H. A., L. S. Levitz, and G. M. Kimbrell. *Eating Is Okay! A Radical Approach to Successful Weight Loss. The Behavioral-Control Diet Explained in Full*. New York: Rawson, 1976.

McGill, Marion, and Orrea Pye. *The No-Nonsense Guide to Food and Nutrition*. New York: Butterick, 1978. A down-to-earth, easy-to-understand guide to nutrition.

Mayer, Jean. *A Diet for Living*. New York: Pocket Books, 1977. An excellent review of current nutrition issues.

Recommended Dietary Allowances. Revised, 1980. Food and Nutritional Board, National Academy of Sciences–National Research Council, Washington, D.C.

Fitness

CHRISTINE E. HAYCOCK, M.D.

Associate Professor of Surgery, New Jersey Colleges of Medicine
and Dentistry, New Jersey Medical School, Newark, New Jersey
Fellow, American College of Sports Medicine

Serious interest in physical fitness and a more than casual involvement in sports for women have become increasingly widespread since the late 1960s. Even before this period health authorities were placing more and more stress on the relationship between physical fitness and improved health. And for the rapidly growing ranks of women who were self-supporting or who were the sole support of their families, good health had become more than a matter of good looks: it was a top priority for compelling economic reasons.

During the 1970s ads for sturdy hiking boots and sneakers for women displaced those for "spectator" sports shoes, and jogging clothes joined dinner dresses in the wardrobe. Across the United States more and more girls and women are spurred on to athletic achievement by the accomplishments of such women as Billie Jean King, Tracy Austin, Nadia Comaneci, Nancy Lopez, and Dorothy Hamill, and those who are not motivated to excel in sports are making a commitment to the goal of good health through fitness. Women of all ages are hiking, playing tennis, dancing, swimming and playing team sports. Women have discovered that the bicycle is a blessing, for exercise, economy, and getting from one place to another conveniently. More and more women are joining physical fitness classes at the Y, spending their vacations at health spas, and banding together to organize community sports programs. And everywhere—in city streets, local gyms, athletic clubs, suburban roads—women are jogging. It is estimated that 6 million American women have adopted this sport as their chief means of maintaining physical fitness.

Much publicity has been given to that aspect of the women's movement which has focused on equal access to athletic facilities for school children of both sexes, on allowing young girls to participate in traditional male sports, and on breaking down sexist barriers to achievement for girls who would prefer to pitch in Little League than go to social dancing class. What is sometimes not emphasized in this situation is how physical activity relates to changing the overall stereotype of the female as nonphysical, helpless, and weak. Increased emphasis on physical activity can allow a young girl to develop the habit of thinking in terms of physical fitness, to acquire an awareness of the capabilities of her body, and to experience the satisfaction that can be derived from achieving competence in any area.

Not every woman, and perhaps only a few, has the ability or the interest to become a star athlete or even a participant in competitive sports. Many see little connection between their overall image of themselves and their attitude toward the condition of their body. You live with your body all the time and feeling awkward, helpless, and weak about such an important aspect of yourself cannot help but affect your total self-image. In more positive terms, to know that your body functions well and to realize that with proper training and discipline you can become competent in physical activity cannot help but contribute to a good self-image, to the habit of thinking of yourself as able to *do*.

There is no question that physical fitness is related to improved health and that specific types of exercise improve the function of specific parts of the body (these will be discussed later). However, in terms of total fitness the benefits of activity seem to derive from more than this direct relation between exercise and improved tissue function. Exercise per se is not the automatic key to fitness. Studies have shown that people who exercise do not need less sleep, eat less, smoke less, or lose weight. But, studies have shown that the percentage of people who score positively on indexes of psychological well-being is higher among those who are highly active than among those who are inactive. The more active report increased self-confidence, better self-image, improved coordination, increased stamina and strength, and fewer illnesses. They feel less tense, more disciplined, less tired, and more productive. Clearly, we cannot separate the physical and psychological aspects of physical activity; they interact and enhance one another in contributing to good health and well-being.

BENEFITS OF PHYSICAL FITNESS

The term physical fitness is defined as the ability to exercise or carry on daily activities without undue distress or fatigue and to be able to respond to occasions requiring physical exertion. A fit individual usually feels good and functions well.

The benefits of exercise fall into two general categories: the physical or physiological improvement of the body itself and the achievement of greater psychological or emotional well-being. Obviously, exercise alone cannot accomplish these goals unless accompanied by other requirements of good health, such as proper nutrition and rest.

For many years it was thought that if women were to lift weights or even engage in a great deal of strenuous physical activity, they would develop bulging muscles and a masculine physique. However, we now know that a normal female will never develop in this way no matter how much she exercises. A male develops bulging muscles because he produces more testosterone. This hormonal difference accounts for the fact that men will always be stronger than women in terms of their ability to lift greater weights, run faster over short distances, and excel in events of sheer muscular development. But this does not mean that the male hormone is necessary for endurance, flexibility, the strength needed to accomplish the tasks a woman wishes to do, or healthy muscle tone.

Exercise contributes to the physiological improvement of the body by increasing muscle strength, increasing the flexibility of the joints, and improving cardiovascular endurance. Exercise, along with suitable diet, increases muscle strength, heightens muscle tone, and reduces the amount of fat. Exercise that strengthens the muscles can also improve cardiac and respiratory function and circulation. The heart muscle is strengthened, and the reduction of the general proportion of fat in the body aids in lowering blood pressure and lessening the amount of cholesterol. Healthier muscle tone makes it possible to perform daily tasks at home or in the office with much less fatigue.

An improvement in flexibility enables women to bend and stoop and reach without undue risk of muscle strains and pulls. Women tend to be more flexible than men because they generally have looser joints. Because of this flexibility and because their muscles are smaller, they can bend their back and touch their toes more easily than most men. Flexibility exercises involve stretching muscles and maintaining the mobility of joints. These are the exercises that have traditionally been encouraged more for women than for men, not only because they are consistent with the woman's physique, but also because they do not produce the muscular development which was assumed would result from other types of exercises. This is gradually changing; men are working to develop more flexibility, while women are lifting weights to become stronger.

Endurance is the ability to persist in an exercise, for example, to engage in long distance running, to play a game for an extended period of time, or, in nonsports terms, to be able to complete or remain at a task that requires physical exertion. Endurance depends in part on cardiovascular function, the ability of the heart to pump blood efficiently through the lungs and the circulatory system, thereby supplying plenty of oxygen to muscles. Cardiovascular endurance can be measured by how far a woman can run, how long she can exercise on her bicycle, or how far she can swim in a specified time, all depending upon her age.

One of the most highly publicized aspects of jogging has been its role in improving cardiovascular endurance. It is believed that vigorous exercise increases the rate of circulation, makes the body more efficient at delivering oxygen to the heart and other body tissue, widens the coronary arteries, and perhaps increases the level of high density lipoprotein, a substance thought to remove cholesterol from the arteries. All these effects contribute to the health of the heart and reduce the heart disease risk factors of high blood pressure and high cholesterol level.

In addition to muscle strength, flexibility, and endurance, there are secondary aspects of physical improvement through exercise: power, agility, and speed. Power determines how far you can throw an object, how far you can jump, or how much you can lift or push. Agility enables you to change directions quickly as you chase a tennis ball, skip a rope, or climb a ladder. Speed enables you to win the race, chase a ball, or run after a child. These three assets are obviously critical for excellence in a particular sport and although they are not critical for general physical fitness, they certainly do contribute to the ability to do everyday activities that anyone might be called on to perform.

Exercise affects other body processes. It enhances the digestive function; it is a reliable and effective aid to normal elimination and thereby reduces the incidence of conditions and complaints resulting from constipation. Doing exercises which produce muscle fatigue also helps us to sleep. Exercise reduces muscle tension caused by stress and is therefore an invaluable, and comparatively simple, way to achieve relaxation. For many women suppressed anger or anxiety seem to be sweated out and away in the act of jogging, swinging a golf club, or hitting a tennis ball. The frictions of the day are easier to handle after an invigorating swim, a few hours of handball seem to make housework less of a bore, and evening calisthenics can minimize the frustrations of the office routine.

All of the physiological benefits, including the reduction of the effects of stress, contribute to psychological improvement. The sense of achievement when you have conditioned your body produces justifiable pride. Knowing that you are in good health produces a general feeling of well-being. With the release of stress and anxiety through exercise comes a specific feeling of personal contentment. The long-term result of the increased participation of women in sports and exercise can only be beneficial. The fit woman can expect to live a longer and healthier life.

TABLE 1.

Calories Burned Per Hour in Various Activities (Body weight, 125 lb)

Daily Activities

Class-work, lecture	84	Hoeing, raking and planting	235
Cleaning windows	207	House painting	176
Conversing	92	Housework	203
Chopping wood	367	Kneeling	60
Dancing (moderate)	209	Making bed	196
(vigorous)	284	Mowing grass	
(fox trot)	222	(power, self-propelled)	203
(rhumba)	347	(power, not self-propelled)	222
(square)	342	Office work	150
(waltz)	257	Personal toilet	95
Dressing or showering	160	Resting in bed	59
Driving	150	Sawing wood	391
Eating	70	Shining shoes	149
Exercise, calisthenics	251	Shoveling snow	389
Exercise, Canadian Air Force		Sleeping	59
(Chart 1A)	415	Standing (no activity)	71
Exercise, 5 BX Exercises		(light activity)	122
(Chart 2A)	521	Walking (2 mph)	176
(Charts 3A, 4A)	733	(110–120 paces/min)	260
(Charts 5A, 6A)	830	(4½ mph)	331
Farm chores or carpentry	193	(down stairs)	333
Floor (mopping)	227	(up stairs)	869
(sweeping)	183	Watching television	60
Gardening	178	Working in yard	177
Gardening and weeding	295	Writing	92

YOUR BODY'S ENERGY

When we work or play we need energy. That energy is produced by our bodies from fuel in the form of the foods we eat. (The importance of proper diet is emphasized in the chapter, "Nutrition and Weight.")

An essential component for all energy production is oxygen. Oxygen is obtained from the air through our lungs. It is absorbed into the bloodstream and carried by our red cells (in hemoglobin) to all parts of the body. Our hormones, such as thyroid, parathyroid, and insulin, play necessary roles in energy production and availability for use. For example, a woman with an over- or underactive thyroid gland would have difficulty exercising. An underactive gland slows down all of her metabolic processes to reduce the role of energy production, while an overactive thy-

Sports Activities

Archery		268	Running (5.5 mph)	537
Badminton or volleyball			(9 mph, level)	777
	(moderate)	285	(9 mph, 4% grade)	959
	(vigorous)	488	(12 mph)	984
Baseball (infield or outfield)		234	(in place, 140 counts/min)	1222
	(pitching)	299	Sailing (calm water)	150
Basketball (moderate)		352	Skating (moderate)	285
	(vigorous)	495	(vigorous)	513
Bicycling (level, 5.5 mph)		251	Skiing (downhill)	483
	(level, 13 mph)	537	(level, 5 mph)	586
Bowling (nonstop)		333	Soccer	447
Canoeing (4 mph)		352	Squash	520
Climbing, hill		488	Swimming	
Climbing, mountain		503	(backstroke, 20 yd/min)	194
Fencing (moderate)		251	40 yd/min)	418
	(vigorous)	513	(breaststroke, 20 yd/min)	241
Golf (twosome)		271	40 yd/min)	482
	(foursome)	203	(butterfly)	586
Handball (vigorous)		488	(crawl, 20 yd/min)	241
Horseback riding (walk)		165	50 yd/min)	532
	(trot)	338	(sidestroke)	418
Horseshoe pitching		177	Tennis (moderate)	347
Ping-Pong		194	(vigorous)	488
Rowing, pleasure		251	Water skiing	391
Rowing, machine or sculling			Wrestling, judo, or karate	643
(20 strokes/min)		684		

SOURCE: Adapted with permission of Universal Fitness Products, 20 Terminal Drive South, Plainview, New York 11803.

roid speeds up the body processes to the degree that energy is used up even when she is not exercising.

Energy is measured in the form of calories. We know that the body requires a certain number of calories per day in order to maintain itself and to carry on normal activities. The number of calories consumed during exercise is variable. Vigorous activity such as jogging, jumping rope, or bicycling obviously will consume more calories than team sports such as softball, and these in turn more calories than less active sports such as golf or bowling.

There are calorie guides available in most book stores as well as texts on nutrition and exercise that indicate just how many calories are produced from different foods and how many are burned in different activities. One handy device is a small slide calculator available from Universal

Fitness Products which indicates how many calories are burned per hour for most sports and daily activities according to your weight. (See Table 1 listing calories burned during exercise for a 125 pound woman.)

THE FIRST STEP—A PHYSICAL EXAMINATION

Before embarking on an active exercise program of any kind, a woman of any age who has been leading a sedentary life or who has been exercising only mildly or sporadically should have a thorough physical examination.

Health problems may exist that a woman is not aware of. For this reason, in addition to the routine general physical, she should have a pap smear, a chemical analysis of the blood that includes a blood count and a basic thyroid screening test, a cardiac evaluation, and a pulmonary evaluation.

Mild cases of iron deficiency anemia (low hemoglobin) are common, due in some cases to poor dietary habits, but more often to the fact that some women lose more iron during menstruation than they get in their diets. An anemic woman is handicapped in exercises requiring endurance or strenuous exertion. When the oxygen-carrying capacity in the bloodstream is reduced, the ability to produce energy is also reduced. Iron deficiency anemia is quickly corrected by taking iron tablets daily.

An electrocardiogram can reveal certain malfunctions of the heart, and if the woman is over 35, a stress cardiac test should be done. In this test electrocardiograph leads are attached to the subject's chest while she runs on a treadmill. The result gives a good indication of the heart's reaction to the extra stress of exercise. It must be done under strict medical supervision at a center properly equipped with the necessary instruments.

Where special conditions such as heart disease, hypertension, diabetes, or pregnancy exist, medical monitoring is a must, but this does not mean you cannot participate. Quite the contrary, exercise can be very beneficial and actually lead to physical improvement.

SUITABLE CLOTHES AND PROPER EQUIPMENT

Clothing and equipment for the exercise of your choice should be selected carefully. Except for leotards, clothing in general should be loose-fitting, have a high cotton content for absorbency, and an open weave to permit sweat to evaporate. These characteristics are especially important in both underclothing and uniforms worn in warm climates or for indoor sports. In the outer garments a higher percentage of synthetic materials is acceptable, but they should be lined in cotton.

Studies indicate that the considerable force involved in breast motion during vigorous exercises can result in chafing, sore breasts, and irritated, bleeding nipples. A properly made bra restricts this abrasive motion and prevents chafing or discomfort caused by bra straps that slip off the shoulders. While a small-breasted woman seldom has problems related to her bra, large-breasted women often do. A bra that is well made and correctly fitted will not slip up over the breast no matter how strenuous the exercise. Bras specifically designed for wear by women engaged in active sports are available.

Shoes and socks should always be selected with care since improperly fitted footwear will result in blisters, foot strains, and sprains. If you have any problems, consult a podiatrist familiar with athletic requirements and get properly made arch supports and correctly fitted shoes. Socks should be absorbent and should be of the proper bulk to help fill the shoe to avoid rubbing.

Equipment such as tennis racquets and golf clubs should be chosen with the advice of a professional or at least with the help of a knowledgeable clerk in a well-equipped sporting goods store. Equipment that is the wrong size or weight or is poorly made may lead to injuries, such as tennis elbow (an inflammation of the tendons in the elbow).

INJURIES

Injuries to women in sports are basically no different from those sustained by men. Injuries seemed more prevalent among women when they first began their active involvement in sports in large numbers, but this was due primarily to poor physical fitness before beginning their play, lack of conditioning, and poor training and coaching. Inadequate preparation caused greater vulnerability not only of women playing on teams, but of individuals who jogged, played tennis, or went skiing before they knew how to handle themselves and their equipment.

Even though it now appears that women in general are no more susceptible to injury than men, it is still true that any individual in poor condition beginning a new activity is especially vulnerable. If no other help is available, read a good book on the sport that interests you. A knowledgeable friend can be a big help. It is often worth the expense of joining a sports club or taking a few private or group lessons before dashing off into a disaster on the tennis court or ski slope.

In general most injuries sustained by women involve the lower limbs. Ankle and knee strains and sprains are especially common, and shin splints (pain in the anterior shin area of the lower leg) and chondromalacia (cartilage inflammation of the knees) occur more frequently in women than in men.

TABLE 2.

Activities Rated According to Physical Fitness Benefits
(Flexibility, Strength, Cardiovascular Endurance)

	Flexibility	Upper Body Strength	Lower Body Strength	Cardio-vascular Endurance	RATING 1 Poor 2 Fair 3 Average 4 Good 5 Excellent
Walking					
slowly			x		1
briskly			x	x	2
Running			x	x	3
Running program*	x	x	x	x	5
Bicycling			x	x	3
Swimming					
(all basic strokes)	x	x	x	x	5
Kayaking		x			2
Canoeing		x			2
Sailing					
small boats	x	x	x		3
large boats					1
Rowing	x	x			2
Horseback riding			x	x	3
Karate (martial arts)	x	x	x	x	5
Bowling		x	x		1
Ballet	x		x		4
Folk dance			x	x	3
Square dance			x	x	3
Modern dance	x	x	x	x	5
Aerobic dance	x	x	x	x	5
Gymnastics	x	x	x	x	5
Backpacking			x	x	2

Women do not suffer severe injuries to the breast and the idea that a blow to the breast will cause cancer is an old wives' tale. Injuries to the reproductive organs of the nonpregnant female are rare. After the first trimester of pregnancy, when the uterus rises up out of the protective bony pelvis, there is a danger of injury as a result of a severe blow. So after the third month the pregnant woman should avoid sports in which there is any possibility of a blow to the abdomen, but other activities, such as swimming, dancing, tennis, may be continued as long as the woman desires.

					RATING
					1 *Poor*
					2 *Fair*
	Upper	*Lower*	*Cardio-*		3 *Average*
	Body	*Body*	*vascular*		4 *Good*
	Flexibility	*Strength*	*Strength*	*Endurance*	5 *Excellent*
Golf					
walking		x	x		2
cart		x			1
Snow skiing					
Alpine	x		x	x	4
Nordic	x	x	x	x	5
Water skiing		x	x		3
Mountain climbing	x	x	x	x	5
Yoga	x				2
Weight lifting		x	x		2
Tennis					
singles	x	x	x	x	4
doubles	x	x	x		3
Badminton	x	x	x	x	4
Racquetball	x	x	x	x	5
Field hockey	x	x	x	x	4
Basketball	x	x	x	x	4
Soccer	x	x	x	x	5
Softball	x	x	x	x	3
Volleyball	x	x	x	x	4

* Running combined with upper body flexibility and strength exercises.

SOURCE: *Total Woman's Fitness Guide,* © 1979 by Gail Shierman and Christine Haycock. World Publications, Inc., Mountain View, California. Reprinted with permission.

Certainly a woman's menstrual period is no reason to discontinue any sport, even swimming.

DEVELOPING A FITNESS PROGRAM TO CONDITION YOUR BODY

You can develop your own fitness program to suit your available time, your activity preferences, and available facilities. It might consist of an exercise routine alone, or sports activities alone, or a combination of exercises and any other vigorous activity, such as jogging, swimming, or whatever you like to do. However, there are certain requirements that your program should meet. First, it should include activities to develop all the components of fitness—flexibility, strength, and cardiovascular endurance. Second, it must be done regularly. Third, it must include adequate warm-up and cool-down periods. Fourth, it must involve a high enough level of exertion of long enough duration to achieve its intended benefits.

Different types of activities develop different components of fitness. In the exercise routine described in the next section, the component for each is listed. Sports also vary in the aspect of fitness they develop. For example, softball is good for strength, but not for endurance. Jogging and bike riding are excellent for endurance and for strengthening pelvic and leg muscles, but do not increase flexibility or exercise the arms. Yoga is excellent for flexibility and relaxation, but does little for strength and endurance. Swimming and dancing, particularly aerobic dancing, develop all components and use all parts of the body. Consider the activity of your choice and then be sure to combine it with other activities to achieve a total conditioning program.

Maintaining a regular routine may be the hardest part of conditioning. Plan the time you intend to devote to it and stick to your schedule. Studies have shown that effective results will not be derived from less than three periods of activity each week. If you find it hard to carry out an exercise routine at home or on your own, try to interest your neighbors or friends in forming a group. Exercises done with a group are generally more pleasurable than those done alone. Some women are too self-conscious to join a group until they have achieved some competence, but eventually they find that the social benefits of the group include many psychological advantages. Join the local Y, see if a local university has an open sports program, or find a community center with exercise classes. Health clubs can be good, but check with members to find out whether the privileges are worth the price. You should also check on the staff to find out whether they are properly trained in the use of the equipment and in handling any medical emergencies that might arise. Find out if the club requires a physical examination prior to admission and what types of exercise programs it has. Don't commit yourself to a year's membership until you have visited the premises as a guest once or twice. Unless you participate regularly in its programs, you will probably waste money. On the other hand, if investing the money in a membership will discipline you into regular participation, it might be money well spent.

Remember that you cannot plunge into vigorous activity directly. If you are just beginning your routine, you must work into it gradually. Even after you are in condition to sustain strenuous activity, your body needs a warm-up and cool-down period of moderate exertion to avoid undue stress. Ten minutes of some of the stretching exercises described below would provide the necessary transition.

The question of how long each period of activity should be depends on the kind of activity. The most fitness benefit is derived from activity which maintains the heart beat at 70 percent of its maximum rate for 30 minutes. For the average woman the maximum is about 180 to 190 beats per minute. If you can maintain your rate at about 125 to 135, you will be achieving fitness. You can measure your heart rate by counting the pulse at the neck (carotid artery) or wrist (radial artery). The less stress your activity places on the heart and muscles, the longer you have to do it to achieve fitness. For example, running produces a steady stress which can sustain the 70 percent heart rate, so that 30 minutes of running is sufficient exercise for one period of activity. Sports which produce less or more sporadic stress have to be done longer to achieve the same results.

THE EXERCISE ROUTINE

The following pages describe various recommended exercises. Following the description is a daily routine suitable for various age groups. To help you choose an exercise routine best suited to your circumstances, I enlisted the aid of two experts: Mervyn Haycock, Director of Physical Education at Bergan High School in Peoria, Illinois and Dr. Gail Shierman, Assistant Professor of Physical Education at the University of Oklahoma, Norman, Oklahoma.

Jumping Jack (endurance)

1. Starting position: stand with feet together and arms down.
2. Move arms overhead, jump, and land with your feet 2 feet apart.
3. Return to starting position.

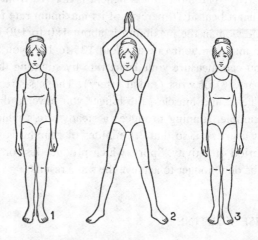

Squat Bender (strength and flexibility)

1. Starting position: stand with legs slightly apart and hands on hips.
2. Bend knees to half squat position and stretch out arms in front of you for balance.
3. Return to starting position.
4. Bend from waist keeping knees straight and touch toes.
5. Return to starting position.

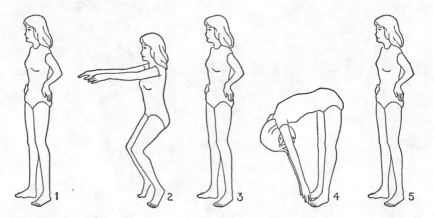

Alternate Toe Touch (flexibility)

1. Starting position: stand with feet spread apart and arms outstretched to the side. Keep legs straight throughout.
2. Touch right hand to left toe.
3. Return to starting position.
4. Touch left hand to right toe.
5. Return to starting position.

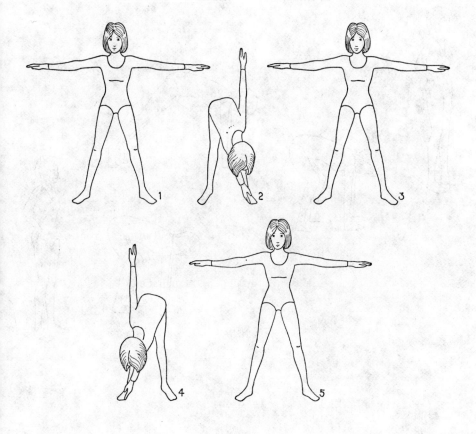

Squat Thrust (flexibility and shoulder strength)

1. Starting position: stand with feet slightly apart and hands on hips.
2. Bend knees to squat position and place palms on the ground.
3. Thrust legs straight out behind you.
4. Return to second position.
5. Return to starting position.

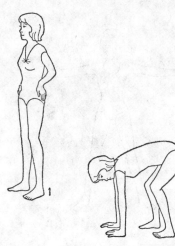
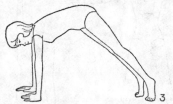
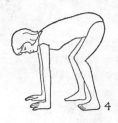
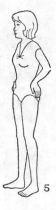

Knee Lift (flexibility)

1. Starting position: stand with feet together and arms down.
2. Raise right knee as high as possible holding leg with hands and pulling knee against body while keeping your back straight.
3. Return to starting position.
4. Repeat with left knee.
5. Return to starting position.

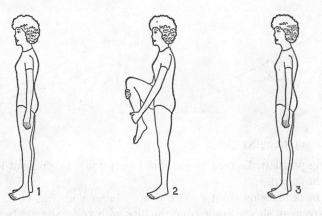

Side Bender (flexibility)

1. Starting position: stand with feet spread shoulder width apart and hands behind neck with fingers interlocked.
2. Bend trunk sideways to the right as far as possible while keeping hands behind head.
3. Return to starting position.
4. Repeat to the left.
5. Return to starting position.

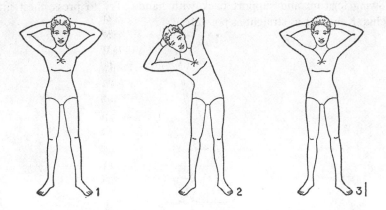

Sprinter's Drive (flexibility)

1. Starting position: squat down with your palms on ground and right leg fully extended to the rear.
2. Reverse position of your feet by bringing right foot under you and extending your left leg backward all in one movement.
3. Reverse feet again to return to starting position.

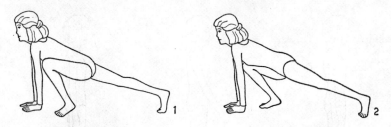

Flutter Legs (strength)

1. Starting position: lie face down, with hands under thighs, and legs 8 to 10 inches apart.
2. Arch back bringing chest and head up. Flutter your legs continuously; the movement should come from the hips with knees slightly bent. Each flutter is counted as one.

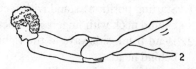
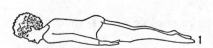

Shoulder Stand (flexibility)

1. Starting position: lie on your back.
2. Swing legs up and support back with hands. Try to press chest into chin. Keep legs as straight as possible.

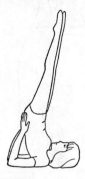

Kickover (flexibility)

1. Starting position: shoulder stand position.
2. Place palms on floor and bring legs over your head until feet touch the ground. If you can't touch your feet to the ground, come as close as you can.

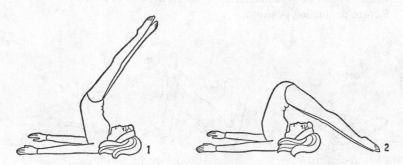

Figure 8 (agility)

1. Place two chairs 6 feet apart.
2. Start at one chair and run in a figure 8 pattern around both chairs five times. Time yourself, if possible, to see improvement.

5-10-15 Agility Drill

1. From a starting line run 5 yards to some mark, turn around, and run back to starting line.
2. Turn around, run 10 yards to a mark, turn around, and run back to starting line.
3. Turn around, run 15 yards to a mark, turn around, and run back to starting line. Time yourself, if possible, to see improvement.

Line Jump (coordination and endurance)

1. Make a short, straight line on floor or ground. Jump back and forth over the line on toes, but just barely off the ground. Do not pace yourself. Go as fast as you can until you run down.
2. Repeat at each exercise session. Time yourself for 30 seconds and count how many you do within that 30-second period. With each repetition, you will improve.

Push-Up, knee (strength)

1. Starting position: lie with legs together and face down; bend your knees with feet raised off the ground; put hands palm down on the floor under shoulders.
2. Push upper body off the floor by straightening arms until arms are fully extended and body is in a straight line from head to knees.
3. Return to starting position.

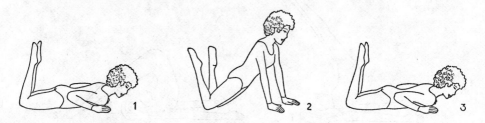

Push-Up (strength)

1. Starting position: lie with legs together, face down, and palms on the ground under shoulders with fingers pointing straight ahead.
2. Push body off the ground by extending arms until the body is in a straight line from head to toes, and weight rests on hands and toes.
3. Lower body until chest touches the floor. Keep the body perfectly straight throughout the exercise.

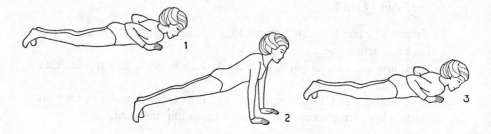

Sit-Up (strength)

1. Starting position: lie on back with legs straight and together and arms extended on floor above head.
2. Bring arms up and forward over head and roll up to a sitting position, extending your arms until you touch your toes.
3. Roll back to starting position.
4. To make this exercise more challenging clasp hands behind head and touch elbows to thighs. A further challenge is to perform sit-ups with your knees bent. An incline bench can also be used to increase difficulty of exercise.

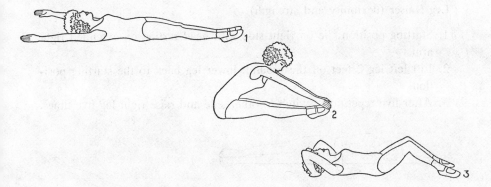

Back-Up (flexibility and strength)

1. Starting position: sit with legs extended and hands on floor behind you with fingers pointing to the rear.
2. With your buttocks tight, press down on hands and lift body off the floor. Keep legs straight and point toes.
3. Return to starting position.

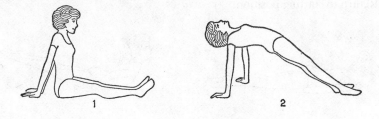

Back Lift (flexibility and strength)

1. Starting position: lie on back with arms at sides and palms down.
2. Arch back, keeping head, elbows, and buttocks on the floor. Hold for 5 seconds.
3. Return to starting position.

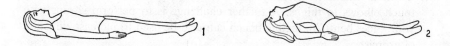

Leg Raiser (flexibility and strength)

1. Starting position: lie on right side with head resting on extended right arm.
2. Lift left leg 2 feet off the ground; lower leg back to the starting position.
3. After five repetitions switch to other side and raise right leg five times.

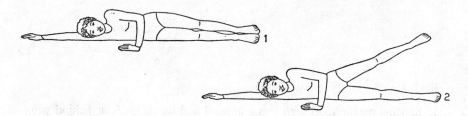

Arch Back (strength)

1. Starting position: lie face down with palms under thighs.
2. Raise head, shoulders, and legs from the ground.
3. Return to starting position.

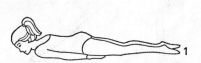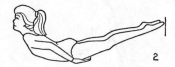

Rocker (coordination and flexibility)

1. Starting position: lie face down; bend knees and grasp ankles.
2. Pull heels away from buttocks, keeping elbows straight to raise your head and chest off the ground.

3. Pull on feet, keeping elbows straight, to get thighs off the floor.
4. Rock forward and backward on stomach.

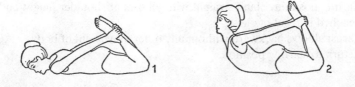

Abdominal Lift (strength)

1. Starting position: stand straight (this exercise can be performed from several positions, but we will describe it in a standing position); take a deep breath and let it out before starting the exercise.
2. Place hands on thighs with hands turned in and head up. Contract abdominal muscles by sucking them in and up. Hold for 4 to 8 seconds.
3. Relax abdominal muscles. Repeat the exercise.

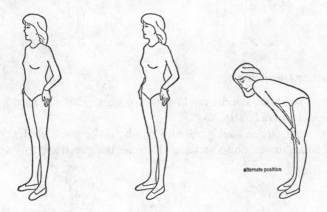

alternate position

Reach and Lift (strength)

1. Starting position: lie on back with hands on thighs.
2. Raise arms, head, chest, and legs a few inches off the floor. Hold 5 seconds.
3. Return to starting position.

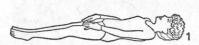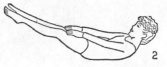

Wing Stretch (flexibility)

1. Starting position: stand straight with elbows at shoulder height and fists clenched in front of chest.
2. Thrust elbows backward without any other movement of body.
3. Return to starting position.

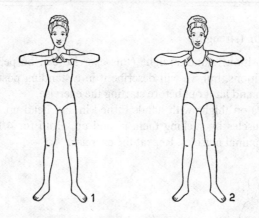

Arm Rotator (flexibility)

1. Starting position: stand straight with arms extended sideward at shoulder height and palms up.
2. Make small circles backward with hands; make small circles forward.
3. With palms turned down make small circles backward and forward.

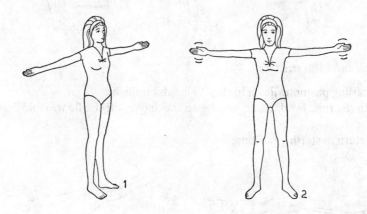

Trunk Rotator (flexibility)

1. Starting position: stand with hands on hips.
2. Bend at the waist and make slow circles clockwise and then counterclockwise.

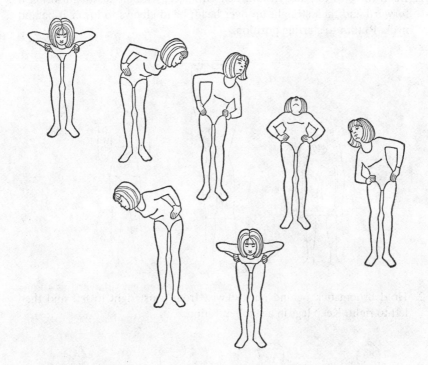

Push-Back (strength)

1. Starting position: stand with arms at sides.
2. Make a fist and bring your arms as far behind you as you can.
3. Return to starting position. Keep your arms straight throughout exercise.

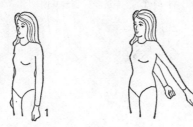

Broomstick Activities (flexibility and strength)

Use a 2-foot long portion of a broomstick; do the activities in a standing position.

1. Bend forward to place broomstick on knees; with arms straight bring it forward and then straight up over head; bend elbows to lower it behind neck. Return to starting position.

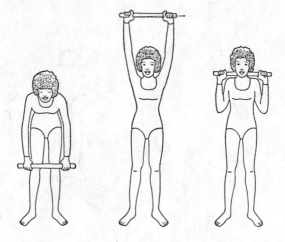

2. Hold broomstick behind neck. Twist from waist right to left and then left to right. Keep legs in a stable position.

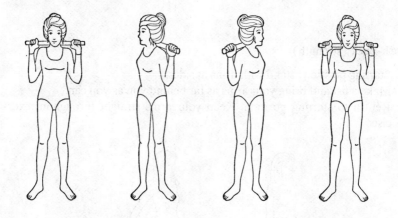

3. Hold broomstick at chest level. Push forward and backward to chest.

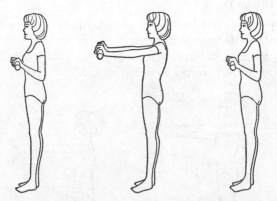

4. Grasp broomstick tightly and hold with arms extended at shoulder level. Using wrists and fingers, roll stick forward 10 times and backward 10 times.

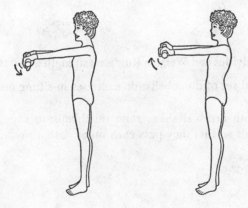

5. Hold broomstick at thighs. With arms extended raise it forward and upward to shoulder level. Return to starting position.

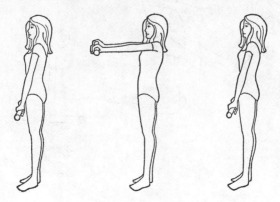

Toe Raise (strength)

1. Starting position: stand with arms straight out in front for balance.
2. Raise heels off the ground and return.
3. If you have good balance, place a large book or block of wood under balls of feet and do exercise in same manner.

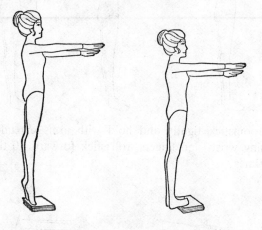

Dumbbell Activities and Weights Routine (strength and flexibility)

Use a 2-pound set of dumbbells; do exercises in sitting and lying positions on the floor.

1. Starting with arms at sides, raise dumbbells to shoulder level, alternating hands so that they pass each other. Use a rhythm to your count.

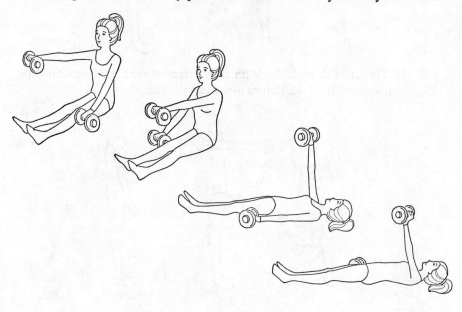

2. Vigorously push dumbbells forward and backward from chest to arm
   outstretched position, alternating hands so they pass each other.

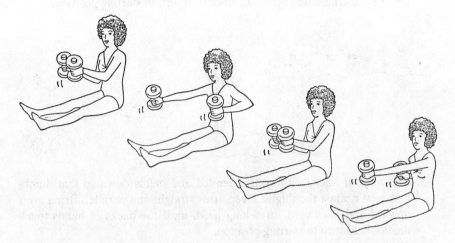

3. Raise dumbbells forward and upward to a vertical position, keeping
   arms straight and close to your ears as you raise them over your head.
   Lower dumbbells to forward position, then to starting position.

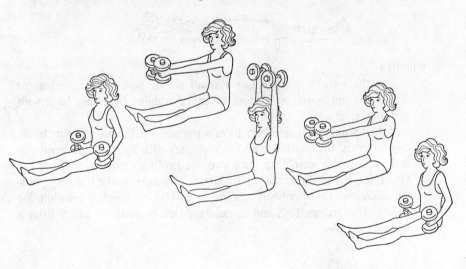

4. Lie on your back with arms extended at shoulder height. Keep arms straight. Raise arms vertically over chest. With palms facing each other lower both arms sideways to the floor to return to starting position.

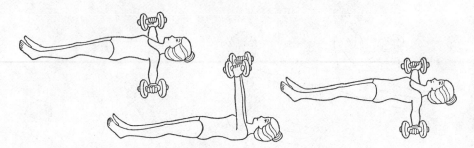

5. Lie on your back, with arms extended and palms down so that dumbbells rest against the thighs. Keep arms straight and parallel. Bring arms upward and backward, stretching hard, until the backs of hands touch the floor. Return to starting position.

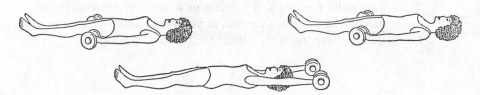

WEIGHTS

For the weights routine use a small set of barbells or weights for dumbbells purchased at a store or make weights by filling bags with dirt, rocks, or sand.

A few points to remember: have a partner work with you for "spotting," that is, for assistance and safety; start with light weights until you feel secure with each lift; since you are probably not training for the Olympics, if you do increase the amount of weight, make it a very gradual increase. Do dumbbell routine first. Use a standing position for dumbbell exercises 1, 2 and 3; do dumbbell exercises 4 and 5 from a table if possible.

6. Wing Lift. Lie on a table on your stomach with arms hanging down, holding weights. Keeping arms straight, lift weights sideways as high up as you can. Return slowly to starting position. Do 3 sets of 10 (30).

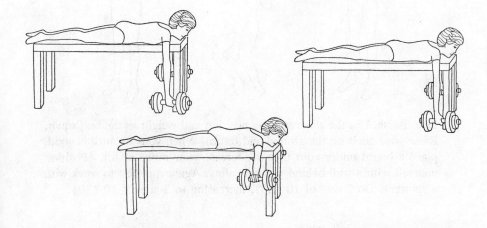

7. Rowing. Bend over from the waist with legs straight and both arms hanging straight down. Bring the weights up to the chest and return to starting position. Do 3 sets of 10 (30).

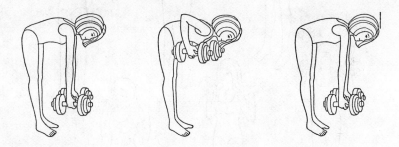

8. Half Squat. Stand with feet shoulder width apart, slightly pointing out, and place barbell behind your neck on your shoulders. Keep heels on ground throughout lift. Squat by bending knees to 45 degree angle. Do NOT let knees bend beyond 90 degrees at any time and do not bounce into full-squat position. The lift must be performed in a smooth manner. Return to starting position. The amount of weight you use will depend upon your strength and balance. Start at 1 set of 10, go to 2 sets of 10, before increasing the weight.

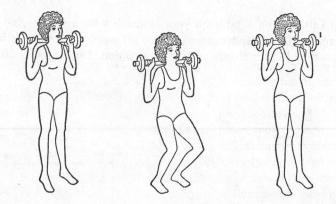

9. Heel Raise. Use the same starting position and weight as the half squat. Raise your heels off the ground and return. When your balance is good, place a board under your toes to increase your range of lift. (Position yourself with a wall behind you for safety. Again it is best to work with a spotter). Do 2 sets of 10 (20), increasing to 3 sets of 10 (30).

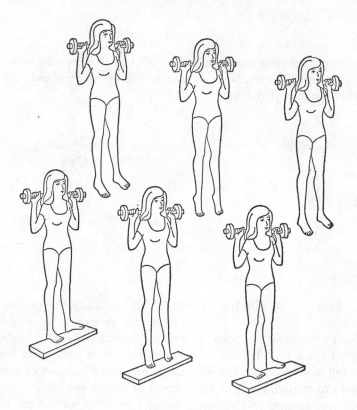

Routines Suitable for Various Age Groups

Some general statements apply to all the routines. The numbers shown are the maximum number to be done in each routine. Start with about a fourth of the number and gradually increase until you are doing the total number daily. Exercises may be increased or decreased in amount and time according to your endurance limit or available time. Start at a moderate pace and move quickly from one exercise to another.

If you have access to barbells or specialized equipment such as a Universal Gym or Nautilus, one of the weight routines is recommended. (Note that the owner or operator of the machine should have an exercise manual on the wall describing all possible exercises and should supervise your workout).

The amount of time for various athletic activities will vary with the type of activity and your ability and condition, but 20 to 30 minutes of active participation in each activity can be taken as a general rule.

How you fit these exercise routines into your schedule will vary. Some women find it easiest to do them in the morning before breakfast, but others fit exercise into their lunch hour or after work. In general it is best to exercise before eating a meal as vigorous exercise within two hours after eating may result in improper digestion and gastrointestinal upset.

Up to Age 25

Jumping jack	25	Shoulder stand	10 sec
Squat bender	10	Kick-over	2
Alternate toe touch	10	Figure 8 or 5–10–15	
Squat thrust	7	agility drill	1
Knee lift	10	Push-up	10
Side bender	10	Sit-up	
Flutter legs	10	(inclined, if possible)	6
Line jump	30 sec	Back-up	5

Athletic activity should be vigorous and regular. Some suggestions are 20 to 30 minutes of jogging, 20 to 30 minutes of bicycling, a set or two of tennis, swimming laps, skating (ice or roller), gymnastics, or racquetball. Team sports such as soccer, softball, and basketball can be substituted, but they are not as easy to fit into a regular routine because you must find other people to participate. Various forms of dance from square dancing to disco, done regularly and vigorously, are also good.

Age 25 to 35

Squat bender	10	Back lift	2 deep breaths
Alternate toe touch	10	Leg raiser	5
Knee lift	10	Arch back	10

Side bender	10	Rocker	1 (hold 5 sec)
Sprinter's drive	10	Push-up	6
Flutter legs	10	Abdominal lift	5 (hold 5 sec each)
Sit-up		Reach and lift	5 (hold 5 sec each)
(inclined, if possible)	6	Line jump	30 sec

Athletic activity should be vigorous and regular. Some suggestions are 20 to 30 minutes of jogging, 20 to 30 minutes of bicycling, a set or two of tennis, swimming laps, skating (ice or roller), or racquetball. Team sports such as soccer, softball, and basketball can be substituted, but they are not as easy to fit into a regular routine because you must find other people to participate. Various forms of dance from square dancing to disco, done vigorously and regularly, are also good.

Age 35 to 50

Squat bender	5	Leg raiser	5
Alternate toe touch	5	Abdominal lift	5 (hold 5 sec each)
Knee lift	10	Reach and lift	5 (hold 5 sec each)
Side bender	10	Wing stretch	15
Line jump	20 sec	Arm rotator	10 each way
Sit-up		Trunk rotator	5
(inclined, if possible)	5	Push back	5

Athletic activity should be vigorous and regular. Some excellent activities are 10 to 20 minutes of jogging if able, rapidly walking up and down a normal flight of steps five times in succession, bicycling, golf, tennis, and swimming laps.

Age 50 to 65

Squat bender	5	Trunk rotator	4
Alternate toe touch	5	Broomstick activities	10 each
Knee lift	8	Full or half sit-up	5
Side bender	8	Toe raise	5
Wing stretch	10	Dumbbell activities	5–10 each
Arm rotator	5 each way		

Athletic activity should be regular. One of the best activities is fast walking for short distances, such as ¼ mile. Walking at a moderate pace for a mile or two is another good activity. Continue whatever vigorous exercise you are accustomed to. Continue to jog if you have been a jogger in the past. Play 18 holes of golf if you are a golfer. Bicycling, swimming, and dancing are other possibilities. Your general physical condition will determine just how much you can do.

Age 50 to 65 (out of condition)

The following exercises are for women over 50 who are totally out of condition and want to work their way back into shape. If you continue these exercises consistently for about six weeks, you should be able to work into the previous list of more difficult exercises and more difficult forms of similar exercises. Each day gradually increase the number of times you do the exercises. Move from one exercise to another quickly once you get into the routine.

1. **Arm circle** (flexibility)   Standing or sitting comfortably, lift one arm at a time up and around to make a complete circle. Do this several times forward and backward.

2. **Knee press** (flexibility)   Lie on your back, bend one knee, grasp it with your hands, and pull it toward your chest. Repeat with the other knee. Repeat several times.

3. **Trunk twist** (flexibility)   Standing or sitting, put your hands on your hips and twist your trunk to the right side, then to the left. Repeat several times.

4. **Head circle** (flexibility) Standing or sitting, move your head forward, to one side, back, to the other side and forward again to make a complete circle. Repeat several times in each direction.

5. **Shoulder shrug** (flexibility)   Standing or sitting, lift your shoulders to your ears, then push them forward and then backwards as far as possible. Keep your head straight. Repeat this exercise in a rolling fashion several times.

6. **Side leg raise** (flexibility)   Lying on one side, lift your top leg as high as possible. Repeat several times and then roll over and repeat on the other side.

7. **Wall push-off** (strength)   Stand 2 feet from a wall, facing the wall. Keeping your body straight, lean forward and place your hands on the wall. Bend your arms so your head almost touches the wall. Then push your body away from the wall. Repeat several times.

8. **Partial sit-up** (strength)   Lying on your back, arms at your sides, raise your head and shoulders off the floor. Repeat several times.

9. **Rear leg lift** (strength)   Lie on your stomach propped up on your elbows. Lift one leg as far as possible and then the other leg. Repeat several times.

10. **Running in place** (cardiovascular endurance)   Bend your arms to about 90 degrees and keep them relaxed as you run in place. Gradually increase the length of time you run.

Age 65 and over

Alternate toe touch	5	Arm rotator	5 each way
Side bender	5	Trunk rotator	4
Sit-up	5–10	Broomstick activities	8 each
Wing stretch	10	Toe raise	5

Those women who have done these exercises in the past can increase repetitions as general conditioning permits. Those who have not should start with a few repetitions and go through the full range of motion before increasing the repetitions.

Broomstick activities can be done in the sitting position if standing is not physically possible. Exercises for the out-of-condition 50 to 65 group can all be used in this age group.

Athletic activity for the 50 to 65 group also applies to the 65 and over group. Your general physical condition will determine just how much you can do.

Exercises on the Job

For women working outside the home, there are often special exercise classes scheduled at local Y's or health clubs, either during the noon break or immediately after work.

Many of the exercises described here can be done while seated at your desk at work, standing behind a counter, or in the restroom during the lunch or coffee break.

Exercises that can be done while sitting down include the wing stretch, arm rotator, trunk rotator, knee lift from a sitting position, and side bender. Some other suggestions for exercising at your desk are:

1. Sit forward in your chair and slowly bend forward with your elbows between your knees and reach for the floor. Hold this position for a count of five and return slowly to your upright seated position.
2. Turn your head in circles, repeating five times each way.
3. Move your shoulders in circles with the arms either outstretched or bent at the elbow, five times in each direction.
4. Grasp arm rests of chair and raise entire body off seat, five times.

FURTHER READING

Darden, Ellington. *Especially for Women.* West Point, New York: Leisure Press, 1977.

Getchell, Bud. *Physical Fitness: A Way of Life.* New York: John Wiley & Sons, Inc., 1976.

Hockey, Robert. *Physical Fitness: The Pathway to Healthful Living.* St. Louis: The C. V. Mosby Co., 1977.

Klafs, Carl, and Joan Lyon. *The Female Athlete.* St. Louis: The C. V. Mosby Co., 1978.

Mirkin, Gabe, and Marshall Hoffman. *The Sportsmedicine Book.* Boston: Little, Brown and Company, 1978.

Shierman, Gail and Christine Haycock, M.D. *Total Woman's Fitness Guide.* Mountain View, Calif.: World Publications, 1979.

Smith, Everett L., M.D. and Karl Stoedefalke, M.D. *Aging and Exercise.* Department of Preventive Medicine, 504 Walnut, University of Wisconsin, Madison, Wis. 53706.

Sexual Health

LONNY MYERS, M.D.

Director of Sexual Health Services,
Midwest Population Center, Chicago, Illinois

SEXUAL STAGES

Born Free—Infancy and Childhood

You were born a sexual being. Infants include their genitals as they explore their bodies. We are just beginning to realize how sexual infants are. Orgasms have been observed in babies of 3 months and are common in childhood before puberty.

Unfortunately, most infants soon learn that "down there" is "dirty." Many mothers who smile while they play with other parts of their babies' bodies frown as they change diapers and wash the genital area. Very early in life most infants get the message that genitalia are off limits for playful fondling. Attitudes toward masturbation vary greatly; many mothers slap infants' hands with a stern "No! No!" Some simply ignore masturbation in their babies, and a small but growing number smile at the activity.

Sexual activity, that comes so naturally to children, has been condemned by religion, creating much guilt and anxiety. Rational discussions of sex are rare, especially in the presence of children. The simplest questions may evoke such negative responses from adults that children may not ask again, and this negativism becomes a significant part of their sex education. Avoidance, too, plays a major part. When the subject of sex is avoided, children receive a strong message that there is something mysterious, exciting, wrong, and upsetting about it. However, an ever increasing number of young parents seem to be able to talk comfortably about sex with their children.

Children also get sex messages from many other sources. A popular message that comes through the media is, "Be sexy; don't have sex!" Radio, television, billboards, magazines, comics, all encourage girls to have sexy eyes, sexy hair, sexy teeth, sexy breath, while the official rules of behavior dictate no sex. Girls are trained to tease men. Traditionally, they are taught to hold out for marriage. That is less common now, but many are still encouraged to extract a price—don't give it away.

Another contradictory message is, "Sex is dirty; save it for the one you love!" Individually, fewer and fewer people seriously regard sex as dirty, yet sexy pictures are dirty pictures, a sexy joke is a dirty joke, and "Don't be dirty" means don't do anything sexual, even tell a sexy story. Why one should save this "dirty" thing for a loved one is a logical question with no good answer.

Adolescence

Although parental negatives may drastically limit children's awareness of sex, by adolescence they are keenly aware of sexual changes in the body. At this sensitive time the relationship with parents usually changes. There is a sudden lack of intimacy; hugging and kissing and most forms of physical contact are greatly diminished. Sometimes children feel guilty, thinking they have done something to displease their parents.

Our society provides few acceptable means for close physical contact during adolescence, and actually encourages unacceptable means. In addition to the media messages that to "Be sexy" is one of the most important standards by which people are judged and also the key to happiness, society provides leisure time, proximity, and highly suggestive books, pictures, music, and dancing. The results are predictable: millions of sexual contacts among adolescents and an epidemic of adolescent pregnancies.

Only a generation ago fear of pregnancy kept many girls virgins. Now, not only are contraception and abortion available to many, but out-of-wedlock pregnancy is no longer the horrible worse-than-death consequence of sex that it used to be. In fact, in at least two ways it may be regarded as positive. First, it appears to be a way of achieving status, and, second, it may be seen as an expression of a principle of radical feminism, that is, a woman does not need a man to rear a child. Although the status of motherhood gets the adolescent a lot of attention she may have lacked, the majority of adolescent mothers are far more harassed by the burdens and responsibilities of motherhood than impressed by the new status. Feminism has less influence than status does on the incidence of adolescent pregnancy and probably even encourages delaying motherhood until adulthood. But the impact of the feminist message is very real to many adolescents. By minimizing the need to be sexually pleasing to men, it counteracts the mainstream media messages. This may create a significant struggle for many sensitive girls. They see power in using sex appeal to help them achieve their goals, while also being tempted by the get-there-on-your-own-performance cry of the women's liberation movement.

Adulthood

Each individual has distinct and unique experiences. You approached your adult sexuality in your own special way. You may have read manuals with explicit pictures and detailed information about sex. You may have seen pornography often. You may be knowledgeable about the details of human sexual response. You may have friends who live alternate life styles, for example, swinging singles, gay world, open relationships, group marriage. On the other hand, you may have chosen to avoid dealing with explicit sex material and nontraditional sexual relationships, preferring to retain a sense of privacy and some mystery about the subject of sex.

Sexual activity may play an important part in your life, its role may be minor, or it may be completely absent. All variations are found in large groups of women with similar socioeconomic and marital status.

You may have a set of moral values and standards that work well for you, or you may be somewhat confused about what is right and wrong about sex, for yourself and for teenagers. Clearly, setting standards in a free and contraceptive society is far more difficult than accepting established standards based on a concept of wrong-doing and a fear of pregnancy. There are no simple answers and we need to think through this highly complex and fascinating aspect of human living. We may be born sexually free, but how much freedom is compatible with responsible adulthood? with intimate marriage? with sensitive parenthood? We have dealt only with the tip of the sexual iceberg.

SEX AND HEALTH CARE

Whatever your response to all these contradictory and confusing influences in your past, sexual activity or lack of it, the type of relationships you have, and your feelings about yourself are factors that contribute to your overall health and well-being, just as much as what you eat, what you breathe, and how you exercise.

What makes sex different from other factors involved in health are society's proscriptions. Although we live in a society in which unhealthful eating habits and environments are not only acceptable, but in many ways encouraged, there is no stigma to seeking healthy alternatives; that is, you may move to a less polluted area or choose to eat unprocessed foods. But when you seek to alleviate anxiety and reach for better health by experimenting sexually, the resultant stigma may create more anxiety than the new sexual experience can relieve.

A woman who recognizes her sexual needs and seeks to satisfy them, even within the bounds of what is considered conventional sex, may be regarded with some suspicion by her partner. And a woman who has any ideas about unconventional sex, such as acting out a fantasy of having sex with another woman, had better keep them a secret. Few of her friends would understand and, most probably, her family physician would be shocked. Both professionals and nonprofessionals might well wonder about her "mental health," describing her curiosity as a "neurotic compulsion." Most medical opinions expressed in professional journals and advice columns in newspapers are very moralistic about sex.

There are only a few outspoken physicians and other professionals who are openly supportive of experimental sex, but these few do speak for many more who choose to remain silent for nonmedical (usually political) reasons. They are rarely quoted in medical journals, but some have written books and some get good coverage in the lay press. This group believes that sexual activity, including sexual experimentation, may be very beneficial to your health—whether within marriage or not, whether with the opposite gender or not, whether with one person or several, whether with love and commitment or not. There is general consensus that many people do not enjoy the health aspects of unconventional sex largely because of the condemnation of sex-for-pleasure they experienced as children and its reinforcement in religion.

One of the most famous spokesmen for experimental sex is Dr. Alex Comfort, who believes that much joy is missed because of irrational taboos on a normal function. He has written two best sellers on the subject, *Joy of Sex* and *More Joy*. Dr. Eugene Scheimann, in *Sex Can Save Your Heart*, emphasizes the physiological benefits of regular sexual activity, for married and unmarried, for young and old. He claims that sexual satisfaction helps maintain the balance of our body chemistries and hormones, thus slowing down the aging process. In addition, in an article entitled "Sex Can Help You Live Longer," the 82-year-old sexually active physician states that "good sex helps to rehabilitate heart attack victims; is good exercise, an antidote for depression, and a form of self-affirmation; and provides hope, optimism, and a positive frame of mind."

Unfortunately, most people do not even think of sexual satisfaction in terms of health benefits or consider possible ill effects of sexual deprivation. And this approach is confirmed by many doctors. Certainly, they would not prescribe sex even if the history of the patient suggested that sexual frustration was contributing to the physical symptoms presented. Suppose you go to your primary care physician complaining of vague symptoms such as headaches, insomnia, or indigestion, and the routine physical examination and laboratory tests are normal. Your complaints will probably be dismissed with a prescription for medication to relieve the symptoms, but it is not likely that the physician will explore or even discuss sexual deprivation as a contributing factor. If your mild symptoms develop into severe and demonstrable problems, such as hypertension or a gastric ulcer, your doctor will then take you seriously and treat your worsened condition with respect and professionalism. The chances are that even after you have developed a serious medical problem, the doctor will not investigate the psychosexual difficulties that may have contributed to it, that may slow or prevent recovery, and that may contribute to recurrence. Doctors' training and the way they practice medicine work against their having time or ability to recognize and deal with the role of sexual deprivation in physical diseases.

Now suppose you go to an enlightened doctor who suspects that sexual deprivation is a significant factor in your health problem. Obviously a doctor cannot write a prescription for a lover for you, for some inventive variation in sex with a monogamous partner, or for experimentation with more unconventional sexual expression. But he or she will probably not even discuss this remedy as first choice and go on to second-best treatments. If your problem were arthritis, and a change of climate were the treatment of choice, your doctor would be equally powerless to change the climate or arrange for your whole family to move, but he or she would be comfortable first stating the advantages of a warm, dry climate and then discussing second-best options. Regarding touching needs, the situation is quite different. How often do patients discuss the need for tender touching with their physicians? And actually, the deprivation may be more of a touch deprivation than a lack of sexual stimulation and response. Unfortunately, there are very few ways in which to enjoy skin-to-skin contact except during sex and satisfactory sex partners are not always available to fulfill needs. Some sophisticated, assertive adults might be able to make clear contracts to cuddle naked without sex, but for most people it is difficult to find such contact outside a pair-bond relationship where the two sleep together often. Fear of sex denies many people many opportunities to touch warmly, with or without clothes. We have only recently learned how important "stroking" is for our psychological and physical good health. It has been proven that babies do not thrive without adequate tender touching, and almost all adults need tender touching, too. Sexual deprivation usually means touch deprivation. The number of orgasms reached per unit time is usually less important. Orgasms reached by masturbation may be highly gratifying "sexually" in one sense and still leave you feeling "sexually" deprived. Imaginative masturbation combined with socially acceptable mutual massages might well help alleviate sex-partner needs, but we can't touch for fear of sex!

So far only the ill effects of sexual inactivity have been discussed. There are possible ill effects from sexual activity as well. It may not only be a contributing factor to physical disease, but may also cause it directly. The dynamics of its indirect effect are the same as for inactivity, that is, sexual relationships may cause anxiety, frustration, hostility, and other negative emotions that contribute to physical disease. Its direct effect is clear: sexual activity is the means by which the sexually transmissible diseases (STD) are contracted.

There is a middle ground between being hysterical about STD and pretending that they do not exist. Every effort should be made to minimize the risks, but contracting STD should not stigmatize a person nor should the fear of STD be used as an excuse to impose religious restrictions on sexual behavior. Thousands of persons have enjoyed multiple sex partners for a lifetime without ever contracting any of the diseases. Apparently, we have far greater tolerance for people who risk cancer by smoking or risk cirrhosis by drinking than we have for people who risk STD by enjoying sexual adventures. My point is to be realistic. Consider that every time you drive to a dinner party or a football game, you do take the very real statistical risk of being in a serious automobile accident. It seems out of proportion to deny yourself an equally enjoyable sex experience because you are afraid to risk contracting STD.

LOVE

Love is equally complex, but less controversial than sex. I think we can all agree that love has a definite positive effect on our physical state, whether we speak of romantic love, friendship love, or family love. All these forms of love help to minimize the development of so-called stress diseases (hypertension, ulcers, coronary heart disease).

Some people insist that a romantic relationship, a pair-bond, is the form of love that is essential to good health. In my opinion, that reflects a limited concept of love. We all know fascinating persons who thrive on various forms of nonromantic love. We also know the sad plight of women who have limited their interests to an exclusive romantic relationship, with very little outside stimulation. The importance of romantic love usually changes several times in a lifetime. Other interests or needs may crowd out the desire for romance temporarily, or you may want romance and not be able to find it. Friendship love and family love can remain more constant. Both are usually available to the outgoing, sensitive person. Loyalty and caring, the foundation of all forms of love, can be exchanged between lovers, friends, and relatives. There are many overlaps with all three types of love.

In general, our society does not regard it as healthy to have sex with friends or co-workers, that is, with anyone outside the pair-bond. The theory is that sex will change the relationship either because a pair-bond will develop or because the ego complications that are involved with sex will interfere with the relationship. However, I know of many cases in which people who have been friends for more than ten years report that their relationship included sex during some periods and not during others, depending on circumstances, other commitments, or the mood of one or both of the friends, and that sex never interfered with their healthy on-going friendship. I know of a few cases where persons who were working together had sex only once and went right back to a normal working relationship, without any of the complications so-called experts would predict.

Society grossly overemphasizes the importance of the sex act, often making it more important than friendship or love. The statement "There is nothing between us" usually means that two people do not have genital sex; it dismisses as "nothing" a relationship which might be one of deep friendship or intense intimacy. Saying "We are *just* friends" represents the same kind of misplaced value. Although sex adds a unique dimension to a loving relationship, it is often not the determinant of whether or not an intimate experience takes place. True friendship love is far more precious, difficult to obtain, and important to your health than a sexual experience.

SELF-RESPECT

Everyone needs self-respect for good health. At the basis of self-respect is a complex system of standards of behavior and expectations we set for ourselves and society sets for us. It is generally accepted that self-respect is enhanced by giving and receiving love, whether it be romantic, friendship, or family love. The relationship of sex to self-respect is much more variable, because it involves so many social and religious proscriptions. At one end of the spectrum are women who need to limit sex to one life-long partner for self-respect. At the other end are women who need to feel respect for their partner(s), but to whom the number or gender of sexual partners is unimportant. In between is a full range of conditions different women need to nurture their self-respect: marriage, but serial monogamy is okay; love and commitment, but marriage is not necessary; singles only, but never involve a married person; no homosexuality; one partner only (no group sex); and so forth.

Some believe that different standards not only can co-exist, but are healthy for a society; others believe that conformity is desirable for a healthy, good society.

Sex, love, and self-respect have a profound influence on our overall health and well-being. A loving sex relationship is somewhat like a strong body constitution: both contribute toward an exuberant sense of good health, but neither can guarantee anything. Remember that whereas you can be healthy, even thrive, without sex adventures, you cannot thrive without love and self-respect.

FEMALE SEXUAL RESPONSE

Although Masters and Johnson have described physiological response to direct sexual stimulation in great detail, they do not deal with the sudden desire to kiss or hug someone who turns you on. This is also a "sexual response." Having dinner, walking along the beach, washing dishes—almost any common activity may be sexual, depending on whom you are with or sometimes depending on your fantasies! Your sexual response can be a way of looking, a way of moving your body, a way of touching, a dream.

Commonly, "female sexual response" means how your body responds to genital stimulation. Masters and Johnson effected a gigantic breakthrough by making these responses legitimate concerns. It is clear that they emphasize variety and that no two persons react exactly alike, but by publishing charts and describing standards, they have inadvertently created goals for many who read their material. Remember that all the charts and descriptions are a compilation of many, many different variations. They should not be taken as a statement of how you should respond.

Physiological Response

The basic female sexual response described by Masters and Johnson consists of a period of arousal, a plateau phase, one or more orgasms, and a resolution to the resting state. But that need not be! You may enjoy just arousal and resolution. You may jump to the plateau stage without a slow gradual arousal. You may have a slow arousal and a long plateau with a gradual release of tension that could never be classified as orgasm, but still leaves you relaxed in your resolution stage. My definition of "good sex" is to be aroused, have a good time, and end up feeling warm, glowing, and contented.

As a matter of information, I will describe the basic response in more detail. During arousal the vagina becomes lubricated. This lubrication is a seepage from the walls of the vagina, not an actual secretion, since structured glands are not involved. This response is considered analogous to the erection of the penis in the male. As stimulation continues (whether direct or indirect), there is generalized vascular engorgement of the entire pelvic area. The swelling includes the clitoris, the labia, and the expansion of the vaginal barrel. Also the nipples become erect and both the areola and breasts themselves enlarge. The uterus begins to elevate.

During the plateau phase the uterus continues to be elevated and may double in size due to vasocongestion. While the deeper vagina continues to expand, the lower third of the vagina decreases in circumference. Color changes occur and may include a flush on the chest and deepening of color of the vulva. In women who have given birth sometimes the vulva reaches a purplish hue. In very dark complexioned females this will not be recognized.

Although most of us think of orgasm as a total body response, the female orgasm, as described by Masters and Johnson, consists solely of a series of contractions of the orgasmic platform, a group of muscles located in the lower third of the vagina. These contractions are 0.7 to 0.8 seconds apart and are usually from 3 to 12 in number. During orgasm, pulse, blood pressure, and respiration are significantly increased, often accompanied by convulsive body movements. With continued stimulation orgasms may occur in succession. The orgasmic phase is followed by the resolution phase. During resolution the engorgement subsides, and breasts and genital area (including uterus) return to their usual state.

Voluntary movements range from minimal hip movements to total body involvement throughout arousal and plateau. During late plateau and orgasm involuntary movements are added, sometimes overwhelming, sometimes small and specific. Individual responses cover a wide range. Some women are always silent, others routinely make gasping or grunting sounds, still others scream out. Also, the same woman may have very different responses (with the same or different partners) on different occasions.

The important thing to remember is that the cycle may take different forms. With direct stimulation of the clitoris an orgasm may occur with none of the ancillary changes, such as enlargement of breasts or color changes in the labia. The resolution phase may be complete within a few minutes of the beginning of stimulation. Or you may experience an arousal and plateau that may last a half hour or more with a very gradual return to complete resolution. It is quite possible to experience engorgement and resolution without ever recognizing a point of orgasm. Instead of a major peak experience you may have a series of small orgasmic releases, each one discharging some of the tension until gradually there is no tension and you feel relaxed and comfortable.

And you can enjoy all these responses without having intercourse. Masters and Johnson report that orgasms during manual and oral stimulation are more intense than orgasms during coitus. But remember that Masters and Johnson measure intensity with laboratory equipment, without regard for the woman's personal response, that is, how she experienced the orgasm.

"Did you come?" may be difficult to answer. How many of us count contractions of the orgasmic platform and check stopwatches to clock them at 0.7 seconds? Far more sensitive questions are "Did you enjoy yourself? Do you feel comfortable?" But if there is good communication, even these questions are usually unnecessary. Whatever your sexual experience, clinical or dramatic accounts of others need not cause anxiety or performance demands. Orgasms need to be put in perspective. Enjoy your sex life with mini-orgasms, the Big O, or just plain close, intimate pleasure.

Questions Often Asked About Orgasm

What is the difference between a vaginal orgasm and a clitoral orgasm? An orgasm, as defined by Masters and Johnson, is a specific physiological response. Most orgasms are produced by direct or indirect stimulation of the clitoris by a finger, a tongue, or a thrusting penis. Indirect stimulation is produced by pulling on the tissue immediately surrounding the clitoris to create friction on the clitoral head or shaft. This is the common way to elicit orgasm during intercourse. However, orgasm may be produced without indirect or direct stimulation of the clitoris. The thrusting penis may not stimulate the clitoris and orgasm may be produced by vaginal stimulation alone. Rarely, breast stimulation or even just a very erotic situation may elicit an orgasm. The orgasm, the response to stimulation, is the same whether or not the clitoris is involved. It is somewhat like tearful weeping. The tears are the same whether produced by an onion or a tragedy, even though the emotional and body reactions may be very different. Similarly, the contractions of the orgasmic platform are the same, whether produced by stimulation of the clitoris or by a more unusual stimulus.

I can have an orgasm by direct stimulation when my husband uses his fingers, but I want to have an orgasm during intercourse. What can I do? First, try to understand *why* this is so important to you. Is this goal something you feel must be accomplished to be "sexually mature"? Are you seeking to experience what so many romantic novels describe, that is, the ecstasy the woman feels while her lover is thrusting within her? Or is it just a curiosity, something you expected and anticipated, but has never happened? If you conclude that it really isn't important, simply cross it off your list of things to worry about. It is possible to have an exciting, fulfilling sex life without having orgasms during intercourse. However, if you conclude this is a "must" for you, try supplementing the penile thrusting with direct stimulation of the clitoris. This can be done by using your finger, or your lover's finger or by either of you applying a small vibrator to the clitoris during intercourse. Another technique is to stimulate your clitoris to a point close to orgasm just before intercourse. At that sensitive phase orgasm may be triggered by coitus. A third method is to try different positions. In addition to the woman-on-top position, there are several sideways positions that afford freedom of movement so that the woman can actively rub the clitoral area against the pubis or thigh to produce the necessary stimulus (see end of chapter for sources of more "how-to" information).

I have read about orgasm, but I have never reached the peaks others describe. Sometimes I wonder if I have ever had one. Can you help me understand? As I have said before, you should not attempt to measure your own responses against the reports of others. What is often omitted from descriptions of the orgasmic response is that it may be a rather dull experience with only the involuntary contractions of the vagina to confirm it. At the point of orgasm your body takes over the sexual response. Movements that had been partly involuntary and partly voluntary become entirely involuntary. But it need not be dramatic. The important part is this lack of control. There may be no waves of energy, no undulating movements of the hips, perhaps a gasp or two, and that's it. This has been proven in the laboratory. Masters and Johnson have recorded physiological orgasms manifested only by specific muscular contractions when the woman was unaware of a peak experience.

Romantic novels and stories often describe the ecstasy of simultaneous orgasm. I've never experienced this. Is it important or very different from nonsimultaneous orgasm? In my opinion simultaneous orgasm has been overrated. It does give the satisfaction of cooperative good timing and a special joy that your partner is climaxing at the same time you are, but what is lost is the sharing of the other's orgasm. During climax your attention is directed to the sensations of your own body. There is no "attention" left to direct toward your partner, other than the general knowledge that he is experiencing his climax at the same time. Separate climaxes allow you to share each other's experience in a much more intimate way. When your partner climaxes, you can empathize, appreciate, almost live through the experience, and when you climax, you can completely abandon yourself to yourself without diverting any attention outside your own body. I am talking about only the few minutes of high plateau phase and climax itself; before and after these stages the feeling of intimacy may be exquisite. Whatever you like best is right for you. If you feel it is important, put your imagination to work figuring how, with your particular pattern of intercourse, this might be possible. But do not allow it to create anxiety. Simultaneous orgasm is not essential to a full and satisfying sex relationship.

SEXUAL ENRICHMENT FOR COUPLES

For a small percent of couples, sex gets better and better. These rare couples report that after twenty or thirty years both excitement and satisfaction surpass their younger years. This may be due to an easier life style, fewer worries about children and finances, and so forth. Often women get a new interest in sex after menopause, and they realize that fear of pregnancy all those years was detrimental to full relaxation and an anxiety-free state. If such a revival is matched by their partners, they're off on a second honeymoon.

However, this storybook crescendo of sexual enjoyment just isn't true for most couples. More common is a gradual decrease in excitement, with or without continued deep satisfaction. Most marriages sustain many ups and downs in the joy, comfort, and closeness that sex offers. Whether you consider your sexual relationship good, mediocre, or bad depends a great deal on your expectations. Some women were taught that they were lucky if it didn't hurt and that "nice" women did not enjoy sex. Other women have been exposed to the fantastic joys possible during sex play and coitus and are disappointed if each encounter is not "the greatest show on earth."

Unfortunately, communication in this area is almost always awkward. Not only have both boys and girls been reared not to be open about sex, but each has had sharply different messages about what sex is all about. So we have two adults with different body rhythms, different social stresses, different needs, yet conventional marriage demands that they satisfy each other's sexual needs decade after decade without ever really being open about their wants, needs, joys and disappointments. No wonder so many married couples have sexual problems. It is a tough assignment.

But there are ways to make it easier. Although most psychologists and marriage counselors advise "honesty," I do not think most marriages could withstand complete honesty about sexual feelings, at least not suddenly after years of withholding. Gradual revelations offered with kindness and consideration would seem preferable.

A good beginning is to expect that your partner has been strongly attracted to other women. After all, it is an unusual person who is capable of intimacy with only one person. Desiring other women and even fantasizing about a romantic sexual adventure is the most natural thing in the world. How to handle the desire and the fantasy is another matter. If it weren't for our oversensitivity to sex, we could discuss such thoughts the same way we can discuss wanting a million dollars or a free trip to the South Seas. A person may like to think about having something, but not really want it; a person may want something, but not really need it or be willing to give up things of more value to get it. In a traditional marriage, the price tag on fulfilling sexual fantasies is sometimes exorbitant.

I do think that this first step is important. Start off knowing that you cannot be all things to anyone and that variety is tempting to most people. But the chances are you can enhance your sexual relationship if the spark is still there and communication lines are open. Here is a list of suggestions that may be helpful in improving a couple relationship. It is designed to suggest other different ideas; the list is open-ended.

Create an atmosphere conducive to tenderness, sensitivity and romance.

When was the last time you really prepared for sex? Have you ever given it the amount of time and energy you devote to a dinner party? Incense, candlelight, your favorite music, uninterrupted time that is planned. Too often sex is relegated to "after everything else" when it is easier to fall into a routine than to be creative about your sexual relationship.

Try a sensuous massage with slightly scented oil; try looking at erotic pictures or reading erotic stories together; take time. Remember how sexy taking each other's clothes off can be. Perhaps a dance in your underwear, or nude. Once in a while make a contract not to have genital sex, but spend time caressing and enjoying sensuality to the fullest. If one or both is experiencing a refractory period following an early orgasm, continue the gentle touching and cuddling, with or without more sex.

Experiment with new techniques. Perhaps you already have a large repertoire, perhaps not. Perhaps you already enjoy oral sex as an experience by itself; perhaps oral sex offends you. It is interesting that we used to tell unmarried couples that it is okay to experiment so long as it does not lead to intercourse, and tell married couples that it is okay to experiment as long as it does lead to intercourse! Too many people think of noncoital sex, such as oral sex, as only foreplay. But for many couples oral sex is a rewarding experience in and of itself, whether or not it leads to orgasm. Oral sex is very different when done simultaneously than when you take turns. Sometimes it feels good to caress your partner during oral sex; other times it may feel good just to lie back and receive. Treat yourself to some time when every iota of energy is directed fully to responding, to feeling the sensations all over your body as well as in your genitals. And you may be surprised at how much you enjoy changing roles, becoming the initiator instead of the receiver.

Explore the use of sexual aids. Two of the most common sexual aids are dildos and vibrators. They may be used in a variety of ways, including dildos during oral sex and vibrators during intercourse. Rejecting sexual aids is another example of an isolated standard for anything sexual. When a male friend pooh-poohed the use of a dildo, one female friend of mine retorted, "You may be talented and possess a magnificent penis, but I don't know any man who can perform oral sex on me when his penis is in my vagina, and I like that as a variation."

You can find all kinds of sexual aids in adult book stores. Though many advertise, "Women Welcome," you may be the only woman inside. Expect the premises to be tacky. Most have peep shows in the back. It is an experience to go in and browse around. Every time I've been in one, I've been treated politely and with respect, sometimes with a bit of amusement. Vibrators may be found in most drug and department stores.

Occasionally emphasize humor, playfulness, and craziness. If you feel better making every sexual encounter a serious matter, skip this paragraph. But if you have suppressed harmless, crazy ideas because grown-ups "don't act like that," read on. I believe that too many times we live under restrictions that serve no purpose and prevent a lot of fun. Haven't you ever felt you wanted to just play like a puppy dog? Is there a law against going to the bedroom to change for dinner and arriving at the table in your birthday suit? Have you had sex at least once in every room in the house? How about a good roll on the living room floor? Do you have a favorite scene in a play you would like to act out? This is only scratching the surface of possibilities. Although someone said of sex, "I never knew you could have so much fun without laughing," you can laugh too!

Get away. There is something about entering a hotel room and closing the door that acts like magic for some couples. A bathroom you didn't clean; a bed you won't have to make up. If the prices in the dining rooms are exorbitant, bring a picnic of your favorite foods or send out for a pizza. Pick a hotel with the services you like, such as a sauna or swimming pool. It will be a change from a dinner and the theatre night and within the same price range.

Talk openly. For some this will be one of the hardest suggestions to follow. Sometimes it is easier just to do something different and not discuss it ahead of time. That's fine. By talking openly I mean discussing your expectations, your wants, and what feels good with your partner. I also mean asking and listening. One way to start is to recognize how difficult it is and question each other about why it is so awkward, always with a sense of perspective. You are only verbalizing about a basic human response!

Attend a sex workshop. Workshops are held in major cities throughout the country. Most show explicit films and use street language for desensitization and resensitization. To find out about workshops in your area, contact ASSECT or the American College of Sexologists (see p. 119). Not everyone might enjoy or benefit from one, but I will never forget one couple who wrote to us after attending, "We've been married 35 years and never enjoyed sex so much as that weekend after the workshop; and it keeps getting better!"

SEXUAL THERAPY

With sex out of the closet more people are becoming more aware of their sexual needs and more interested in sexual health. These new attitudes help explain the steady increase in the number of people seeking sexual therapy.

Among sexual therapies there is a definite trend toward treating couples even though only one partner appears to have a problem. In females the usual complaint is lack of orgasm, especially orgasm during intercourse. In males the most common complaints are impotence and premature ejaculation.

One form of couple therapy begins with a complete sex history and thorough physical exam. The couple is instructed in the importance of touch and instructed to practice at home specific exercises in sensual intimacy. These usually include overall tenderness with an initial proscription against touching the breasts or genital area. The couple discusses the exercises at the next session. This process is very helpful in encouraging the partners to express themselves about what pleases and does not please them. Being instructed to tell your lover what feels good removes much of the embarrassment and fear of being critical and leads to improved communication. After several assignments, genitals may be caressed, but no intercourse is permitted. This is especially helpful to the male, as it allows for intimate, sensuous massage with no demand to perform. Since anxiety is a major cause of sexual problems, being relaxed and understanding goes a long way toward a satisfying sexual relationship.

Sexual Dysfunction—Physical Conditions

Most sex therapists are not physicians, and most will ask you to be checked for any physical abnormality that might relate to your sexual problem. For example, a complaint of painful intercourse (dyspareunia) may be due to any number of physical conditions including: an intact hymen, skin or mucous membrane irritations of the vulva, vaginitis (infectious or atrophic), adhesions of the clitoral hood, insufficient vaginal lubrication, a severely retroverted uterus (tipped way back), pelvic infection, ovarian tumor, endometriosis, and a disturbance in the lower bowel. If there seems to be no evidence of organic abnormality, psychological causes must be explored. For example, dyspareunia might be traced to religious proscriptions or sexual trauma in childhood, such as rape or incest.

One cause of dyspareunia is vaginismus, a severe spasm of the perineal muscles and lower third of the vagina. Vaginismus is a classic example of a psychosomatic disorder. It is a physical condition that has its origin in psychological trauma; the physical condition is entirely involuntary and no amount of will power can relax the muscles. The treatment consists of a combination of psychotherapy and dilation with Hegar dilators. Masters and Johnson send the couple home with dilators and instructions after the initial dilation in the clinic. It is essential that both partners understand both the physical condition and the psychological origin for the best therapeutic results. The spasticity of vaginismus is very distinct from the spasmodic contractions of the same muscles during orgasm. Vaginismus and various physical causes of dyspareunia generally can be diagnosed only by a careful pelvic examination.

Despite the general statements that vaginas accommodate to all sizes of penises, a significant number of cases of dyspareunia are due to the inability of a small vagina to receive a large penis comfortably. Some penises are simply too big for the woman's introitus (opening) or vaginal barrel. The dyspareunia may be caused by the penetration or by the thrusting. A short, very thick penis may cause pain only on penetration, whereas a long, moderately thick penis may cause no pain on penetration, but be extremely painful on deep thrusting. Thrusting pain may be alleviated by trying positions that do not utilize the entire shaft of the penis within the vagina. Penetration pain may be relieved by lubrication and dilation or in rare cases surgery.

Some of the less common physical conditions that may influence sexual behavior are hormonal imbalances and nervous system disorders, which cause interference with the normal pathways between sensory and motor components of sexual response, and diabetes, which may cause impotence in the male and affect female response. Diabetes, alcohol, and anti-hypertensive drugs are common in our society and should always be considered as possible causes of sexual dysfunction.

Sexual Dysfunction—Psychological Causes

The actual prevalence of physical causes for sexual dysfunction is in the realm of 3 percent. Most female and male sexual problems can be traced to psychocultural roots. Traditionally, our sexual training has been one of restraint. To be "good" we had to train our bodies not to respond to sexual stimuli. Then, suddenly, this body, thoroughly conditioned over many years not to respond to sexual stimulation, is supposed to respond enthusiastically. Sexual restraint, which used to be good, is now bad, and sexual response, which used to be bad, is now good! Unfortunately, our nervous system is very complex, and we cannot compel our bodies to reverse their carefully developed patterns of restraint. Much of sex therapy is "unlearning" the proscriptions of the past.

Some of these proscriptions are sexist and restrict females to a lower status, thus diminishing self-respect. The nonphysical causes for inadequate sexual response in women include: fear of consequences (pregnancy or disease); low self-esteem (self-depreciation); anxiety about doing the right thing (fear of failure); ignorance about what is healthy (fear of perversion); guilt about experimenting (feeling only penis-vagina penetration is proper); inability to communicate (silent sex and hope for the best); being unable to receive (trained only to nurture others); inability to accept sex-for-pleasure (cannot defy early proscriptions).

Sometimes these handicaps to sexual fulfillment exist when there is adequate libido; the woman wants to enjoy sex to the fullest, but just can't. Other times the desire for sex is lacking. Loss of libido may be general, relating to all men, or specific, relating only to the spouse or partner. General loss of libido may be voluntary or involuntary. Some people make an effort to turn off sexual desire. They find the hassles of sex outweigh the joys and they intentionally train themselves not to respond to sexual stimuli. With disuse, the neural pathways will indeed become less responsive, but still remain functional. An ideal situation with an ideal partner can almost always revitalize this basic human response.

Involuntary loss of libido may stem from a series of rejections, multiple unsatisfactory experiences, lack of opportunity, or some conflict with a partner. Within the pair-bond, boredom, hostility, and disappointment are common causes of loss of libido. You may be turned off at night because your partner was too critical, too flattering, or too dull during the day. You may have a feeling of distance because he doesn't understand you or your needs, and your desire for sex may depend on feeling intimate with someone who empathizes with you. Or you and your partner may have reduced sex to such a mechanical level that you just can't stand going through antics, once joyful and meaningful, now just dull routine.

Excitement is an important factor in libido. (I have suggested possible ways to inject excitement into a partnership in the section on couple enrichment.) Often age is used as an excuse to allow libido to wane. Finding a partner may be difficult for an older woman, and rather than admit defeat, she may use the excuse, "I'm too old for that."

Many women are aware of the psychocultural source of their problems, but are unable to get their emotions and bodies to catch up with their minds. They intellectually accept and understand, but need and want help in overcoming old habits. These women are highly motivated and have a high success rate with modern couple therapy.

In addition to individual therapy and couple therapy, group therapy is also effective. These groups stress both education and self-assertion. Women learn basic female anatomy and physiology and receive training in assertive behavior. Honesty and self-revelation are encouraged, but the dynamics are supportive rather than based on confrontation as in the encounter groups. Although groups directed at therapy are led by professionals, it is quite possible to start your own support group, if only to share experiences and gain confidence in the process.

For help in finding therapists in your area, I suggest consulting your local medical society, organizations dealing with marriage counseling, or professionals trained in various schools of humanistic psychology, such as transactional analysis, rational emotive therapy, gestalt. If you have difficulty finding someone locally, you might write to:

- American Association of Marriage and Family Counselors, 41 Central Park West, New York, New York 10023
- American Association of Sex Educators, Counselors & Therapists (AASECT), 5010 Wisconsin Avenue, Washington, D.C. 20016

- American College of Sexologists, 1523 Franklin Street, San Francisco, Calif. 94109
- Association of Humanistic Psychology, 325 Ninth Street, San Francisco, Calif. 94103

If you are just given a name or look in the classified section of your telephone book, be sure to get references. Be sure to find out the average length of therapy and the cost range. There are many competent sex therapists, but there are also quacks and, unfortunately, there is no single clearinghouse or any uniform licensing process. Check credentials in terms of both training and current membership in reputable organizations, such as those listed above. Help is available, even if hard to find.

SEX AND NONSEX FOR SINGLE WOMEN

Many legally single women are in a committed couple relationship, but many more are not. Society's attitude toward sex and the single woman has changed dramatically. In the past single women were either celibate or secretly sexual. Now, although women are "allowed" to be sexual, most women restrict their behavior far beyond what they would fantasize as ideal. Some of these self-imposed restrictions relate to the image they present to others, to parents, children, bosses, neighbors. When I ask single parents "What do you want your children to think about your sexuality?" I find much confusion. Most want their children to view them as sexual, but are uncomfortable bringing sex partners home to share the bedroom and stay overnight. Having a man be there for breakfast is somehow far more embarrassing than "dating" and coming home alone at 3:00 AM.

Even when the children do not have to confront the partner there is difficulty between parents and children. This appears to be true whether the children are 5, 15, or 25. Some parents are seriously upset about *their* parents' sexual behavior, and don't know how to explain grandmother's sexual behavior to her grandchildren.

A very practical problem is, of course, finding suitable partners. Even among those authors who extol the health benefits of sexual activity, I sometimes get the impression that they imagine that finding a satisfactory partner is as easy as calling for room service: "I'll have one male, 30 to 40 years old, attractive, bright, and sensitive to the sexual needs of a woman." However, even if available, most women would not use such a service, because most women do not think of sex in terms of physical gratification with strangers, regardless of health benefits. They cannot or do not want to separate sex from a relationship with love and commitment. Many believe that high moral standards and good mental health cannot possibly include sex with casual partners.

Regardless of age, there is much more acceptance of sex if it occurs within an on-going serious relationship. Medical experts continue to write about why casual sex for women is always sick and destructive, the neurotic desire of some women for sex without love and commitment, and the painful regrets that follow the temporary joy of an affair. It is accepted that normal men have the desire for casual sex, but that moral convictions will encourage them to use restraint. The truth is that biologically females can enjoy both limited love and casual sex as much as males, but in order to do so women must openly contradict the mores or act secretively and contribute to the sexual hypocrisy that pervades our society.

A growing number of respected professionals believe that it is not only normal, but even a sign of maturity to be able to enjoy sex whenever you want to, providing that you make a clear contract with your partner and that you don't allow it to interfere with other responsibilities. Unfortunately, many women who think that they are making a clear contract find themselves feeling empty and regretful after casual sex. These cases are paraded out by the traditionalists as a warning for *all* women. Actually, we don't know what percent of the total these cases constitute. How many satisfied cases are there for every regretful case? We do know that many women can and do enjoy casual sex, particularly those in sophisticated metropolitan areas, where anonymity is made easy. We also know that these case histories are conspicuously absent in professional articles on sex and marriage.

In our mobile, contraceptive, affluent society, the modern single woman of all ages has many options regarding her sex life. Although older women are still lower on the "sex-appeal ladder," the time is ripe for them to be assertive. In many European countries the experience and sensuousness of the older woman is regarded as more desirable than the youthful beauty of less experienced women. So what can you expect if you are single? Certainly a lot depends on your community. Your options may be very limited if you live in a very small town without access to a large city. In large cities it depends mostly on you. However mature or liberated you feel your views are, if your partner does not share the same views, you may find yourself in an exploitative sexual situation. Thousands of single women are hurt every day and many become very frustrated: "Is there no such animal as a sensitive, decent man?" Many conclude that the price of sex is too high. They prefer to go without sex until they can enjoy a solid commitment on the man's part.

On the other hand, if you are single and want a more active sex life, I strongly suggest that you begin to talk openly about sex when you date, and I am including the grandmothers here, too. One easy way to break into the subject of sexual values is by talking about role stereotypes: Do you believe women and men should continue to have different roles (the man taking the initiative, picking you up, paying for dinner)? What do you think of changing social roles over the last decade? Do you believe in the double standard?

And don't be angry if your date is honest and says he wants sex. Do you want to be so unattractive that, even though he is horny, he doesn't want to have sex with you? What is important is that he doesn't pressure you with his wants and that he is sensitive to your wants, whether that involves the opera, swimming, or sex. If you've been burned, tell him. Be as honest as possible about your feelings and what you want. And don't be afraid to say that you are confused, if that is true. Take some risks, but always weigh what you are doing against the realistic alternatives. You may decide you would rather be home with a good book. If so, gently excuse yourself early and go home.

Finally, some support for those singles who want a vacation from sex, temporary or permanent, sometimes referred to as "the new celibacy." This implies celibacy by desire or design, not by fear or default. Sometimes it is much simpler to make a decision to abstain from sex than to weigh the pros and cons on each date or in each relationship. The declaration need only be to yourself. If a fantastic man appears on the scene, you can certainly change your mind. In the meantime you have avoided the decision-making process regarding the average man you will meet. Sex becomes nonnegotiable. You are temporarily choosing abstinence. You may or may not include masturbation in your pact with yourself. You may experience a sense of relief. No more struggling with, "Shall I or shall I not?" "If he takes me to dinner, will he expect me to go to bed with him?" "I wonder if he really likes me or just wants sex." "If I go to that party and do meet someone very attractive, do I want to have sex?" If sexual encounters have been troublesome for you, maybe a clean break will be more helpful than "I'll give it one more try." For some, one reason for experimenting with the new celibacy is political, a way of demonstrating independence. For most, I believe, it is far more personal.

If you decide to experiment with the new celibacy, you may want to get the no-sex message across loud and clear before accepting a date. You can then accept the dinner without implying any sexual trade off. Given our traditional role playing, you may have a hard time convincing men you are serious. If they are surprised, let them chalk it up to a lesson in understanding the new woman: She means what she says!

EXTRAMARITAL SEX

If your husband is a bore, never shows affection for you, puts you down in public, and is mean to the children, he is not guilty of infidelity; nor has he broken any marriage vows. Women have been educated to regard brutality and degradation as more tolerable than sexual infidelity in an otherwise super husband! This was confirmed for me when I spoke to a large audience of women and specifically asked, "What would you do if you found out that your husband was having an affair?" They shouted, almost in unison, "I'd kill him!" For a moment, at least in fantasy, murder and widowhood were more acceptable than the shame, betrayal, and horror of extramarital sex.

Granted this was a dramatic response, granted many women would not react this way in the privacy of their homes, still the idea of being beaten by their husbands evokes no such response. Physically abused women tend to be submissive and resigned to months or years of suffering before rebelling. This attitude continues to be maintained despite the fact that in terms of your well-being, your health is far less threatened by a husband who is loving and kind and has experienced extramarital sex, than by a husband who is mean and cruel and has never experienced extramarital sex.

But the medical profession never deals with the health aspects of extramarital sex, even if one partner has been in an institution or incapacitated for ten years. The medical profession prefers to reflect the religious-moral position of our society rather than to concern itself with the sexual health of the deprived marriage partner. One eminent medical consultant suggested that long separations could be used for spiritual growth. Maybe so, for some people, but this expert offered no other options, not even masturbation.

In my opinion, marriage partners are entitled to a more realistic approach to extramarital sex. I have observed the harm that results from placing such enormous emphasis on the "badness" of extramarital sex. We are pressured into perceiving it as universally bad, even though no actual harm was done. Sexual possessiveness is so ingrained that it affects any long-standing pair-bond, marital or not, even though in an unmarried couple it does not have the same kind of legal, social, and religious reinforcement.

Women who are neglected by their husbands may find joy and renewed energy in an affair. Too bad we are not trained to be logical in such a situation. It would seem reasonable (even if radical) for these husbands to be happy that their wives are more cheerful, less complaining. But a sudden improvement in mood may cause anger and suspicion of that ogre, sex. Better to be bitchy, frustrated, and "faithful."

Part of this overreaction is caused by possessiveness. We are programmed to include a sense of ownership in our concept of marriage—a sense of gaining a part of a person and giving up a part of ourselves to that person. This promotes a deep fear of loss, for we are now dependent on one particular person to feel secure, especially in regard to sex, and a sense of jealousy stems from our insecurity. We are encouraged to be financially, socially, and professionally secure, but a little sexual insecurity in marriage is often endorsed to "keep us on our toes." Many women have told me that they actually enjoy their husband's jealousy; they perceive it as flattering. Many couples find a certain amount of possessiveness desirable, but too often possessiveness in the sexual area grows way out of proportion.

It is true that extramarital sex may be seriously harmful to the marriage relationship. Thousands of case histories substantiate this fact. The problem is that the medical journals and most newspaper advice columns strongly suggest that in all cases of extramarital sex one or both partners are sick or bad. In fact, the published medical data are so convincing that some professionals sincerely believe that it is impossible for a woman to have an extramarital affair that will enhance her marriage or increase her self-esteem. They simply discount the work of sociologists and take comfort in the cases presented by psychiatrists and marriage counselors. Moreover, your own personal experience may reinforce this view. Everyone learns about affairs that end in tragedy. Persons enjoying successful affairs often don't risk talking about them, and their cases probably will not reach your ears or get recorded in doctors' files.

This bias continues into the study of spouses who are frustrated, want to have extramarital sex, and don't. The medical profession will quote cases where exercising self-control and turning away a potential love experience end up in greater appreciation of one's spouse, a greater love for family, and so forth. Cases where sexual frustration results in resentment, contributes to alcoholism, and worsens family life are ignored.

By taking this one-sided stance, we eliminate the possibility of diminishing the harmful effects of extramarital sex, such as rejection, jealousy, low self-esteem, self-pity, resentment, hostility, and ultimate break-up of the marriage. We really know a great deal about what makes an affair constructive and what makes it destructive. Suppression of this information increases the risk of disastrous results. Apparently, we have a compelling need to deny the existence of extramarital sex among "nice" people who "deserve" help in avoiding its pitfalls. If health professionals offered guidelines for extramarital sex, they would probably be accused of promoting serious immorality.

My message to the nonparticipating spouse is far less controversial. First, understand that your spouse's adventures may have nothing whatsoever to do with your adequacy, your attractiveness, your love, with *you* at all! Many persons can and do love more than one person at the same time. Many persons can enjoy sexual fun without further commitment. Many women and men would enjoy many sex partners in a lifetime were it not for social and religious pressure.

Limiting sex to one partner is a difficult imposition on women and men who have not accepted the absolute virtue of sexual monogamy. However, very often the effort to conform is worthwhile. Many couples prefer the security of sexual monogamy with a lifetime partner and sometimes the relationship becomes more meaningful because of the restraint each partner has exercised. On the other hand, we are all familiar with serial monogamy, which is socially more acceptable, but not necessarily more humane than a stable marriage that sustains one or more affairs.

Before reinforcing society's current social, religious, and moral rejection of all extramarital sex, let's take a look at the evidence. Evidence from sociological studies (Kinsey, Hunt, Cuber, Newberg) shows that (1) extramarital sex is widespread among normal mature people as well as among neurotic immature people, (2) extramarital sex may disrupt the family, have no effect on the family, or benefit family relations, (3) the guilt and anxiety of the participant and the response of the spouse usually cause more harm than the act itself, (4) the nonparticipating partner may be a charming, adequate, mature adult, (5) though some are "driven" to extramarital sex, others choose to enjoy it as an added source of excitement, tenderness, and intimacy. The purpose of this section is to remove from extramarital sex its inordinate power to destroy something which is far more meaningful and important to us than sex could ever be.

ALTERNATIVES IN SEXUAL EXPRESSION

We have been considering options in sexual expression that include experimenting within and outside traditional monogamous relationships. Sexual health can also mean an understanding of forms of expression that have been considered unconventional or that have been tabooed by our society. We should be able to consider in an objective and open way alternative forms that might be desirable for others or for ourselves.

Masturbation

Current attitudes toward masturbation range from an unwavering position that it is unnatural and sinful to the position that it is a healthy, pleasurable activity to be enjoyed throughout life. The most prevalent attitude is probably just about in the middle: Masturbation is a natural aspect of child development. It should not be encouraged or punished. It should be accepted, but kept subdued. In adulthood masturbation is an acceptable substitute for sexual intercourse for those without a partner or when the partner is unavailable.

A growing number of professionals in the field of human sexuality assume the pleasure-throughout-life position. Many adults regard it as a different kind of sexual expression that may be desired at a particular time, even when they are having a satisfactory sexual relationship. During masturbation you need not concern yourself with the other person's needs, but simply focus on your own. Perhaps you have never thought about taking time to prepare yourself for a "masturbation session," that is, enjoy your body in a bath or shower, make yourself comfortable, make sure you won't be interrupted, turn on your favorite music, and take plenty of time to pleasure yourself. One technique is to start with the less erotic zones and gradually work up to the more sensitive clitoral area. Many consider the prolonged techniques selfish and narcissistic, but others consider it no different from treating themselves to a gourmet meal or a new dress—except it's cheaper! Traditionally, we have been taught that it is all right to make your body feel good by taking a bath, by applying lotions, by an exhilarating sport followed by rest and relaxation, by sunning, by eating your favorite food, but not by sex. You can get a massage to make every part of your body feel good, except one, your genital area.

In workshops in human sexuality masturbation is discussed routinely. Some of the women remember masturbating to climax as a small child. Some say they have never masturbated, but with increased awareness they begin to recall certain activities they did, such as "riding" on the arm of a chair, which produced friction in the area of the clitoris. Many women are surprised to find others masturbate in front of their partners. It is common for men to be turned on by watching their partners masturbate. Many partners want to learn just what makes you feel good.

Now, on a subject such as this it is difficult to address more adventurous readers without frightening those for whom the idea of masturbating in front of their partners or in front of a mirror or perhaps under any circumstances would be disturbing. Maybe you do not want to examine attitudes in such depth. Perhaps what you have been taught seems right to you and you are comfortable sticking to the rules set down for you. No one is suggesting that anyone ought to change. But many do want to be free from old rules, including rules about masturbation, especially because it may be very private and not involve anyone else. My approach is to apply to masturbation exactly the same standards for behavior one applies to other activities. Do you want to? Will it hurt someone? Will it interfere with your other obligations? Will it make you feel good? Will it cause guilt and anxiety?

Although this chapter is not designed to advocate any particular behavior, but rather to give support to various options in human sexual expression, I cannot write about masturbation without defending the right of children to masturbate without guilt or physical punishment. I do not endorse the right of parents to punish children for masturbating; in my opinion it constitutes a form of child abuse.

Masturbation is a universal practice throughout the world. Some cultures condemn it, some encourage it, and some, like ours, sustain a variety of views. Without being taught that it is sinful or harmful, all children would enjoy masturbating and probably would regard the genital area as just more fun to play with than other parts of the body. But negative messages are received very early in life. For parents who would like to avoid the negative message, but still find it difficult because of their own background to discuss masturbation with their children, I suggest making a book about it available to the child. Then, if the child is curious, the information is there. Not all children accept the serious approach of their mentors. When one small girl was told that masturbation would make her blind, she asked "Can I do it at least until I need glasses?"

Sexual Fantasies

A significant contribution to the understanding of female sexuality relates to the sexual fantasies of women. Recent reports affirm the capacity of females to have dramatic, exciting fantasies during sex, just reading about sex, looking at sexy pictures, lounging on their couches, sunning at the beach, or whatever.

In my experience interviewing women and men, I find a definite difference in the incidence of male and female fantasy. Many more males have experienced fantasies and more regularly than females. But among the females who fantasize, the imagination and extent of fantasy is comparable to males.

There is a tendency for some females to be anxious about the "wildness" of their fantasies or to feel guilty if they fantasize about someone else while making love to their partners. Most professionals would be supportive of the fantasies. Let go! Enjoy whatever fantasies come into your head. Unfulfilled dreams acted out in fantasy often relieve tension and anxiety. It is understandable that some people might be judgmental about fantasizing about other people while making love, especially if sharing the fantasy would be upsetting to the partner. However, no matter how much honesty there is about physical activities, it is a rare person who can share every dream with her mate—not impossible, but rare.

It is important for most women to have a private, unshared segment of life. For some it may function as a boost toward independence, helping to get away from the total belonging to another person. For others, whose independence is more secure, fantasies can be shared as an option, what they *want* to do, not what they *need* to do.

We can conclude that the fantasy world is one where you can try all sorts of extremes without criticism or consequences. You can fantasize hundreds of lovers; bondage where you are helpless and revel in the lack of responsibility; total control where you demand exactly what you want; exotic environments such as floating on a flying carpet; or seducing the president on the floor of the Oval Room in the White House. The fantasy world is yours to use with *imagination unlimited!*

Lesbianism and Bisexuality

We don't know how prevalent lesbianism is. Kinsey estimated that homosexual experiences to the point of orgasm occur in from 10 to 12 percent of women. The *Hite Report* indicates a slightly lower incidence. Lesbians who do not advertise the erotic aspect of their relationships are rarely distinguished from good friends. Most lesbians stay "in the closet" because of jobs, family, and neighbors. But a small radical group not only has come out of the closet, but has adopted anti-male standards. These radicals consider anyone who has sex with a man a traitor to the cause. To them, bisexuality is wishy-washy, not liberated.

There are probably thousands of secret lesbians who never act out their sexual preference and many who repress knowledge of that preference. These women get married (because they are supposed to), have children (because they are supposed to), and never find the right circumstances to express their true inclinations.

And then there is a group of women who are heterosexual, but have a curiosity about making love to another woman. Some interest in loving women is really quite logical in our society, where "sexy" is equated with a provocative female body. Although the image of the sexy woman is used to appeal to men, women are exposed to the same message. In addition, most female bodies are softer, more graceful, generally more conducive to caressing than male bodies. Women are allowed to have tender, warm feelings for each other, and the idea of making love could be construed as a reasonable extension of that. I am convinced that it is common for women to fantasize having sex with a dearly loved female friend. Perhaps most never make these feelings known because they do not want to risk offending or hurting the people they love.

In studying human sexuality, Kinsey did not categorize individuals as either homosexual or heterosexual; rather he tried to determine the proportion of each preference within the individual. He devised a scale to measure the proportion in a person's actual behavior and a person's inclinations. The scale ranges from 0 to 6 with 0 meaning 100 percent heterosexual and 6 meaning 100 percent homosexual. Thus, a woman with a strong homosexual preference who leads a completely heterosexual life would be rated 0 on the behavior scale and perhaps 5 on the inclination scale, assuming she did indeed have some inclination toward heterosexuality. A person who has an equal number of experiences with women and men and who has no preference between the genders would be a 3 on both scales. Double 3's are rare. Most people have a preference for one gender or another, though they may be active with both genders. The word bisexual loosely applies to all who even have fantasies about sex with both genders, even though their behavior is limited to one gender, such as the secret lesbian rated 0-5. In a more restricted sense the word bisexual would apply only to persons who, in adult life, have experienced sexual relations with both genders.

It seems to me illogical to consider a bisexual woman less mature in her sexual attitudes than an exclusive heterosexual. If she can make love the way heterosexuals do and also make love to another woman, in what way is she less good, less sexual, less of a person, and, most of all, less lovable?

Because little research has focused on female homosexuality and because women with such inclinations tend to keep them secret, many myths about lesbians and bisexual women remain current. We can contribute to debunking a few of them.

In any lesbian couple, there is always a butch and a fem. Most lesbian couples do not consist of a masculine type (butch) and a feminine type (fem). They are commonly women without such specific characteristics who happened to be attracted to each other and enjoy satisfying each other sexually. Of course, as in any couple there will be differences in assertiveness but generally couples do not follow the traditional male-female model of primary breadwinner and primary homemaker.

Women are lesbians because they can't get a man. Many men regard lesbians as making the best of second-best and express the belief that they would not be lesbians if they were able to find a man to love them. This is simply not true. Lesbians *prefer* women and would choose a woman rather than an equally attractive, compatible man. They have no trouble describing how much better women make love.

Lesbians always use penis substitutes. Although most lesbians have experimented with dildos, few use these penis substitutes as a regular part of love making. Rather, they enjoy caressing each other, including oral stimulation.

All lesbians are unfit mothers. Few heterosexual mothers could pass the psychological tests given to lesbian mothers seeking custody of their children. Many of these mothers have been judged by professionals to be psychologically healthy and their homes described as loving, supportive environments for children, only to have the legal system deny them custody. This same legal system is far more hesitant to demand that children be separated from heterosexual women, even though they may be far less competent and less loving. With limited foster homes and other alternatives available, a heterosexual drug addict, alcoholic, or known childbeater has less chance of having her children taken away from her than a responsible out-of-the-closet lesbian. Only within the last decade are the courts finally beginning to consider the welfare of the child. Too often the "unfitness" of the lesbian mother exists only in the bias of the judge, without regard to the actual nurturing the child is receiving.

Lesbians and bisexual women are basically different. Lesbians and bisexual women have no special qualities that set them apart from other women, except their choice of sex partners. Some are smart, some are dull; some extroverts, some introverts; some leaders, some followers; some creative, some not. They do live in a different environment than their exclusively heterosexual sisters however. Our society is actually quite tolerant of their behavior, so long as it remains private and discrete. It is when they create a relationship or household parallel to the conventional family that society regards lesbianism as a threat and seeks to penalize them. They cannot attain the status of conventionally married women, they must endure social rejection, and their job opportunities are extremely limited.

Many women feel that heterosexual relationships are never equal, that an imbalance of power always exists, and that only through sex with another woman can they enjoy a truly equal partnership. For some bisexuality seems to provide the best of both worlds. However, the majority of lesbians and bisexuals are not involved in equal rights. Like their exclusively heterosexual sisters, they are more interested in paying the rent, buying groceries, keeping their jobs . . . and finding and maintaining love.

SEX AND EDUCATION FOR PARENTHOOD BY CHOICE

Why don't we stress to children how important it is not to have a baby unless and until they are prepared for parenthood—intellectually, emotionally, socially, and financially? Although we cannot set up standards for adults without dangerous encroachment on individual freedom, we can generalize that girls under 18 years of age are not qualified to be independent mothers. Mothers 17 and under could be required to be supervised and to attend classes in nutrition, child care, etc. Details of such a program are beyond the scope of this chapter, but I believe that there is a real need to get out of our current paradox. Namely, girls who are denied birth control because they are too young for sex may become mothers with no education in either responsible sex or responsible parenthood.

Despite the fact that some teenagers get pregnant intentionally, grade school teachers would have no trouble convincing most pupils that the burdens of parenthood are great and that it is most important to avoid accidental pregnancy at a young age. Sounds so reasonable, so why not? I have concluded that the major reason is that teaching parenthood by choice validates recreational sex. Apparently this is so abhorrent to our mores that it is better to put up with ignorance and millions of accidental pregnancies among teenagers. All teenagers are sexually active: some in fantasy only, some in masturbation only, some in necking and petting, some in coitus, some in homosexual sex. Our need to ignore this reality and to continue to outlaw practical courses in responsible sexual behavior is basic to our problem of children having children.

And it's not just children. Many adults do not have adequate birth control information or services. True, many doctors provide contraception and Planned Parenthood has centers in all major cities, but birth control is still a taboo subject in television, radio, and newspaper ads. Our ostrich-like attitude toward sex is the culprit. Contraception is medically accepted, yet newspapers can advertise cigarettes, but not contraception. Radio and television can encourage the consumption of junk foods, but not voluntary sterilization. We should demand the right of every woman to have knowledge of and access to birth control.

The desire to bolster the social directive that people ought to "get married and have children" in that order links parenthood more closely to marriage than to sex and makes us unwilling to deal with the problem of the thousands who do not follow that directive. We seem to ignore the fact that marriage does not cause parenthood, sex does!

When we do offer sex education, we do relate it to parenthood, but parenthood in marriage. Too often sex is described as "something mommies and daddies do when they feel close and want a baby." What other course could be taught that dealt with such an infinitesimal portion of the subject matter? Questions about satellites can be answered to the best of our knowledge, but accurate knowledge about sex had best wait until later.

One last point. The religious proscriptions against birth control are not really against birth control; they are against sex, especially sex for women. Babies that are denied birth because of abstinence are not lamented. It is all right not to have babies, as long as you do not have sex. We need to endorse nonprocreational sex in order to teach responsible sexual behavior. So long as we deny the right of women to be sexual except when they want to become pregnant, we are doomed to random reproduction, irresponsible parenthood, and all the social tragedies that follow. It is clear that our attitudes toward sexuality reach far beyond our personal lives into the realms of education, politics, and sociology.

FURTHER READING

There are so many books on female sexuality it is difficult to recommend just a few. Probably you know as many of the best sellers as I do and are fully aware of the wide range of material available.

I mention here only a few unusual books that might have escaped your attention. For book lists, I recommend you send for the *Multi-Media Resource Center Book List,* which is conveniently organized by subject matter. Write to MMRC, 1525 Franklin Street, San Francisco, Calif. 94109.

For excellent pamphlets about all aspects of sexuality write SIECUS, 84 Fifth Avenue, New York, N.Y. 10011.

For readers interested in the development of our current sexual mores, I strongly recommend *The American Way Of Sex, An Informal Illustrated*

History, by Bradley Smith. The book is a review of how Americans have reacted to the legal and social restraints imposed on sexual behavior throughout our history. If some of the new freedom is distasteful to you, do examine this book to get a glimpse of how Americans actually behaved in "the good old days."

For factual material and explicit pictures of nudity at all stages of female and male development, I suggest *The Sex Book, A Modern Pictorial Encyclopedia,* by Martin Goldstein, M.D., and Erwin J. Haeberle, Ph.D. This book allows children to look up any common word pertaining to sex and read an understandable explanation, often with pictures. The pictures are most sensitive and the book has an overall serious tone.

For the same solid facts in humorous style, I recommend that you write to Ed-U-Press, 123 Fourth St. NW, Charlottesville, Va. 22901, for a catalog of their publications. The Ed-U-Press series, by Sol Gordon, Ph.D., introduces humor to sex in a unique way. Instead of jokes that distort reality, Dr. Gordon uses a comic book style to present medical information based on the latest scientific data. He also conducts sexual workshops and offers audiovisual aids, for example, a filmstrip on "HERPIE, the New VD Around Town."

For those readers who have some conflict about how to integrate a liberated sexual attitude with religion and to any who would appreciate a sensitive, reverent, pictorial description of human sexuality, I highly recommend *Meditations on the Gift of Sexuality,* text by Ted McIlvenna and photographs by Laird Sutton, Specific Press, 1523 Franklin Street, San Francisco, Calif. 94109. The text states, "Finding God in sex is the theme of this symphony." All persons photographed are "sharing a portion of their most intimate relationships because they want to help others feel good about themselves sexually."

For more about deemphasizing sex, especially extramarital sex, see *Adultery and Other Private Matters,* by Lonny Myers and Hunter Leggitt, Chicago: Nelson-Hall, 1975.

REFERENCES

American Medical Association. *Human Sexuality.* Chicago: American Medical Association, 1972.

Clark, Vincent E. *Human Sexuality in Medical Education and Practice.* Springfield, Ill.: C. C. Thomas, 1968.

Comfort, Alexander. *Joy of Sex.* New York: Crown, 1972.

Cuber, J., and P. Harroff. *The Significant Americans.* Englewood Cliffs, N.J.: Prentice-Hall, 1965.

Francoeur, Robert. *The Future of Sexual Relations.* Los Angeles: Spectrum Productions, 1974.

Hunt, M. *The Affair*. New York: Harcourt Brace Jovanovich, 1969.

Libby, Roger W., and Robert M. Whitehurst. *Marriage and Alternatives*. Chicago: Scott Foresman, 1977.

McCary, James Leslie. *Human Sexuality*. New York: Van Nostrand, 1967.

Mazur, Ronald. *Commonsense Sex*. Boston: Beacon Press, 1968.

Myers, Lonny, and Hunter Leggit. "A New View of Adultery," *Sexual Behavior* (February 1972).

Neubeck, G. *Extra-marital Relations*. Englewood Cliffs, N.J.: Prentice-Hall, 1969.

O'Neill, Nena, and George O'Neill. *Open Marriage*. New York: Evans, 1972.

Otto, Herbert A. *The New Sexuality*. Palo Alto, Calif.: Science & Behavior Books, 1971.

Scheimann, Eugene. *Sex Can Save Your Heart*. New York: Crown, 1974.

Scheimann, Eugene. "Sex Can Help You Live Longer." *Forum* (January 1978).

Contraception and Abortion

ELIZABETH B. CONNELL, M.D.

Associate Professor, Department of Obstetrics and Gynecology,
Northwestern University School of Medicine, Chicago, Illinois

Throughout most of history the continued existence of society—families, communities, nations—depended on producing enough children to survive against the great odds of infant mortality, famine and drought, pestilence, and war. But even in this struggle for survival both men and women had reasons to want to control fertility and devised methods to plan their families.

With the development of modern technology, survival was no longer as tenuous or as dependent on numbers as in the past, and people were able to turn more attention to private reasons for family planning. As the dependence of the social unit on numbers decreased, cultural expectations changed and peer pressure to have many children decreased. Whereas at one time economic benefits were derived from the large family, modern cost factors encouraged fewer children.

Added to these changing social and economic factors was the emergence at the beginning of this century of the women's movement—their attempts to establish their identity in the world outside their role in the home. Increased education, opportunities for employment, and development of role models outside the family tradition resulted from and further stimulated the movement. It became clear that in order to pursue these expanded goals, women had to be able to control their fertility—to reduce the number of children they had and to be able to plan when they would have them.

Most recently, survival has again begun to influence ideas of family planning. People have become increasingly aware of the many dangers associated with overpopulation, such as pollution of our environment and depletion of our natural resources. We now recognize that our environment can suffer irreversible damage and that we may not find ways to replace the resources we are consuming at an ever increasing rate. For these and many other reasons, people are concerned about the need to limit reproduction of ourselves.

Virtually every type of fertility regulation we have today has been used in some form or other in the past. Many of the earliest methods—chemicals taken to prevent conception or induce abortion, physical means of abortion, and so forth—were dangerous or actually lethal. In recent years much effort has been made to understand the various steps involved in reproduction in both men and women and to learn what can be done to control human fertility. The result has been the development of a number of new forms of contraception. We now have what is called the "contraceptive cafeteria," a group of techniques for both the female and the male which we will consider in greater detail below.

RISK-BENEFIT RATIO

The question is often asked, "What is the best method of family planning?" At the present time there is no single best method, and there will be none until the "ideal contraceptive" is discovered. The attributes of the ideal contraceptive are that it be totally safe, effective, and reversible, that it be inexpensive, easy to distribute, and easy to use, and that its use not be related to the actual time of sexual relations.

With the development of the oral contraceptives and subsequently the IUDs, it was believed in each case that an ideal contraceptive method had been found. Unfortunately, with time and continued study, it has been discovered that neither of them is entirely safe or entirely effective. Since there seems to be little chance of discovering a perfect method, at least for quite some time, we are forced to continue to deal with what is known as the risk-benefit ratio.

We have learned that any medication which is powerful enough to have a desired effect on the human body will, almost of necessity, carry with its use a certain amount of risk. Today's medications, taken according to instructions, are, in general, safe and effective. The risk-benefit ratio of most drugs in proper dosages is heavily weighted on the side of the benefits. The level of risk which is acceptable varies with the intended use of a particular drug. For example, when one is looking at drugs to be given for the treatment of advanced cancer, one is willing to accept a relatively high degree of risk. However, when one is dealing with contraceptive methods which are given by and large to normal, healthy women to prevent a possible pregnancy rather than to treat an existing disease, it is essential that the risks be very low.

SELECTION OF METHODS

A woman should carefully consider several factors when deciding which birth control method she prefers. First of all, medical factors must be considered. It has been shown that the risk of death for any woman in good health up to the age of 30 to 35 is lower using any of the currently available methods than becoming pregnant and carrying a child to term. Furthermore, after the age of 30 to 35 any method except the oral contraceptive is much safer than becoming pregnant and having a baby. In the

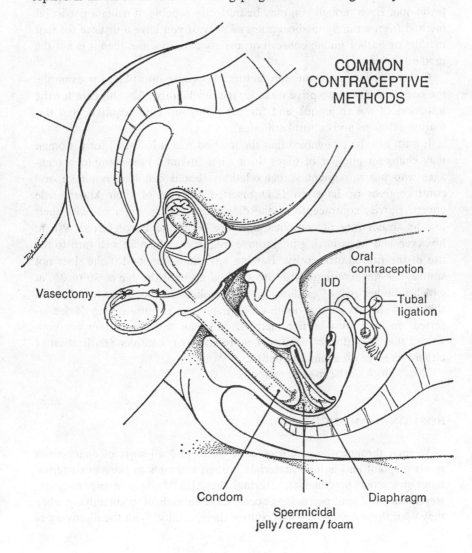

COMMON CONTRACEPTIVE METHODS

Vasectomy

IUD

Oral contraception

Tubal ligation

Condom

Spermicidal jelly / cream / foam

Diaphragm

current climate of great anxiety about the side effects of pills and IUDs, these two facts are often ignored. These comparisons are valid in developed countries where the health care is excellent; they are infinitely more important in developing countries. In areas of the world where health care is minimal or absent the risks associated with pregnancy and childbirth far outweigh any possible danger associated with contraceptive use. When a woman is not in perfect health, it is necessary to look at the specific contraindications to the use of any particular form of family planning. These will be considered below under the various methods.

In addition to purely physical factors, emotional and psychological factors must also be taken into consideration when selecting a contraceptive technique. Even though you may be perfectly capable of using a particular method from a purely medical point of view, if you have a distaste for that method or harbor undue concern or anxiety about its use, then it is not the method for you.

Certain social and economic factors also come into play, for example, the cost of the contraceptive method, the availability of health care for the initiation of the technique and for the follow-up care required, and numerous religious and cultural attitudes.

It must also be recognized that the method which is "best" for a woman may change a number of times during her lifetime. For example, a teenager who has infrequent sexual relations should definitely not take oral contraceptives or have an IUD inserted because of their known side effects. Barrier contraceptives—the diaphragm and spermicides—with their low to absent rate of complications, are by far to be preferred. When, however, she starts having intercourse frequently, she may well turn to the use of the oral contraceptive. Barring any difficulties and if she does not smoke, she may continue with this method up until the age of 30 or 35, at which time her risk of cardiovascular complications begins to increase. At this point she has several options. She may have an intrauterine device inserted, go back to a barrier method, or if she and her partner are convinced that they do not want any more children, consider sterilization of either one as an excellent alternative.

Now to look at the specific methods.

HORMONAL METHODS—FEMALE

Women through the centuries have swallowed all sorts of concoctions made of plant and animal materials in their attempts to prevent or terminate unwanted pregnancies. During the Middle Ages many mercury, strychnine, and lead poisonings occurred, thousands of women dying when they used these agents to try to control their fertility. With the discovery of oral contraceptives, women for the first time had a technique which, if taken as directed, was virtually 100 percent effective.

The combined oral contraceptives (estrogen plus progestin) have been in use for approximately two decades and the mini-pill (progestin alone) for more than ten years. These agents have been more widely studied than any medication in the history of mankind. At the present time it is estimated that 54 million women are using the pill, 10 million of them living in the United States. In addition, there are another 50 million women who have used an oral contraceptive at some time in the past.

The combined estrogen and progestin pills (those with dosages of 50 micrograms and above) prevent pregnancy by stopping ovulation, the monthly release of an egg by an ovary. Their use as a contraceptive method is based on the fact that during pregnancy these hormones, made by the ovaries and placenta, block the production of the hormones which are responsible for ovulation, thus preventing the establishment of an additional pregnancy. In the case of the mini-pill (progestin alone) and the low estrogen combined pills, the mechanism is somewhat more complicated. Studies have shown that not all women who use these pills stop ovulating. The mechanism (or mechanisms) of action in this instance appears to be the effects of the hormone on the cervical mucus, the lining of the uterus, and the cervix, along with certain other anatomical changes. These changes probably all combine together to block the migration of the sperm or perhaps the implantation of the fertilized ovum. While similar effects occur with the higher dose combined pills, their effectiveness is achieved mainly by the blocking of ovulation.

Major Severe Side Effects

Not long after widespread use of the pill began, it became clear that certain complications were occurring in a small number of women. Considerable unhappiness has been voiced over the years about the fact that these side effects were not recognized earlier. However, it must always be remembered that with any drug when complications are rare, say once in every quarter- to half-million users as in the case of the pill, thousands of women must be carefully followed for a number of years in order to detect those complications.

In addition, because of the complexities of civilization today, it is very difficult to be able to relate any particular adverse reaction to a particular medication. To link a given side effect with a specific drug—given the number of drugs in common use, the various food additives, and all of the other pollutants in our environment—takes wide usage of that drug over a considerable period of time.

CARDIOVASCULAR

The first side effects noted (and the ones which are still the most serious) are related to the cardiovascular system. It was shown a number of years ago in both British and American studies that oral contraceptives increase the risk of forming blood clots (thromboembolism) which may break off and go to the lung or brain. The original estimate of the increase in risk was felt to be 3 per 100,000 women per year. Somewhat later it was found that there is also an increased risk of stroke associated with the use of oral contraceptives. However, more recent studies with lower dose pills show that the risk today is considerably less.

Originally it appeared that the chances of developing either of these complications were in the range of four- to tenfold greater in users than in nonusers. However, many of these calculations were made when the dosage of the pill was considerably higher; as the amounts of hormones in the pill have continued to drop, the estimates of risk have been somewhat lower. Whereas the amount of estrogen in the original combined pill was 100 micrograms, today we are using pills with 50 or 35 micrograms or even less.

More recently it has been found that the danger of heart attack is also increased by the use of oral contraceptives. This complication is rare before the age of 30; prior to that age there is virtually no difference in the rate of heart attack between users and nonusers of the pill. It is essential to note that the risk of heart attack associated with the use of oral contraceptives is considerably greater in those women over 30 who smoke, particularly those who smoke heavily.

Women who have major surgery, particularly abdominal surgery, also have a four- to sixfold increase in thromboembolic complications. Pills should be stopped at least four weeks prior to major elective surgery and another contraceptive prescribed. The alternative contraceptive should be continued after surgery for about another month. The same rule holds true for women who are immobilized, for instance, because of serious fractures, for a long period of time. Thus it can be seen that women who take the oral contraceptives run a small, but real risk of vascular complications.

The annual death rate from cardiovascular conditions in pill takers is currently estimated at 25.8 per 100,000 women as compared to 5.5 per 100,000 in non-pill takers. This rate, however, is only a general figure. The risks are greater for older women, especially smokers. Women between the ages of 35 and 44 have an annual death rate of 42.6 per 100,000 woman-years as compared with 9.0 under 35. Smokers have an annual death rate of 39.5 per 100,000 women as compared to 14.0 in nonsmokers. Moreover, older age and smoking taken together have a much higher risk than simply adding the two risks would imply—a fact which suggests that pills not be used at all under such circumstances.

METABOLIC

A number of metabolic changes occur in women taking the oral contraceptives, related primarily to the sugar and fat metabolism of the body. Blood sugar levels are elevated as are a number of blood lipids (fats).

A very few women have a profound elevation in their blood pressure when they first start taking the oral contraceptives. This hypertension disappears promptly when the pill is stopped. A certain number of other women develop a mild increase of blood pressure as they continue to take the oral contraceptives. However, their blood pressures usually remain within normal limits and usually return to pretreatment levels upon stopping the pill.

It has been shown that certain of the liver function tests change during pill use, reverting quickly to normal after discontinuing its use. There is also a rare benign liver tumor which is apparently associated with the use of the oral contraceptives. It regresses after the pill is stopped, but because these tumors are vascular, bleeding has occasionally occurred, necessitating emergency abdominal surgery.

In addition, it has been noted, after several years of use, that there is a slightly increased incidence of gallstones in women on the oral contraceptives. There is still some question as to whether these women would have developed gallstones in any event, but perhaps the pill, because of its effect on the liver, precipitated their formation.

FETAL

There have been many studies to determine whether oral contraceptives taken early in pregnancy have any effect on an unborn baby. Early in the study of the oral contraceptives, when higher dose pills were being used, it was noted that a certain type of chromosomal abnormality occurred which caused miscarriage. However, as lower dose pills began to be used, this problem virtually disappeared. The discovery of the serious effects on a small percentage of daughters of mothers who took large doses of the estrogen diethylstilbestrol (DES) during pregnancy (discussed below) raised many questions and considerable anxiety about possible, unknown fetal effects of regular doses of any form of estrogen.

High-dose oral contraceptives have also been used as tests for pregnancy, but this is no longer an acceptable medical practice. First of all, they are not particularly reliable tests, and secondly, there is an outside chance that the fetus might be damaged by the exposure to the hormones. Because of uncertainties in this area, women should not use oral contraceptives when there is any question that they might be pregnant.

MALIGNANCY

One of the major reasons given by women today for either not starting or for stopping the pill is the fear of cancer. Thousands of unplanned and unwanted pregnancies have occurred because of this fear, when women panicked and stopped using the pill, but did not substitute any other method. Whereas a cause-and-effect relationship between cardiovascular complications and oral contraceptives has been established, there are still no data to suggest that any such relationship exists between oral contraceptives and cancer of any part of the female reproductive tract or elsewhere.

Actually, there is evidence to suggest that quite the opposite may be true. British and American studies have both shown that there is a lower incidence of benign breast and ovarian tumors and possibly malignant ovarian tumors in women taking the pill. Moreover the combined pill may well exert a protective effect against endometrial cancer which can be caused by preparations that contain only estrogen. The progestin in the combined pill provides the protective effect.

Despite tremendous amounts of adverse publicity resulting in great anxiety, there is no proof today that oral contraceptives cause cancer. However, since we know that it takes a considerable period of time for cancer to develop, careful observation of women taking oral contraceptives is being continued.

Contraindications

At the present time the U.S. Food and Drug Administration lists a number of absolute contraindications to the use of the pill. The list is based on proven major adverse side effects, as in the case of the cardiovascular disorders, and on conditions for which a relationship is suspected, but not necessarily proven.

1. Known cardiovascular conditions or a past history of these conditions, including thrombophlebitis and thromboembolic disorders (formation of blood clots and embolisms), cerebrovascular disease (stroke), myocardial infarction (type of heart attack), or coronary artery disease.
2. Markedly impaired liver function.
3. Known or suspected carcinoma of the breast.
4. Known or suspected estrogen-dependent neoplasia (abnormal tissue growth).
5. Undiagnosed abnormal genital bleeding.
6. Known or suspected pregnancy.

Smoking, although not currently listed by the FDA, should be considered a relative contraindication. As we have mentioned, more and more evidence is being accumulated showing that the combination of increasing age and heavy smoking raises the risks of heart attack and stroke considerably higher than either age or smoking alone. In fact, current data indicate that the two factors have a synergistic effect, that is, one in the presence of the other increases the risk that each could produce separately, that their combined effect is greater than the sum of their effects simply added together.

Therefore, women of any age, but particularly those over 30 and those with additional risk factors, should be encouraged not to take the pill if they smoke or not to smoke if they take the pill. Obviously, as a general health measure, women should be encouraged not to smoke whether they take the pill or not. Indeed it has been suggested, not entirely facetiously, that, given the differences in relative risks, pills should be put in vending machines and cigarettes placed on prescription!

Minor Adverse Side Effects

There are a number of side effects which are annoying, but not serious or life-threatening. Among the most frequent of these are alterations in the menstrual flow. Most often the change is a decrease (a change considered to be desirable by many women). There may also be irregular spotting and bleeding between periods, heavier bleeding at the time of the menses, and on occasion a total absence of menses. Breast tenderness may be observed, and there is often an increase in the amount of vaginal discharge. Weight gain is noted by some women, but this is much more apt to be related to changes in dietary intake than to the pill. Pigmentation over the forehead and cheeks, the same type seen in pregnancy, may also occur with use of the oral contraceptives.

Beneficial Side Effects

Too often only the bad side effects of the pill are presented in all forms of media. The beneficial side effects of the pill are only rarely discussed in the same context.

A number of salutary changes have been noted, such as the decreases in breast and ovarian tumors. In addition, women whose cycles are extremely irregular or who have heavy menstrual bleeding resulting in anemia may be virtually assured that these problems will be solved by the use of the oral contraceptives. Premenstrual symptoms and menstrual discomfort are also often relieved, and acne often improves markedly. One fascinating side effect which was noted in a British study is a 25 percent decrease in ear wax, although it is unclear what major advantage this may have for women.

Injectables

For a number of years researchers have sought a long-acting hormonal preparation which could be given by injection to block ovulation. Such a method would have its greatest application in certain areas of the world where medication is not felt to be significant or helpful unless it is given by injection, but it would also benefit any women who, because of medical, social, or psychological reasons, cannot cope with the demands of pill-taking or the use of barrier methods. Moreover, when health care personnel and facilities are limited, a technique which requires a single act of motivation on the part of the patient and infrequent professional follow-up is obviously highly desirable.

At present there is no injectable contraceptive available in the United States. A number of hormones, given once every one to six or more months, have been evaluated. One progestin preparation, Depo-Provera, has been extensively studied for more than 10 years and is currently being marketed and widely used in almost 70 other countries. Side effects of Depo-Provera include irregular bleeding, temporary stopping of menses, and in some instances a slower return to fertility. Because of concern about these effects, about laboratory tests in which beagle dogs given the drug in large doses developed breast tumors, and about the possible development of cancer of the cervix in women (which was subsequently disproved), Depo-Provera has been disapproved by the FDA for marketing in this country for purely contraceptive purposes.

"Morning After" Pill

Considerable research has been directed toward finding a substance, a so-called "morning after" pill, which will prevent pregnancy after unprotected sexual relations at the time of ovulation. It was shown many years ago in monkeys and then in the human female that the use of sufficient doses of any estrogen at this time will prevent implantation.

The major work in this area has been done using diethylstilbestrol (DES). This drug is not used in any of the oral contraceptives. At the present time DES is the only drug approved by the FDA as a morning after pill—and then only in emergency situations including rape. However, to date there is no evidence of a relationship between malignancy and DES used as a morning after pill. Research is now being undertaken to see if other estrogens will produce the same beneficial effects without producing adverse side effects.

HORMONAL METHODS—MALE

Pressure to develop male contraceptive methods has increased in recent years, particularly by activist women's groups, but even an ideal male contraceptive would in no way replace female contraception. Many women feel that men should share in the responsibility for preventing unwanted pregnancy, but at the same time they would not be willing to surrender their own fertility control to their sexual partner, even in a monogamous situation. It is even more unlikely that women with multiple sex partners would want to depend entirely on the males to use contraceptives to protect them against pregnancy. Thus, although male methods would not supplant all female methods, they would certainly be an excellent addition to the total contraceptive cafeteria.

Male methods have been studied for many years. It has been found much more difficult to completely block male fertility than female. There is a growing body of evidence, based on some recent studies, that a man may produce a pregnancy even though his sperm count is very low.

A number of hormonal preparations have been tested as male contraceptives. Some of the earlier studies were done with estrogens. While these agents effectively depressed the development of sperm in the male, they were quickly abandoned when it was found that they also produced a number of unfortunate side effects such as breast enlargement, impotence, and the lack of desire for sex.

Research is now being done combining estrogens with progestins or male hormones. These agents are either taken by mouth or given by injection. Thus far it appears that these newer techniques may be successful in reducing the sperm count to zero, while allowing the continuation of normal sexual desire and performance. It seems quite possible that sometime in the next few years, after sufficient data have been collected, these agents will be approved for use by the male.

INTRAUTERINE CONTRACEPTIVES

The second major form of female contraception, introduced more recently than the pill, is the intrauterine device (IUD). We know from history that the first intrauterine device was a pebble placed in the uterus of a camel to keep her from getting pregnant on long trips across the desert. Metal devices have also been used by women in the past. However, because of concerns about infection, their use flourished briefly and then disappeared.

In the last decade or so this form of family planning has once again become very popular. Today there are roughly 3 to 4 million American women using IUDs and 10 to 15 million women using them worldwide. These figures include the older plastic devices as well as the newer medicated IUDs. When IUDs are compared with oral contraceptives, the data currently available show that IUDs cause fewer deaths, but more illness. The current mortality rate for IUD wearers is 3 to 5 deaths per million women annually, mainly due to infection. With regard to overall effectiveness, the IUD has never quite equaled the pill, the general range of effectiveness for most IUDs being somewhere between 96 and 98 percent.

For a while it was felt that intrauterine devices prevented pregnancy either by speeding the egg through the tube so quickly that it could not be fertilized or by producing a mild and otherwise insignificant uterine infection that prevented implantation. Continued study has shown that neither of these mechanisms is the one that prevents pregnancy. It is now believed that the presence of the intrauterine device induces some histochemical change in the endometrium (lining of the uterus) which makes it hostile to the sperm going up and, more importantly, hostile to the blastocyst (developing embryo) coming down. In the case of the medicated devices, there is also a direct action of the metal or the hormone in the device which makes it extremely unlikely for implantation to occur.

Intrauterine devices are inserted through the cervix into the uterus using special instruments. All IUDs inserted today have a string which protrudes through the cervical os. These strings are used for identification and removal of the devices. Following insertion, it is quite common to have cramping and spotting, but this usually disappears over a few hours or days. IUDs may be inserted at any time, but it is easier to do so during a menstrual period because the cervix is dilated slightly. Also there is no chance of the woman's being pregnant. It has been shown that IUDs may be inserted immediately following early abortion without increasing the risk of side effects. IUDs inserted immediately after delivery have had high expulsion rates, and there is also an increased risk of perforation of the uterus at that time. Therefore, it is usually advised that the insertion be postponed six to eight weeks after delivery. Newer devices, which look quite promising, are being studied for this particular use.

Currently Marketed IUDs

The first of the widely used intrauterine devices was the Lippes loop; this was followed by the Saf-T Coil. Both of these IUDs are made out of plastic. The loop comes in four sizes and the coil in two in order to fit properly in uteri of varying size. During the studies carried out with these and a number of other devices, certain generalizations were formulated. First, devices which were larger were more effective in preventing pregnancy and were not readily expelled, but they had higher rates of cramping

INTRAUTERINE CONTRACEPTIVE DEVICES

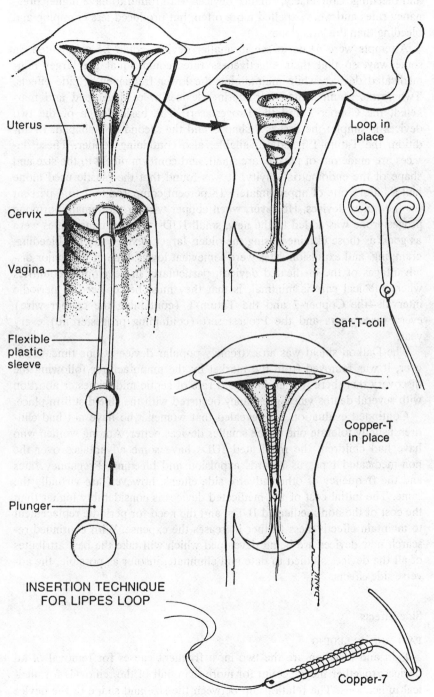

Uterus

Cervix

Vagina

Flexible plastic sleeve

Plunger

INSERTION TECHNIQUE FOR LIPPES LOOP

Loop in place

Saf-T-coil

Copper-T in place

Copper-7

and bleeding. Conversely, smaller devices were found to have higher pregnancy rates and were expelled more often, but produced less cramping and bleeding than the larger ones.

Attempts were made to see if smaller devices could be augmented, in some way, so that their effectiveness rates could equal the larger non-medicated devices while maintaining the lower frequency of side effects. Two forms of medicated intrauterine devices were developed and marketed, the Copper-7 and the Progestasert. The basic design of the two devices is simple; the first is 7-shaped and the second is T-shaped. In addition, the Tatum-T is now available, also containing copper. These devices are made out of plastic, are small, and conform nicely to the size and shape of the endometrial cavity. It was found that the plastic used alone had a failure rate of approximately 18 percent compared to 2 to 4 percent for the larger devices. However, when copper wire or the female hormone progesterone was added to the new, small IUDs, the pregnancy rates were as good as those obtained using the older, larger devices and the bleeding, cramping, and expulsion rates were somewhat lower. One of the major disadvantages of the medicated devices, particularly in developing countries where medical care is minimal, is that they must be replaced at periodic intervals—the Copper-7 and the Tatum-T (containing the copper wire) every three years and the Progestasert (containing progesterone) every year.

The Dalkon shield was an extremely popular device at one time. However, it was removed from the market by the manufacturer following the discovery that there was an increased rate of septic mid-trimester abortion with several deaths when pregnancy occurred with the shield still in place.

Continued evaluation has revealed that women who have not had children usually tolerate one of the smaller devices better. Among women who have had children, the medicated IUDs have some advantages over the non-medicated types as regards expulsion and bleeding. Pregnancy rates and the frequency of other adverse side effects, however, are virtually the same. The initial cost of the medicated devices is considerably higher than the cost of the non-medicated IUDs, and the need for periodic replacement to maintain effectiveness further increases the expense. With continued research new devices are being developed which will take the best attributes of all the devices studied to date and eliminate, insofar as possible, the adverse side effects.

Side Effects

PAIN AND BLEEDING

Pain and bleeding are the two most frequent causes for removal of all devices; together they account for more than half of the removals for medical indications. The relationship between the size and shape of the device and the dimensions of the uterine cavity are extremely critical. This is one reason that the newer, smaller IUDs have somewhat lower rates of pain and bleeding, especially in women who have never been pregnant. The larger, older devices are better tolerated by women who have had children.

However, it is interesting that when one looks at both national and international data on IUDs, one finds that factors other than medical indications create a tremendous variation in the removal rate of the same device. Primary among these is the motivation of the patient. Women who have had a larger number of children usually are better motivated and tolerate side effects better than those with fewer children. Also, the attitude toward and degree of acceptance of side effects depends greatly upon social and cultural attitudes toward bleeding. Finally, the attitude of those giving medical care to women, how supportive they are, and their insertion skill make a major difference in removal rates.

It has been shown that the older plastic devices produce the largest amount of blood loss and the copper devices somewhat less. With the progesterone-bearing devices, because of the effect of the hormone on the lining of the uterus, there is actually less blood loss than with a woman's normal period.

PREGNANCY

If an IUD fails to prevent conception, there may be undesirable side effects during the pregnancy that results. It has been found that intrauterine devices protect quite well against intrauterine pregnancy (99.5 percent), less well against ectopic, or tubal, pregnancy (95 percent), virtually not at all against that rare form of gestation, pregnancy occurring in the ovary. Because of this varying degree of protection against different forms of pregnancy, it is important to consider that a woman with an IUD who does become pregnant may have an ectopic pregnancy. There is some new evidence that the presence of an IUD in a uterus may actually slightly increase the risk of ectopic pregnancy, not just reduce the probability of uterine pregnancy. Because ectopic pregnancy is possible, although the incidence is extremely low, any woman who has not yet completed her family should discuss this issue carefully with her physician when she is choosing a form of family planning. Women who have had a prior ectopic pregnancy and want more children would probably be well advised not to use this form of contraception.

If a woman does become pregnant in her uterus with her IUD still in place, it is extremely important to remove the IUD as quickly as possible. It was originally felt that removal of an IUD would almost inevitably precipitate an abortion. We now know that quite the opposite is true—the rate of spontaneous abortion drops from 50 percent if it is not removed to 25 percent if the IUD is removed early in pregnancy.

One of the more serious hazards of pregnancy with an IUD in place is the development of severe, overwhelming, and occasionally fatal infection in the mid-trimester. Women with this type of infection often become sick very quickly, and deaths have been reported within two to three days of the onset of remarkably mild symptoms. Prompt removal of the device in a woman who wishes to carry her pregnancy to term will not only decrease her chance of early spontaneous abortion and the risk of mid-trimester infection, but it will also decrease the likelihood that she will have a premature delivery.

In most cases the IUD is easily removed by pulling on the string. However, if the IUD cannot be removed by the string, the only other way to remove it is by an abortion procedure. In view of the risks of leaving the IUD in place, careful consideration must be given as to whether or not to continue the pregnancy. It may be advisable to remove the IUD and terminate the pregnancy at the same time.

PERFORATION

One of the complications which may result from the use of the intrauterine device is perforation of the uterus. This is an unusual complication, occurring in less than 1 percent of cases. It usually happens during the insertion of the device. However, there are instances in which, at some time after insertion, part or all of the device has apparently been pushed by the contractions of the uterus out through the uterine wall, or part of it has perforated through the cervix into the vagina. In many instances this occurs without any symptoms.

If a plastic device has perforated the uterus and entered the abdominal cavity, there is a general feeling now that it should be removed, although this still remains a somewhat optional procedure. However, if a copper device is found to be free in the abdominal cavity, it is important that it be removed as soon as it is medically feasible, since the copper ions coming from the device cause an intense reaction inside the abdomen. Its continued presence may produce dense adhesions and may cause serious infection.

Any device that has a closed configuration must also be removed immediately, since it has been shown that a loop of bowel may become trapped in the closed part of the device, causing intestinal obstruction which is a surgical emergency.

EXPULSION

All devices developed to date have been expelled from the uterus. The percentage varies from 1 to 20 percent, with the older, non-medicated devices being expelled somewhat more often than the newer, medicated IUDs. If a woman can no longer feel the string and if she is not aware of the device having been expelled, it must be determined where the device is. If it has been expelled, she is unprotected against pregnancy. If it has not, but is no longer in place, the possibility of perforation or partial expulsion must be considered. Before attempting to locate the position of the device, it is important first to find out if the woman is pregnant. If she is not pregnant, then ultrasonography and X-rays may be used to determine the presence or absence of the device and its precise location. If she is pregnant, careful thought must be given about how to proceed, as described above.

INFECTION

For years it was felt that most of the infections which occurred with the use of intrauterine devices were gonorrheal in origin and would have occurred whether or not the patient had an IUD. Critics of the IUD stated that the device increased the likelihood of spreading gonorrhea because people were no longer using barrier methods such as spermicides and condoms, which helped to prevent the spread of sexually transmitted diseases.

It now appears that there is indeed an increase in the risk of infection in IUD wearers, but not all of it is due to gonorrhea. The incidence of infection is quite low overall. However, the woman who has not completed her desired family size should give careful consideration to the fact that infection may affect, temporarily or occasionally permanently, her future fertility.

Pelvic infection may involve one or more organs, starting with the uterus, going to the tubes and ovaries, and spreading out into the pelvic cavity and abdomen. The symptoms from these infections vary from none at all in the case of extremely mild infections to severe, sometimes fatal disease with high fever, chills, abdominal pain, and bloody and foul-smelling vaginal discharge.

When the infection is mild, it is frequently diagnosed only by finding a small tender mass involving the tube or ovary on routine examination. A mild infection may in some cases also produce a vaginal discharge. A culture is taken to attempt to learn which organism is responsible for the infection, and antibiotic therapy is begun. If considerable improvement has not occurred within 24 hours or if the infection is initially very severe, the IUD must be removed. The women who are most frequently at risk from these infections are those who have more than one sexual partner, which increases the likelihood of their acquiring a sexually transmitted disease.

MALIGNANCY

Considerable concern has been expressed, as in the case of the oral contraceptive, about whether or not the continued presence of an intrauterine device could stimulate malignancy. Once again, careful prolonged study of thousands of women has failed to show a connection between the presence of an intrauterine device and the subsequent development of a malignancy of the cervix or the uterus.

Contraindications

At the present time the FDA lists the following contraindications to the use of the IUD.

1. Known or suspected pregnancy.
2. Acute, chronic, or recurring pelvic inflammatory disease.
3. Acute cervicitis.
4. Postpartum endometritis and infected abortion.
5. Abnormal genital bleeding.
6. Gynecologic malignancy.
7. Anomalies of the uterus which grossly distort the uterine cavity.
8. Submucosal or intramural leiomyomata (tumors beneath or within the wall of the uterus) that grossly distort the uterine cavity.
9. Known or suspected allergy to copper (for copper IUDs only).

BARRIER CONTRACEPTIVES

Barrier forms of contraception—the condom, the diaphragm, and spermicides—were for many years the only relatively effective techniques available. Their use decreased considerably when the oral contraceptives and the intrauterine devices were introduced. Barrier methods have long been criticized by both users and the medical profession. Terms such as "greasy kid stuff" have been applied to the various vaginal preparations. Men have been disenchanted with the use of the condom because of its interruption of and interference with sexual response.

This negative view is, however, undergoing considerable change. Now, because of concern over the side effects of the newer methods, people are once again turning to the barrier forms, an intense search is under way for better barrier methods, and the entire field has once again become a subject of great interest. Studies have shown that various spermicides (foams, jellies, creams, suppositories, foaming tablets) and diaphragms, when used properly and consistently with each act of sexual intercourse, actually have a far higher rate of effectiveness than thought by the general public and, in fact, by many physicians. The key to this, of course, is absolute adherence to proper and consistent usage. Each barrier method has its own special instructions for use on the package which must be followed carefully if these levels of effectiveness are to be attained.

In addition to being highly effective forms of contraception, when used properly, the various barrier methods have been shown to have an added advantage in that they lower sexually transmitted disease rates. The physical barrier blocks the transmission of infecting organisms, and the

BARRIER CONTRACEPTIVES

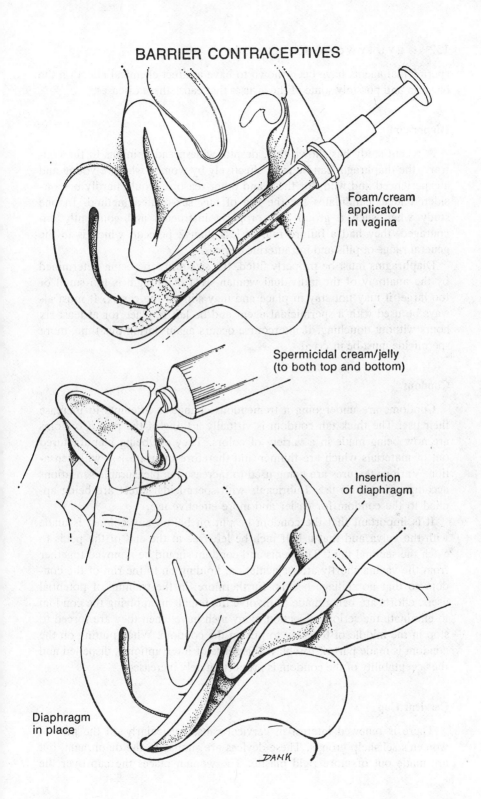

Foam/cream applicator in vagina

Spermicidal cream/jelly (to both top and bottom)

Insertion of diaphragm

Diaphragm in place

DANK

spermicidal agents have been shown to have a direct chemical effect on the bacteria and possibly some of the viruses that cause these diseases.

Diaphragm

A recent study has shown that, despite widespread opinions to the contrary, the diaphragm can be used effectively by women who are young and inexperienced and who, for these and other reasons, would hardly be considered ideal candidates for the use of any sex-related method. In one study when such a group was properly instructed and constantly encouraged, they had a failure rate of less than 2 percent, which is in the general range of pills and intrauterine devices.

Diaphragms must be properly fitted, the size and type being determined by the anatomy of the individual woman. If a diaphragm is too small or too large, it may not stay in place and may slip off the cervix. It must always be used with a spermicidal agent and be left in place for at least six hours without douching. If intercourse occurs again during this time, more spermicide must be inserted.

Condom

Condoms are undergoing a tremendous change in attempts to increase their use. The thick tan condom is virtually a thing of the past. Condoms are now being made in a variety of colors. They are being manufactured out of materials which are thinner and therefore interfere less with sensation. Various textures are being used to increase the pleasurable sensations accompanying their use. Lubricants with spermicidal effect are being applied to the condom for easier and more effective use.

It is important that the condom be put on before any contact is made with the vulva and that a half inch be left free at the end of the penis to catch the seminal fluid. The penis and condom should be removed together from the vagina shortly after ejaculation, holding on to the rim of the condom so that no spillage occurs. Furthermore, in the training of potential users, efforts are being made to involve the female in applying the condom to eliminate the serious objection many men have when they are forced to stop in the middle of foreplay to put on the condom. When putting on the condom is made part of foreplay, this sense of interruption is dispelled and the acceptability of the condom is proportionately increased.

Cervical Cap

There is renewed interest in cervical caps, particularly on the part of women's self-help groups. These devices are similar to the diaphragm, but are made out of more rigid plastic. The woman places the cap over the cervix, and it remains in place because of suction. She should remove it for cleaning regularly and during menstruation.

At the present time cervical caps are not being made in this country, their use having stopped when the more convenient pill and IUD became available. However, it is possible that if this interest continues, further research could result in the development of more practical and acceptable cervical caps.

Methods in Combination

Combining two barrier agents considerably decreases their overall failure rates. It is now being increasingly appreciated that the combination of a male and a female method, for example, condom plus spermicide, has a very high rate of effectiveness with a failure rate of approximately 1 percent. The lack of any serious side effects of the various barrier methods makes them extremely attractive for those individuals who have sexual relations very infrequently, who have contraindications to the pill and the IUD, and who are looking for maximum safety in the use of a form of contraception.

It has been repeatedly shown that the safest method of family planning today is the use of one or preferably two (male and female) barrier methods backed up by early suction abortion, since both of these techniques have a very low complication rate and virtually no death rate.

Many attempts are currently under way to make the barrier methods more attractive and thereby increase their use. New agents are being tested, and efforts are being made in both packaging and the physical nature of these preparations to make them easier and more pleasant to use.

NATURAL FAMILY PLANNING

New attention is also being paid to methods of "Natural Family Planning," largely because these techniques are the only ones acceptable to the Roman Catholic church. They are all based on the premise that sexual intercourse must be avoided during that period of each menstrual cycle when ovulation is occurring. There are a number of these techniques currently in use.

The first of these methods of natural family planning is calendar rhythm; a woman keeps track of her menstrual periods, attempts to predict the day of ovulation based on her previous cycles, and avoids intercourse for several days before and after the time of presumed ovulation.

Temperature rhythm is a much more effective form of natural family planning and is based on the fact that at the time of or just after ovulation the basal body temperature goes up about ½ a degree. A woman takes her basal (resting) temperature every morning before getting out of bed and does not have intercourse following her menses until her temperature rises, indicating ovulation has occurred and has been sustained for several days.

Both of these techniques suffer from the disadvantage of moderate to severe curtailment of the frequency of sexual relations. Furthermore, if a woman's cycles are grossly irregular, it is extremely difficult to predict the actual time of ovulation and therefore the number of days she must abstain from sexual intercourse is increased proportionately.

Other forms of natural family planning are the symptothermic methods, based on varying combinations of records of the temperature changes which occur at the time of ovulation and observation of signs typical of various stages of the menstrual cycle. For example, the Billings method is a technique in which a woman examines her cervical mucus every day, since at the time of ovulation the mucus is thin and watery, while at all other times in the cycle it is thick and viscous. Sexual intercourse is avoided at the time of the presumed ovulation. These methods also suffer from the problem of difficulty in pinpointing the exact time of ovulation, particularly in women who have irregular cycles, and the fact that there are major blocks of time when sexual relations are forbidden.

These family planning techniques work well (over 90 percent effective), particularly temperature rhythm, if a couple is highly motivated and totally conscientious about following all the rules. However, these techniques generally have not been well accepted around the world because of the necessity to impose artificial regulations on sex life and because of the high pregnancy rates which result when they do not follow all the rules. Furthermore, recent studies have suggested that when failures occur in couples using these methods, there is a higher than average rate of fetal abnormalities in the pregnancies which result and an increased number of male fetuses. It has been suggested that this may be due to the fact that because of the attempt to delay intercourse until well after ovulation, any egg which is fertilized is likely to be old, and thus more apt to produce a male or a defective offspring. Further research must be done to clarify this issue.

COITUS INTERRUPTUS

Coitus interruptus is an ancient method of birth control and one which is still widely used. There are three major problems with its use. First, it requires absolute control on the part of the man, so that he always withdraws from the vagina prior to ejaculation. Second, both men and women have psychological aversions to interrupting love-making at a critical moment. Third, a few sperm may escape prior to ejaculation and cause a pregnancy.

LACTATION

Lactation is also an ancient form of family planning. Many years ago women discovered that the likelihood of their becoming pregnant was considerably less when they were nursing their children. However, it has been found that breast-feeding is only partially effective. Lactation does suppress ovulation to some degree, but the longer one goes from the time of the delivery, the more apt one is to have a return of ovulation. This can occur even before the first postpartum menses. Full lactation (nursing at all feedings with no supplementary food) suppresses ovulation and menses considerably longer than partial lactation.

STERILIZATION

Sterilization of both the male and the female is now the most frequently used method of family planning, both in the United States and around the world. There are a number of reasons for this. There is growing concern, as we have seen, about the side effects of the two most effective forms of family planning—the oral contraceptives and the IUDs. There is still considerable distaste for barrier methods. There is general disenchantment with the natural family planning techniques.

Many couples are now limiting their families to fewer children than in the past. They are tending to have only two children, fairly close together, in their mid to late twenties. This leaves them with perhaps 25 years of having to use some form of contraception, choosing among methods which are neither totally safe nor totally effective. Sterilization of either the male or the female becomes, therefore, a reasonable and practical alternative.

Female Sterilization

Sterilization of women has been made much easier in recent years by the development of new instruments and new techniques. Prior to the last decade or so, sterilization was most often performed after delivery while the woman was still in the hospital. It was also often done immediately under the same anesthetic which was administered for the delivery of the baby. Interval sterilization (between babies) was not done very often since it meant admission to a hospital, a general anesthetic in an operating room, a major operation, a number of days in the hospital, and several weeks of recovery.

A number of techniques are used for female sterilization. The oldest of these is laparotomy, that is, the surgical opening of the abdomen. Once this has been accomplished, the fallopian tubes can be ligated in any number of ways—by tying, cutting or clipping. It makes no difference how it is done provided that a segment of each tube is blocked. The tubes can also be occluded using the vaginal route (colpotomy), and, still experimentally, via the uterine route (hysteroscopy).

With the development of the laparoscope and other more sophisticated forms of equipment, the entire scene changed radically. Procedures may now be done at any time during a woman's reproductive life. Moreover, a steadily larger percentage of these procedures are now being carried out in hospital and free-standing outpatient clinics and often under local rather than general anesthesia. Many patients come in, have their procedures done, and go home the same day or, at most, stay one night in the hospital.

Most recently, the mini-lap procedure has been developed. This method is even simpler than the laparoscopic techniques. A small incision is made near the top of the pubic hair, the tubes are grasped under direct vision and ligated. The entire procedure takes only a few minutes and the patient is able to rest for a few hours and then go home.

There has been considerable discussion in recent years as to whether elective hysterectomy should be carried out purely for sterilization purposes, when no medical indications are present. One school of thought says it should. It cites studies which show that some women having tubal ligations later develop abnormal bleeding or cancer of the uterus. It claims that hysterectomies for sterilization would prevent both. The other school cites data showing no increased abnormal bleeding. It contends that the added risks of major surgery are not justified. The outcome of this debate awaits the results of more and better studies evaluating the situation.

While some of the new techniques are much easier, faster, and less expensive than the older ones, no method has been developed to date which is completely effective and totally safe. The failure rate in most female sterilization procedures is extremely low, being less than 1 percent. However, since the tubes are intra-abdominal organs, even the simplest procedure involves opening the abdomen. This inevitably carries with it some degree of risk, though very small, of complications such as hemorrhage and infection. The chances of repairing the tubes varies directly with the amount of the tube destroyed at the time of surgery.

Male Sterilization

Male sterilization, or vasectomy, is now performed as often as female sterilization. It has always been and remains an extremely simple technique since the vas are in the scrotum. It is simple to identify the vas under local anesthesia and to perform either cauterization or removal of a piece of both of the vas. There are virtually no serious complications, and in this country no deaths have resulted from vasectomy. The infrequent minor

PERMANENT CONTRACEPTIVES

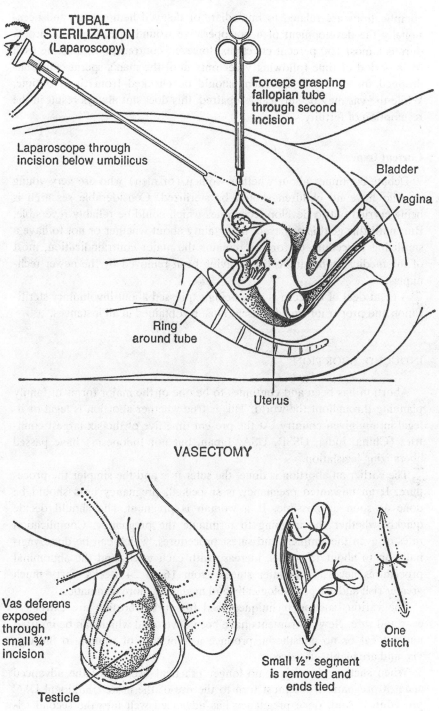

TUBAL STERILIZATION
(Laparoscopy)

Forceps grasping fallopian tube through second incision

Laparoscope through incision below umbilicus

Bladder

Vagina

Ring around tube

Uterus

VASECTOMY

Vas deferens exposed through small ¾" incision

Testicle

Small ½" segment is removed and ends tied

One stitch

complications are related to immediate or delayed hemorrhage and occasionally the development of a postoperative wound infection. The procedure is almost 100 percent effective. However, contraception must be used for a period of time following vasectomy until the man's sperm count has dropped to zero, and the count should be checked from time to time. While the vas may be surgically repaired, this does not always result in the resumption of fertility.

Current Issues

Debate continues about whether women (or men) who are very young or who have no children should be sterilized. Considerable research is being carried out to develop techniques which could be reliably reversible. But, until this goal is achieved, uncertainty about whether or not to have a sterilizing procedure performed remains the major contraindication, most of the medical contraindications having been removed by the newer techniques.

A great deal of concern is now being expressed about involuntary sterilization and proper informed consent must be obtained in all instances.

INDUCED ABORTION

Abortion has been and continues to be one of the major forms of family planning throughout the world. This is true whether abortion is legal or illegal in any given country. At the present time five of the six largest countries (China, India, USSR, USA, Japan, but not Indonesia) have passed liberalizing legislation.

The earlier an abortion is done, the safer it is and the simpler the procedure. If an unwanted pregnancy is suspected, pregnancy tests should be done as soon as possible. If a woman is pregnant, she should decide quickly whether she is going to terminate the pregnancy. Complication rates of even the simplest and safest procedures, which can be done vaginally up to about 15 weeks, increase with each week, and the abdominal procedures necessary at later stages, from 16 to 24 weeks, carry much greater risk and are psychologically and medically more traumatic.

The various suction techniques used for early abortion are extremely easy and safe. New instruments have been developed which can be inserted under local or no anesthesia, produce a minimum of trauma to the cervix, and are highly effective.

When suction abortion is no longer practical because of the advanced state of pregnancy, one must turn to the use of the more traditional D&C procedures. And, once pregnancy has advanced well into the second trimester, an entirely different approach must be used. The uterus may be emptied by the induction of labor, using one or more chemical agents such as prostaglandins, saline, or glucose, or the products of conception can be removed by surgical procedure, a hysterotomy or hysterectomy.

Techniques

MENSTRUAL EXTRACTION

Menstrual extraction is a term applied to abortions usually done within six weeks of the last menstrual period. It is also commonly referred to as menstrual regulation, endometrial aspiration, endometrial extraction, preemptive abortion, and a variety of other terms. The original menstrual regulation was carried out simply to cut down on the length of time a menstrual period took. It removed all of the tissue at one time rather than have it flow out over a period of several days. The same name and the same technique were subsequently applied to the termination of early pregnancy, usually before a positive diagnosis was made. The term has been maintained for several reasons. First, in those areas of the world where abortion is illegal, these procedures are carried out as therapy for the delayed onset of menses. Since pregnancy is not diagnosed, there can be no legal consequences. Secondly, women who find themselves in these situations very often do not wish to know whether they were pregnant or not.

DILATATION AND EVACUATION (D&E)

As more experience has been gained in doing early abortions, dilatation and evacuation (suction abortion, suction curettage, vacuum curettage) has come to be used for the majority of the first trimester procedures. More recently, it has been found possible to terminate pregnancy in this way up to fourteen weeks. The instrument most frequently used is a suction curette (vacurette) made out of a soft material, inserted into the uterine cavity after dilatation of the cervix. This reduces the possibility of perforation of the uterus. The procedure is usually done under local anesthesia, the woman being given a tranquilizer or a short-acting intravenous barbiturate.

The advantages of these procedures are that they are relatively easy to do, the complication rates are very low, the amount of blood lost is minimal, and the effectiveness in totally removing the pregnancy is very high. The procedures can usually be done in less than one minute in early pregnancies, but require somewhat more time when the pregnancies are more advanced.

Patients recover rapidly from these procedures; they usually return to their home within a matter of hours and resume their normal activities almost immediately. Complications are rare. They include perforation of the

DILATATION AND EVACUATION
(SUCTION ABORTION)

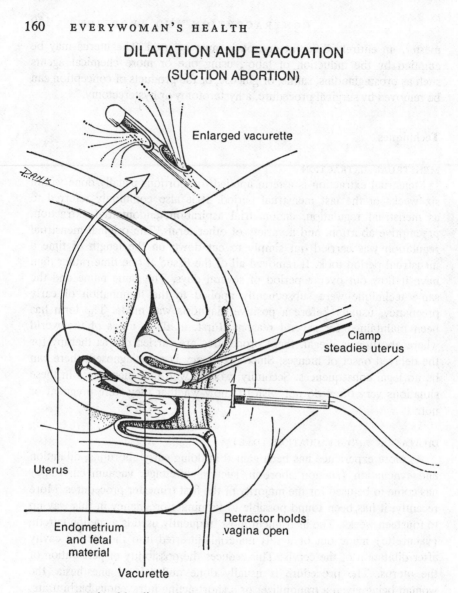

Enlarged vacurette

P.ANK

Clamp
steadies uterus

Uterus

Endometrium
and fetal
material

Retractor holds
vagina open

Vacurette

uterus, excessive bleeding, postoperative infection, and on occasion not all
of the tissue is removed, thus requiring a repeat procedure.

DILATATION AND CURETTAGE (D&C)

This procedure has been carried out for the diagnosis and treatment of
uterine conditions for many years and is also used for first trimester abortions. In most instances, it is carried out under general anesthesia. However, dilatation and curettage can also be done using paracervical block,
backed up with tranquilizers, sedatives, and other drugs.

Before doing the curettage, it is necessary to dilate the cervix in order to introduce the curette. This may be done by progressively enlarging the size of the endocervical canal using metal dilators. It may also be done by inserting laminaria (a form of seaweed) and leaving it for several hours, usually overnight. This technique allows for the gradual dilatation of the cervix. Studies are currently under way to see whether this gradual dilatation may produce less long-term damage such as premature delivery and spontaneous abortion than the more rapid dilatation with metal dilators.

Once the cervix has been dilated, a surgical curette, usually made of metal, is introduced into the uterus through the cervical canal. The entire surface of the uterine cavity is then scraped with the curette, removing all the fetal and placental tissues.

In this procedure, the complications are also rare. They include perforation of the uterus, excessive bleeding, and the development of postoperative infection.

INTRA-AMNIOTIC INFUSION

Abortion can also be induced by the introduction of various fluids into the amniotic sac. Preparations that have been used are hypertonic saline, hypertonic glucose, urea, and prostaglandins. These techniques are indicated when the pregnancy has advanced beyond the fourteenth week of pregnancy. The skin is sterilized, a local anesthetic is injected, a needle is put through the abdominal wall into the amniotic cavity, amniotic fluid is withdrawn, and then the solution is introduced into the cavity. Contractions generally begin twelve to twenty-four hours later and the patient then proceeds to deliver the dead fetus and the placenta.

There are a number of complications which have been noticed with these techniques. With the use of saline, patients may develop abdominal pain, vomiting, hypertension, and a rapid heart rate. In rare instances they may develop problems with blood clotting. Patients receiving prostaglandins often have the side effects of lowering of blood pressure, nausea and vomiting, and diarrhea. Inasmuch as these are surgical procedures, there is always the risk of hemorrhage. Incomplete evacuation of the uterus, delayed hemorrhage, and infection may also occur although they are not frequently encountered.

HYSTEROTOMY AND HYSTERECTOMY

Hysterotomy (the surgical opening of the uterus) is also employed as a form of abortion, but only in late pregnancy. The abdomen and the wall of the uterus are opened surgically, and the fetus and the placenta are removed. The uterine wall is sewed back together. On rare occasions the uterus and the fetus may be removed by hysterectomy, usually because of some uterine abnormality.

These two surgical techniques are much more complicated and therefore have a higher rate of complications than the simpler techniques described earlier.

Counseling

Effective counseling is one of the most important aspects of abortion services, and any facility that does not provide it must be viewed as inadequate. A counselor can explain and answer questions about the procedure to reduce fears and clear up any misunderstanding about what is about to happen. It is almost inevitable that the woman will have some feelings of guilt and anxiety; the counselor can give support for the decision to have the abortion and give the woman a chance to express these feelings. Given current knowledge about contraception and its wide availability, the question of why the pregnancy occurred can be explored. Perhaps the woman simply did not know enough about contraceptive methods, a situation which the counselor can remedy easily. Bringing out into the open more complex reasons for having an unwanted pregnancy—social factors, personal relationships, or even just lack of forethought—may not eliminate the reasons, but awareness of them may help her to avoid another unwanted pregnancy.

Whatever the reasons, a discussion of future contraception is essential, even though the abortion procedure is safe and most women overcome the psychological trauma associated with it.

Newer data now becoming available suggest, although the conclusions are still controversial, that women who have more than one abortion, regardless of the type of procedure that was performed, may in the future have higher rates of spontaneous abortion, fetal death in utero, and premature delivery than women who have had one abortion or none. Even if there is only a possibility that this medical conclusion is true, it is important to counsel women to use contraception to prevent future abortions.

AVAILABILITY AND FURTHER DEVELOPMENT
OF EFFECTIVE CONTRACEPTION

Despite the many developments in all forms of birth control and sterilization and abortion procedures, the benefits of these advances are not uniformly available. There is a tremendous variation, particularly in the availability of sterilization and abortion, from one section of this country to another and from one area of the world to another. Society has placed varying degrees of emphasis on the importance of these techniques. In some areas their use has been facilitated, even encouraged, in others such services have been totally discouraged, and in still others they are impossible to obtain without breaking the law.

The problem arises from many areas—religious and ethical objections to some or all forms of fertility regulation, inadequate health care personnel and programs, lack of economic support for these services for people who cannot otherwise afford them, and the influence of political pressures on decision-makers. The complex social and political factors obscure a direct analysis of the medical and economic benefits for the woman, her partner, and her family. From a purely economic point of view, it is clear that effective contraception has every advantage over unwanted pregnancy. This is equally true of the health implications. When one views the medical problems wrought by large numbers of unwanted pregnancies in terms of illegal abortion, the increased infant and maternal illness and death, the increase in psychological problems (in both parents and children) there are compelling reasons for making contraceptives freely available to all those who need and wish to use them.

Looking at today's research, it is fairly clear that there will be no major breakthroughs in contraceptive technology within the next few years. This is not to say that our techniques will not change during that time. There is every reason to believe that there will be improvements in all of the methods we are currently using. The hormonal contraceptives for both males and females will probably be improved; there may well be an approved injectable agent for women and possibly for men. More acceptable and effective barrier methods should become available. Abortion techniques will also undergo considerable improvement.

More radical changes, if not possible within the next few years, can at least be foreseen. Considerable work is being done on reversible sterilization, a procedure by which fertility could be blocked and then restored. New ways of administering hormones, by vaginal rings and subcutaneous implants, seem entirely possible.

Dramatically different forms of family planning are many years in the future. For example, the immunologic techniques (making people allergic to some portion of the reproductive system) for both men and women are currently being studied. These are complicated methods with tremendous potential for effectiveness but also for the production of complex side effects. Therefore, it is unlikely that any of these will become available for widespread use any time in the next decade.

We have seen the development of the safest and most effective fertility regulation methods the world has ever known, but we still do not have a perfect method. It is therefore essential that we use the methods currently at our disposal in the best possible manner to protect against unplanned and unwanted pregnancy, always keeping in mind the risk-benefit ratio. If this is done, the payoff, both to individuals and to society, is probably one of the highest ever to be offered to mankind.

FURTHER READING

Boston Women's Health Book Collective. *Our Bodies, Ourselves.* New York: Simon & Schuster, 1971.

Demarest, R. J., and J. J. Sciarra. *Conception, Birth and Contraception.* New York: McGraw-Hill, 1976.

Garcia, C. R., and D. L. Rosenfeld. *Human Fertility: The Regulation of Reproduction.* Philadelphia: Davis, 1977.

Jorgenson, V. "The Gynecologist and the Sexually Liberated Woman." *Amer. J. Obstet. & Gynec.* 42 (1973): 607.

Rugh, R., and L. B. Shettles. *From Conception to Birth: The Drama of Life's Beginnings.* New York: Harper & Row, 1971.

Pregnancy and Childbirth

KATHRYN SCHROTENBOER, M.D.

Assistant Attending Physician, Obstetrics and Gynecology,
New York Hospital–Cornell Medical Center
Clinical Instructor, Cornell Medical School

As an obstetrician-gynecologist I had taken care of pregnant women for several years and thought that I knew a lot about pregnancy. But when I became pregnant myself, I found that there was much more to learn. Early in my pregnancy I was surprised at how badly I felt with nausea and heartburn and even more surprised at how tired I was. I didn't want to talk about my pregnancy until it became obvious, so I forced myself to smile and keep on going. Fortunately, most of the unpleasant early side effects quickly passed.

During the rest of my pregnancy I felt quite well. I was able to work hard in surgery and in the delivery room and to see patients for their routine checkups. I ran up and down stairs, traveled, and rode my bicycle. Though my pregnancy was uncomplicated and I was not high risk in any way, like most prospective mothers, I had private worries. Would any complications develop? Would the child be normal? Would I make it through labor? Would I be a good parent? I found that I was moody and would cry easily.

When the last month arrived I was eager to have the baby. Although I wasn't overly uncomfortable, I was tired of being pregnant and probably more apprehensive about labor and delivery than I would admit. Although much has been said recently about alternative methods of childbirth, I personally never cared whether the delivery room had curtains or carpeting or whether the birth took place on a delivery table or a bed. I knew, however, that I didn't want it to be at home. I hoped that I would need little or no medication, but I reserved the right to decide about that during labor. I knew that there would be a fetal monitor and an IV (intravenous feeding). I also knew that if the baby was breech or if there were fetal heart rate abnormalities, I might need to have a cesarean section. In short, I wanted to have my baby where the best possible medical attention for any situation was available.

One evening after a long day at work, I went into labor. Labor was much different from what I expected—faster and more intense. Labor pain was not at all like any pain I had felt before. It was more like hard and physically exhausting work than like pain. I became so absorbed in that work that I no longer was aware of the appearance of the labor room; I did my Lamaze breathing while staring at a fleck of paint on the wall. My husband and I were fortunate to have our son's birth attended by some of our best friends (the obstetrician, the labor nurse, and the resident).

The days in the hospital were happy ones—filled with a whirl of phone calls, visitors, cards, and flowers and with amazement and wonder at this new life. The night before I went home, I became teary and I didn't know what was the matter. Though not really depressed, I began to wonder what I would do if the baby cried. After going home, I found that a little common sense could solve most of the problems. Being at home with a newborn baby is not without its difficulties (although years as an intern and resident had prepared me well for being awakened in the middle of the night). Breast-feeding was easier and more enjoyable than I had imagined. I cooked simple meals and let the dust accumulate a little more than usual. The three of us seemed to survive quite well.

My son seems to grow and develop before my eyes and I have found that the first few years are quite amazing. I sometimes am very reluctant to leave him to go to work and I cherish the hours we have together. Being involved with the childbirth process has always been thrilling to me and now, because of my own experience, I feel even more excited about sharing it with other women.

DECIDING TO HAVE A BABY

The birth of a first child is a major milestone in a woman's life; it marks the end of one stage and the beginning of a new one. The decision to have a child or not is one that must be weighed carefully. It is not uncommon today for a couple to decide that for them the burdens outweigh the rewards. On the other hand, a couple who wait until they know they are ready for the responsibilities of a child often find that the commitment which results from such a decision increases their enjoyment of parenthood. A conscious decision that now is the right time for you to have a baby will help you to see beyond the problems and permit you to focus on the joys of pregnancy and parenthood.

CONCEPTION AND EARLY DEVELOPMENT

The reproductive process begins as your body hormones make the necessary changes to ripen an egg (ovum) in one of your ovaries. If you have a 28-day menstrual cycle, this will take place in the first 14 days of the cycle. As the egg ripens, it moves to the outer surface of the ovary. On about the fourteenth day ovulation occurs—a surge of hormones causes the egg to burst forth from the ovary. In a woman with a shorter or longer cycle the day of ovulation will be sooner or later, as described below.

The menstrual cycle may be divided into two parts by ovulation. From the first day of the menstrual period to ovulation is the preovulatory (also called the proliferative or follicular) phase. From ovulation until the next menstrual period is the postovulatory (also called the secretory or luteal) phase. Regardless of the length of the menstrual cycle the postovulatory phase lasts approximately fourteen days. The variation in women with shorter or longer cycles takes place in the first part of the cycle. For example, in a woman with a 21-day cycle the first part of the cycle lasts 7 days, ovulation takes place on the seventh day, and the second part of the cycle lasts 14 days. In a woman with a 35-day cycle the preovulatory phase lasts 21 days, ovulation occurs on the twenty-first day, and the postovulatory phase lasts 14 days.

During sexual intercourse semen is deposited in the vagina, usually near the cervix. The sperm move first through the cervical canal and then through the uterus to the fallopian tubes. The sperm are best able to fertilize an egg in the first 48 hours after intercourse, although there are reports of sperm living as long as a week before fertilization.

After ovulation the egg begins traveling down the fallopian tube toward the uterus. The sperm usually meet the egg in the outer third of the fallopian tube where one sperm penetrates the egg to fertilize it. The egg is generally fertilized within 4 to 20 hours after ovulation, but there are exceptions to this as well. After the egg has been fertilized, no other sperm can enter it. The egg and the sperm each contribute to the child half of its genetic material.

Each egg carries an X chromosome. Half of the sperm carry Y chromosomes and the other half carry X chromosomes. If an X-bearing sperm fertilizes the egg, the resulting child is female (XX). If, instead, a Y-bearing sperm fertilizes the egg, the resulting child is male (XY). Therefore, the sex of the child is determined by the sperm.

Recent laboratory studies have shown that there are biochemical differences between the X-bearing and the Y-bearing sperm. These differences may allow either the X or Y sperm to survive longer or move faster in certain environments. Books and articles have been written which

FEMALE GENITAL TRACT
OVULATION, FERTILIZATION AND IMPLANTATION

CROSS-SECTION OF UTERUS

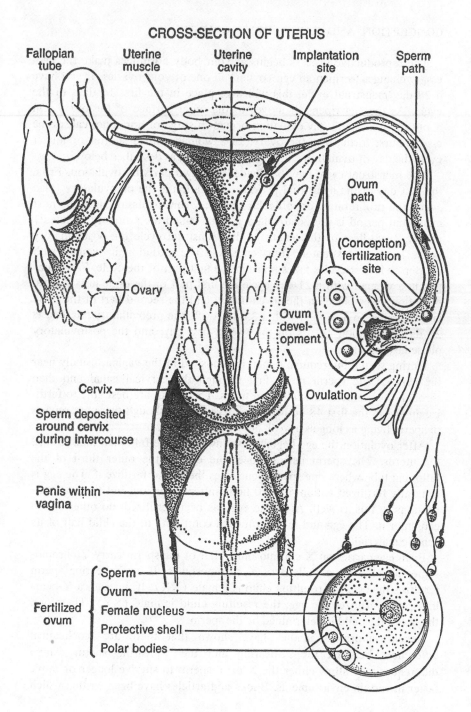

suggest that using acid or alkaline douches or changing the position, frequency, or timing of intercourse may help you alter the odds of having a boy or a girl. Unfortunately, the reproductive tract is more complex than the test tube, and many studies have given conflicting results. It is difficult to say whether future research will allow couples to control the sex of their child.

Twinning may occur by two separate alterations in the reproductive process. Fraternal twins result when a woman produces two eggs during the same month and they are fertilized by two different sperm. Identical twins result when a single fertilized egg splits in half at an early stage of development. Identical twins are much less common than fraternal twins, occurring in about 1 out of 250 pregnancies. Fraternal twins occur in approximately 1 out of 90 pregnancies, but the percentage is increased with the use of fertility drugs or when certain racial or hereditary factors exist. For example, twins are more common in the United States than in Japan and are more common in black families in the United States than in white families. A woman who herself is a twin has an increased chance of having twins.

The endometrial lining of the uterus is prepared every month by hormonal changes to receive a fertilized egg. If no fertilized egg is received, the endometrium is shed as the monthly menstrual flow. During the cycle in which conception occurs, the fertilized egg continues to travel down the fallopian tube and implants in the endometrium. The implantation takes place about seven or eight days after the egg has been fertilized. The area on the ovary where the egg developed forms a small cyst (called the corpus luteum of pregnancy). This cyst produces a hormone (progesterone) which sustains the pregnancy in the early weeks until the placenta (afterbirth) has developed sufficiently to take over this function.

Nestled in the endometrial lining of the uterus, the cells divide. Some of the cells will develop into the fetus. Other cells begin forming the placenta. Besides producing hormones necessary to maintain a pregnancy, the normal placenta acts as an organ of exchange between mother and fetus. Oxygen and nutrients are removed from the mother's blood, absorbed by the fetal blood, and delivered to the developing fetus through the umbilical vein. The fetal waste products return to the placenta via the umbilical arteries and are then transferred into the mother's bloodstream.

In the early weeks of pregnancy the embryo is too small and underdeveloped to be recognizable as human. After 7 weeks have elapsed from the last menstrual period, the fetus is approximately 1 inch long. There is a recognizable head and body, but there are only thick buds where the arms and legs will form. By 10 weeks the fetus is about 2½ inches long and is taking more recognizable human form as the arms and legs are lengthening. At 14 weeks the fetus is about 4½ inches long and may weigh 3 ounces. By this time the placenta is normally well-developed. By

UTERINE-FETAL RELATIONSHIP

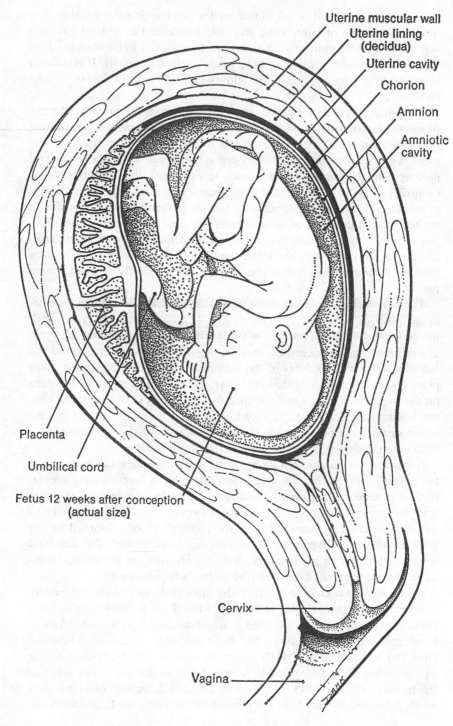

Uterine muscular wall

Uterine lining (decidua)

Uterine cavity

Chorion

Amnion

Amniotic cavity

Placenta

Umbilical cord

Fetus 12 weeks after conception (actual size)

Cervix

Vagina

18 weeks the mother may feel slight movements. At 28 weeks the fetus weighs an average of 2½ pounds and measures about 14 inches. In the last few months of pregnancy, the fetus grows rapidly. At 40 weeks, the end of the average pregnancy, the fetus is usually about 20 inches long and weighs 6 to 9 pounds.

Your doctor will measure your pregnancy in weeks from your last menstrual period. The reason for this is that most women know the date of their last menstrual period, but few know the exact date of conception. The average pregnancy lasts 40 weeks from the last menstrual period. To make a quick calculation of the "due date," subtract three months and add one week to the first day of your last menstrual period.

DIAGNOSIS OF PREGNANCY

Signs and Symptoms

Many women think that a missed period, morning sickness, and fatigue are necessary signs of early pregnancy. However, even these classic symptoms may not always be present, and their presence does not always indicate pregnancy. There are other reasons for missing a menstrual period including emotional stress, illness, thyroid disease, and the recent use of birth control pills. For example, if you recently stopped taking birth control pills, it may be several months before your body readjusts and you resume having regular monthly periods. On the other hand, many women who are pregnant have a light "menstrual period" during the first month or two of pregnancy.

Nausea or inability to tolerate certain foods or tobacco smoke is common during early pregnancy. Often the nausea can be relieved by eating a few crackers in the morning before getting out of bed. Sometimes, however, vomiting is such a problem that medication is required to control it.

Breast tenderness is a very reliable sign of pregnancy which starts about the time of the missed menstrual period or a week or two later. Since breast tenderness also occurs premenstrually, however, it is possible to be fooled by this sign. Some women begin producing excessive saliva, others experience fatigue. Some have constipation, others have diarrhea. Still others experience a large increase in appetite. Every person is slightly different. You may experience all of these symptoms or you may experience none of them.

Pregnancy Tests

There are many different types of tests to confirm pregnancy, and they vary widely in their accuracy and their sensitivity. Some family planning centers offer free pregnancy tests. Check with your local medical society or health department to find out where an inexpensive pregnancy test may be obtained.

The simplest test, often called the slide test, is done by mixing urine with a testing solution on a slide. This method usually cannot detect a pregnancy until about four weeks after conception or about six weeks after the last menstrual period. Even later, this test sometimes gives either false negative or false positive results. The advantage of the slide test is that it is simple and quick to perform.

Slightly more accurate, although results take longer, is the test called the hemaglutination inhibition or tube test. This test is also done with a urine sample mixed with a testing solution. The many available home pregnancy tests are tube tests. Though the home tests have become quite popular, they can give inaccurate results if not done properly. It should be remembered that, like the slide test, the tube test is often not positive until six weeks after the last menstrual period. Performing the test too soon may give a false negative result. Also, the home test may be more expensive than a test done in a local laboratory or clinic.

The advantages of a home test are that the results can be obtained day or night, weekday or weekend, and that it is completely confidential. However, some physicians require a laboratory test to confirm the results of the home test.

More accurate is a recently developed blood pregnancy test, the radioreceptor assay (RRA) for HCG (human chorionic gonadotropin). If a woman is pregnant, this test may be positive as early as the time of the missed menstrual period. Some medical centers have facilities to refine this test even further so it can detect a pregnancy only a few days after conception. The RRA may be helpful in special situations when early diagnosis of pregnancy is important or when an ectopic pregnancy might be expected.

WHO WILL DELIVER YOUR BABY?

In America babies are delivered every day by obstetrician-gynecologists, family practitioners, nurse-midwives, and lay midwives. Depending on the state in which you live and the size of your community, some or all of these choices may be available to you. Whichever type of professional you select, the most important thing is to find someone with whom you are comfortable and in whom you have confidence. This person will share with you an important event in your life.

Obstetrician-Gynecologist

To become an obstetrician-gynecologist, in addition to obtaining a medical degree, a physician must spend a minimum of three or four years in an approved residency program working in the field of obstetrics and gynecology under the supervision of specialists in that field. After completing this training, most become certified in obstetrics and gynecology by passing difficult examinations given by the American College of Obstetrics and Gynecology. Obstetrician-gynecologists and residents in obstetrics and gynecology deliver approximately 70 percent of the babies born in the United States. At the present time approximately 9 percent of the obstetrician-gynecologists in the United States are women. This percentage is increasing as more women are graduating from medical schools and selecting a career in this specialty.

Obstetricians vary in their attitudes toward childbirth as well as such specifics as medications during labor, breast-feeding, role of the father, episiotomy, rooming-in, and length of hospital stay. If any of these things are important to you, discuss them with your obstetrician early in pregnancy.

Family Practitioner

Many babies are delivered by family practitioners, particularly in rural areas or small towns where such a doctor may be the only one available. Many women enjoy having the family doctor, who takes care of the entire family for all medical problems, care for them during pregnancy, labor, and delivery. Many family practitioners have had some advanced training in obstetrics. A family doctor trained in obstetrics can handle a normal pregnancy and childbirth, but he or she may refer you to a specialist if you have serious complications at any time during pregnancy.

Nurse-Midwife

Certified nurse-midwives deliver approximately 1 percent of the babies born in the United States. These midwives are registered nurses (RNs) who have had an additional one or two years of training in obstetrics. Almost all are women. There are less than 3000 certified nurse-midwives involved in clinical practice throughout the United States, but that number is increasing and is expected to continue to increase.

According to the American College of Nurse-Midwives, the nurse-midwife's management of labor and delivery may differ from that of some physicians. Nurse-midwives are less likely to use fetal monitors or use forceps. They often prefer deliveries in a bed instead of on a delivery table. An episiotomy, an incision to enlarge the vaginal opening prior to delivery, is often not done by nurse-midwives. Some nurse-midwives do home deliveries, although many deliver babies only in hospitals. Many offer family planning and postpartum checkups. Typically, they try to encourage breast-feeding and rooming-in. (Of course, there are also a substantial number of physicians who would be willing to deliver your baby and care for you in this manner.)

Because nurse-midwives generally have fewer patients than either obstetricians or family practitioners, they may have more time to spend with each patient during prenatal visits or during labor. Nurse-midwives handle uncomplicated pregnancies quite satisfactorily. However, if complications arise, the patient may have to be transferred to the care of a physician.

The licensing of medical personnel varies from state to state, and a few states still have very restrictive laws regarding nurse-midwives. By law in most states there must be an obstetrician available to the midwife in case of emergency. Most midwives today practice with obstetricians or use obstetricians as consultants. If you would like to know whether there are any nurse-midwives practicing in your area, contact the American College of Nurse-Midwives, 1012 14th Street, NW, Washington, D.C. 20005.

Lay Midwife

Lay midwives are people without nursing degrees who are trained to deliver babies. As a group lay midwives are the most willing to perform home deliveries. Many states recognize only nurse-midwives and do not allow lay midwives to practice. Some states which permit lay midwives to practice have little or no regulation. Because of this wide variation in regulation by states, the level of training required of a lay midwife also varies enormously. Before you select a lay midwife, you should inquire thoroughly into the level of his or her training.

WHERE WILL YOU HAVE YOUR BABY?

Hospital Delivery

Approximately 99 percent of all babies born in the United States today are born in hospitals. The birth of a baby is a normal physiological process and is usually uncomplicated. However, when complications do occur, they often happen very quickly and with little or no warning. Labor may be progressing well when vaginal bleeding begins and the baby's heartbeat starts to slow. Even a healthy mother with an uncomplicated pregnancy and a normal labor and delivery may have a baby that has difficulty breathing and needs to be given oxygen and receive immediate pediatric care. Similarly, a woman with a totally uncomplicated labor and delivery may have a postpartum hemorrhage ten minutes later. While these complications are not common, they can be catastrophic if proper medical care, including needed blood, oxygen, or medications, is not available. Most women opt for a hospital birth to have the assurance that any necessary treatment is immediately available if any complications do occur.

Home Delivery

Some women choose to have their babies at home. They object to the cold and sometimes impersonal environment of the hospital and prefer to share the intimate joyous experience of birth with their families and friends rather than with doctors and nurses in masks and gowns. Labor and delivery are normal processes, not diseases.

If you are considering home delivery, discuss it thoroughly with the person who is overseeing your prenatal care and delivery (your clinician, whether it be physician, nurse-midwife, or lay midwife). During the course of your prenatal care the clinician can tell you if any condition indicates a likelihood of complication. In such a case you may be advised that hospital delivery would be much safer.

Even if it is assumed that delivery will be normal, arrangements must be made for emergency transportation and additional medical aid in case of unexpected difficulty. Even if arrangements have been made, there is still a risk that complications may develop too quickly to be treated adequately. In many European countries home delivery is safer than in the United States because of an extensive system of back-up ambulances and emergency teams that can be dispatched at a moment's notice. Here, comparable systems have been developed in only a few communities.

Maternity Center Delivery

Some women have a third option open to them. There are several maternity centers in the United States which combine a homelike environment with the availability of medical personnel and equipment in case of emergency. Because there are a significant number of women who would like to deliver at home, but do not want to accept all of the risks associated with home delivery, more of these centers may open in the next few years.

Ideally, a maternity center is located in or near a hospital. Only women with uncomplicated pregnancies are accepted for delivery. Anesthesia and fetal monitoring are usually unavailable. If complications develop during labor, the patient is transferred to the hospital.

Some maternity centers are not located in or near a hospital. If you are interested in having your baby at such a center, be sure to investigate the arrangements for transfer to a hospital in case of emergency. If hospital facilities are not readily accessible, many of the same risks that pertain to home delivery will be present.

HEALTH CARE DURING NORMAL PREGNANCY

As soon as you think or know you are pregnant you should begin your prenatal care. The early visits are important to identify any problems or potential problems. If you are healthy, early visits will probably be infrequent, usually only once a month. By the end of pregnancy your visits will probably be weekly.

The first visit will most likely be the longest. It will include a medical history and a physical examination. Blood tests will be taken to determine your blood type, whether you are Rh-negative or Rh-positive, and whether you are anemic. Other tests will be taken to see if you have syphilis, gonorrhea, or a urinary tract infection. You may also be tested for immunity to German measles and toxoplasmosis. If you are healthy and your pregnancy is uncomplicated, subsequent visits will be simple. They will include an examination of the size of the uterus, a measurement of your blood pressure and weight change and perhaps a urine test. Blood tests may be repeated later in pregnancy. Although these checkups are simple, they can detect many of the problems that can occur during pregnancy.

Now that you are pregnant you will undoubtedly want to learn as much as possible about the process which you are about to experience. Recently there has been an increase in the availability of "preparation for childbirth" classes. These classes may be given in hospitals, doctors' offices, community meeting places, or private homes. Although the format may vary, the basic goal of these classes is to educate a pregnant woman and her partner about what to expect during pregnancy, labor, and delivery. The more you understand about what is happening and why it is happening, the more comfortable you will feel. If tours of the labor and delivery area of your hospital are offered, take one. Such a tour will make your surroundings seem more familiar to you when you arrive for your delivery. You owe it to yourself to learn as much as possible about childbirth before it happens.

Emotional Changes

For many women pregnancy is a pleasant, happy time; it may also be a time of psychological stress and mixed emotions. Much of what a woman expects of pregnancy is a result of what she has heard over the years from her mother, sisters, friends, and relatives. A woman who has heard repeatedly of the horrors and terrible pain of labor may face childbirth with fear and apprehension. A woman who has grown up in a neighborhood where many families had five or six children may assume it must be easy.

An unplanned pregnancy, in or out of wedlock, may bring with it considerable emotional stress. Even a couple who has planned and waited for years for a family will still probably have some doubt and ambivalence. You don't know in advance how the baby will affect your life and whether or not you will like the changes. You may worry about how much everything will cost. If you have been working, you may be concerned about how you will find a baby-sitter and may wonder how having a baby will affect your career.

Though often a time of closeness between a husband and wife, pregnancy can also be a time of friction in a marriage. Men's attitudes toward childbirth vary as much as women's. Some men cannot relate to the pregnancy at all, while others feel every wave of nausea and every contraction personally. The important thing to remember is that these attitudes don't make them better or worse as husbands or as fathers.

Most psychologists consider pregnancy a crisis time. Your feelings about your own parents, your childhood experiences, your relationship with the father of the child, your friends, and your job are all changing. Your body is going through rapid physical and hormonal changes and it is sometimes hard to believe that you will ever return to a nonpregnant size and shape. It is not at all surprising that there are times of emotional fluctuations during pregnancy.

Diet

If a woman is healthy and has good eating habits, it may be unnecessary for her to make any major diet changes during pregnancy. Many women are surprised that there is not a great increase in the amount of food required during pregnancy. Although a pregnant woman's caloric intake may not be greatly increased, it is important that the calories be obtained from foods that will provide the proper protein, vitamins, and minerals for her baby's development. If you have not been eating a well-balanced diet, it is essential that you correct that once you become pregnant. Your baby is totally dependent on you to supply it with the necessary nutrients for proper growth and development. For advice on proper nutrition and weight gain during pregnancy, see "Nutrition and Weight," pp. 36–65.

Occasionally women develop cravings for strange substances during pregnancy. These include such things as clay, starch, and baking soda. While eating small quantities of these substances probably will not be harmful, eating larger amounts may dangerously reduce your intake of foods that benefit your baby's growth and development.

Smoking, Alcohol, and Drugs

Anytime is a good time to stop smoking, but pregnancy is an especially important time for you to stop. In women who smoke there is an increased

WEIGHT GAIN DURING PREGNANCY

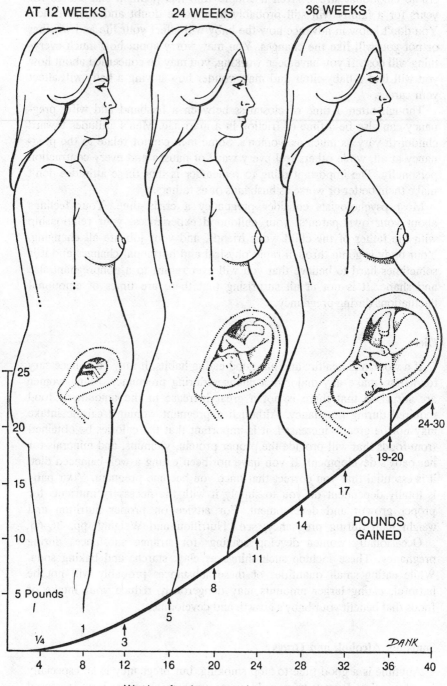

AT 12 WEEKS   24 WEEKS   36 WEEKS

25

20

15

10

5 Pounds

POUNDS
GAINED

24-30

19-20

17

14

11

8

5

3

¼

1

DANK

4   8   12   16   20   24   28   32   36   40

Weeks after last normal menstrual period

likelihood of premature, low-birthweight, and stillborn babies. Complications of pregnancy including bleeding, placenta previa, and premature rupture of the membranes are also more frequent in smokers. Many of these complications are thought to be caused by higher levels of carbon monoxide and lower levels of oxygen in the blood of women who smoke. Nicotine and small amounts of carbon monoxide circulating in the mother's bloodstream also may have adverse effects.

The harmful effects of smoking on the baby probably do not all end at the time of delivery. Nicotine is transmitted through breast milk and the consequences of this are unknown. Also, bronchitis and pneumonia are more common in small children who live in a family where one or more family members smoke.

Alcohol also has recently been shown to affect the fetus adversely. Babies of alcoholic mothers are more likely to have birth defects including mental and growth retardation. The fetal alcohol syndrome consists of a small baby with a smaller than normal head, characteristic facial appearance, heart defects, and mental retardation. These serious problems are usually associated with heavy drinkers and not with women who confine their intake of alcohol to two or fewer drinks a day. Nevertheless, some medical researchers feel that even smaller amounts of alcohol may have a harmful effect on a developing fetus.

Studies have shown that very few women go through an entire pregnancy without taking a single drug. This, of course, includes such things as vitamins, iron, or an occasional aspirin. Unfortunately, in our society many drugs are used more from habit than actual need—a decongestant for every stuffy nose or a sleeping pill that is not always necessary. Pregnant women should try to break this habit and avoid the use of any medications that are not truly essential.

Most drugs taken by a woman during pregnancy can cross the placenta and reach the fetus. The effects on the fetus of most drugs have not been tested (because of FDA restrictions and potential dangers involved in such testing) and are therefore unknown. Although many drugs probably will not exert any unfavorable influence on the fetus, there are unfortunately several examples of drugs which were incorrectly believed to be safe when used during pregnancy. Among the best known of these are thalidomide and the estrogen diethylstilbestrol (DES), which were both later shown to cause serious harmful effects on the children.

The FDA has issued warnings on certain medications because they are thought to be harmful to the fetus if taken by the mother during pregnancy. Tranquilizers such as Valium and Librium may cause cleft lip and palate or other defects in a small percentage of babies if taken by the mother during the first three months of pregnancy. Lithium, a drug used in certain psychiatric conditions, is thought to cause a significant increase in congenital cardiovascular malformation if taken during early pregnancy.

Hormones, including progesterones, estrogens, androgens, and birth control pills, if taken during early pregnancy perhaps may endanger the fetus and cause genital or limb abnormalities. The FDA recommends that all women discontinue birth control pills at least three months before becoming pregnant, though recent studies have challenged the necessity of this. Anticonvulsant medications, though necessary for most epileptic mothers, cause a significant increase in congenital malformations including cleft lip and palate and other defects.

A pregnant woman must be concerned about other substances besides drugs. Artificial sweeteners cross the placenta and reach the developing fetus. Any live-virus vaccines should also be avoided. Chemicals, pesticides, and other toxic sprays may be absorbed into the mother's bloodstream. Because the effects of such substances on the fetus are unknown, it is best to limit contact with them.

Activity

Keeping active during your pregnancy is very important. However, because of cardiovascular, weight, and posture changes many pregnant women find that they tire more quickly during exercise. In moderation most activities, sports, and exercises that you enjoyed before you became pregnant can be continued. Exceptions include sports such as water or snow skiing or motorcycling where a sudden fall may occur. Swimming, bicycling, running, and walking are all safe. In fact, walking is one of the best exercises for a pregnant woman.

Many women wonder if they should travel while they are pregnant. This question usually can be answered with a bit of common sense. It would normally not be wise to travel to an underdeveloped country or one where there was an epidemic. In general, the greatest risk in traveling is that you could develop a complication in a place where it would be difficult to obtain adequate medical care. Since complications are fewest during the middle three months, that is the safest time to travel. During the first three months there is always a possibility of a spontaneous abortion; during the last three there is a chance of premature labor or of ruptured membranes.

Many factors contribute to the change in sexual relations that most couples experience during pregnancy. A woman may feel extremely feminine during pregnancy or she may feel that she is totally undesirable. A man's feeling about the attractiveness of his pregnant lover may be just as variable. Some couples find that pregnancy is a time of increased sexual intimacy. Others find that their previously good sexual relationship has deteriorated. Some men express anxiety about possible trauma to the developing fetus during intercourse. Women often experience uterine cramping after orgasm which may lead to fear of inducing abortion in early pregnancy or inducing labor later on. The pregnant woman's expanding shape may cause difficulty in finding comfortable positions.

Certain conditions may cause your doctor or midwife to recommend limitation of sexual relations during pregnancy. Among these conditions are a history of several early or midtrimester spontaneous abortions or of premature labor, multiple pregnancy, polyhydramnios (excess amniotic fluid causing overdistention of the uterus), low-lying placenta, or placenta previa. Sexual relations should be discontinued if you have been told that your cervix has started to dilate, if your membranes have ruptured, or if you are having vaginal bleeding.

If the pregnancy is uncomplicated, I have always advised my patients that they could continue sexual relations until I find, by vaginal examination, that the cervix has started to dilate. Because this often occurs during the last month of pregnancy many physicians routinely recommend discontinuance of sexual intercourse a month before the baby is due. Some recent studies have questioned the safety of intercourse in uncomplicated pregnancies, pointing to a small number of spontaneous abortions, infections, and premature deliveries occurring after sexual intercourse. More definitive studies need to be done in this area. In spite of the questions raised by these studies, the evidence doesn't seem conclusive enough to recommend limitation of sexual relations during the first eight months of a normal pregnancy.

COMPLICATIONS OF PREGNANCY

Though pregnancy is usually uneventful and results in the birth of a normal healthy baby, complications sometimes arise. These complications include bleeding and spontaneous abortion, ectopic pregnancy, preeclampsia and eclampsia, chronic and genetic disease, infections, Rh disease, intrauterine fetal death, and hydatidiform mole.

Bleeding and Spontaneous Abortion

Vaginal bleeding in early pregnancy is not uncommon. However, you should see your doctor promptly if it occurs. Until then, limit physical activity as much as possible and avoid sexual intercourse. Often the bleeding stops spontaneously and is no further problem. In cases like these, usually no cause for the bleeding is found.

Vaginal bleeding may be one of the first signs of a possible spontaneous abortion. You may pass blood clots and perhaps some tissue and you may have severe cramps. If, as often happens, some tissue from the pregnancy remains in the uterus, that tissue must be removed by a dilatation and curettage (also called a D&C or a completion: see chapter on abortion for a description of the procedure). If this tissue is not removed, you could continue to bleed or an infection of the uterus could develop.

A spontaneous abortion is often a very upsetting experience. It is important to realize that spontaneous abortions are very common, occurring in about 1 out of 10 pregnancies, and usually cannot be prevented. Furthermore, recent studies on the aborted tissue have shown that many of these pregnancies were not developing normally. Thus, spontaneous abortions help to assure that most pregnancies that reach the sixth month will result in normal, healthy babies. Having one spontaneous abortion does not mean that you will experience difficulty with your next pregnancy nor does it mean that there is anything wrong with you or your partner. However, if a woman has repeated spontaneous abortions, further studies may be necessary to look for uterine or chromosomal abnormalities or hormone imbalances.

Bleeding later in pregnancy may have several causes. One relatively uncommon problem is placenta previa. The placenta normally attaches to the side or the top of the uterine cavity. In placenta previa it attaches instead to the lowest part of the uterus and covers all or part of the cervix, thus possibly blocking the baby's exit through the birth canal. Bed rest will decrease the likelihood of bleeding, although extensive bleeding may nevertheless occur. The baby must be delivered by cesarean section if the placenta is blocking the entire cervix.

Another cause of bleeding in pregnancy is separation of a portion of the placenta from the uterine wall (placental abruption). If the detached portion is large, labor may begin. If the placenta detaches completely, the fetus will be unable to receive oxygen and nutrients from the mother and will die. Fortunately, the amount of separation is often small enough to allow the pregnancy to proceed normally.

If you have any bleeding during pregnancy, you should contact your physician. Keep in mind that not all bleeding during pregnancy means that something is wrong. Some women bleed during the first few months of pregnancy at the time they would have had their menstrual period. Sometimes an irritation on the cervix can cause bleeding after intercourse. During the last few weeks of pregnancy many women have some spotting after a vaginal examination. Also, a small amount of bleeding sometimes occurs near the end of pregnancy as the cervix begins to dilate.

Ectopic Pregnancy

In less than 1 out of 100 pregnancies the fertilized egg does not implant in the uterus, but in an ectopic (abnormal) location. By far the most common type of ectopic pregnancy is the tubal pregnancy. Other types include abdominal, ovarian, and cervical pregnancy.

Some women with an ectopic pregnancy exhibit all of the normal symptoms of pregnancy; others have none because of the lower hormone levels associated with ectopic pregnancies. Spotting is quite common in tubal pregnancies. As the embryo grows and pushes on the walls of the fallopian tube, pain can develop. Because the diameter of the tube is small, the pregnancy may rupture through the side of the fallopian tube, causing extensive intra-abdominal bleeding. In some cases the first sign of an ectopic pregnancy is a fainting spell caused by this sudden loss of blood internally.

The chances of developing an ectopic pregnancy are greater among women who have a history of pelvic infections, an infection after an abortion, who have had an ectopic pregnancy in the past, or who use intrauterine contraceptive devices (see chapter on contraception for the relationship between IUDs and ectopic pregnancy). However, ectopic pregnancies often occur in the absence of any of these factors.

In rare cases an early tubal pregnancy may be removed and the fallopian tube repaired, but often the tube is irreparably damaged and must be removed. However, if the other tube is normal, future pregnancies are possible.

Pre-eclampsia and Eclampsia (Formerly Called Toxemia of Pregnancy)

An abnormal elevation of blood pressure developing during the latter half of pregnancy (gestational hypertension) may occur in up to 5 percent of all pregnancies. A mild increase in blood pressure without any other symptoms is common. Though bleeding during pregnancy and placental abruption are more common in women with gestational hypertension, in most cases there is no ill effect. If the increase in blood pressure is significant, bed rest may be recommended in an attempt to prevent complications.

However, a rise in blood pressure, when accompanied by edema (fluid retention) and protein in the urine, indicates the onset of a condition called pre-eclampsia. Rapid weight gain caused by the fluid retention, severe headaches, and visual disturbances may occur. Pre-eclampsia is more common with first pregnancies. When mild, it can be treated by bed rest and sedation. Severe cases may require large doses of sedatives and medications to lower the blood pressure. In its most severe form pre-eclampsia can be life-threatening to both mother and baby and delivery may be necessary even if the infant is premature. Severe pre-eclampsia is rare and with proper treatment is usually not a problem after delivery.

Eclampsia is an intensification of the symptoms designated as preeclampsia and is also characterized by convulsions. Eclampsia may develop from untreated pre-eclampsia or it may occur without preliminary milder symptoms. No matter when in pregnancy eclampsia occurs, the pregnancy must be terminated after appropriate anticonvulsive-antihypertensive medication has been given. In women without chronic high blood pressure or kidney disease, pre-eclampsia or eclampsia usually does not recur during subsequent pregnancies.

Chronic and Genetic Diseases

Because of medical advances, successful pregnancy is now possible for women who in past years might not have been able to have children. This includes women under treatment for diabetes, high blood pressure, heart disease, epilepsy, and many other diseases. However, since proper treatment during pregnancy may be quite complicated, a woman with any of these problems should consult a doctor before she becomes pregnant.

If you have a mild form of diabetes which is controlled by diet or by constant amounts of insulin, your diabetes probably will not prevent you from conceiving. However, pregnancy is not always easy for a diabetic woman. Blood sugar levels must be followed closely and the insulin dosage adjusted frequently during pregnancy. Hospitalization is often necessary, especially late in pregnancy. If your diabetes has been difficult to control or if it has affected your kidneys or vision, pregnancy could seriously worsen your diabetes and threaten your life.

Diabetic mothers have an increased chance of needing a cesarean section, since babies born to diabetic mothers may be large, sometimes over 10 pounds. Also, many babies of diabetic mothers are delivered early to avoid complications during the last few weeks of pregnancy. A baby of a diabetic mother may have hypoglycemia (low blood sugar) for the first day or two of life, but this can usually be treated by prompt feeding or intravenous feeding of sugar solutions.

Medication for high blood pressure may have to be adjusted during pregnancy. Some drugs are safer than others during pregnancy, and you should be on the safest possible drugs in the lowest dosage which will control your blood pressure. Some complications, such as bleeding and separation of the placenta, are more common in patients with high blood pressure. Babies born to mothers with severe high blood pressure may be smaller than average.

There are many changes in your heart and circulatory system during pregnancy. Some, but not all, heart problems may be worsened.

Pregnancy may be complicated by epilepsy. The risk of having a baby with a serious congenital defect is three to four times higher in epileptic women. Many of these birth defects, including cardiac anomalies, facial anomalies, and cleft lip and palate, are thought to be caused by the drugs used to control epilepsy, yet studies have shown that epileptic mothers who did not take medications during pregnancy also had an increased incidence of birth defects. At present there is no test for these specific defects during pregnancy. However, even with these problems and despite the substantially greater risks, most babies born to epileptic mothers (whether they are taking medication or not) are completely normal.

If there is any history of congenital malformation, mental retardation or known genetic disorders in your family, you should see a qualified genetic counselor before you become pregnant. Some birth defects are hereditary, while others are not, and a counselor can advise you in advance about your chances of having a normal child. During pregnancy some of these conditions are detectable by amniocentesis (described below).

Infections

A woman may be exposed to a variety of infections during pregnancy. The most frequent of these is the common cold. A cold is a viral infection and the usual routine of adequate rest and fluids is also appropriate for a pregnant woman. In addition, your doctor may recommend small doses of aspirin or an aspirin substitute. In large doses even aspirin may not be completely safe at certain times, and some nonprescription cold remedies contain drugs that may or may not be safe during pregnancy. You should check with your physician before you take any medication.

If you have a bad cough or a fever, you should notify your doctor promptly. What begins as a cold may progress to a more serious infection such as tonsillitis, sinusitis, or pneumonia. These infections are often bacterial and should be treated with antibiotics. Some antibiotics, such as tetracycline and chloramphenicol, should usually be avoided during pregnancy, but others, such as penicillin and erythromycin, are commonly used without any known side effects to the baby.

Urinary tract infections, such as bladder and kidney infections, may also occur in pregnant women. The symptoms of a bladder infection are burning urination and foul-smelling urine. The symptoms of a kidney infection are low back pain and a high fever. If you have any of these symptoms, notify your doctor promptly. Your urine can be examined microscopically and cultured for bacteria to determine whether you have a urinary infection. A mild infection can usually be treated by an oral antibiotic, but a severe infection may require hospitalization and intravenous antibiotics.

Some infections during pregnancy can cause dangerous side effects to the fetus before birth or to the baby as it passes through the birth canal. These include rubella (German measles), syphilis, gonorrhea, and genital herpes.

Rubella in a woman during the first three months of pregnancy can cross the placenta and cause congenital rubella syndrome, that is, fetal blindness, deafness, brain damage, growth retardation, or death. Although not every baby whose mother has German measles during early pregnancy develops these abnormalities, the percentage that show some damage is high, perhaps up to 50 percent. After the rubella epidemic of 1964 there were over 20,000 babies born in the United States with congenital rubella syndrome. Because of widespread vaccination against the disease and improved diagnostic techniques, the number of affected babies born has decreased to about 25 a year.

A simple blood test can confirm if a woman is immune to rubella. If she is not immune, she should have an immunization against the infection before she becomes pregnant. Because the vaccine contains a mild strain of live rubella virus, it should be given at least three months before a woman becomes pregnant; it should never be given to a woman who is already pregnant.

Unfortunately, many women first realize that they are not immune to rubella during pregnancy. In this case exposure to anyone with the infection should be avoided. If you are not immune to rubella and think that you may have been exposed, notify your doctor so that the appropriate blood tests may be taken to see if you develop the disease. Postpartum rubella immunization should be given to prevent this problem during subsequent pregnancies.

Syphilis is a bacterial infection usually transmitted through sexual relations (see the chapter on sexually transmissible diseases for a description of syphilis, gonorrhea, and herpes). If a pregnant woman is or becomes infected with syphilis, the bacteria can travel through her bloodstream and across the placenta to infect the baby. If she is treated promptly with antibiotics, the baby has a good chance of being completely normal. For this reason blood tests for syphilis are done routinely during pregnancy. If you think you may have been exposed to syphilis after your initial blood test, let your doctor know promptly in order that the test may be repeated and your baby protected.

In the early stages of gonorrhea a woman may notice a foul-smelling yellow vaginal discharge, although often there are no symptoms at all. In early pregnancy the infection may spread into the uterus and the fallopian tubes causing a generalized pelvic infection, which if not treated promptly, can cause spontaneous abortion. During the second half of pregnancy, gonorrhea is less likely to spread, but may remain in the cervix and infect the baby at delivery.

In the past, babies exposed to gonorrhea while passing through the birth canal often developed gonorrheal eye infections which caused blindness. Today the routine administration of silver nitrate eye drops or penicillin usually prevents blindness.

A third sexually transmitted infection is herpes genitalis (herpes type II), caused by a virus closely related to the virus which causes cold sores (herpes type I). The initial symptoms of this disease may be painful blisters in the genital area, often accompanied by fever and swollen lymph nodes in the groin. Exposure to the virus as it passes through the birth canal can lead to severe infection and death. A woman who has herpes genitalis near the end of pregnancy should be delivered by cesarean section before the membranes rupture to prevent exposure of the infant to the infection.

Rh Disease

Your routine blood tests will determine whether your blood type is A, B, AB, or O and whether you are Rh-positive or Rh-negative. If an Rh-negative mother has an Rh-positive fetus, any leakage of fetal blood into the mother may cause the formation of Rh antibodies in the mother's blood. This leakage most commonly occurs at the time of delivery. For this reason the first pregnancy with an Rh-positive fetus is almost always unaffected by the incompatibility. But, if in a subsequent pregnancy the fetus is again Rh-positive, the antibodies previously formed in the mother's blood may react with the fetus's blood to cause Rh disease. The damage to the fetus's red blood cells may cause severe hemolytic anemia or death. If amniocentesis reveals that the fetus has this disease, premature delivery may be necessary to prevent further destruction of the fetal blood. An exchange transfusion at birth of Rh-negative blood, which is not affected by the antibodies, may control the anemia.

Fortunately, since the mid-1960s Rhogam (Rh-immune globulin) has been available to prevent Rh disease. An Rh-negative mother who has an Rh-positive baby is given an injection of Rhogam shortly after delivery to stop the formation of the dangerous antibodies and thereby to prevent Rh disease in subsequent pregnancies.

An abortion may also result in the passage of a small amount of fetal blood into the mother and the formation of Rh antibodies. Because the fetal blood type is not known, Rhogam is given to all Rh-negative women who undergo spontaneous or induced abortion. Rhogam may also be given to an Rh-negative woman during pregnancy after amniocentesis or after a bleeding episode.

Intrauterine Fetal Death

Sometimes for no apparent reason in a normal, uncomplicated pregnancy the fetus will die. Fortunately, this is an uncommon occurrence. A mother may notice that the baby has stopped moving. An examination by her doctor will fail to detect a fetal heart beat, and other tests, such as X-rays or sonograms (see discussion of fetal health below), may confirm that an intrauterine fetal death has occurred.

In the past after such a diagnosis the woman was sent home to wait for labor to begin spontaneously, which might take as long as a month or two.

With better labor-inducing medications available today, labor is often induced shortly after the diagnosis of intrauterine fetal death.

After delivery, the fetus is examined to determine the cause of death. The umbilical cord may be wrapped tightly around the fetus's neck or may be knotted. It may be abnormal, or there may have been a problem with the placenta. However, in a significant number of cases no cause at all is found. You should ask your doctor if there is any evidence that the cause of death might be repeated if you become pregnant again. Fortunately, these problems usually do not recur and subsequent pregnancies generally result in normal healthy babies.

Hydatidiform Mole

Another complication of pregnancy is hydatidiform mole (also called molar pregnancy). It is not common in the United States, occurring in approximately 1 out of 2000 pregnancies. It is more common elsewhere, for example, occurring as frequently as 1 out of 125 pregnancies in Taiwan.

Early in pregnancy the placenta becomes a "tumor," with the appearance of a large cluster of grapes. Usually no fetus develops. Though usually benign, a hydatidiform mole has the potential for becoming malignant. In early pregnancy there may be no unusual symptoms. Eventually, it may be diagnosed by bleeding and passage of characteristic tissue, by an abnormally large or small uterus with no fetal heart beat, or by X-ray studies.

Hydatidiform mole is usually removed by a dilatation and curettage or a suction curettage. If it occurs in a woman who has completed her family, hysterectomy may be recommended. Because the hydatidiform mole produces pregnancy hormones, any remaining growth or a recurrence can be detected by blood or urine pregnancy tests. Such tests are taken on a regular basis for 9 to 12 months or longer following removal to make sure that the condition does not recur or become malignant. If frequent testing reveals a recurrence or a malignant change, it is treatable and almost always curable by chemotherapy. In many women future pregnancies are still possible even after chemotherapy and a suitable waiting period to ensure there is no recurrence.

EVALUATING FETAL HEALTH

There have been many advances in the field of obstetrics over the past few decades including the development of new techniques to study the fetus before birth, including amniocentesis, sonography, fetal monitoring, and chemical and hormone studies. The development of these techniques has helped to reduce infant mortality and the incidence of serious complications such as brain damage and cerebral palsy.

Amniocentesis

The fetus can be tested for chromosomal abnormalities and other problems by amniocentesis, performed ideally between the fifteenth and eighteenth week of pregnancy. The most common chromosomal abnormality is Down's syndrome (mongolism) which is caused by the presence of one extra chromosome. The risk of having a child with Down's syndrome is 1 in 1500 if you are under age 30. Between age 30 and 34 the risk is 1 in 750. Between age 35 and 39 the risk is 1 in 280. By age 40 the risk increases to 1 in 130, and over age 45 the risk is 1 in 65. When amniocentesis was a new procedure, few facilities were available to perform it, and since the risks had not yet been determined, it was offered only to women over 40. Today it should be considered by all women 35 and over who would consider abortion if they knew they were going to have an abnormal baby or who want to know for other reasons.

The procedure is fairly simple. The lower abdomen is cleaned with an antiseptic solution. After a local anesthetic is given, a long, thin needle is inserted through the abdominal and uterine walls into the amniotic sac. Amniotic fluid is then removed with a syringe. The fetal cells in the fluid are cultured and examined microscopically for chromosomal abnormalities. Amniocentesis must be performed by a specially trained physician and requires the availability of specialized laboratory equipment for the culturing and examination of the cells. If your local hospital does not have the facilities to perform the procedure, it may well be worth a trip elsewhere.

The risks of amniocentesis include infection, injury to the fetus or the placenta, Rh-sensitization, leakage of amniotic fluid, and bleeding. Some of these complications may lead to spontaneous abortion. Rhogam is given to Rh-negative women to prevent Rh-sensitization after amniocentesis. In expert hands the overall complication rate of amniocentesis is approximately 1 percent.

The amniotic fluid drawn by amniocentesis can be tested for certain other problems in addition to chromosomal abnormalities. If you have a hereditary disease in your family or have had a previous baby with a serious disease or malformation, you should check with your doctor to see if this disease can be tested for. The sex of the fetus can be determined and this information is helpful if there is a family history of a disease that would affect only children of one sex, as for example, hemophilia and males. However, because of the risks of the test, it should not be performed simply because the parents are curious about the sex of their baby.

Amniocentesis may also be used near the end of pregnancy to determine whether the baby's lungs are mature. If an infant is to be delivered prematurely, vaginally, or by cesarean section, perhaps because of a medical problem of the mother, this test can help to determine whether to treat the fetus

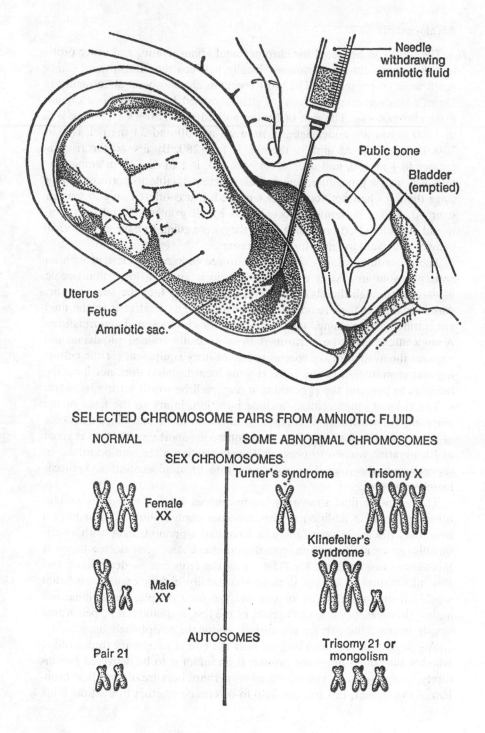

AMNIOCENTESIS IN EIGHTEENTH WEEK

Needle withdrawing amniotic fluid

Pubic bone

Bladder (emptied)

Uterus

Fetus

Amniotic sac.

SELECTED CHROMOSOME PAIRS FROM AMNIOTIC FLUID

NORMAL	SOME ABNORMAL CHROMOSOMES

SEX CHROMOSOMES.

Turner's syndrome   Trisomy X

Female XX

Klinefelter's syndrome

Male XY

AUTOSOMES

Trisomy 21 or mongolism

Pair 21

and the best time to deliver it and to alert the pediatrician to possible respiratory problems. Amniocentesis may also have to be done many times to check on the condition of a fetus of a woman with Rh-negative blood who has been sensitized to Rh antigen.

Sonography

Another new technique which has been used with increasing frequency over the last few years is ultrasound or sonography. This procedure produces an image on a screen (sonogram) by bouncing sound waves through the abdomen. It locates the fetus in a manner similar to radar locating a submarine. This test is painless and although it is often performed in the X-ray department of a hospital, the fetus is not exposed to X-rays. Sonography can locate the placenta, diagnose twins, and measure the fetal head to estimate the baby's gestation age and therefore its due date. Sonography can also detect certain congenital anomalies. In many medical centers sonography is done routinely prior to amniocentesis to guide the physician to the best site for obtaining amniotic fluid and to avoid injury to the placenta and the baby.

Fetal Monitors

Many hospitals now have fetal monitors which record the fetal heartbeat and contractions of the uterus during labor. In some hospitals monitors are used for all patients in labor; others have monitors only for patients who have a higher than normal risk of developing complications.

Fetal monitors can be attached either externally or internally. In external monitoring the monitor is placed on the mother's abdomen by means of adjustable bands. In internal monitoring a wire is inserted through the vagina and attached to the fetal head. A catheter may also be inserted through the vagina into the amniotic sac adjacent to the fetus.

The use of a fetal monitor should not prevent the woman from finding a comfortable position in labor whether that be sitting or lying on her back or side. Although some women do not like the idea of being attached to a machine, it is important to realize that valuable information may be obtained which may protect the life of the baby, and many women are reassured to be able to "see" the baby's heartbeat on the monitor during labor.

There are no known risks of external monitoring and studies are inconclusive as to whether internal monitoring may increase slightly the risk of uterine infection. There is a small risk with internal monitoring that the baby may develop a temporary localized scalp infection similar to a boil at the site where the scalp electrode has been placed.

Monitors are used, among other things, to test for abnormalities in the fetal heart rate. For example, a drop in the fetal heart rate may signal that the fetus is not receiving adequate levels of oxygen because of an abnormal decrease in blood flowing to the baby during contractions. The decrease might be caused by a twisted or knotted umbilical cord. This problem can sometimes be improved by changing the position of the mother or by giving her oxygen. Depending on how serious the drop is, how long it lasts, and when it occurs in relation to the mother's contractions, if the drop in fetal heart rate continues, your doctor may recommend cesarean section.

Monitoring may also be used for patients who are not in labor if the pregnancy is complicated, if the baby is overdue, or if the mother has a medical problem. For example, a fetal monitor can be used to perform the nonstress test, which determines whether the baby's heartbeat accelerates after the baby kicks or moves. A temporary increase in the fetal heart rate after movement is an indication that the baby is in satisfactory condition.

Similarly, a fetal monitor is used for the oxytocin challenge test (generally referred to as OCT or contraction stress test). Mild contractions are started by a dilute intravenous solution of oxytocin, the hormone that is released by the body during labor. A healthy fetus will exhibit a stable heart rate during and after the contractions. On the other hand, a decrease in the fetal heart rate following the contractions may indicate that the fetus is not receiving sufficient oxygen.

Another fairly recent procedure, now available in some large medical centers, is a test to see if a baby is receiving sufficient oxygen by actually taking a sample of the baby's blood. This test, called a scalp pH, is usually done only during labor and only if the membranes are ruptured. It may be performed if fetal heartbeat abnormalities are noted or if there are other reasons to believe that the baby may not be receiving adequate oxygen. In a manner similar to the way a blood sample is obtained by sticking a finger with a lance, a small puncture is made in the baby's scalp and a few drops of blood are drawn into a capillary tube. The pH of the blood indicates the amount of oxygen being received.

If these tests indicate that the baby is in jeopardy and delivery is not imminent, it will be necessary to induce labor or to deliver the baby by cesarean section. These tests have undoubtedly prevented the deaths of some babies who would not have lived if prompt action had not been taken.

Chemical and Hormone Studies

A set of new techniques used to monitor high-risk pregnancies are blood and urine tests for certain pregnancy hormones such as estriol and placental lactogen. These tests evaluate the functions of the placenta. They may be necessary if the mother has diabetes, high blood pressure, or any other medical problem which may potentially harm the fetus. However, in some situations they are less helpful than it was originally hoped they would be.

LABOR AND DELIVERY

Natural Childbirth

Natural childbirth has become quite popular in the United States over the last few years. Its popularity began after Grantly Dick-Read wrote *Childbirth Without Fear* in 1944. He wrote that labor pain could be eliminated by education in the process of labor and delivery. Despite the substantial contribution of this new theory, it soon became apparent that Dick-Read was not entirely correct, since even with extensive knowledge about labor and delivery many women still felt pain.

The next step in the popularity of natural childbirth was the Lamaze or psychoprophylactic technique. Psychoprophylaxis is the psychological and physical preparation for childbirth. This technique originated in Russia and was brought to France by Dr. Ferdinand Lamaze in the early 1950s. Its popularity in the United States followed the publication in 1959 of *Thank You Dr. Lamaze* by Marjorie Karmel, an American woman who became familiar with the Lamaze technique during her pregnancy in France.

The Lamaze technique combines education about labor and delivery with breathing and relaxation exercises. The exercises must be practiced in the months and weeks prior to labor. The partner has an important role as coach. Using the Lamaze breathing techniques, many women are able to go through labor needing little or no medication. Though a purist may insist that a true Lamaze birth means no medication at all, many people believe that the concept is broad enough to include the use of a small amount of medication to relieve pain.

With my observations as an obstetrician and as a woman who has experienced labor, I feel that the Lamaze technique has something to offer to every pregnant woman. I believe that the knowledge of what is happening to your body in labor and delivery can reduce your apprehension and fear and therefore reduce the pain of your labor. I also feel that the Lamaze breathing and relaxation techniques reduce, though not necessarily eliminate, the need for medication in labor.

First Stage of Labor—Dilatation of the Cervix

No two labors are alike. Labor may be long and difficult or it may be short and uncomplicated. Unfortunately, there is no way to predict what your labor will be like or how you will respond to it. When labor begins, you may feel the contractions as mild cramps or they may be very uncomfortable. As labor progresses, the contractions become stronger and more frequent. In active labor the contractions usually occur about every 2 to 3 minutes and last from 45 to 90 seconds. Usually the membranes rupture spontaneously either before or during labor, but if they do not, they are ruptured artificially before the delivery.

The cervix, the lowermost portion of the uterus, must open so that the baby may be born. During most of pregnancy the cervix is firm, thick, and long, with only a very small opening in the center. Late in pregnancy the cervix becomes softer, thinner, and may begin to open before the onset of labor. When labor begins, the changes in the cervix take place much more rapidly. The contractions of the uterus push the baby's head against the cervix and cause it to open. In order for the baby to be born, the cervix must be fully dilated to 10 centimeters (about 4 inches).

The first stage of labor is the time from the onset of labor to the time when the cervix is fully dilated. The length of this stage of labor varies greatly from woman to woman. It averages 8 to 12 hours in most women having their first child, but it can be much shorter or much longer. In subsequent pregnancies it is usually shorter.

Near the end of the first stage of labor, when the cervix is almost fully dilated, the contractions are usually quite strong and the woman begins to feel the urge to push with them. This part of labor is called transition. After complete dilatation, with pushing and the force of the contractions the baby descends in the pelvis, usually turning to the most favorable position as it descends.

It is sometimes necessary to induce labor instead of waiting for it to start spontaneously. For example, if the mother develops severe preeclampsia or has diabetes, if the baby is long overdue, if fetal monitoring indicates that the baby's life is in jeopardy, or if labor does not begin spontaneously after the membranes rupture, labor may have to be induced. In some cases it is induced by the artificial rupture of membranes. In most cases an infusion of a solution of pitocin (oxytocin), which causes the uterus to contract, is necessary. Intravenous pitocin may also be administered to stimulate spontaneous labor that is progressing very slowly. This solution is given intravenously in gradually increasing amounts. Induced labor may be both faster and stronger than spontaneous labor.

Anesthesia

A difficult and painful labor may require some anesthesia or analgesia. Anesthesia may also be required for medical reasons or for a forceps delivery.

The most commonly used medications for labor are pain-killing drugs such as Demerol. With small doses many women are less uncomfortable, but still wide awake and able to participate in and enjoy the delivery of their child. However, some women find that even small doses of these medications make them drowsy or nauseated.

Twilight sleep is an anesthetic technique that has declined greatly in popularity in recent years. The technique combines large doses of pain medications with a drug that has the effect of temporary amnesia (scopolamine). Women who have this medication often say that they have no memory of the labor and delivery.

Epidural anesthesia involves the insertion of a needle in the mother's back and the injection of a novocaine-type drug into the space next to the spinal canal. An epidural will normally eliminate pain from approximately your waist to your toes and will make it difficult to move your legs. This technique allows you to be completely awake, but free from pain. Caudal anesthesia is similar to an epidural but the needle is inserted at a point much lower on your back.

Epidural or caudal anesthesia requires a specially trained anesthesiologist and is not available at all hospitals. These anesthetics do not always work perfectly and they may have undesirable side effects. Some women are numbed on only one side of their body or not at all. Sometimes this type of anesthesia can cause the contractions to become less frequent and it often interferes with the mother's urge to push during the second stage of labor. By lowering the mother's blood pressure, epidural or caudal anesthesia can even cause a temporary slowing of the baby's heartbeat.

Unlike epidural or caudal anesthesia, which can be used to provide pain relief during labor, spinal anesthesia is used to provide relief only for delivery. Saddle block is a type of spinal anesthesia. A needle is inserted into the mother's back and the medication is injected into the space which contains the spinal fluid. Under spinal anesthesia most women are completely numbed from their waist to their toes. When spinal anesthesia is given for a cesarean section, the numbness usually extends to the lower part of the mother's ribcage. The numbness may last for several hours after delivery depending on the type of anesthetic used and the individual's sensitivity to it. A small percentage of women may have a severe headache for several days after spinal anesthesia.

Local anesthetics can be used in various ways during labor and delivery to provide pain relief. Paracervical block is the injection of local anesthetic into the tissue adjacent to the cervix during labor. Pudendal block involves the numbing of the nerves that supply the lower vagina and perineum (the space between the vagina and the rectum). This technique is often used in order to perform a forceps delivery. Finally, local anesthesia may be injected directly into an area where an episiotomy is to be cut or a tear is to be repaired.

Second Stage of Labor—Delivery

The second stage of labor extends from full dilatation to the delivery of the baby. The length of this stage also varies. It may last two hours or more with the first baby, but is usually much shorter in subsequent pregnancies.

In a typical United States hospital delivery you are taken from the labor room to the delivery room and put in the lithotomy position (on your back with your legs in stirrups as for a pelvic examination). In other countries the mother's normal position for delivery may be on her side or in a squatting position. The area around the vagina is washed off with an antiseptic solution and cloth or paper drapes are placed over your abdomen and legs.

If an episiotomy is necessary, it will be done after the top of the baby's head becomes visible. An episiotomy is an incision made in the perineum to expand the vaginal opening to allow the baby to be born without extensive stretching or tearing of the muscles and tissues in this area. Some physicians and midwives believe that an episiotomy should be performed as infrequently as possible since it's not always necessary and may be uncomfortable. Others believe that it should be done in most cases to avoid the stretching and tearing. In countries where episiotomies are seldom used, there is an increased incidence of protrusions of the bladder or rectum into the vagina in older women who have had several children. This problem is thought to be related to the damage to the tissues that sometimes occurs if no episiotomy is done. However, many women who deliver without an episiotomy do not have this problem. Much depends on the strength and flexibility of your muscles and tissues and the size of your baby.

The first part of the baby to emerge is usually its head. Then the shoulders are delivered and the rest of the body slips out easily. After emerging, the baby will take a first breath and cry a first cry. When the baby begins breathing, oxygen is received through the lungs rather than through the placenta and the umbilical cord. At this time the cord is clamped and cut.

There is no need to become alarmed if forceps are used to assist in the delivery of your baby. Forceps are metal instruments, shaped somewhat like a pair of large spoons, which fit against the sides of the baby's head and are used to guide it through the birth canal. Marks commonly caused by the forceps may remain on the baby's cheeks for several days and are not indicative of any problem. Forceps are often used if an emergency delivery is necessary as in the case of "fetal distress" or bleeding. However, if these problems occur early in labor, before the cervix is fully dilated, a cesarean section may be necessary. Sometimes forceps are used because the mother is too exhausted to push the baby out or because the baby's head is tilted in a position that makes spontaneous delivery very difficult. Some doctors believe that premature babies should always be delivered with forceps to protect the head from the pressure of the birth canal.

A device sometimes used as a substitute for forceps is a vacuum extractor, a plastic or metal suction cup that is placed over the baby's head to guide it through the vagina. While a vacuum extractor does not leave

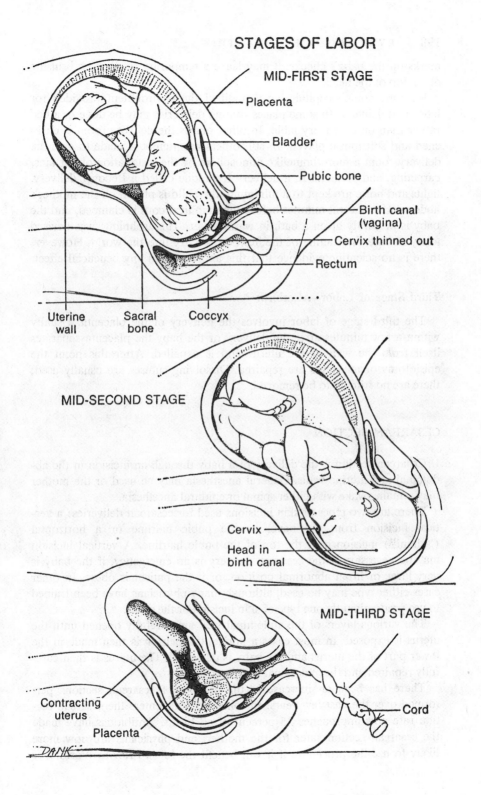

STAGES OF LABOR

MID-FIRST STAGE

Placenta

Bladder

Pubic bone

Birth canal (vagina)

Cervix thinned out

Rectum

Uterine wall

Sacral bone

Coccyx

MID-SECOND STAGE

Cervix

Head in birth canal

MID-THIRD STAGE

Contracting uterus

Placenta

Cord

DANK

marks on the baby's cheeks, it may leave a temporary swelling or bruising of the top of the head.

Recently some hospitals have modified the environment provided for labor and delivery. In some places routine deliveries may be done in a bed rather than on a delivery table. In other places the delivery room is darkened and soft music played. In still others an attempt is made to give the delivery room a more homelike atmosphere by the installation of curtains, carpeting, and pictures. In a delivery technique called a Leboyer delivery, lights and noise are kept to a minimum, the child is placed on the mother's abdomen for several minutes before the umbilical cord is clamped, and the baby is promptly given a bath in warm water. This technique was devised to try to ease the trauma of the newborn's entry into the world. However, there is no scientific evidence that this approach has any beneficial effect.

Third Stage of Labor—Afterbirth

The third stage of labor involves the delivery of the placenta. Usually within a few minutes after the delivery of the baby the placenta separates itself from the wall of the uterus and is expelled. After this point the episiotomy or any tears are repaired. Dissolving sutures are usually used; there are no stitches to be removed.

CESAREAN SECTION

Cesarean section is the delivery of a baby through an incision in the abdominal and uterine walls. General anesthesia may be used or the mother may remain awake with either spinal or epidural anesthesia.

There are two types of skin incisions used for cesarean deliveries: a vertical incision from the navel to the pubic hairline or a horizontal ("bikini") incision near the top of the pubic hairline. A vertical incision may be necessary if the cesarean delivery is an emergency, if the baby is very large or in an abnormal position, or if the patient is obese. In other cases either type may be used, although many physicians have been trained to use predominantly one type of skin incision or the other.

The various layers of the abdominal wall are carefully opened until the uterus is exposed. In most cases a horizontal incision is then made in the lower part of the uterus and the baby is delivered. The uterus is then carefully repaired and the abdominal wall is closed.

There has been an increase in the number of cesarean sections performed over the past few years. In some medical centers the cesarean section rate now approaches 25 percent of all births. Antibiotics have made the cesarean section safer for the mother, and physicians are now more likely to use the procedure if it will benefit the fetus. Prior to World War

II the dangers involved in the operation often outweighed other risks for the mother or the baby in a long and difficult vaginal delivery.

Cesarean section may be necessary if the baby is in a position that makes vaginal delivery difficult or potentially dangerous. For example, 4 percent of all babies are in the breech position (either buttocks or feet first) at the end of pregnancy. The baby's head is the largest part of the baby that must pass through the mother's pelvic bones. When a baby is born head first, the head has a chance to elongate and thus decrease in diameter in order to pass through the pelvic bones. When the baby is breech, the head does not have a chance to accommodate itself to the mother's pelvic bones, and some babies born breech suffer permanent damage. For this reason many doctors now advise a cesarean section in all cases of breech babies unless there is specific evidence that the mother's pelvic bones are large enough to accommodate the baby's head. The evidence of adequate pelvic bones could come either from the history of a previous delivery of a large baby, from a physician's examination of the mother and fetus, or from pelvic X-rays. Even if the pelvis is large, other factors involving the position of the breech baby's arms or legs may influence the physician to recommend a cesarean section.

A position that makes vaginal delivery impossible is a transverse lie (across the pelvic opening, neither the head nor buttocks down). Unless the baby can be turned into a normal position, it cannot be born vaginally and must be delivered by cesarean section.

Sometimes a cesarean section must be done for the safety of the mother. If the mother has severe pre-eclampsia, severe high blood pressure may be life-threatening to her. If labor cannot be quickly induced, a cesarean section may have to be done. Similarly, any danger to your baby, as evidenced by a drop in the baby's heart rate, may cause your doctor to recommend a cesarean section.

After a cesarean section, you will probably be in the hospital for about a week. As with most abdominal operations, you will receive intravenous fluids for a few days. Moving around will be difficult, but forcing yourself to get up and walk will probably speed your recovery. You will need more rest than if you had a vaginal delivery. Not only is your body going through the adjustment of getting back to a nonpregnant state, but it must also recover from a major abdominal operation.

Until recently most physicians in the U.S. have done repeat cesarean sections routinely on all women who have had a previous one, because of concerns about the uterus rupturing during labor. Now many physicians feel that if neither the reason for the previous section(s), nor any other reason for doing one, is present, a vaginal delivery may be safe. For example, if a past cesarean section was done for a breech baby but this is a vertex baby, vaginal delivery may be possible. On the other hand, if the woman has a small pelvis, cesarean section must always be done. If a vaginal de-

POSITIONS OF THE FETUS

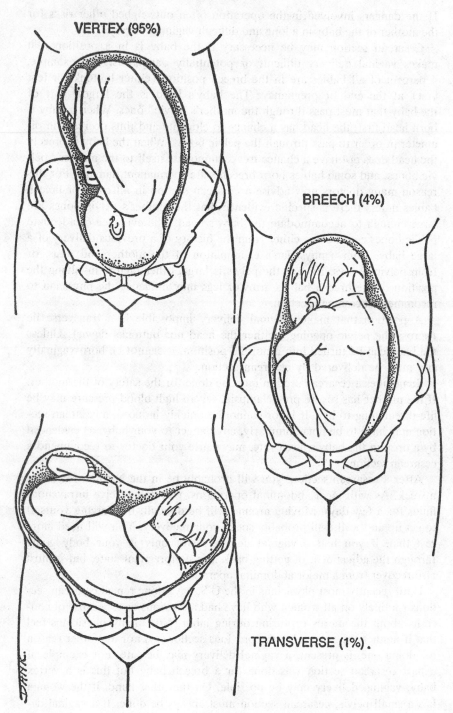

VERTEX (95%)

BREECH (4%)

TRANSVERSE (1%)

livery is planned for a woman who has had a previous section, it is essential that she be in a hospital where a section can be done immediately if it becomes necessary. If you have had a cesarean section, talk with your doctor early in your pregnancy about how your baby will be delivered.

AFTER THE DELIVERY

Your baby has been born and you are probably elated. You hold your baby in amazement at this new life. But labor has been aptly named and you have been working very hard and are exhausted. You very likely have missed a night's sleep and you will probably sleep soundly for a few hours after the baby is born.

Rooming-in

Many hospitals have made "rooming-in" available to mothers. Perhaps you have just had a baby girl. Rooming-in allows you to be with her, care for her, feed her, bathe her, and change her under the supervision of the hospital's nursing staff. Some hospitals offer a modified rooming-in where you can take your baby during the day, but have her cared for in the nursery at night. Others allow you to rest for the first day or two before you take the baby both day and night. The baby is usually taken out of the room when you have visitors.

If you are at all apprehensive about caring for your new baby, rooming-in provides excellent practice with trained people to answer your questions and to give you assistance. Recent experimental evidence, mostly from animal studies, seems to show that prolonged early contact between mother and child (called bonding) may be beneficial to the health and well-being of both mother and child. Rooming-in allows more contact between mother and child during these important early days.

However, you should consider your feelings and physical condition after the delivery. When you leave the hospital, you will be returning to your care of the household with the additional attention and energy the baby requires. If you're very tired and want to take advantage of your days in the hospital to recover your strength, rooming-in is not essential.

The "Baby Blues"

After the first day or two of excitement, many women experience some form of postpartum depression, the "baby blues." Many things contribute to it—the letdown after nine months of anticipating the birth, hormonal changes accompanying the start of the flow of milk, fatigue from labor, anxiety about the realities of having a baby who needs taking care of. This depression is usually very short-lived—a few bouts of tears and you are on your way home.

However, this depression may recur periodically in the first few months after birth as your body continues to make major adjustments in returning to the nonpregnant state, as you deal with your new role and activities, especially if it is a first child, and as you simply go through the physical stress of not having an uninterrupted night's sleep. Again, the feelings of depression usually pass quickly.

A few women do find that these feelings persist and intensify. If you even begin to feel that they are overwhelming, talk to your physician and consider getting some help in coping with them.

Physical Recovery

After delivery you will have vaginal bleeding. The blood comes from the uterus and is called lochia. Lochia will be heavy and bright red for the first few days after delivery. Thereafter the flow decreases, but may persist as a brown staining lasting for several weeks. If you are breast-feeding, there may be an increase in lochia at feeding time. You may also feel cramps during feedings. You may feel your uterus as a firm grapefruit-sized or larger mass in your lower abdomen. The uterus will return to almost normal size within a month.

If you do not nurse, your first menstrual period may come in six to eight weeks, although it may be delayed for several months. If you do nurse, your first menstrual period will normally be later. Some women have no menses while they nurse; others resume having menstrual periods after four to six months.

The return of fertility is also variable and unpredictable. Some women ovulate within a month after delivery and before their first menstrual period, while in others it takes much longer. Though breast-feeding may reduce your chances of becoming pregnant, you cannot count on this alone to prevent pregnancy. Many women ovulate and become pregnant while nursing. Whether you are nursing or not, if you do not wish to have another baby right away, it is important to use some form of contraception as soon as you resume having sexual relations. Most physicians recommend waiting at least two weeks before resuming sexual relations. Some recommend waiting until after the postpartum checkup, four to six weeks after delivery.

If you have had an episiotomy you may find the stitches quite uncomfortable, especially for the first day or two, and you may be given a mild pain medication. The pain will gradually decrease, although it may last for several days or weeks. Pain with sexual intercourse may last for several months after the episiotomy is healed. Conscious tightening and relaxation of the perineal muscles surrounding the episiotomy both aids in healing and in decreasing the pain of the episiotomy. This exercise also helps a normal tone to return to these muscles.

Hemorrhoids are varicose veins in the rectal area and are very common in pregnant women, even those who have no evidence of varicose veins in any other place. They develop during pregnancy because of the pressure on the veins from the growing uterus and are aggravated by the constipation that is common in pregnancy. Hemorrhoids often worsen at the end of pregnancy and during labor. In the first few days after delivery you may need an anesthetic cream to help reduce the discomfort. Fortunately, in most women hemorrhoids disappear or become asymptomatic within a few months after delivery.

Some women experience difficulty in urination after delivery. The baby's head presses against the bladder while moving through the birth canal, and this pressure can result in a decrease in the normal sensation in this area for a time after delivery. Anesthetics used in labor and delivery can also decrease the sensation of the bladder. The reduced sensation can cause difficulty in control of urination or difficulty in knowing when the bladder is full. Sensation and control gradually return to normal after delivery.

If you weigh yourself on the day after delivery, you will probably find that you have lost only about 12 to 16 pounds. The weight gained in pregnancy is more than just the weight of the baby, the placenta, and the amniotic fluid. For example, the breasts normally increase by about 1 pound, blood volume increase accounts for about 3½ pounds, and the uterus increases by 2½ pounds. The mother's body also retains fluid and a small amount of fat is deposited. Most mothers shed an additional 5 pounds in the first two weeks after delivery. Since mothers who nurse use up some of the additional fat that has been deposited during pregnancy, mothers who do not nurse may have to go on a more restrictive diet than nursing mothers in order to return to their normal prepregnancy weight.

The stretch marks (striae) that may have developed on your abdomen or breasts will gradually fade, but will not disappear completely. In spite of many available ointments and home remedies, there is no prevention or cure for a stretch mark.

Breast-Feeding

During pregnancy the glands in your breasts develop in order to produce milk after the baby is born. During the last few months there may be leakage of a small amount of colostrum, a thin yellow fluid. Shortly after delivery the amount of colostrum increases substantially and colostrum is the only food that breast-fed babies receive during the first few days of their life. On the third or fourth postpartum day, production of milk begins. The amount of milk that is produced depends on the amount of stimulation and sucking by the baby. The repeated emptying of the breasts increases the milk supply to meet the needs of a growing baby.

Breast milk is the ideal food for a baby. The Committee on Nutrition of the American Academy of Pediatrics recommends that every mother breast-feed her baby unless there is a specific medical reason why she cannot. I would urge every woman who thinks she might be interested in breast-feeding to give it a try. Almost all women who really want to can do so if given the proper support and encouragement. I would recommend that every pregnant woman read one of several excellent books available on the subject (see Further Reading at end of chapter). If you have not yet decided about breast-feeding, try talking with a woman who has nursed her baby.

The good nutritional habits of pregnancy must be continued during breast-feeding. Most women require more calories each day during nursing than they did during pregnancy. For advice on nutrition while breast-feeding, see "Nutrition and Weight," pp. 36–65.

Breast infections are not uncommon in nursing mothers, but if promptly treated they need not be serious. A breast infection may result from a clogged milk duct or from a small crack in the nipple. The infected breast is hot and tender to touch, and the woman may have a fever or feel weak and generally ill. Notify your physician promptly if you have any evidence of a breast infection. Usually antibiotics can be given and nursing can continue when the infection improves. If the infection is not treated soon enough, an abscess may develop (a localized collection of pus in the breast). An abscess may respond to antibiotics or may require surgical drainage. Even after this complication breast-feeding may be continued if desired.

One of the most difficult problems for a breast-feeding mother is not knowing the amount of milk that her baby is receiving. In the early weeks of life babies often cry for unexplained reasons. The bottle-feeding mother knows how much formula the baby took at the last feeding and can feel with confidence that hunger is not the problem. A breast-feeding mother may worry that the baby is hungry and that her milk supply is inadequate. These doubts may lead her to substitute a bottle at the next feeding or give a supplementary bottle. The baby then nurses less and as a result her milk supply is decreased. If a mother's milk production is insufficient, continued stimulation by frequent nursing will usually increase the supply. It is important to remember that for thousands of years before infant formulas were available, all babies were raised on breast milk alone.

Alternatively, many women prefer and enjoy the many advantages of bottle-feeding their babies. Perhaps they are planning to return to work in a short time or they are afraid that they will be tied down. To some mothers the idea of breast-feeding is simply not appealing. If you feel this way, it is better to make your choice and abide with it. A woman who breast-feeds only because her friends or doctor have urged her to do so is rarely successful.

If you decide not to breast-feed you will experience a few days of discomfort from about the third to sixth day after delivery. Your breasts may feel full and may leak a small amount of milk. Your breasts should be tightly bound to maintain pressure on them in order to decrease the production of milk and to relieve the discomfort that you may experience. If the breasts are not emptied, the production of milk ceases and the milk already in the breasts is eventually absorbed.

This, then, is the story of childbirth. Too often when I was pregnant, I thought of the labor and delivery as an endpoint. So many thoughts during pregnancy are directed toward that long awaited day. Of course, I knew that I would go home from the hospital with a baby, but when I was pregnant it was difficult to think of the growing, kicking lump in my abdomen as a real person. I soon found that instead of being the end, delivery is only the beginning of much more. I'm continually amazed at how quickly a child grows and develops. To laugh with a child, to play with him on the floor, to watch as he struggles to crawl or stand is a genuine pleasure. My son is still young and there are many things we haven't faced yet such as toilet training or nursery school, let alone adolescence and summer camp.

It's not always easy with a busy career and a growing child. The living room furniture has been crowded into a corner to make way for a playpen and baby swing. The coffee table often has little fingerprints on it. There are many things that I don't have much time for any more—needlepoint, dinner parties, the movies and museums—but I enjoy spending as much time as possible with my son. He has brought many changes into our lives, but most significantly he has given us great joy and happiness.

FURTHER READING

Bean, Constance A. *Methods of Childbirth*. New York: Dolphin, 1974.

Brewer, Gail S. and Tom Brewer. *What Every Pregnant Woman Should Know: The Truth About Diet and Drugs in Pregnancy*. New York: Random House, 1977.

Campbell, A. *Your Pregnancy Year*. New York: Doubleday, 1979.

Colman, Arthur and L. Colman. *Pregnancy: The Psychological Experience*. New York: Bantam, 1977.

Eiger, Marvin and Sally Olds. *The Complete Book of Breast Feeding*. New York: Workman, 1973.

Parfitt, Rebecca R. *The Birth Primer*. Philadelphia: Running Press, 1977.

Infertility

KATHRYN SCHROTENBOER, M.D.

Assistant Attending Physician, Obstetrics and Gynecology,
New York Hospital–Cornell Medical Center
Clinical Instructor, Cornell Medical School

Infertility is usually defined as one year of intercourse without contraception that does not result in pregnancy. Various studies have shown that from 65 to 90 percent of all couples who conceive spontaneously will do so within the first year of trying, and 90 to 95 percent will achieve pregnancy within the first two years. However, fertility and infertility are not always absolutes. "Reduced fertility" would be a better term than infertility in those cases where pregnancy is possible, but takes longer than an average time to achieve.

At least one couple out of ten will experience some difficulty in becoming pregnant. This may be a trying experience as their friends and neighbors are having children and relatives keep asking questions, while month after month goes by without any sign of pregnancy. Unwanted infertility can put a tremendous strain on a marriage as well as on the individual partners.

A professional evaluation of infertility may add to the humiliation and sense of failure. The reproductive capacity of both partners will be examined and their sexual relations timed to comply with a doctor's suggestions. There is often an emotional toll when a man is told that his sperm count is below normal or a woman learns she does not produce enough of the necessary hormones. It may be particularly difficult for a woman to find herself infertile if she had a previous pregnancy voluntarily terminated because it was unplanned or inconvenient.

Great advances have been made in the study of infertility in the last twenty years. There are improved diagnostic techniques, such as blood hormone tests and laparoscopy. There are improved surgical techniques and better treatment for medical problems, chronic illnesses, and infections.

Since there are many causes of infertility, there are many tests to evaluate an infertile couple. Often there is more than one contributing factor. Most infertility problems in women are handled by obstetrician-gynecologists; the male partner may be referred to a urologist. In larger cities or at a university hospital, there may be an infertility clinic or a physician who specializes in infertility problems.

CAUSES OF MALE INFERTILITY

Male factors are estimated to cause about 40 percent of all infertility problems. The production of sperm may be affected by congenital and genetic abnormalities, injuries to the genital tract, heat, age, acute and chronic infection, malnutrition, previous surgery, allergies, chronic illness, stress, radiation, varicocele, or certain medications. Sexual dysfunction—impotence or inability to ejaculate—may result from stress, alcoholism, or drug addiction, or certain medications.

Varicocele, a varicose enlargement of the veins of the spermatic cord, is a potentially curable cause of male infertility. Varicocele occurs in many men with normal fertility, but infertile men have a much higher percentage of varicocele, up to 40 percent. Half of all men with varicoceles have decreased sperm count or sperm motility or other changes in the semen analysis. Theories of the cause of these changes include heat, pressure, and toxic substances from the dilated vessels.

Permanent or temporary damage to the male testis can occur as a result of a genital infection or a systemic infection. Gonorrhea may do enough damage to the male genital tract to temporarily cause a marked decrease in the sperm count. Mumps in an adult male may involve one or both testicles, resulting in severe testicular damage. Fortunately, usually only one testicle is involved severely and the sperm count, though possibly reduced, is usually compatible with fertility. Any systemic viral or bacterial infection may cause a temporary depression in the sperm count.

TESTS FOR MALE INFERTILITY

Since many of the infertility tests for women are more complicated and involve more risk than those for men, infertility testing often begins with the man. A semen analysis is a simple test that can provide a great deal of information. The male is asked to submit a recently ejaculated semen specimen to the physician or laboratory. This specimen is then examined mi-

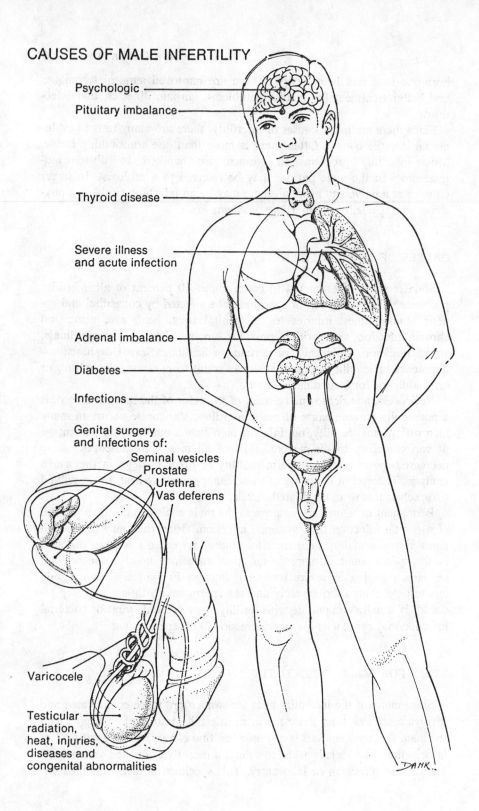

CAUSES OF MALE INFERTILITY

Psychologic

Pituitary imbalance

Thyroid disease

Severe illness
and acute infection

Adrenal imbalance

Diabetes

Infections

Genital surgery
and infections of:
    Seminal vesicles
    Prostate
    Urethra
    Vas deferens

Varicocele

Testicular
radiation,
heat, injuries,
diseases and
congenital abnormalities

DANK.

croscopically to count the number of sperm and to determine if they are of normal size and shape and if they are able to move normally. There is no sharp line of demarcation between fertility and sterility in the sperm count. Counts of less than 20 to 40 million per cubic centimeter are often correlated with decreased fertility, although men with counts of 5 to 10 million have fathered children. A high percentage of sperm with abnormal shape, size, or decreased motility is also correlated with decreased fertility.

TREATMENT FOR MALE INFERTILITY

Some causes of male infertility are sometimes correctable. A varicocele may be surgically treated to improve fertility. Treatment of a chronic infection can allow a previously infertile man to become fertile. In some situations decreasing the intake of alcohol or certain drugs or modifying medications given in treatment of a chronic illness can improve a man's fertility. In other cases administration of various hormones can increase a borderline sperm count enough to make conception possible. These hormones include testosterone, thyroid hormone, and cortisone. In some situations clomiphene citrate, a medication that is used to induce ovulation in infertile women, may also be given to a man.

CAUSES OF FEMALE INFERTILITY

Fifty to 60 percent of fertility problems are attributable to women. Abnormalities of the fallopian tubes, including scarring from endometriosis or previous infections or surgery, or swelling from a current infection account for about 20 to 30 percent of all infertility problems. Problems with ovulation are thought to be the cause of infertility in about 10 to 15 percent of all cases. Chronic diseases such as thyroid disease, uncontrolled diabetes, or liver disease usually cause infertility by interfering with the complex mechanism of ovulation. In approximately 5 percent of the cases there is a problem with the cervix or cervical mucus. The cause for at least 10 percent of all infertility is unclear.

Endometriosis is a condition where tissue that looks like endometrial tissue (the tissue which lines the uterus and is shed each month in menstruation) is located outside of the uterus. Whether this develops from a backflow of endometrial tissue during menstruation into and beyond the fallopian tubes or an "embryological mistake" whereby endometrial cells develop in an incorrect location is uncertain. Endometriosis is usually located only on the pelvic organs surrounding the uterus, but in rare instances it can be found in other places such as the upper abdomen or lung.

These areas of endometriosis may bleed at the time of the menstrual pe-

CAUSES OF FEMALE INFERTILITY

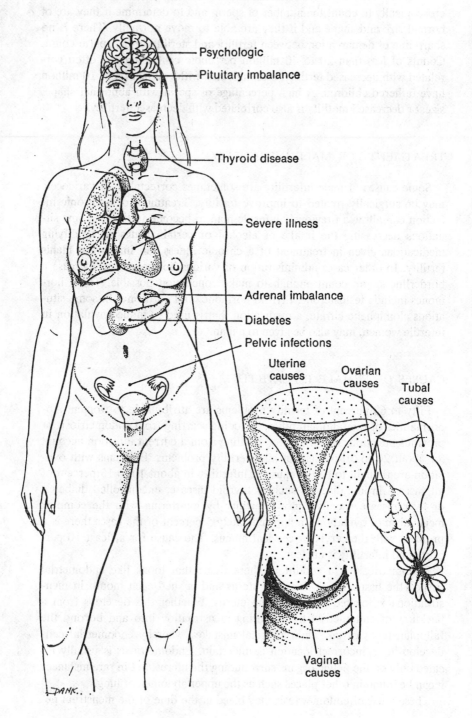

Psychologic

Pituitary imbalance

Thyroid disease

Severe illness

Adrenal imbalance

Diabetes

Pelvic infections

Uterine causes

Ovarian causes

Tubal causes

Vaginal causes

DANK.

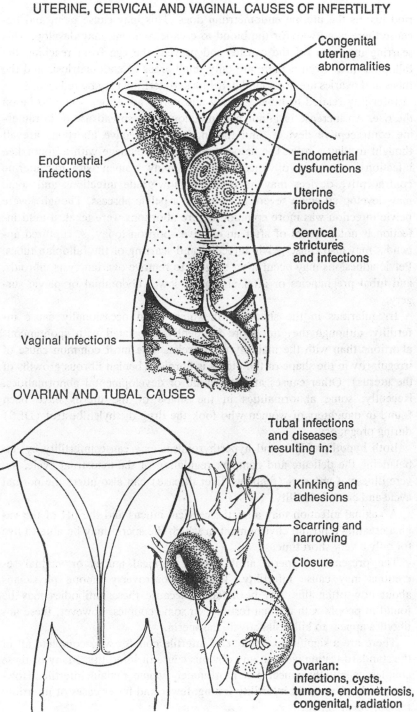

UTERINE, CERVICAL AND VAGINAL CAUSES OF INFERTILITY

Congenital
uterine
abnormalities

Endometrial
dysfunctions

Uterine
fibroids

**Cervical
strictures
and infections**

Endometrial
infections

Vaginal Infections

OVARIAN AND TUBAL CAUSES

**Tubal infections
and diseases
resulting in:**

**Kinking and
adhesions**

**Scarring and
narrowing**

Closure

**Ovarian:
infections, cysts,
tumors, endometriosis,
congenital, radiation**

riod just as the uterine endometrium does. This may cause pain, and because there is no way for the blood to escape, scarring may develop. This scarring may seal off the ovaries and prevent the egg from reaching the fallopian tube. Even if there are only small areas of endometriosis and the tubes and ovaries are not completely blocked, fertility may be reduced.

Infertility related to tubal scarring and pelvic adhesions seems to be on the rise. An increase in gonorrhea infections, widespread use of intrauterine contraceptive devices, and the increase in elective abortions are all thought to play a role. The association of tubal damage with a gonorrhea infection is the most obvious. However, many women with intrauterine contraceptive devices may have chronic low-grade infections and some may develop an acute severe infection or a pelvic abscess. Though severe pelvic infection was more common before abortions were legal, a mild infection is not unheard of after an elective abortion today. A ruptured appendix may also cause pelvic infection and scarring of the fallopian tubes. Pelvic adhesions may occur after surgery to remove ovarian cysts, fibroids, and tubal pregnancies or after any other lower abdominal or pelvic surgery.

Irregularities in the shape of the uterus can occasionally cause infertility, although they are more frequently associated with spontaneous abortions than with the inability to conceive. The most common cause of irregularity in the shape of the uterus is fibroids (benign fibrous growths of the uterus). Other causes are congenital or developmental abnormalities. Recently, some abnormalities in the shape of the uterus have been found in daughters of women who took the drug diethylstilbestrol (DES) during pregnancy.

Both hypothyroidism and hyperthyroidism may cause infertility by unbalancing the delicate and complex regulation of the menstrual cycle. Severe illness of any sort (diabetes, liver disease) can also affect the normal cycle and cause infertility.

A vaginal infection may alter the cervical mucus and the pH of the vagina creating a hostile environment in which the sperm may be able to live for only a very short time.

The presence of sperm antibodies in cervical mucus or vaginal secretions may cause infertility. There is controversy among physicians about how often this may be a factor because these antibodies may be found in people with normal fertility. In some couples, however, these antibodies appear to kill or inactivate the sperm.

There are a significant number of infertile couples who complete all of the standard testing without any obvious cause of infertility. Many of these couples eventually conceive. Unfortunately, some remain infertile. However, with advances in infertility testing, fewer and fewer cases of infertility remain unexplained.

TESTS FOR FEMALE INFERTILITY

Basal Body Temperatures

Keeping a record of basal body temperatures can be helpful in establishing whether or not a woman ovulates. Every morning, immediately after waking up and before any activity, the woman takes her temperature. Special thermometers are available for this purpose which are somewhat easier to read than regular thermometers. Before ovulation morning oral temperatures usually range from 97.0 to 97.5° Fahrenheit (morning temperatures can be a degree lower than those taken later in the day). After ovulation, because of the effect of increased levels of progesterone, morning temperatures are usually 98.0° Fahrenheit or above until menstruation occurs. Ovulation usually occurs during the day before the temperature rise. Therefore, an accurately recorded temperature chart which shows low temperatures in the early part of the menstrual cycle and higher temperatures for the last 14 days is presumptive evidence that ovulation has occurred.

Endometrial Biopsy

Another test to help determine if ovulation is occurring is an endometrial biopsy. This test is usually performed on the first day of the period or in the week before a period is expected. An endometrial biopsy normally can be done in the physician's office without the use of anesthesia. A speculum is inserted into the vagina and the cervix is grasped with an instrument called a tenaculum which may cause a slight pinching sensation. Then a small, thin instrument is inserted into the uterine cavity to take the biopsy. This procedure may cause a brief cramping sensation. The removed tissue is sent to a laboratory to be examined microscopically. As well as confirming whether ovulation has occurred, this test sometimes can identify other causes of infertility such as infection and certain rare causes of infertility. Though rarely a problem, this test has the theoretical risk of interrupting an early pregnancy, so if there is any chance that the patient may be pregnant, it should not be done.

Hormone Tests

Measurement of blood and urinary hormone levels can help to give evidence whether or not a woman is ovulating. For example, progesterone levels in the blood rise after ovulation and a blood test taken after ovulation will reflect this. However, many authorities still consider the endometrial biopsy the most accurate proof that ovulation has occurred.

TESTS FOR INFERTILITY

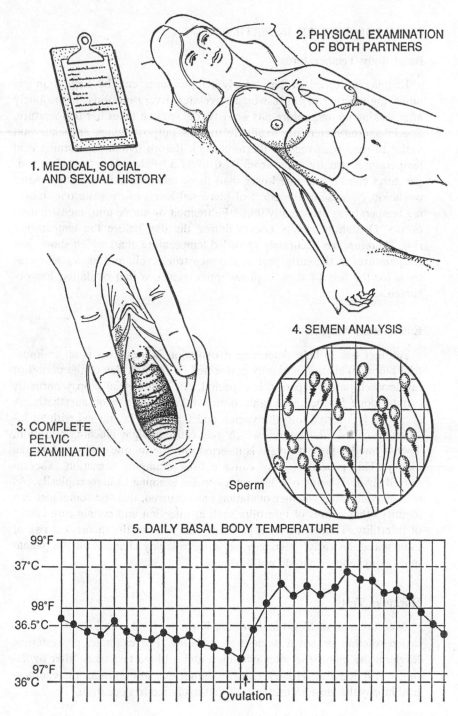

1. MEDICAL, SOCIAL AND SEXUAL HISTORY

2. PHYSICAL EXAMINATION OF BOTH PARTNERS

3. COMPLETE PELVIC EXAMINATION

4. SEMEN ANALYSIS

Sperm

5. DAILY BASAL BODY TEMPERATURE

99°F
37°C
98°F
36.5°C
97°F
36°C

Ovulation

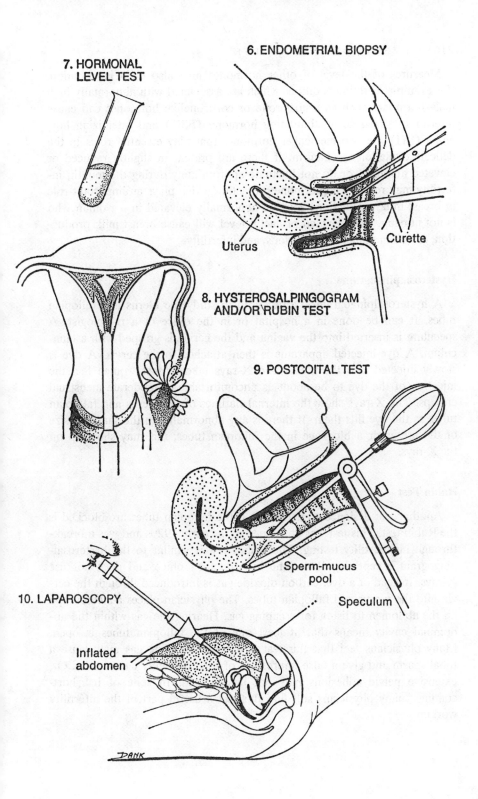

7. HORMONAL LEVEL TEST

6. ENDOMETRIAL BIOPSY

Uterus

Curette

8. HYSTEROSALPINGOGRAM AND/OR RUBIN TEST

9. POSTCOITAL TEST

Sperm-mucus pool

Speculum

10. LAPAROSCOPY

Inflated abdomen

DANK

Measures of the level of other hormones may also yield information. For example, certain conditions which are associated with abnormally high male hormones such as testosterone or cortisonelike hormones can cause infertility. Also follicle-stimulating hormone (FSH) and luteinizing hormone (LH) are two messenger hormones that play essential roles in the delicate ovulation mechanism. If these are present in slightly reduced or elevated amounts, or do not fluctuate appropriately during the month, infertility may result. The hormone prolactin (which plays an important role in breast milk production) may be abnormally elevated in a woman who is not nursing. The elevated prolactin level will cause breast milk production, cessation of menstrual periods, and infertility.

Hysterosalpingogram

A hysterosalpingogram is a test used to study the uterus and fallopian tubes. It can be done in a hospital or in the office of a radiologist. A speculum is inserted into the vagina and the cervix is grasped with a tenaculum. A dye-injected apparatus is then attached to the cervix. A dye is slowly injected into the uterus and X-rays taken. Most women feel the injection of the dye to be about as uncomfortable as moderate menstrual cramps. The X-rays show the internal outlines of the uterus and fallopian tubes as the dye fills them. If there is any abnormality in the shape or size of the uterus or a blockage in the fallopian tubes, this may show up on the X-rays.

Rubin Test

Another test designed to determine if the fallopian tubes are blocked is the Rubin test. This test was developed in the early 1920s and was a breakthrough in infertility testing. The Rubin test is similar to the hysterosalpingogram except that it is done in a doctor's office and does not use X-rays. Instead of a dye, carbon dioxide gas is introduced through the cervix into the uterus and fallopian tubes. The physician places a stethoscope on the abdomen to listen for escaping gas. Hearing the gas within the abdominal cavity means that at least one of the fallopian tubes is open. Many physicians feel that this test is not reliable. The gas may cause a tubal spasm and give a false impression of a permanently closed tube. Or, extensive pelvic adhesions may not be detected. In spite of its shortcomings many physicians still find this test a useful part of the infertility workup.

Postcoital Test

A postcoital test (PC test) is a painless, simple test that often can yield important information in the evaluation of an infertile couple. This test is done around the time of ovulation. You must come to the physician's office within a specified number of hours after intercourse. A speculum examination is done and a small sample of the cervical mucus and vaginal fluid are taken and examined microscopically. This examination will show if the cervical mucus is normal, if the sperm are active and alive, and if there is any evidence of sperm antibodies.

Laparoscopy

Laparoscopy is often the final step in an infertility workup. This is done in a hospital, usually with general anesthesia, though local anesthesia can be used. A small incision is made just below the navel and a long needle is inserted into the abdominal cavity. The abdominal cavity is filled with carbon dioxide gas. The laparoscope, a long, narrow, lighted tube, is inserted into the abdominal cavity and the pelvic organs can be seen. Dye is injected into the uterus. The physician can look through the laparoscope and see whether the dye spills out of the ends of the fallopian tubes, thus determining if the tubes are open or blocked. In addition, laparoscopy can diagnose endometriosis, pelvic adhesions, and previous pelvic infections.

TREATMENT FOR FEMALE INFERTILITY

Once the probable causes of infertility have been identified, treatment can begin. If irregular ovulation or lack of ovulation is the problem, ovulation may be induced with medication. These medications are the well known fertility drugs. It is important to remember that these fertility drugs are helpful only if the infertility is caused by a problem with ovulation and cannot help at all if the infertility is caused by something else.

The most commonly used medication to induce ovulation is called Clomid (clomiphene citrate). Through its effect on the hypothalamus clomiphene citrate stimulates a release of FSH and LH from the pituitary. FSH and LH are the hormones that act on the ovary to cause the ripening and release of eggs. The medication is taken in the form of a pill for five days during the month. Minor side effects include hot flashes and lower abdominal discomfort. Clomiphene citrate substantially increases the chances of having twins by stimulating two eggs to ripen instead of one. It increases the chances of having triplets and quadruplets only minimally.

In rare cases a second type of fertility medication must be used. This medication is called Pergonal (or human menopausal gonadotropin) and must be given by injection every day until ovulation occurs. This treatment is both costly and time-consuming, and a woman must be closely watched for any adverse side effects. By causing several eggs to ripen at one time, this medication can cause triplets or quadruplets. Serious side effects of Pergonal include large ovarian cysts and massive shifts in body fluids.

Problems with the fallopian tubes usually must be treated surgically. The fallopian tubes may have been blocked as a result of a congenital abnormality, of scarring subsequent to a previous pelvic infection or to endometriosis, or of previous pelvic surgery. Sometimes the fallopian tubes themselves are normal, but adhesions surrounding them prevent the egg and sperm from meeting.

There is a reasonable chance that the surgical removal of the adhesions will improve fertility. Unfortunately, when repairing the fallopian tube requires major reconstructive surgery (tuboplasty), the success rate is much lower. Even when it is possible to open the fallopian tubes, tubal function does not always return to normal, and the infertility may persist. It is possible that recent developments in microsurgery, delicate surgery done with the aid of microscopes and very fine instruments, may improve the success rate of tubal surgery.

Treatment of endometriosis may improve fertility. In some cases the treatment is surgical; large areas of endometriosis are removed and adhesions that have formed by the scarring are opened. In other cases the treatment is medical. Endometriosis is known to improve during pregnancy and after menopause, and medication may be given to induce a pseudopregnancy or pseudomenopause state. Female hormones, such as progesterone or combinations of estrogen and progesterone, can be given in high enough doses to prevent menstruation for six to nine months, causing a regression of the endometriosis over this period of time (pseudopregnancy). Alternatively, the regression can be caused by giving danazol, a new antiestrogen drug, which can prevent menstrual bleeding for six to seven months (pseudomenopause). After the medications are stopped, normal menstrual cycles begin again and pregnancy may occur.

Other treatments are available for other specific causes of infertility. For example, treatment of a vaginal infection may correct the infertility. Sometimes problems with the cervical mucus may be treated by the administration of low doses of estrogen. Sperm antibodies may disappear if no sperm are present for six months, so the use of a condom or sexual abstinence may make future fertility possible. If there is a medical problem, such as thyroid disease, treatment of the medical problem may itself correct the infertility.

ARTIFICIAL INSEMINATION

Artificial insemination can be accomplished with sperm from the male partner or a donor. If there is an anatomic defect in either partner preventing the depositing of sperm near the cervix, artificial insemination with the man's semen may be attempted. These defects include hypospadias (abnormal position of the urethral opening) in the man and the abnormal position of the cervix in the woman. This may also be necessary in certain types of sexual dysfunction.

If the man's problem is not correctable, but his partner is fertile, artificial insemination with sperm from an anonymous donor can be attempted. The donor, usually matched to the man in coloring and body build, is found personally or through a sperm bank by the woman's physician. At the time of ovulation the donor sperm is injected into the woman's vagina at the cervical os with a syringe.

With few children available for adoption today, artificial insemination is the only way that some couples can have a child. However, artificial insemination with donor sperm is not something to be undertaken lightly. It raises countless psychological, moral, religious, and legal questions. Some men cannot cope with the fact that they are not the biologic father of their child, while other men feel that a child which has their wife's genes and which they have raised is as much theirs as any child can be.

Couples who choose artificial insemination do not always have the support of others. In fact, some major religious groups feel that artificial insemination with donor sperm is the equivalent of adultery. Many couples who choose artificial insemination do not tell even their families or closest friends.

Over 100,000 children are estimated to have been born by artificial insemination with donor sperm, yet there are many legal questions about these children that have not yet been answered. Some courts in the United States, England, and Canada have held that these children are illegitimate, while other courts have held that a husband who agrees to the artificial insemination of his wife has an obligation to support the child. A few states have passed laws to attempt to clarify the legal position of these children, but further legislation is sorely needed.

Some new developments in infertility treatment may be even more controversial than artificial insemination. In some situations when the man is fertile, but his partner is not, a "surrogate mother" is used. This surrogate mother is impregnated with the man's sperm, becomes pregnant, and after delivery the child is adopted by the infertile couple.

In another new procedure, called in vitro fertilization, a woman's egg is removed surgically from one of her ovaries and fertilized in a glass dish ("test tube"). This fertilized egg is placed in her uterus several days later. To date several women have had babies, all healthy, by this method. It is used for women who have an obstruction of both fallopian tubes but have at least one normally functioning and surgically accessible ovary. These conditions exist in about five to ten percent of infertile women. It is difficult to say what will be the ultimate impact of in vitro fertilization, which at present can be done in only a few medical centers. So far there have been many more attempts than successes.

Though recent advances in infertility have been great, there is much more to be learned. There are still couples whose infertility is unexplained and there are couples with known causes of infertility that cannot be cured. Research continues in this field and solving these problems is part of the goal for the future. Though the testing and the therapy may sometimes be difficult and time-consuming, for many lucky couples it will all be worthwhile when they are finally able to have their long-awaited son or daughter or even both.

FURTHER READING

Harrison, Mary. *Infertility: A Couple's Guide to Its Causes and Treatments.* Boston, Mass.: Houghton Mifflin, 1977.

Menning, Barbara E. *Infertility: A Guide for the Childless Couple.* Englewood Cliffs, N.J.: Prentice-Hall, 1977.

Silber, Sherman, M.D. *How to Get Pregnant.* New York: Scribners, 1980.

Gynecologic Diseases and Treatment

MARY JANE GRAY, M.D.

Professor of Obstetrics and Gynecology,
University of North Carolina Medical School,
Chapel Hill, North Carolina

Gynecology, the medical care of women with special emphasis on problems relating to the reproductive system, becomes of concern to a few women with the onset of menstrual periods, to most women with the beginning of sexual activity, and to all women with recognition of the need for regular examinations and cancer tests. Women need help with menstrual problems, sexual problems, contraception or pregnancy, vaginal infections, sexually transmissible diseases (STD), the menopause, and other problems. Since these conditions concern normal functions as well as disease, the person treating you should be one with whom you can talk comfortably about these conditions and from whom you receive clear and full information.

Most women would like to know more than they do about how their reproductive system functions and what commonly goes wrong with it. Because of dissatisfaction with the care that they have received, some women have left the mainstream of medical care for self-help groups. These groups are excellent for education in normal function and health maintenance and for emotional support; however, they are sometimes short on medical expertise. This chapter is intended to help women understand common gynecologic problems and their treatment (excluding STD and sexual dysfunction, discussed in other chapters) and to give women the knowledge they need to communicate more effectively with their physicians. A review of the anatomy of the female reproductive system and the physiology of normal menstruation will be helpful to the reader at this point (see illustrations pp. 22–23; 27).

FINDING CAUSES OF COMMON PROBLEMS

History

Every physician must depend on the patient's story or history of what has happened in order to be alert to areas of possible problems or to find the cause of an existing problem. Some women are more comfortable talking about headaches or indigestion than about menstrual periods and sex. Nonetheless, if the doctor is to be able to make a good medical evaluation of the health of a patient, he or she must find out as much about the patient as possible. Therefore, the gynecologist will ask about the onset of periods, their previous and present character, pregnancies, and your complete sexual history. It is very important to be honest in answering all questions. If your doctor seems uncomfortable with your life style, find a different doctor.

Pelvic Examination

In order to reach a diagnosis for a gynecologic problem, the woman must be examined. The examination will usually include height, weight, and blood pressure, feeling the thyroid gland, listening to the heart and lungs, and examining the breasts and abdomen before proceeding to the pelvic examination. Laboratory tests will be based on the woman's history and whether the examiner is assuming primary responsibility for this woman's health.

The first part of the pelvic examination is an inspection of the external genitals for lumps, sores, inflammation, and general hormonal status. The folds of skin forming the labia will be separated in order to expose the urinary and vaginal openings. A woman who has had children will often be asked to "bear down" or "strain as if moving your bowels" to demonstrate any weakness of the supporting tissues of the vagina.

Next comes the vaginal examination. After a finger locates the vaginal opening, a speculum is placed inside and opened. The speculum is a metal instrument a little like two shoe horns hinged together. When opened, it holds the vaginal walls apart and allows the examiner to see the vagina and cervix and check for inflammation or signs of infection, damage or growths, lesions, and so forth. A scraping of tissue and samples of discharge are taken for examination under a microscope and for cultures and a pap test. Sometimes the woman may be given a mirror to follow this part of the procedure.

After the speculum is removed, the examiner does a bimanual vaginal examination. By placing two fingers in the vagina and the other hand on the abdominal wall he or she can locate the uterus and ovaries between the

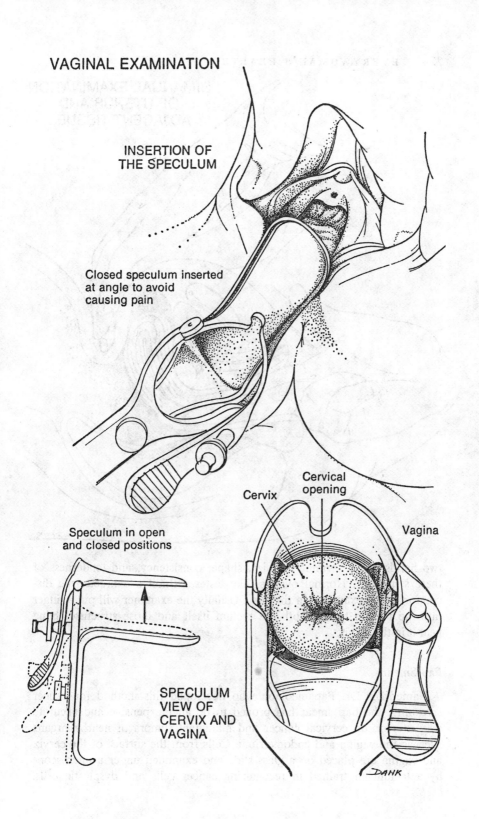

VAGINAL EXAMINATION

INSERTION OF THE SPECULUM

Closed speculum inserted at angle to avoid causing pain

Cervix

Cervical opening

Vagina

Speculum in open and closed positions

SPECULUM VIEW OF CERVIX AND VAGINA

DANK

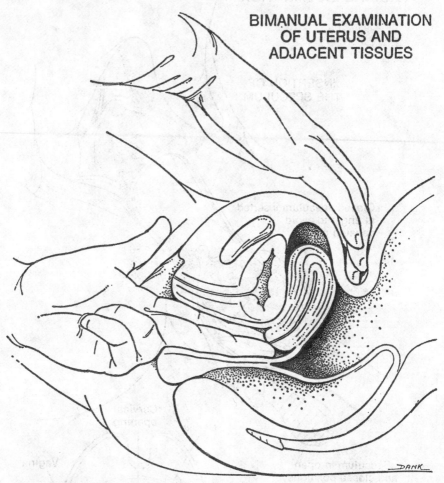

BIMANUAL EXAMINATION OF UTERUS AND ADJACENT TISSUES

two hands and determine the size, shape, consistency, and tenderness of these structures. Normal ovaries, like testes, exhibit a characteristic discomfort when examined in this way. Usually the examiner will put a finger into the rectum to feel both the rectum itself and those structures lying near it in the pelvis.

Pap Smear

Named for Dr. Papanicolaou who developed this method for cancer screening, the pap smear has proved to be an inexpensive and accurate way to pick up cervical cancer and malignant tumors of nearby organs such as the vagina and endometrium. Cells from the surface of the cervix and vagina are placed on a glass slide and examined under a microscope by a technician trained in recognizing cancer cells and dysplastic cells.

Dysplastic cells are cells showing evidence of changes which indicate they might at some time become malignant; dysplasia is the abnormal growth created by the aberrant cells.

Because the pap smear selects a random sample of cells, false negative results are possible when abnormal cells are present, but not sampled. Similarly, false positive readings are obtained when suspicious cells are seen which represent infection and not cancer. Abnormal pap smears must be confirmed by a repeat smear. An abnormal smear suggesting the possibility of cancer must be clarified by a biopsy.

Cytologists (professionals who specialize in detecting cancer cells under a microscope) classify smears as follows:

Class I. Normal smear. Repeat at intervals suggested by your doctor.

Class II. Cells indicative of inflammatory changes, but no evidence of cancerous changes. Inflammation should be treated and the pap smear repeated in six months.

Class III. "Suspicious" cells present indicating dysplasia with no evidence of cancer. Inflammation, if present, should be treated and the pap smear repeated after the next menstrual period.

Class IV. Cells strongly suggest cancer. A biopsy is always taken to confirm or rule out cancer.

Class V. Cancer cells present. Following biopsy, surgery or other treatment is carried out immediately.

A pap smear taken once a year is usually sufficient for early recognition of conditions which require treatment. However, certain conditions, such as previous dysplasia of the cervix, a history of prenatal estrogen medication, or a previous herpes infection, indicate the necessity for more frequent evaluation.

Women are sometimes confused by statements such as one recently issued by the American Cancer Society that a pap smear every three years is enough. In part this reflects an opinion that it would be more cost effective to take a pap smear from every woman in this country every five years than to continue to screen the 20 percent of women who now have the test every year. But this statement is concerned with how to detect the most abnormalities given a limited amount of money for testing. It does not reflect the view of many physicians that women should be screened annually for cancer.

X-ray, Sonography, Laparoscopy, and Colposcopy

If the general examination or pap smear indicates the presence of a problem, but further information is required for an accurate diagnosis, several other diagnostic procedures may be followed.

X-rays may be taken to study the structure and location of organs within the pelvic cavity. X-ray is most effective in showing hard tissue, such as bone or in outlining the urinary and gastrointestinal tracts after the use of contrast material.

Sonography is a technique in which sound waves are sent across the abdomen and their echoes recorded on a screen. The image on the screen is a sonogram. It provides a picture of soft tissue and can be used to determine the size and placement of organs and to detect any abnormal tissue mass, swelling, or fluid collection. The procedure is usually done in the X-ray department of a hospital, but no radiation is involved.

Laparoscopy is a minor surgical procedure in which a lighted viewing tube (a laparoscope) is inserted into the abdomen through a small incision. It allows the visual examination of internal structures. Anesthesia is required, but the procedure can be done without an overnight stay in a hospital.

Colposcopy is the examination of the cervix and vagina with a magnifying device (a colposcope) in order to see details not visible with the naked eye. It is used to identify any cervical or vaginal abnormalities, to examine abnormal surface areas, and to locate specific sites for biopsy if a pap smear indicates the presence of abnormal cells. Since the device enters only the vagina no anesthesia is required and the procedure can be done in a doctor's office.

Biopsy

The biopsy, a surgical procedure, consists of taking a sample of tissue for examination under a microscope to determine whether the tissue is malignant or to identify an unusual growth or infection. In many cases the sample can be taken in the doctor's office with local anesthesia, but biopsies of internal structures or biopsies that involve the removal of a large amount of tissue require full hospitalization and surgery. For example, hospitalization is necessary for a biopsy of an ovary or for a cone biopsy of the cervix, in which a large "cone" of tissue is removed for extensive evaluation.

PROBLEMS AND DISEASES

Menstrual Problems

Too much has been made of the regularity of menstrual periods. No woman starts her first period at 12 and then menstruates every 28 days for 5 days until she reaches the menopause at 49. The magic numbers 12, 28, 5, and 49 are all averages which are not indicative of the wide normal variation. An onset between 9 and 16, an interval from 25 to 35 days, a length from 2 to 7 days, and menopause from 45 to 55 are completely normal. Each woman sets up a pattern that is normal for her. It is also normal for an individual to skip periods in the early teens and again in the years just before the menopause. Periods will not necessarily be the same at 16 as at 26, 36, or 46. Nonetheless, periods can be too heavy, too light, too frequent, or too infrequent. Some of these deviations from normal will be considered.

Delayed onset of periods. Failure to start menstrual periods is termed primary amenorrhea. If a girl has not had a menstrual period by the age of 16, a medical investigation is warranted. A complete history of previous illness is important. The first point to be noted on physical examination is whether breast development shows that the ovaries are secreting estrogen. Then one must discover whether the hymen has an opening and if the vagina and uterus are normal. Other genetic and hormonal tests may follow in an effort to uncover and correct the cause.

Skipped or delayed periods. Skipped periods are common in the early teens before the complicated interactions between the hypothalamic area of the brain, the pituitary gland, the ovaries, and the uterus settle into the patterns that they maintain for almost 40 years. Usually nothing need be done unless these irregularities continue beyond the first year or two.

Pregnancy is one of the most common causes of secondary amenorrhea, or the absence of periods after the initial onset of menstruation. Whenever a period is delayed a week in a sexually active woman whose periods follow a regular pattern, this possibility should be considered. Other symptoms of early pregnancy may include breast tenderness, nausea, and an increased frequency of urination. At such an early stage a pregnancy test is necessary for confirmation because examination is often inconclusive.

Stress, either physical or emotional, and excessive dieting (leading to a weight loss of 15 to 25 percent of body weight) can also cause skipped or delayed periods by affecting the pituitary gland through the hypothalamic portion of the brain. Periods are often delayed one to six months in women discontinuing oral contraceptive pills. Many different problems with the pituitary, adrenals, thyroid, and ovaries also may delay periods. In the absence of pregnancy, it is usually reasonable to wait at least three months before seeking professional advice about the absence of periods.

Light periods. The old wives' tale that a heavy period is necessary to rid the body of poisons runs against the facts that wastes are excreted through the kidney and the bowel and that menstrual discharge contains only old endometrium (the lining of the uterus) and a small quantity of blood. Light periods lasting one to three days are normal for many women. Almost all women on birth control pills have decreased blood loss and a shorter flow, regarded by many of them as "good" side effects of the pill. However, a sudden change to a very light period may mean that the period has been skipped and that bleeding from some other cause is mistaken for a period. This sometimes occurs in early pregnancy.

Frequent periods. Periods that come every three weeks or less usually take place in the absence of ovulation. If they are regular and not heavy and if pregnancy is not desired, this condition is not serious. Periods without ovulation are more likely to occur during the early teens and premenopausal years.

Heavy periods. Some women have heavy periods with clots lasting seven or eight days throughout their menstruating life. These heavier than average periods may be considered normal and not a medical problem. However, the blood lost each month with the menstrual period may lead to anemia in women who do not eat a diet containing sufficient iron. Most women between the onset of menstrual periods and the menopause have less hemoglobin in the blood than men. Heavy periods easily push a woman into iron-deficiency anemia and such women require supplemental iron to be taken as pills.

Bleeding that requires a super tampon or pad that must be changed more than once an hour and continues for more than a few hours is considered unusually heavy and may indicate the presence of a medical problem.

Estrogen from the ovary stimulates growth of the lining of the uterus; progesterone, produced by the ovary after ovulation, matures the endometrium so that breakdown and bleeding is controlled at the time of menstruation. Teenagers and premenopausal women, who often have periods without ovulation and therefore without progesterone, may have very heavy periods with serious blood loss and anemia. In young women these heavy periods may be controlled by giving progesterone. In older women hormones can be used safely only after cancer has been ruled out by curettage or biopsy.

Often pregnancy is not suspected until heavy bleeding occurs after a period is delayed. At least one out of every ten pregnancies ends in spontaneous abortion or miscarriage, usually because of abnormal development of the fetus. Removal of the fragments of the pregnancy which are left in the uterus by suction or D&C (dilatation and curettage; see below) stops the bleeding.

In older women heavy periods are often caused by fibroids (benign muscle tumors of the uterus).

Midcycle bleeding. At the time of ovulation, approximately midway between menstrual periods, there is a transient dip in estrogen levels. In some women this is enough to start the endometrium breaking down and bleeding. If, as is usual, estrogen levels rise again, the bleeding stops. Careful attention to the timing of the bleeding usually clarifies the cause of this symptom.

Painful periods. Pain with menstrual periods is termed dysmenorrhea. The most common type of dysmenorrhea starts within a year or two of the beginning of periods, is relatively constant, and tends to decrease with age and after pregnancies. This characteristic cramping pain is associated with normal cycles in which ovulation occurs and is considered normal if it is not incapacitating. Recent studies have shown that this primary dysmenorrhea is caused by newly discovered substances called prostaglandins. These substances are released when the endometrial tissue breaks down. They cause the uterine muscle to contract and can also stimulate the alimentary canal causing nausea and diarrhea. Incapacitating menstrual periods often can be alleviated either by taking hormone medication, such as the oral contraceptive pill, which stops ovulation, or new compounds which counteract prostaglandins (called antiprostaglandins).

Menstrual pain which begins after years of pain-free periods is usually due to gynecologic causes such as endometriosis, polyps, or fibroids. Dysmenorrhea is a frequent accompaniment of the IUD, making this method of contraception a poor choice for women who already have severe cramps. Whenever previously normal periods become painful, a cause should be sought.

Pain with ovulation. Mittelschmerz, literally "middle pain," is pain that occurs when the egg breaks through the tiny cyst on the ovary where it has been growing. In most women this process is painless, in a few it is always painful, and in many it is occasionally painful. At times the pain may be severe, mimicking the pain of appendicitis or other abdominal crises. The pain is characterized by an abrupt onset and usually clears within a few hours, although it may last a day or two. It is necessary to know when the last period occurred and what the woman's normal interval is between periods in order to label an episode of abdominal pain as being mittelschmerz.

Menopausal problems. The menopause, the cessation of menstruation, is the objective evidence that the ovaries are aging and secreting less estrogen. Hot flashes, frequently accompanied by sweating, and painful intercourse, which is the result of thinning of the vaginal lining and decreased lubrication, are the two clear-cut symptoms that respond to estrogen administration. Other symptoms such as emotional fluctuations and depression are not as readily explained by our current knowledge and may in part reflect the changing life patterns of middle age. Skipping periods near the menopause is normal, but irregular or heavy bleeding is not, and a cause must be sought because cancer of the endometrium is common in women of menopausal age. Hormonal therapy for menopausal symptoms is discussed later in the chapter (see also "Midlife Transitions").

Other Vaginal Bleeding

Bleeding after intercourse. Bleeding which follows intercourse either results from injuries sustained during intercourse or, more commonly, from tissue made sensitive by inflammation or tumors of the vagina or cervix which were without symptoms until irritated by intercourse. Bleeding from tears in the hymen or vagina may occur in children, in those who are having intercourse for the first time, or in postmenopausal women who have not recently been sexually active. Sutures may be required to control heavy bleeding. Intercourse may cause spotting in the woman with vaginitis, but pain is more often the chief problem. An inflamed cervix or one with polyps or tumors is likely to bleed when touched by the thrusting penis. Such tumors can be either benign or malignant. Sometimes blood can come from the ejaculate of the male. Careful evaluation is always necessary.

Irregular bleeding. Bleeding which occurs at random without regard to the menstrual cycle or is unrelated to sexual activity may be a symptom of endometrial cancer (cancer of the lining of the uterus), benign endometrial conditions, or hormonal fluctuations. Bleeding with an IUD in place is usually not serious, but requires careful evaluation to distinguish it from other causes. Irregular bleeding in women on oral contraceptive pills is also sometimes hard to evaluate. Occasionally a D&C needs to be done to find the cause.

Lower Abdominal Pain

In addition to menstrual and ovulation pain, other problems with the female reproductive tract can cause acute or chronic pain. Pelvic infection or pelvic inflammatory disease, often abbreviated PID, is a frequent cause of pain. Gonorrhea, chlamydia, and other infectious organisms can cause PID. Such infections are five times as common in women using IUDs as in others. Whenever there is suspicion of PID, antibiotics should be used to minimize damage to the tubes.

Ovarian and uterine tumors, benign and malignant, may cause pain, as may the uterine contractions of a threatened abortion. Psychological stress may lead to abdominal pain through many different mechanisms, but often many tests are required to eliminate organic causes.

Vaginal Discharge

The increased levels of female hormones which begin to circulate at puberty stimulate the glands of the cervix and increase the thickness and cellular activity of the vaginal wall. Together these changes cause increased vaginal moisture which collects at the vaginal opening as a completely normal "discharge." Observant women notice that this discharge is thickish and profuse about the time of ovulation. A marked increase in vaginal fluid occurs as the first phase of the female sexual response and serves as a lubricant to facilitate intercourse. This reaction occurs whenever the woman is sexually aroused regardless of whether the source of stimulation is dreams, sexual fantasies or thoughts, or actual touching of the genitals and regardless of whether or not the further phases of sexual response are reached.

If the discharge is increased in amount, changed in color or odor, and produces itching or irritation of the surrounding tissues, a vaginal infection is likely to be the cause.

Prolapse of the Uterus

During childbirth the ligaments which support the uterus are often stretched and weakened. This allows the uterus to "fall" (lower) into the vagina, often causing discomfort. Weakness of the bladder and rectum often occurs at the same time, causing difficulty holding urine, especially during the stress of coughing or sneezing or moving the bowels. Surgery is often necessary to correct these problems. Prolapse should not be confused with a "tipped womb," which is a uterus which tips back toward the rectum. This is now known to be a normal position for the uterus in about one third of women.

Infections

Although not all infections of the female genital tract are sexually transmitted, a majority of them are. As in the case of all infections, a search must be made for the organism responsible. Such a search involves cultures, smears which are stained for bacteria, and wet preparations in which a bit of discharge is placed on a slide and examined for organisms.

Cystitis and Urethritis   Increased frequency of urination coupled with pain on voiding usually means a bacterial infection of the bladder or urethra (cystitis or urethritis). Blood in the urine is a common symptom of infection. Often the bladder is so inflamed that the woman has difficulty holding her urine even briefly. If the infection originates in the kidneys (pyelonephritis), there is likely to be fever and pain in the side.

The diagnosis is made by obtaining the history, by a physical exam, and by a urine culture to find out which bacteria are present and to which antibiotic they are sensitive. If the discomfort is severe, the treatment may be started before the results of the culture are known and changed later if indicated. Treatment must be continued for approximately 10 days after the symptoms are gone so that all bacteria are killed and the infection does not recur with bacteria that are partially resistant to antibiotics. "Honeymoon cystitis" is a term used for cystitis which occurs after intercourse. It is thought that intercourse may push bacteria up into the bladder. Voiding promptly after intercourse may help to prevent this.

Since antibiotics kill the normal vaginal bacteria as well as those causing infections in the bladder or elsewhere, a yeast or monilia infection often follows treatment. If these infections are a problem, antimonilial drugs can be used during antibiotic treatment.

Infected Bartholin's glands   On either side of the vaginal opening, there is a gland called Bartholin's gland that contributes to sexual lubrication. If the opening of the gland is blocked, the gland becomes distended and cystic and very easily becomes infected. An infected Bartholin's gland, called a Bartholin's abscess, is extremely painful. Treatment consists of heat, antibiotics, and cutting into the collection of pus so that it can drain. Mere swelling of these glands without infection does not require treatment. Rarely do glands of the urethra or other glands in the vulvar area become infected.

Vaginitis   Vaginitis is an inflammation of the vagina that may cause pain and soreness of the vagina and vulva, burning (especially with urination), itching, abnormal vaginal discharge, and odor. The discomfort may in some cases be severe enough to warrant emergency treatment.

Vaginitis is usually caused by an infection, but may also be caused by irritation or an allergic reaction. Infections are most commonly caused by monilia (a yeastlike fungus), trichomonas (a parasite), and various bacteria and viruses. These organisms are frequently transmitted sexually, but some infections are nonsexual. Changes in the woman's physical condition and changes in the chemical balance of the vagina may allow organisms which are normally present with no adverse effect to produce symptoms. (See "Sexually Transmissible Diseases" for a more complete description of types of organisms.)

Since there are so many different organisms and conditions which may result in vaginitis, it is necessary to find the cause by physical examination, cultures, and microscopic examination of the vaginal discharge before attempting treatment. Because the urethra and bladder are so close to the vulva and vagina, an infection in one area may cause symptoms in the other, making diagnosis difficult.

The most frequent vaginal infection is due to a yeastlike fungus commonly called monilia; its proper name is *Candida* and it is often referred to as "yeast." This organism is present in damp areas of the environment and frequently finds conditions in the human vagina favorable for growth. Antibiotics that kill the normal bacteria responsible for maintaining the acidity of the vagina predispose to the growth of this organism. Pregnancy, the contraceptive pill, diabetes, synthetic fabrics, and tight pants and wet bathing suits also predispose to infection with this organism. Itching, rash, and inflammation are symptoms of the infection which is often characterized by a white, thick discharge. The diagnosis is made by examining a portion of this discharge under the microscope or by growing the organism in a tube. Although many preparations can alleviate the infection, recurrences are common. Monilia is not generally sexually transmitted, but sexual partners may complain of itching or a rash and sometimes harbor the organism.

The term nonspecific vaginitis is used to designate vaginal inflammation caused by miscellaneous abnormal bacteria. The symptoms are often caused by the bacteria *Hemophilis vaginalis* or by *Chlamydia,* but frequently the bacteria cannot be identified. Thinness of the lining of the vagina in a child or postmenopausal woman makes the vagina more susceptible to infection. The discharge with nonspecific vaginitis is usually white or yellow and may be streaked with blood. An unpleasant odor and swollen glands in the groin may be present. Nonspecific vaginitis is often treated with sulfa creams or suppositories. Oral antibiotics may be used, especially for patients sensitive to sulfa drugs or those with recurring infections. Consideration must be given to treatment of sexual partners.

The vagina depends on a balance of normal hormone effects and normal bacteria to maintain its acidity and health. Strong douches can interfere with this balance. Some women are allergic to soaps, deodorants, and other preparations used around the vagina.

Not all organisms capable of producing vaginal irritations have been discovered and, therefore, one should be careful about attributing symptoms to psychosomatic interactions. However, it has been found that for a number of reasons, including inadequate sexual lubrication, women with sexual and relationship problems have an increased incidence of vaginitis. Conversely, almost all women with vaginitis have dyspareunia.

Certain precautions can be taken to prevent vaginitis.

1. Condoms can help prevent the spread of sexually transmitted diseases. They should be used if one has intercourse while being treated for vaginitis. If the area is sore, don't attempt intercourse.
2. Keep the genital area as dry as possible because organisms that cause vaginitis grow well in a moist environment. Cotton crotch underwear allows for more absorption and helps keep the genital area dry. Avoiding tight jeans or pantyhose may also help. Sitting for long periods of time in a wet bathing suit is conducive to yeast infections.
3. Practice good general hygiene; washing the external genitalia thoroughly with regular soap and water is sufficient. Be sure to rinse thoroughly after bathing. Avoid bubble baths and perfumed soaps which may be irritating.
4. Avoid perfumed tampons, vaginal sprays, and frequent douching, especially with over-the-counter products, since they can be harsh and may kill normal bacteria and alter vaginal acidity.
5. An occasional douche (not more than twice a week) with mild vinegar solution (2 tablespoons to 1 quart water) can be used prophylactically

if recurrent vaginitis is a problem or if a woman feels the need for internal cleansing.

6. Do not use other people's towels.

Tumors

The word tumor means growth or swelling, but does not differentiate between malignant growths or cancers which can spread into surrounding tissues and from which pieces can break off and travel to other parts of the body, and benign or nonmalignant growths which may cause problems because of size or pressure, but which do not spread.

Vulvar tumors Most lumps which women find on the external genitals or vulva are benign and may be warts, infections, or cysts. Sores or ulcers which do not heal in two to three weeks could be malignant and should be called to a doctor's attention. The folds of the vulva are made up of skin and are subject to a variety of problems much like skin in other parts of the body.

Vaginal tumors Until the advent of a generation of women exposed before birth to high doses of estrogens such as DES, vaginal tumors were very rare. Now they are somewhat less rare. Most vaginal tumors consist of benign changes in the lining of the vagina, but cancer can occur. The colposcope is used to localize areas for biopsy.

Cervical polyps Small benign growths called polyps are the most common cervical tumors. These start in the cervical canal and appear at the cervical opening. Polyps are small, red mushroomlike growths which bleed easily and irregularly. They are removed by a minor operation called a polypectomy, which often can be done in the doctor's office.

Dysplasia Early changes in the cells of the surface of the cervix which may become malignant are called dysplasia. These changes can be mild or severe, sometimes disappear spontaneously, are usually discovered by a pap smear, and can best be evaluated by a combination of colposcopy and biopsy. Treatment consists of destroying the abnormal cells by means of hot cautery or freezing cryosurgery.

Carcinoma-in-situ More advanced changes in the cells covering the cervix are called carcinoma-in-situ (cancer in place). The term cervical intraepithelial neoplasia (CIN) is also used. These cells appear malignant, but are confined to the covering layer of cells. An area with such cells may become truly malignant at any time, but on the average remains quiescent for about five years before it begins to spread. Carcinoma-in-situ may be treated by cryosurgery, cautery, or excision biopsy if future child-bearing is desired or by a hysterectomy if it is not (see below). Follow-up with frequent pap smears is necessary to be sure all the abnormal areas have been removed.

Cancer of the cervix Invasive cancer of the cervix is one of the most common of the female malignancies, but has dropped in frequency with the advent of pap smears. These smears permit detection and treatment of premalignant lesions. Cancer of the cervix can be treated by a radical hysterectomy or by radiation. A radical or Wertheim type of hysterectomy is one in which the tissue adjoining the uterus—the pelvic lymph nodes, tubes, and ovaries—are removed as well as the uterus. It is generally performed by specially trained gynecologic cancer surgeons.

Benign uterine tumors   Polyps may appear on the endometrium or lining of the uterus and are removed by D&C. Another type of irregular growth of the endometrium is called hyperplasia. Hyperplasia is benign, but if the condition is severe, it is sometimes considered to be premalignant. These conditions are diagnosed and treated by a D&C. A hysterectomy may be recommended for severe hyperplasia.

Fibroids or fibromyomata uteri   Fibromyomata uteri (sing., fibromyoma) or fibroids are very common benign tumors of the muscle of the uterus. Small muscle tumors occur in almost half of all uteruses, but only a small percentage grow and cause symptoms such as heavy menstrual periods and pressure on the bladder and rectum. If treatment is needed, it consists of either removal of the tumors (myomectomy) or hysterectomy.

Endometriosis   Endometriosis is a condition in which normal, benign cells of endometrial tissue break away from the uterus and implant and start to grow in other locations in the pelvic cavity—the tubes, ovaries, and surface of the bladder and rectum. Endometriosis can produce many types of pelvic discomfort or none at all, but most typically causes pain which begins two or three days before the start of a menstrual period, possibly caused by changes in the endometrial tissue similar to those occurring in the uterus. Infertility is increased in women with endometriosis. The diagnosis can be made accurately by laparoscopy. Mild endometriosis, which produces no symptoms or effects, may not require treatment. Hormones and surgery both have a place in the treatment of endometriosis. Hormonal treatment with progestational agents and synthetic steroids such as danazol is based on the observed fact that endometriosis decreases when ovulation is prevented for three to six months. Surgery may be required for removal of benign endometrial growths from the ovaries. Since this condition is often improved by pregnancy, physicians sometimes suggest pregnancy, ignoring the radical upheaval in a woman's life that such a suggestion can make.

Cancer of the endometrium   Malignant growth of the lining of the uterus is called carcinoma of the endometrium. It is one of the most common cancers in women and has been increasing in frequency in recent years. An association with estrogen stimulation, either that produced by the woman's own body or that taken in treatment, has been noted. The chief symptom is irregular bleeding usually during or after the menopause. Diagnosis is by endometrial biopsy or D&C and sometimes by a pap smear.

Treatment is primarily surgical removal of the uterus, often preceded or followed by radiation. The cure rate is excellent (80 to 90 percent) if diagnosed early.

Cancer of the tube Cancer of the fallopian tubes is very uncommon, hard to diagnose, and difficult to cure.

Benign ovarian tumors Because the ovary is a complex structure containing many types of cells including ova (which have the potential of making every type of cell), many different types of tumors can form in the ovary. The most common benign ovarian tumor is the simple cyst which occurs when the small cyst containing the ovum does not rupture at the proper time in the cycle and expel the ovum, but continues to grow. Such cysts usually disappear in one or two months, but if they rupture, they may cause pain or internal bleeding and sometimes require surgery. Dermoid cysts, containing hair, fatty material, and often teeth, are common in young women and are thought to be embryonic remnants present from birth. Although benign, they require removal. There are other benign ovarian tumors, both cystic and solid, which may cause symptoms and require removal. If an ovarian tumor persists, it must be removed to find out whether or not it is malignant.

Ovarian cancer There are many types of cancer of the ovary. The long-term outlook depends on the type, but all are difficult to diagnose early because symptoms do not occur early. Final diagnosis depends on removal of the tumor at the time of exploratory surgery for microscopic examination. Treatment consists of surgical removal of as much tumor as possible followed by chemotherapy.

Endocrine Problems

The gynecologic problems considered up to this point have been those for which a specific abnormal tumor or an abnormal response in a normal tissue has been responsible. Because of the complex interrelationship between the ovary, the hypothalamus, the pituitary gland, the thyroid, and the adrenal glands, many abnormalities of the menstrual cycle are caused by dysfunctions or malfunctions of these endocrine glands. These abnormalities may include heavy, irregular menstrual periods, called dysfunctional uterine bleeding. Lack of periods and lack of ovulation are also endocrine problems.

Unraveling the complexities of endocrine malfunction requires many expensive and complex hormone tests to discover the level of a particular hormone in the body and to find out how one endocrine gland responds when hormones from another gland are administered.

Some pituitary malfunctions are caused by the effect of severe dieting or physical and emotional stress on the hypothalamus of the brain. Other problems are genetically determined. Treatment will depend upon the particular abnormality found.

TYPES OF GYNECOLOGIC TREATMENT

Treatment of Infection

Gynecologic infections may be caused by viruses, bacteria, fungi, spirochetes, and protozoan. Infection caused by each of these types of organisms requires a different type of treatment. Viruses, such as herpes, are impossible to destroy effectively with current drugs. However, symptoms can be relieved and some effects of their presence can be treated. For example, warts, which are virally induced, can be removed by cautery.

Different types of bacteria can be treated effectively with different types of antibiotics, although treatment becomes more difficult when bacteria develop strains resistant to particular antibiotics. Specific agents are available to treat monilia and trichomonas, common causes of vaginal infections. Effective treatment requires knowledge of what is being treated; the telephone management of vaginitis and urinary tract infections is risky and likely to fail.

Hormone Therapy

The vast publicity given to problems associated with the use of the oral contraceptive pill has clouded the fact that the discovery of orally effective estrogen and progesterone compounds has revolutionized the treatment of bleeding problems in women, reduced the number of D&C's required, and often permitted an alternative to hysterectomy for control of hemorrhage. Surgery is no longer the first therapy for heavy bleeding problems. The use of progesterones to bring on a period in women with infrequent periods and those who do not ovulate reduces the likelihood of cancer of the endometrium.

Estrogens have been used successfully in menopausal women for many years to relieve hot flashes and painful intercourse due to the thinning of the vagina. No other treatment works so well. In addition, estrogen slows osteoporosis, the thinning of the bones that occurs with aging. The recent linking of the use of estrogen during and after menopause with an increased rate of cancer of the endometrium has reminded us that relative risks are always difficult to assess. At present the answers are not all known, but it seems prudent to use these hormones only when there is a good reason to do so.

Androgens, male hormones, are produced in small quantities in the female by the ovaries and the adrenal gland. Androgens are occasionally used in the treatment of endometriosis, but newer synthetic hormones, such as danazol, are proving more effective. Hormones of the thyroid, pituitary, and adrenal glands are used to treat problems related to these glands.

Cautery

Cautery refers to the limited destruction of diseased tissue by the use of chemicals, heat, or cold. The use of heat is termed electrocautery; the use of cold, cryosurgery. It is used to treat venereal warts and to destroy the abnormal cells of dysplasia and carcinoma-in-situ of the cervix.

Surgery

Excision biopsy. Cone biopsy or conization, described as a diagnostic technique, may also have therapeutic application. The removal of abnormal tissue for diagnosis may be treatment as well. Drawbacks are the need for hospitalization and anesthesia and the possibility of heavy bleeding and infection.

Incision and drainage. Antibiotics cannot get into the center of a cyst or cavity where blood vessels do not penetrate. Whenever there is a collection of pus which does not drain on its own, it is necessary to cut into the cavity to allow it to do so. This minor operation is called incision and drainage. If the abscess re-forms, the incision must sometimes be sewed open to insure long-term drainage. This procedure is frequently used to treat Bartholin's abscesses. Drainage of a major infection of the tubes and ovaries which does not respond to antibiotics requires abdominal surgery.

Polypectomy. The removal of a cervical or uterine polyp is called polypectomy. Cervical polyps can usually be removed in a doctor's office. Because the removal of endometrial polyps involves dilatation of the cervix, anesthesia is required, either local in an office or out-patient operating room or general anesthesia in the hospital.

Dilatation and curettage (D&C) and dilatation and evacuation (D&E). The cervix can be stretched wide enough to permit a 10 pound baby's head to pass through it, but at other times it is closed so that only a narrow tube ⅛ inch in diameter can be passed into the uterus. If larger instruments are required for an operation inside the uterus, the cervix is opened by passing metal tubes of increasing diameter through the opening until the cervix will allow the passage of the required instrument. This is called dilatation of the cervix.

In order to remove tissue from the uterus, an instrument called a curette, a loop with a sharp edge, is used to scrape the endometrium off the muscular part of the uterus. This procedure is called curettage. The tissue may be removed for examination and diagnosis or it may be done as part of treatment for heavy or irregular uterine bleeding.

Dilatation and curettage (D&C) may also be performed to terminate pregnancy as may a similar procedure, dilatation and evacuation (D&E), which uses a suction curette, that is, a hollow tube connected to a vacuum pump to remove tissue by suction. Usually local anesthesia suffices for both the D&C and D&E.

Myomectomy. The removal of a smooth muscle tumor (fibromyoma or fibroid) of the uterus is called a myomectomy. Because fibroids are usually multiple and small ones continue to grow even though the largest ones are removed and because a myomectomy is technically more difficult to perform and associated with more blood loss than a hysterectomy, these tumors are generally removed by a hysterectomy. The myomectomy is usually reserved for women who want future pregnancies.

Hysterectomy. Hysterectomy is a common operation, often needed and currently embroiled in controversy. Women must understand what the operation is and is not and what the issues are. The term hysterectomy refers to the removal of the uterus. A total or complete hysterectomy is the complete removal of the uterus including the cervix. A partial or subtotal hysterectomy is one in which the cervix is not removed. Most hysterectomies currently performed are complete because the cervix is a frequent site of dysplasia and cancer and therefore should rarely be left behind. A radical hysterectomy involves removal of the uterus with a large amount of surrounding tissue and lymph nodes and is reserved for some types of cancer.

Note that the term hysterectomy says nothing about the removal of the ovaries and tubes. Decisions regarding the removal of these organs must be made separately. Many gynecologists prefer to remove the ovaries whenever they are performing a pelvic operation on a woman at or near the menopause because the ovaries produce relatively little estrogen thereafter and ovarian cancer which develops in 1 out of every 100 women is hard to detect and hard to cure. Sometimes the ovaries must be removed before the menopause because of disease. In this circumstance estrogens should be given at least until the age of normal menopause.

The uterus can be removed through an abdominal incision, either vertical or crosswise, or through a vaginal incision around the cervix at the top of the vagina (see illustration). The operations are called abdominal and vaginal hysterectomies, respectively. Many factors influence the route chosen. The vaginal route is chosen if repair work is required for injuries to the bladder and rectum sustained in childbirth, and occasionally for other reasons. Frequently, with the patient's permission, the surgeon will take out the appendix at the time of an abdominal hysterectomy (it takes only five minutes longer) to prevent future appendicitis. Surgery for cancer is more extensive than other types and is always modified by the extent of the tumor found at the time of the surgery. Ovarian surgery and general exploration of the abdominal organs is easier with the abdominal incision.

Most of the reasons for hysterectomy involve abnormal bleeding, pain,

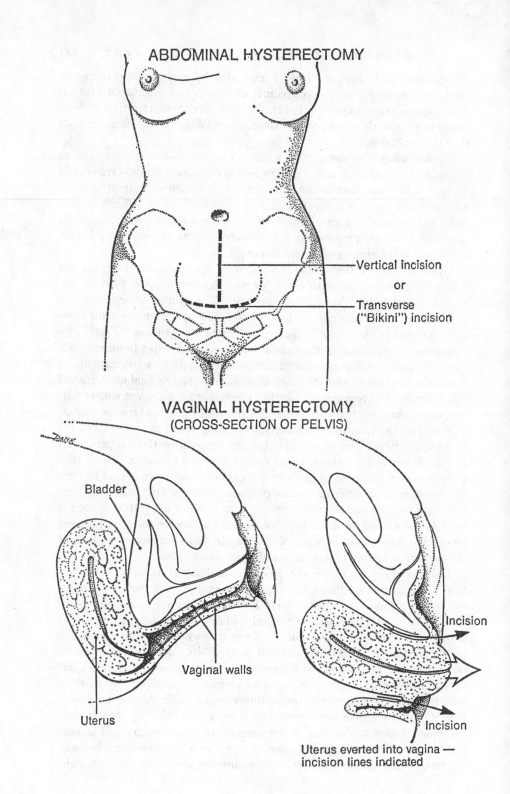

ABDOMINAL HYSTERECTOMY

—Vertical incision

or

—Transverse ("Bikini") incision

VAGINAL HYSTERECTOMY
(CROSS-SECTION OF PELVIS)

Bladder

Vaginal walls

Uterus

Incision

Incision

Uterus everted into vagina —
incision lines indicated

CROSS-SECTION OF PELVIS AFTER HYSTERECTOMY

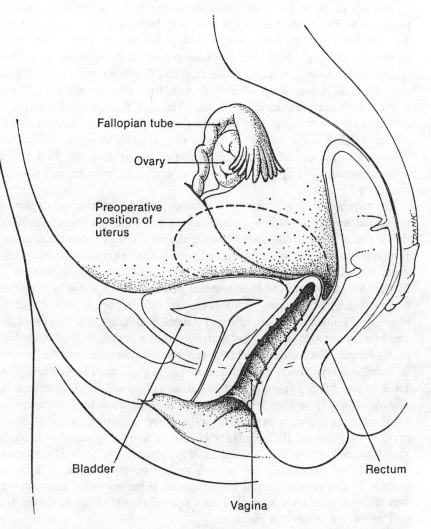

Fallopian tube

Ovary

Preoperative position of uterus

Bladder

Rectum

Vagina

cancer, or potential cancer. Every gynecologist should be willing and able to explain the necessity for the operation as well as why a lesser procedure (such as a D&C) will not suffice. Sometimes a hysterectomy will seem like a good solution to a combination of lesser problems such as severe menstrual cramps, very heavy periods, and a desire for sterilization. It is in this gray zone that a controversy lies. Such operations are not strictly "necessary" and hospital tissue committees may question these procedures when there is no evidence of life-threatening disease. The woman must understand and consider all alternatives in such situations. The final decision is hers. On the other hand, no physician should be forced to perform an operation that he or she does not think is in the patient's best interest.

The loss of the uterus ends both childbearing and menstruation. The capacity to bear children has always been very important to women, and the loss of this potential may be threatening. Many old wives' tales have emerged regarding a hysterectomy. One is that the physiologic sexual response is decreased. Actually, sexual response is affected little if at all, and the vagina is just as deep afterwards as before (see illustration). Some women anticipate the onset of obesity. The fact that physical activity is curtailed for a few weeks may confirm their fear and start them on an inactive, weight-gaining course. If the ovaries remain, estrogen production continues to the age of the expected menopause, so that hot flashes and other menopausal symptoms do not occur until then, even though periods are absent.

The psychological aftermath of a hysterectomy depends on the degree to which the woman regards her uterus as her feminine identity. If she feels that her femininity resides in her womb, she may find the postoperative adjustment hard. If she understands and accepts the operation, she may welcome the relief of symptoms that the operation affords. The adjustment is hardest for the young childless woman; often counseling will be required to help her come to terms with this major crisis in her life. The speed of recovery is influenced by attitude and general health; age can also be a factor. Most women go back to full activity within a month, but still have lingering fatigue. They usually feel fully recovered within three months.

Tubal surgery. The most common operation performed on the fallopian tubes is the tubal ligation for sterilization (discussed in "Contraception and Abortion"). A little less common is the operation necessitated by a tubal or ectopic pregnancy. If the other tube is normal, it is usual to remove the tube and the pregnancy because a scarred tube, if left behind, may become the site of a second tubal pregnancy. Occasionally, women who have had tubal ligations for sterilization request reversal of the procedure. The tubes can be put back together using operating microscopes and microsurgical techniques, but such operations are difficult, expensive, and only about 50 percent effective.

Ovarian surgery. Ovarian surgery involves removing part or all of an ovary because of cysts or tumors. Removal of an ovary is termed oophorectomy. In the case of benign cysts and tumors as much normal ovary is saved as possible. Pregnancies can occur in women with only half of one ovary. If an ovarian or uterine tumor is malignant, all of the reproductive organs are removed together because the cancer tends to spread to the nearby uterus and the opposite tube and ovary. Severe pelvic infections and abscesses involving the tubes and ovaries which do not respond adequately to antibiotics often require extensive surgery for cure.

Surgical complications. Fifty years ago surgery was so dangerous that no one needed to be told that there were risks involved. Now risks may be overlooked. This is a mistake. All anesthesia, whether general or local, involves a small risk of death. Hemorrhage and infection are potential hazards in almost all surgery, although blood banks and antibiotics have greatly reduced these risks. Adhesions, the attachment of one bit of injured tissue to another, occur after most abdominal surgery as part of the healing process and may cause pain or obstruct the bowel. Other specific risks can best be explained by the one performing the surgery.

Radiation Therapy

Radiotherapy involving X-rays or radioactive isotopes is reserved for the treatment of malignancies in which either the tumor has spread to areas which cannot be safely removed or those where experience has shown that the tumor responds better to radiation or a combination of radiation and surgery than to surgery alone. Cells which are dividing rapidly are destroyed by irradiation more easily than are normal resting cells so that growing tumors can be treated with minimal damage to the surrounding tissue. Complications involving skin, bowel, bladder, and rectum do occur, but have decreased with more powerful sources of radiation which can be more precisely directed to the involved area as well as with increasing experience with the use of these tools.

Chemotherapy

The term applied to the use of a variety of drugs for cancer treatment is chemotherapy. Most of these drugs depend for their effectiveness on the susceptibility of rapidly growing tumor cells to toxic substances. The choice and use of these agents is a very complex, specialized field.

Counseling

Many problems seen by the gynecologist involve sexual functioning, interpersonal relationships, and questions concerning contraception and abortion and are aided by detailed discussion of the issues involved. Often this can be done by the gynecologist at the time of a regular visit, but sometimes a more leisurely appointment needs to be scheduled. With some problems the physician may know another counselor who can handle the issue better. Such a referral should not be interpreted as rejection, but as evidence that the referring doctor is trying to find the person who can be' most helpful in dealing with the area of concern.

FURTHER READING

Burchell, R. Clay. "Decision Regarding Hysterectomy," *Am. J. Obstet. & Gynec.* 127 (1977): 113.

Clay, Vidal S. *Women: Menopausal and Middle Age.* Pittsburgh: Know Inc., 1977.

Gifford-Jones, W. *What Every Woman Should Know About Hysterectomy.* New York: Funk & Wagnalls, 1977.

Gross, Harriet Engels. "Women's Changing Roles—The Gynecologists' View," *Women and Health* 2 (1977): 9.

Llewellyn-Jones, Derek. *Every Woman: A Gynecological Guide for Life.* London: Faber & Faber, 1971.

Lansen, Lucienne. *From Woman to Woman.* New York: Knopf, 1975.

Morgan, Suzanne. "Sexuality After Hysterectomy and Castration," *Women and Health* 3 (1978): 5.

Richards, Bruce C. "Hysterectomy: From Woman to Woman," *Am. J. Obstet. & Gynec.* 131 (1978): 446.

Sloan, Dan. "The Emotional & Psycho-Sexual Aspects of Hysterectomy," *Am. J. Obstet. & Gynec.* 131 (1978): 598.

Sexually Transmissible Diseases

LOUISE TYRER, M.D.
Vice-President for Medical Affairs,
Planned Parenthood Federation of America, Inc.

The specter of venereal disease (VD), long kept in the closet, has emerged in epidemic proportions. Last year alone, over 6 million Americans were infected with a sexually-contracted disease, and the number keeps growing. As we learn more about diseases that can be transmitted from one sex partner to another, it has become apparent that the term VD is outmoded. VD covered the "Big Five" diseases reported to most state health departments in the United States—gonorrhea, syphilis, chancroid, lymphogranuloma venereum, and granuloma inguinale. However, there are many other diseases that can be sexually transmitted, and there are also diseases that may be contracted as a result of low systemic resistance, altered body metabolism, or other causes and are then transmitted to a sexual partner. Therefore, the term *sexually transmissible diseases* (STD) has been adopted to cover this broad spectrum of conditions.

As long as people communicate through touching—and let's hope that this is forever—STD will be a potential problem. So, rather than deny ourselves sexual expression, we should learn about STDs, how to prevent them, and how to recognize their symptoms so early treatment can be obtained. Now that we have the antibiotics and other drugs, all STDs can be cured or arrested with the exception of those caused by viruses. But this fact should not foster carelessness, either in protecting against STD or in seeking early diagnosis and treatment. The commonly held belief that a "dose" of gonorrhea is no worse than a bad cold, and just about as common, can have disastrous consequences. Gonorrhea is still a severe disease which can make a woman sterile and has the potential for rare, but very serious complications.

There are about 20 diseases that may be transmitted by sexual contact. Many ask why, with more knowledge about STD and readily available treatment, haven't STDs been eliminated or at least contained? As with other complex problems, there is no single simple answer. Some of the factors responsible are:

Increased sexual expression. All types of intimate contacts, including sexual, are increasing, particularly among the young. Changing sexual partners or having multiple partners greatly increases the risk of contracting an STD.

Shift in contraceptive practices. Today the most commonly used methods of contraception are the pill, the IUD, and sterilization. None of these offers any protection against STD as does the condom and to some extent the vaginal barrier methods such as the diaphragm and spermicides.

Social disgrace. Many people, including health professionals, still attach strong negative judgments to a person with an STD. This person then reacts with shame and fear and delays diagnosis and treatment. Also, he or she may be unwilling to disclose his or her sexual contact(s), making it impossible to break the chain.

Asymptomatic carriers. Six of the STDs, including the most serious, syphilis and gonorrhea, may occur without any symptoms. People may be highly infectious and be completely unaware of their condition.

Resistant strains. Certain bacterium, particularly the one causing gonorrhea, may become resistant to the usual antibiotics. Since most people believe that one magic shot will cure them, they may not return for "tests of cure" and may still harbor the infection.

World travel. The mobility of our population today accounts for an increased rate of spread of STDs. Also, rare diseases, once indigenous to specific areas of the world, are now spreading globally.

Complacency. Public health agencies no longer commit as much time and money to identifying cases and contacts. This is coupled with an attitude held by many people that reporting of cases and tracing contacts is unimportant since treatment is so readily available.

Underreporting of cases. By law syphilis and gonorrhea (in most states), and recently herpes type II (in some states) must be reported to health departments. These diseases can represent a considerable threat to health. However, only about one out of nine cases of these STDs in the United States is reported. This is frequently related to physician negligence, often because the professional is overly concerned about "protecting" the patient.

Education. There is insufficient education at all levels regarding STD's frequency, prevention, recognition, diagnosis, and treatment. Also, educators need to dispel the stigma associated with STD so that it is considered with the same nonjudgmental attitude as other diseases requiring urgent treatment, such as appendicitis.

WHAT WOMEN NEED TO KNOW ABOUT STD

A woman has a built-in awareness of her bodily functions. Education about symptoms of the STDs can increase that level of sensitivity so that she can notice subtle changes that may indicate the onset of an STD. But what can she do to protect herself against infection and what should she know if she suspects she may have been infected?

There is no way to know in advance that a sexual partner is free of STD. Abstinence is the only guarantee against exposure. Of course, if it is apparent that the partner has a genital lesion or a discharge or admits exposure to an STD, avoidance of sex is the only safe course. A woman must not be bashful about querying her partner or even inspecting his genitals for lesions or urethral discharge, nor should she be offended if he wishes to do the same.

Assuming one is sexually active, the greatest protection against contracting an STD is to develop a monogamous relationship with a partner who is also monogamous. The general rule is: the more partners, the greater the risk of exposure and of contracting disease.

If neither partner is monogamous, insisting that the male use a condom affords a woman the best possible protection against her getting or giving STD. She would do well to carry condoms with her, in case her partner does not have one available, and should hold firm to the premise "no condom, no sex."

A woman can supplement this protection if she uses a vaginal barrier (for example, diaphragm with jelly or cream; foam; and possibly suppositories). This is not to recommend that she should use these as her primary method of birth control as their failure rate in general use is about 15 pregnancies per 100 women per year. However, the woman who takes the pill or has an IUD can, by the use of a spermicide preparation, not only slightly increase the protection her contraception affords, but at the same time can have some protection against STD.

It is important that the genital area be cleaned prior to and after sex. Also, urination prior to coitus may wash some of the bacteria that cause STD from the urethra.

If you have had sexual contact with someone you have reason to suspect may have STD, there are some things you can do right away. Urination immediately after sexual contact may "flush out" of your urethra bacteria such as gonococci that can cause urethritis, and when the urine is acid it serves to discourage the growth of these sensitive organisms. This approach, however, will not reduce the occurrence of infection in the vagina or the cervix. Immediately wash the vulva with soap and water. Avoid strong medicated or highly perfumed soaps and deodorant sprays as they may be irritating. Insert an applicator or two of contraceptive foam, cream, or jelly high into the vagina and rub it on the external genitals as well. Although the protective effect of after-the-fact use of a vaginal contraceptive has not been documented, its prior use is known to be somewhat effective, so it couldn't hurt.

Douching is not effective and may even encourage bacteria to enter the cervical canal. Also, if you have a chemical vaginal contraceptive in place, douching would remove this effective barrier.

If there is a good possibility you have been exposed—say, your partner tells you of his prior exposure to someone with STD or you were raped—call a clinician (physician, hospital clinic, public health facility) and make an appointment to be seen right away. There are antibiotics that can be given that provide effective prophylaxis against gonorrhea and syphilis when taken shortly after such sexual contact. (Antibiotics should be taken only after a known or possible exposure. They should never be taken before expected contact.) The clinician can recommend a plan of follow-up examinations to assure you of proper diagnosis and, if indicated, treatment.

Anxiety about having STD is common. Many people think they have STD when they do not. The only way to be sure is to have an examination and diagnostic tests. If the proper testing procedure is followed and the tests are negative, you can put the matter from your mind, while vowing to be more careful in the future. Some women, however, become so obsessed that they imagine all sorts of symptoms, such as itching and abnormal discharge. This is an unhealthy attitude, and if examination, testing, and reassurance does not solve the problem, psychological help may be necessary.

Certain important considerations are applicable to all STDs. The specific diseases are discussed in the next section.

1. A woman should ask her clinician to examine and test her for STD, most particularly for gonorrhea and syphilis, at the time of her annual health checkup.

2. Certain STDs or their treatment create a special risk for a fetus or a newborn. Therefore, a pregnant woman should familiarize herself with those STDs that may place her and her child at risk; she should talk with her obstetrician about the need for special tests and discuss appropriate options, if certain tests are positive.

The type of therapy and the dosage of many medications must be made consistent with protection of the fetus. For example, pregnant women should not take tetracyclines as they can affect dental development in the fetus.

3. A woman may have more than one STD. Therefore, it is important that tests to determine whether several diseases are present, particularly syphilis or gonorrhea, should also be considered and done if indicated.

4. The sexual partner(s) often require examination and treatment in conjunction with the woman to ensure a cure.

5. If a woman masters the technique of internal vaginal and cervical examination, using a speculum, a good light source, and a mirror, and practices it routinely at least once a month (usually best done shortly after the menstrual period when the hormonal influences are at a low level), she may observe changes suggestive of the onset of STD. This will enable her to seek earlier diagnosis and treatment. For example, she may notice a change in the character of the vaginal discharge or an inflammation of the cervix.

6. If a woman has recurring bouts of vaginal infection, with irritation of the surrounding skin, the local reaction can be reduced and sometimes virtually eliminated by not wearing restrictive and nonabsorptive clothing, such as tight pants or nylon panty hose. Dryness is a very important part of the healing process. During this phase it is best to wear either skirts and no underpants or cotton panties, changed daily, washed with a mild soap (avoid detergents), and thoroughly rinsed. Deodorant sprays should never be used on the sensitive vulvar skin. They can only cause problems.

7. A woman must inform the clinician prior to therapy as to whether she has any drug allergies, particularly to penicillin or sulfa.

8. Follow-up examinations and tests to assure cure are mandatory following treatment of any STD. The return visit needs to be scheduled at the time of the initial visit.

DESCRIPTION OF SPECIFIC STDs

Each STD is discussed below alphabetically (not by frequency of occurrence) with symptoms, diagnosis, and treatment explained.

Chancroid

Symptoms. The first symptom is a small, painful boil most commonly found on the external genitalia. It does not heal like the usual pimple and becomes a running sore. The causative organism, *Hemophilus ducreyi*, moves through the lymphatics into the groin and, if untreated, these infected glands break down and exude pus. It is fairly common in the tropics, rare in the United States.

Diagnosis. Often the diagnosis can be made by inspecting the lesion, but microscopic examination of the pus will reveal the causative organism. A microscopic examination to rule out syphilis must also be performed.

Treatment. Therapy usually consists of oral sulfa drugs or tetracycline combined with intensive compressing of the lesion(s).

Chlamydial Infections

Chlamydia are organisms that cause a variety of infections, some of which are sexually transmitted. The infections are difficult to diagnose. Chlamydia are neither viruses nor bacteria, but are called elementary bodies. These bodies are incorporated in cells where they dwell and can be identified upon microscopic examination of stained smears of the infected tissue.

There are several groups of chlamydial infections, one of which affects the urogenital tracts of both the female and the male.

Symptoms. Burning and frequency of urination occur most commonly in the male, but females can also suffer from this problem. Chlamydia can cause chronic infection of the cervix; urethra (urethritis), with even obstruction or destruction of it; and infection of the tubes and ovaries, commonly known as pelvic inflammatory disease (PID). Trachoma, a chlamydial infection of the eye, may occur simultaneously. Therefore, there is a considerable risk that chlamydial infection may be transmitted to the eyes of a newborn as it passes through the birth canal, causing serious disease. The eyes of the newborn so infected require prompt treatment to avoid extensive scarring and blindness.

Diagnosis. These chlamydial infections may be diagnosed by special cell culture, by serological testing for antibodies, or by a microimmunofluorescence test (micro-IF test) using the electron microscope.

Treatment. The usual treatment is tetracycline; sulfa is the alternative.

Cytomegalovirus (CMV)

Symptoms. This infection, caused by the cytomegalovirus, is usually asymptomatic. It may be acquired, though rarely, through blood transfusion. Its serious implications relate to an active infection occurring during pregnancy. The fetus may develop CMV infection from the mother through their common blood supply or by direct contact in the birth canal. The nursing child may acquire it from breast milk. About 50 percent of infants born to women who have this infection during pregnancy are infected, and 5 to 15 percent of these infants have serious central nervous system abnormalities.

Diagnosis. A blood serum test will be positive for CMV antibodies. The virus may also be discovered on the pap smear.

Treatment. There is no known treatment. Since there is no cure and the effect on the fetus may be severe, it is important, though not often done routinely, for a woman to be tested for this infection in early pregnancy so that she may make a considered decision as to whether she wishes to continue her pregnancy.

Fungal Infections (Tinea Cruris)

Symptoms. This fungal infection, related to the one causing athlete's foot, may be sexually transmitted, but is not generally classified as an STD. It produces itchy, reddish patches in the groin with vesicles that tend to heal with formation of crusted lesions as its borders extend.

Diagnosis. Microscopic examination of scrapings of the skin lesions mixed with a solution of potassium hydroxide will reveal the strands of fungus.

Treatment. Treatment is the local application of benzoic acid compound ointment or other fungicides.

Gonorrhea

Symptoms. This common STD is caused by *Neisseria gonorrhoeae*. It has an average incubation period of 3 to 5 days. There is an 80 percent chance that a woman infected with gonorrhea will have no symptoms because the infection is located in the cervix, high up in the woman's vagina. In males the infection is in the urethra and causes a pussy discharge. However, 10 to 20 percent of infected men have no discharge and no other symptoms. Asymptomatic carriers explain why this disease is almost impossible to eradicate. When symptoms are present in a woman, any combination of the following, with their accompanying complications, may occur as the disease spreads and causes inflammation and infection throughout the system.

1. A green or yellow-green vaginal discharge.
2. A distinctive mushroomlike odor, not previously present, from the genital area.
3. Lower abdominal pains.
4. Continuous low back pains.
5. Burning and frequency of urination, sometimes associated with a drop of pus or blood.
6. Swelling and tenderness (abscess) of the Bartholin's gland located near the opening of the vagina.
7. Pleurisy-type pains in the right upper abdomen (perihepatitis) or in the shoulder area.
8. Severe pain in the pelvic area as gonorrhea moves up into the fallopian tubes (pelvic inflammatory disease).
9. Severe generalized abdominal pain as the infection spreads from the tubes to the abdominal cavity (pelvic peritonitis).
10. Pelvic pain and masses, as the pelvic infection walls off in the pelvis (pelvic abscesses).

11. Sterility, resulting from blocked tubes or surgery necessary to remove abscesses.
12. Other serious complications, such as gonorrheal arthritis and gonorrheal pericarditis.

The eyes of the newborn are particularly susceptible to gonorrheal infection. If prophylactic measures, such as instillation of silver nitrate solution or penicillin injection, are not taken at birth and the infection develops, blindness may result.

Diagnosis. In women gonorrhea is diagnosed by a culture taken from the cervix. Other sites of possible infection, such as the throat, urethra, or rectum need to be cultured as well, if history and examination should indicate possible exposure at these sites. A positive culture provides a firm diagnosis of gonorrhea. However, a negative culture does not necessarily rule out the possibility, particularly if the infection has spread into the tubes or is at a site other than one that was cultured.

Treatment. Injectable penicillin that is short-acting but gives a high blood level concentration is the preferred treatment. It should be combined with the penicillin-enhancing drug probencid. Higher than usual doses of penicillin for longer periods are required when the infection is in the tubes or causing peritonitis.

The presence of a rare strain of gonorrhea that is resistant to penicillin can be revealed by antibiotic sensitivity tests done on the cultured gonococci bacteria. In such cases another antibiotic, spectinomycin, can be used for treatment.

Infertility (sterility) is higher with each infection. About 13 percent of women are infertile after their first infection involving their pelvic organs. This rises to as high as 75 percent with three attacks. If abscesses have formed in the tubes and ovaries, surgery may be required, frequently leaving a woman sterile. Early diagnosis and treatment can practically eliminate the need for surgical management.

It is hoped that sometime in the future there will be a vaccine against gonorrhea.

Granuloma Inguinale

Symptoms. This disease, caused by an intracellular organism (*Donovania granulomatis*), is rare in the United States, is generally found in tropical climates, and is usually associated with lack of personal cleanliness. A woman infected with this disease may note an unusual cyst, papule, or nodule in the genital area 3 to 8 days, or as long as a few months after exposure. The cyst eventually breaks down, forming an ulcer with a granular base (a granulation is one of the tiny, red granules of new capillaries that form on the surface of an ulcer). Another type of early lesion is a clean, raised, velvety tuft of granulation tissue with a sharply defined margin that bleeds easily. These early lesions are not painful. They do not heal readily and they spread, so that, if untreated, they eventually may involve most of the vulva and even extend onto the buttocks or lower abdomen. Late in the course of the disease there is interference of lymphatic drainage and elephantiasis may occur.

Diagnosis. Microscopic examination of tissue smears will reveal Donovan bodies included within the cell to confirm the diagnosis based on the appearance of the lesions.

Treatment. The preferred treatment is tetracycline until all lesions are healed. Ampicillin, an oral penicillin derivative, is an alternative therapy. In the late stages surgery may be necessary. However, if the disease is of long duration, it is often progressive, even with surgery.

Hemophilus Vaginalis (HV); Corynebacterium Vaginale

Symptoms. Heavy and unusual vaginal discharge, with or without irritation, is the most common symptom. Often, the discharge has an unpleasant fishy odor, is grayish, and may be frothy.

Diagnosis. On a wet mount of vaginal secretions examined under the microscope, the causative organism will be seen, identified as "clue cells." It may also be identified in a pap smear or a stained smear examined under the microscope.

Treatment. Use of sulfa creams or suppositories, alone or in combination with ampicillin, should be curative if the sexual partner(s) is also treated or wears condoms for about six weeks.

Herpes Simplex Virus Infection

Symptoms. Herpes simplex is a virus. Its two variants are herpes labialis, also known as herpes simplex virus type I (HSV-1), and herpes genitalis, or herpes simplex virus type II (HSV-2). Herpes labialis (type I) infection affects primarily the area of the head and neck where it causes what are commonly called cold sores or fever blisters. However, about 25 percent of genital infection is also type I, and it can be transmitted by oral or anogenital sex. Herpes genitalis (type II) is a distinctly different virus that affects primarily the genital area, often causing intensely painful lesions.

A woman infected for the first time in the genital area with type II is usually asymptomatic (75 to 90 percent). The symptomatic woman generally will notice one or more small, painful, fluid-filled blisters on the external genitalia within 3 to 20 days after exposure. They may occur also or only in the vagina or on the cervix and may not be noticed, but they can be seen on examination or be identified by a pap smear. These soon rupture and, when located externally, form soft, extremely painful, open sores. Secondary infection with bacteria can further aggravate the situation. The lymph glands in the groin may become enlarged and tender.

The herpes viruses have a tendency to remain in the body and may reactivate with such factors as stress or illness. The initial infection usually heals in about 10 to 12 days. Recurrences heal faster and are less painful.

An acute herpes infection of the genital area (both types) during pregnancy may have adverse effects, such as abortion, still birth, or infection of the newborn as it passes through the birth canal. When active infection is present at term, delivery by cesarean section greatly reduces the chance of infecting the baby. There is an additional concern that remains to be proven, and that is the possible relationship between herpes type II infection and development, years later, of cancer of the cervix.

Diagnosis. Herpes type II infection is usually diagnosed clinically by inspection of the lesions or by pap smear where a typical giant cell is identified. In addition, viral cultures may be taken from the sores for positive identification, or a fluorescent antibody study (micro-IF test) may be done.

Treatment. There is no specific treatment that cures herpes. Therapy is directed toward relief of discomfort and prevention of secondary bacterial infection of open genital lesions, usually with compresses and sitz baths; sometimes prescription pain medication is required. Although it is not known whether use of the condom will, with certainty, prevent transmission of the virus from an infected male, its use is recommended to prevent exposure, particularly if a woman is pregnant.

Molluscum Contagiosum

Symptoms. The very large virus of molluscum contagiosum affects the skin. In addition to being an STD, it may be transmitted by other forms of close body contact. It causes a very small, pinkish-white, waxy appearing polyplike growth appearing in the genital area and on the thighs. The incubation period varies from 3 weeks to 3 months.

Diagnosis. Usually the diagnosis is made clinically. Microscopic examination of the stained contents of the lesion reveals the inclusion bodies of the virus contained within large ballooned cells.

Treatment. Each lesion must be destroyed by hot or cold cautery or cauterizing chemicals. New lesions may occur 2 to 3 weeks following the initial therapy and require additional treatment.

Pelvic Inflammatory Disease (PID)

Symptoms. PID is an infection of the tubes and ovaries and has multiple causes, some of which are STDs. The gonococcus organism is the commonest cause of this disease, at least of the first episode of PID. Other bacteria, chlamydia, or fungi also cause it. It is now known to occur without the history or findings of an STD among some IUD users. In such cases, if the infection does not respond promptly to treatment, it is best to remove the IUD.

Infectious organisms travel up through the cervix and uterus and cause inflammation and even abscess of the fallopian tubes, the ovaries, and the pelvis. Typically, a woman who has PID is acutely ill with fever and lower abdominal pain.

Diagnosis. The diagnosis of PID is made by history, abdominal and pelvic examination, and laboratory testing. At times the interior of the abdomen is viewed with the laparoscope to differentiate between PID and appendicitis, ectopic pregnancy, or other intra-abdominal emergencies, these conditions being surgical emergencies while PID usually is not.

Treatment. The treatment is a combination of antibiotics, orally or intravenously. If abscesses have formed which cannot be eliminated with antibiotics, surgery may be required. If so, the chance of sterility resulting is high, as often the uterus, both tubes, and the ovaries must be removed to effect a cure.

Pubic Lice

Symptoms. An infestation with pubic lice (crab lice) is almost always an STD. However, lice or their eggs may be transmitted through infected clothing, bedding, and toilet seats. The adult organisms infest immediately, while their eggs hatch after 3 to 14 days. The most common symptom is intense itching in the pubic hair as a reaction to the bites of the lice.

Diagnosis. The pubic louse is yellowish-gray in color, but after it is swollen with blood it becomes dark in color. It can be found attached to pubic hairs. The eggs are white and give the appearance of a "growth" near the base of the hair shaft.

Treatment. An infestation of pubic lice can be cured readily with the application of gamma benezene hexachloride, commonly known as Kwell. It is available as a cream, lotion, or shampoo. In order to prevent recurrence, the sexual partner(s) must also take treatment, and clothes and bed linen must be washed or dry cleaned.

Scabies

Symptoms. Scabies may or may not be an STD and is readily transmitted by intimate contact. It is caused by a mite called *Sarcoptes scabies.* The characteristic lesion is the burrow of the mite under the skin. It appears initially as a small, wavy line, usually located between the fingers, on the wrists, armpits, breasts, buttocks, thighs, and rarely on the genitalia.

The face is not usually involved. Itching is present wherever the burrowing parasite is found and is aggravated at night. Scratching can cause second-ary infection of the lesions.

Diagnosis. Scabies can be diagnosed by clinical history and the presence of characteristic lesions. Additionally, the burrow can be scraped to obtain the mite, eggs, and larvae which can be identified under the microscope.

Treatment. After a prolonged bath, with thorough cleansing of the affected areas, an emulsion of 25 percent benzyl benzoate, available with-out a prescription, is applied from the neck down. The treatment needs to be repeated in 24 hours. Often, the best way to diagnose scabies is to take the treatment. Continued itching after the treatment is related to secondary infection and should be treated symptomatically. Bedding and clothing must be washed or dry cleaned.

Syphilis

Symptoms. Syphilis is the most serious of the STDs as it is life-threaten-ing, not only to the woman herself, but to her future children. It is caused by a spirochete organism known as *Treponema pallidum*. It dies very quickly outside the human body and is killed by soap and water if present on the skin—a good reason for thorough washing after sex. The organism passes from the chancre or skin of an infected individual who is in the pri-mary or secondary stage to an uninfected person through the latter's mu-cous membranes or a break in the skin. Since symptoms can simulate many other disease conditions or the disease may be asymptomatic for many years, the discussion of symptoms will be divided into the stages of the disease—primary, secondary, latent, and late—and other special situ-ations. The stages describe the untreated course of this disease.

Primary Syphilis The primary sore of syphilis is the chancre. It ap-pears where the organism entered the body, usually on the genitals, and may appear as early as 10 days or as long as 3 months after infection. The chancre is usually a solitary, painless ulceration that feels firm and has a slightly elevated border. In the woman it is commonly located on the cer-vix or in the vagina hidden from view. The chancre exudes the spirochete and is highly infectious. Often the associated lymph glands are swollen. Even without treatment the chancre heals within 1 to 5 weeks, concluding the primary stage.

Secondary Syphilis The onset of the secondary stage occurs anywhere from 6 to 24 weeks after the untreated primary phase. It is often heralded by a general feeling of ill health. This may include any combination of the following general symptoms: headache, muscle or joint aches, pain in the long bones, loss of appetite, nausea, constipation, and a lowgrade, persist-ent fever. Swelling and tenderness of the lymph glands are often present, and the hair may fall out in patches.

The most classical visible symptom of a secondary infection is a nonirritating, highly infectious rash. It may appear anywhere on the body. If the extremities are involved, it is symmetrically distributed. It may also affect the mucous membranes of the body and in women is commonly found around the labia. On the mucous membranes it appears initially as a grayish-white surface that breaks down into sores with a dull red base which ooze a clear fluid loaded with the infectious spirochete. Syphilitic warts may also develop on the genitals. Unless secondary infection occurs, these lesions are not usually painful. Without treatment the secondary phase usually passes in 4 to 12 weeks.

Latent Syphilis Latent syphilis is asymptomatic, beginning at the conclusion of the secondary phase. It is not infectious to a sexual contact, but the spirochete can spread within a pregnant woman to her fetus. Early latent syphilis has a duration of less than 4 years, while late latent syphilis extends from 4 years to the development, if it occurs, of late syphilis.

Late Syphilis Approximately one-third of individuals develop manifestations of late syphilis. The other two-thirds do not, but we do not yet know what determines into which group they will fall. The most common manifestations of late syphilis are gumma (syphilitic tumors) in any affected organ, cardiovascular syphilis, and neurosyphilis. Late syphilis can cause insanity and death.

Syphilis in Pregnancy The spirochete of the mother's untreated syphilis at whatever stage invades the placenta and eventually the fetus between the tenth and eighteenth week of pregnancy. If untreated, the risk of stillbirth or of congenital syphilis affecting the newborn is high. It is important for every pregnant woman to be tested for syphilis early in pregnancy so that the disease may be treated before it can damage the fetus.

Congenital Syphilis Most children born to women who have untreated syphilis during their pregnancies will have congenital syphilis. Its effects range through blindness, deafness, crippling bone disease, and facial abnormalities. Special blood tests combined with other diagnostic measures are essential when congenital syphilis is suspected.

Diagnosis. There are several tests used to diagnose syphilis; their performance and accuracy are related to the phase of the disease. Part of the diagnostic process is a complete physical examination, not limited to the genitals. Laboratory tests that are diagnostic are as follows:

DARKFIELD MICROSCOPIC EXAMINATION. Fluid obtained from a chancre or other open sores is examined under a microscope to identify the spirochete.

SEROLOGIC TESTS FOR SYPHILIS (STS). A number of different tests are done on blood serum to see whether an individual has a pathologic level of antibodies to the spirochete *T. pallidum*. It takes about three weeks following the appearance of the chancre for STS to become positive. Certain tests measure antibodies which show a declining titre concentration in blood serum with treatment and are indicators of successful therapy. Others measure antibodies which remain permanently elevated and thereby indicate whether a person has ever had the disease.

SPINAL FLUID EXAMINATION. With latent or late syphilis it is necessary to have a serologic test done on the cerebral spinal fluid to determine whether the infection has invaded the central nervous system since neurosyphilis requires special treatment.

Treatment. The treatment of choice is long-acting penicillin. The dosage and duration of treatment vary with the stage and manifestations of the disease. Follow-up to ensure cure or arrest is absolutely essential. In the event of penicillin allergy, alternative therapy is tetracycline or erythromycin.

Trichomoniasis

Symptoms. This is one of the most common vaginal conditions. It is caused by a simple, one-celled, motile organism called *Trichomonas vaginalis.* The condition may be asymptomatic, and a woman may not know that she is infected until the organism is identified as part of the pap smear procedure. Usually, however, infected women will notice, within 4 to 28 days after exposure, a greenish-yellow, often frothy, vaginal discharge associated with itching and an unpleasant musty odor. The discharge frequently causes irritation and redness of the vulva, and a spotting of blood may be mixed with the discharge. Inspection of the vaginal mucous membranes and cervix may reveal small red dots, commonly referred to as "strawberry marks." The lymph glands in the groin may become enlarged. The infection can spread to the urinary tract where it may be asymptomatic or may cause symptoms of urinary frequency and urgency. Trichomoniasis is frequently associated with other STDs and may mask their symptoms.

Diagnosis. Clinical diagnosis can be made by identifying the strawberry marks on the vaginal wall and cervix. Microscopic examination of the vaginal discharge mixed with saline will reveal the presence of the organism. Diagnosis on a pap smear in the absence of clinical symptoms or microscope confirmation does not constitute an indication for treatment.

Treatment. Metronidazole, marketed as Flagyl, is a specific cure for *T. vaginalis.* Alcoholic beverages must be avoided during therapy. Flagyl should not be taken during at least the first four months of pregnancy. Sexual partner(s) also need to be treated simultaneously. Vaginal creams, suppositories, and douches may relieve symptoms, but are seldom curative.

Vaginitis (Nonspecific)

Symptoms. Because, as the name implies, a single causative organism or agent is seldom responsible for this condition, the symptoms vary widely. However, the condition is almost always associated with a vaginal discharge. This may be accompanied by itching or irritation of the vagina or vulva. It may also cause urinary symptoms of urgency and frequency. There are three general causative categories, two of which cannot be considered STD, but must be considered in the differential diagnosis.

CHEMICAL. Irritation often occurs from using products for "feminine hygiene," for example, sprays, perfumed soaps, and douches. If the condition is chemically induced, it should subside when the use of such products is stopped.

MECHANICAL. A foreign body, such as a tampon, inserted in the vagina and "lost," frequently accounts for vaginitis with a particularly unpleasant odor. Removal and use of local antibiotic preparations bring about prompt subsidence of symptoms.

BACTERIAL. Many bacteria that are not normal inhabitants of the vagina may cause vaginitis and be sexually transmitted. Those known to be responsible for causing vaginitis are as follows: T-strain mycoplasmas, fusobacteria, *Escherichia coli,* and other coliform organisms (normal inhabitants of the bowel), clostridia, actinomycetes, and group B streptococci. Of these, the group B strep infection has the greatest potential of producing serious problems, particularly for a child born while a woman is harboring this infection as well as for post pregnancy infection for the woman.

Diagnosis. A culture will usually reveal the causative organisms.

Treatment. Treatment varies with the diagnosis, the severity of the symptoms, the sensitivity of the organisms to antibiotic therapy, and whether pregnancy coexists. For such nonspecific bacterial infections, local vaginal therapy with creams or suppositories containing sulfa is generally the treatment of choice. This may be combined with antibiotic therapy if the infectious organism is group B strep and particularly if the woman is pregnant and near term.

Venereal Warts (Condyloma Acuminata)

Symptoms. Soft, cauliflower-appearing warts, caused by a virus, develop anywhere from 6 weeks to 8 months after sexual exposure. In a woman these warts may be located in and around the vagina and rectum and may be single, multiple, or even confluent. They thrive in warm, moist areas. They grow even more rapidly when associated with vaginal infections and also with pregnancy. There is a tendency for recurrences.

Diagnosis. The diagnosis is usually made on the basis of appearance.

Treatment. Since this is a viral infection, there is no specific cure. Two of the most important adjuncts to therapy are to treat any associated vaginitis and to keep the affected areas dry. Venereal warts usually can be treated successfully by applying a chemical called podophyllin. The medication must be used with care. Because it is very irritating to normal skin, it should be applied to the surface of the warts only, and within 6 to 8 hours after treatment a warm sitz bath should be taken to remove excess medication. This chemical generally is not recommended for use during pregnancy, because if too much is used and some is absorbed, it is toxic to the fetus. The warts can also be removed by cold or hot cautery or surgical excision.

Yeast Infections (Monilia)

Symptoms. Monilial infections of the vagina and vulva are caused by a yeastlike fungus known as *Candida albicans.* This organism and other similar related organisms are, to some extent, normal inhabitants of the mouth, intestinal tract, and vagina of most healthy women. An upset of the normal symbiotic balance among these organisms can result in a marked overgrowth of the Candida organisms, leading to infection. Conditions that predispose to such an imbalance are diabetes, lowered systemic resistance, use of drugs such as antibiotics or cortisone, altered metabolic states such as pregnancy, use of birth control pills, and estrogen deficiency of the vaginal tissues in postmenopausal women. Acquiring Monilia under such conditions is not considered an STD. However, once infection occurs, it can be transmitted to others through sexual contact.

The major symptoms in women consist of a white, cheesy vaginal discharge, vulvar itching and irritation, and a "yeasty" odor. If there is also associated yeast overgrowth in the gastrointestinal tract, it can produce symptoms of bloating, abdominal distress, and altered bowel patterns.

When the infection occurs in the mouth, it is known as thrush. White, cheesy patches appear on the tongue and then may spread inside the mouth and to the throat. Infants may acquire it following birth if the mother has the infection in her vagina.

Diagnosis. The identification of the white, cheesy patches, adhering to the vaginal wall or in the mouth, is suggestive of a yeast infection. Microscopic examination will show the characteristic long chains of budding yeast organisms. Cultures can also be diagnostic.

Treatment. Underlying causes, that is, the conditions leading to the symbiotic imbalance, should be sought and treated if possible. Treatment is designed to reduce the number of causative organisms and restore a more normal vaginal flora. If the infection is not too severe, the use of a mild, acidic douche about 2 or 3 times a week may control it. A recommended douche is 2 tablespoons of white vinegar to 1 quart of warm water to which has been added 2 tablespoons of acidophilus culture. This culture (similar to normal vaginal flora) can be obtained from most health food stores; when kept refrigerated, the acidophilus bacteria survive for some time.

Specific therapy consists of vaginal and vulvar applications and of pills taken by mouth. A course of treatment is usually carried out for 14 days and, if being re-treated, through a menstrual period. A male partner with symptoms of genital irritation or itching should be treated simultaneously.

If monilial infections are resistant or recurrent, a thorough medical evaluation should be done to determine appropriate steps most likely to effect a cure. For example, a course of oral medication may be instituted to reduce gastrointestinal moniliasis and its associated spread to the genital areas. Or, if oral contraceptive pills seem to be the aggravating factor, a different prescription or another method of contraception might be recommended, at least temporarily.

OTHER STDs AND SEXUAL PRACTICES

Because sexual practices other than vaginal intercourse are not uncommon, certain diseases not generally considered as STDs may be acquired through sexual contact. Therefore, if one also practices oral or anal sex, it is important that the clinician know this so that appropriate tests can be taken to evaluate the possibility of disease of the pharynx or gastrointestinal tract. Gastrointestinally transmitted STDs are much more common among homosexual and bisexual males and, through this route, their female partner(s) may contract any one of the following diseases.

Amebiasis

Symptoms. This infection is caused by a single-cell amoeba known as *Endamoeba histolytica.* Symptoms consist of diarrhea, often containing blood and mucus, associated with abdominal distress, low-grade fever, and a general feeling of illness. Infection can occur in the liver and other organs. Carriers of the disease, although asymptomatic, may have cysts in their stool or around their rectum that are highly infectious with oral contact.

Diagnosis. Microscopic examination of the stool reveals the organism or the cysts.

Treatment. Individually determined by a physician.

Shigellosis

Symptoms. The shigella bacteria cause a serious form of dysentery shortly after infection. The dysentery is associated with frequent stools containing blood, pus, and mucus, ulcerations of the bowel, rectal pain, abdominal cramps, fever, and dehydration.

Diagnosis. The shigella bacteria can be identified by microscopic examination of smears or by culture.

Treatment. Individually determined by a physician.

Viral Hepatitis

Symptoms. Viral hepatitis occurs in at least two forms, known as A and B. Their incubation periods are approximately 1 and 3 months respectively. Although they particularly affect the liver, they start with symptoms resembling flu. Jaundice may develop in severe cases and last 2 or more weeks. In the presence of jaundice, one usually notices dark "cola-colored" urine, light stools, and bodily itching. A person harboring one of these viruses may have no symptoms, yet the virus is highly infectious with oral-anal contact.

Diagnosis. Special blood tests, along with the findings on history and physical examination, give the diagnosis.

Treatment. As with other viral diseases, the treatment is symptomatic and supportive. Medical care must be obtained.

Confronting this alarming array of diseases that may be sexually transmitted, one might be inclined to exclaim, "No more sex ever again!" However, the sex drive is a powerful part of human nature and so is a short memory for the unpleasant things described in this chapter. But, to be forewarned is to be forearmed. Remember to take precautions to protect yourself against STD, have regular checks at least annually that include examinations to detect the presence of such diseases, be alert for unusual symptoms that may suggest the onset of a disease, and seek early diagnosis.

REFERENCES

Brecher, E. "Prevention of the Sexually Transmitted Diseases," *J. Sex. Res.* 11 (1975): 318–328.

"Chlamydia Infection," *J. Infect. Dis.* 11–12 (1975).

Cutler, J. C., B. Singh, V. Carpenter, O. Nickens, A. Scarola, N. Sussman, M. Wade, L. Volkin, A. Marsico and H. Balisky. *Vaginal Contraceptives as Prophylaxis against Gonorrhea and Other Sexually Transmitted Diseases.* Pittsburgh, Pa.: University of Pittsburgh and Allegheny County Health Department, 1976.

Dritz, S. K. "Patterns of Sexually Transmitted Enteric Disease in a Metropolitan Center." Unpublished, San Francisco, July 1976.

Edwards, R. G. "Research in Reproduction," *International Planned Parenthood Federation* 7 (no. 4) (1975).

Eschenback, D. A. "Myths of the Woman with Asymptomatic Gonorrhea," *Medical Aspects of Human Sexuality* 10 (1976): 118–126.

"Flagyl," G. D. Searle & Co., 1979 (package insert).

Holvey, D. N., and J. H. Talbott. *The Merck Manual of Diagnosis and Therapy.* Rahway, N.J.: Merck & Co., 1972.

Jordan, G. R. "Other Venereal Diseases," *Urban Health* 5 (October 1975): 31–34.

Keith, L. and J. Brittain. *Sexually Transmitted Diseases.* Aspen, Colorado: Creative Informatics, 1978.

Lucas, J., E. G. Price, J. D. Thayer, and A. Schroeter. "Diagnosis and Treatment of Gonorrhea in the Female." *N. Engl. J. Med.* 276 (1967): 1454–1459.

Melish, M. E. and J. B. Hanshaw. "Congenital cytomegalovirus infection," *Am. J. Dis. Child.* 126 (1973): 190.

Morton, B. M. *V.D.: A Guide for Nurses and Counselors.* Boston: Little, Brown, 1976.

Packin, G. S. "Herpes Genitalis," *JAOA* 75 (1975): 324–328.

Plain Talk About Crabs and Lice. Young's Drug Products Co., Piscataway, N.J.: 1975.

Rein, M. F. "Attacking Vaginitis, Therapeutic Strategies Against the Big Three Offenders," *Current Prescribing,* July 1976.

Rodgerson, E. B. "Diagnosis and Treatment of Trichomonas Vaginalis," *Medical Aspects of Human Sexuality* 10 (no. 4) (April 1976): 127–128.

American College of Obstetrics and Gynecology. "Sexually Transmitted Diseases—Gonorrhea and Syphilis," *ACOG Technical Bulletin* no. 50 (June 1978).

American College of Obstetrics and Gynecology. "Sexually Transmitted Diseases—Other than Gonorrhea and Syphilis," *ACOG Technical Bulletin* no. 51 (July 1978).

Tietze, C., J. Bongaarts, and B. Schearer. "Mortality Associated with the Control of Fertility," *Fam. Pl. Persp.* 8, no. 1 (January–February 1976).

U.S. Department of Health and Human Services. *Criteria and Techniques for the Diagnosis of Gonorrhea.* Atlanta, Ga.: Center for Disease Control, 1974.

U.S. Department of Health and Human Services. *Recommended Treatment Schedules for Syphilis.* Atlanta, Ga.: Center for Disease Control, 1976.

VD Statistical Letter. (U.S. Department of Health and Human Services, Public Health Service, Center for Disease Control). No. 126 (May 1977).

Weller, T. H., and J. B. Hanshaw. "Virologic and clinical observations on cytomegalic inclusion disease," *N. Engl. J. Med.* 266 (1962): 1233.

Wright, R. A. "Pelvic Inflammatory Disease," *Medical Aspects of Human Sexuality* 10, no. 7 (July 1976): 139–140.

FURTHER READING

American College of Obstetrics and Gynecology. "Sexually Transmitted Diseases—Gonorrhea and Syphilis," *ACOG Technical Bulletin* no. 50 (June 1978).

American College of Obstetrics and Gynecology. "Sexually Transmitted Diseases—Other Than Gonorrhea and Syphilis," *ACOG Technical Bulletin* no. 51 (July 1978).

American Foundation for the Prevention of Venereal Disease, Inc. *The New Venereal Disease Prevention for Everyone*. (6th rev. ed.). New York: American Foundation for the Prevention of Venereal Disease, 93 Worth Street. 8 pp. 1978.

Carroll, D., M.D. *The Love Bugs; Los Bichos de Amor* (Spanish edition) Daly City, Calif.: Physicians Art Service, Inc. Patient Information Library, 1976. 15 pp.

Judson, F. N., M.D. "Update in Sexually Transmitted Diseases," *Amer. Med. Women's Assoc.* 31, no. 1 (January 1976): 11–19.

Keith, L. and J. Brittain. *Sexually Transmitted Diseases*. Aspen, Colo.: Creative Informatics, 1978. 100 pp., paper.

National Institute of Allergy and Infectious Disease. *Sexually Transmitted Diseases*. Pueblo, Colo.: Public Documents Distribution Center, 1976. 24 pp.

Wright, R. A. "Pelvic Inflammatory Disease." *Medical Aspects of Human Sexuality* 10 (July 1976): 139–140.

Breast Care

MARGARET A. NELSEN, M.D.
Associate Medical Director for Utilization Control,
Surveillance Utilization Review and Education Program,
Electronics Data Systems–Federal, Raleigh, North Carolina;
Assistant Professor of Surgery (1975–1979), University of
North Carolina School of Medicine, Chapel Hill, North Carolina

Not only are a woman's breasts a graceful compliment to her womanhood, but they are also symbols of her individualism and sexuality. It has been some time since the human breast was thought of as a mere milk gland, primarily useful for nourishing the species. The average woman, however, has little understanding of normal breast structure and function. The two facts which are generally known are (1) breast cancer is a leading cause of death in women and (2) therapy often involves removal of the breast. Therefore, it is not surprising that the perception of any abnormality of the breast leads to anxiety and fear. Some women respond to this anxiety by seeking immediate attention for what often are normal physiologic changes. Other women respond by ignoring a significant abnormality which should be seen promptly for effective treatment.

It is the purpose of this chapter to alleviate unnecessary anxiety and fear and to encourage all women to participate in their own breast care. By becoming aware of the normal structure and function of your breasts, you can deal more confidently with any needed treatment. The attitudes of women patients and the capabilities of physicians are changing. No longer is the woman willing to be the ignorant recipient of treatment, and no longer are physicians limited to a single form of treatment.

GROWTH AND DEVELOPMENT OF THE BREAST

Throughout your life your breasts reflect changes in your endocrine system as well as changes related to age. Your breasts are formed during gestation and by the time of birth consist of a branching system of ducts which empty into the nipples. In the newborn, due to the influence of the hormones of pregnancy, there is often evidence of a clear milky secretion from the nipple. After a few days this secretion ceases. The breasts then remain dormant throughout the remainder of childhood, consisting chiefly of the nipples and rudimentary duct systems. Occasionally, a mass is noted during infancy or childhood which most often disappears. There is no cause for concern, although there is no satisfactory explanation for such masses.

At the time of puberty, as your ovaries begin to manufacture estrogen, several changes begin to take place. Between the ages of 9 and 15, the first changes are noticeable. At first the areola, the pigmented skin surrounding the nipple, begins to enlarge and darken. Beneath the nipple and the areola the previously quiescent duct system enlarges and grows. Branches also begin to form. Usually by the time of your first menstrual period the normal protuberant and firm adolescent breast is well developed. As the ovaries produce progesterone and the breast continues to develop, ducts begin to bud at the end of their branches, producing groups of glands. The essential components of the adult breast are now present (see illustration).

Let us take a more detailed look at the normal adult breast. The breast normally extends from the second to the sixth or seventh rib and from the sternum (breast bone) to the side of the chest wall and into the axilla (arm pit). Although quite variable, the average breast extends 1 to 2 inches out from the chest wall, is 4 to 5 inches in diameter and weighs about ½ pound. The weight may almost double during lactation. It is very common to have one breast larger than the other, and most often it is the left breast which is larger. There is no explanation for this sometimes striking difference. The overall size of the breast is greatly influenced by the fat content.

Under the upper portion of the breasts are the muscles of the chest wall and some of the shoulder muscles which are attached to the chest wall. These muscles are the pectoral muscles. The breast itself normally glides smoothly over all of these muscles and is supported by ligaments called Cooper's ligaments which rise from the deep portions of the breast to the skin, like guy wires.

The nipple and areola are covered by a modified membrane which is lubricated by special glands which appear as little rough areas in the areola. These glands are called the glands of Montgomery and are similar to your other oil-producing glands. Situated in the center of the areola is the conically shaped nipple which has 15 to 25 tiny openings. These openings come from the ducts of the breasts and are very hard to see without magnification. Beneath the areola and nipple are tiny muscles which are responsible for erection of the nipple when stimulated. They are quite similar to the muscles which cause fine skin hairs to stand on end. The tiny openings on the nipple connect to the duct system of the breast which radiates away from the nipple like the spokes of a wheel. Just underneath the nipple and areola these ducts enlarge somewhat to serve as a reservoir for milk. As each duct extends toward the chest wall there are multiple branchings. At the end of these branchings are the secretory glands of the breast. Each grouping of glands and duct tissue is called a lobe; the smaller branches and glands themselves are called lobules. Between the lobes and lobules is fat and connective tissue, including Cooper's ligaments. The lining of the ducts and glands consists of two layers of cells. Around the glands themselves are tiny cells which are like muscles and help to move milk toward the major duct system and nipple.

Blood is supplied to the breasts by arteries branching from beneath the sternum and between the ribs as well as branches from the large axillary artery. Blood is drained from the breast by veins which follow the same routes. Often the veins in and just under the skin of the breast are very visible. Lymph drains from the breast to five major lymph node areas. These areas are in the axilla, just above the collar bone, under the sternum, across to the opposite breast, and through passages that lead to the lymph nodes in the upper abdomen.

The nerve supply to the skin of the breast and the nipple-areola complex is generous and specialized at the microscopic level. The nerves are thought to play a role in stimulating milk production. They are also the explanation for the increased sensitivity of your breast, skin, and nipple to stimulation of all sorts. These nerves originate low in the neck and from the nerve supply to the ribs.

During early pregnancy the first noted breast changes occur in the areola, which darkens and begins to enlarge. Subsequently there is increased budding and growth of the glands as well as the duct system. For more detailed discussion of these changes, see "Pregnancy and Childbirth."

With the onset of menopause your breasts will become less firm due to the regression of the glandular structures. Frequently, too, the supporting ligaments relax and the breast becomes more pendulous. It is not unusual to be able to actually feel the breast ducts themselves in an elderly woman. If, however, a woman is taking estrogens after menopause, there may be less regression of the glandular and ductal structure. Such women will have breast tissue more like the younger adult, although there is still some relaxation and "drooping" due to lax ligaments and skin.

DEVELOPMENT OF THE BREAST

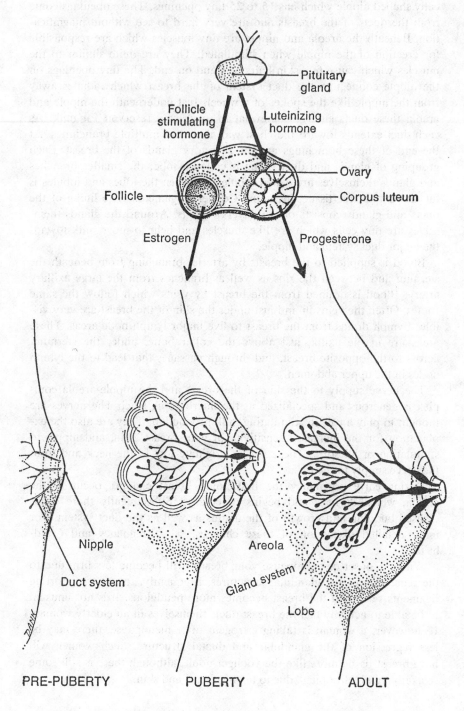

Pituitary gland

Follicle stimulating hormone

Luteinizing hormone

Follicle

Ovary

Corpus luteum

Estrogen

Progesterone

Nipple

Duct system

Areola

Gland system

Lobe

PRE-PUBERTY

PUBERTY

ADULT

CROSS-SECTION OF THE BREAST

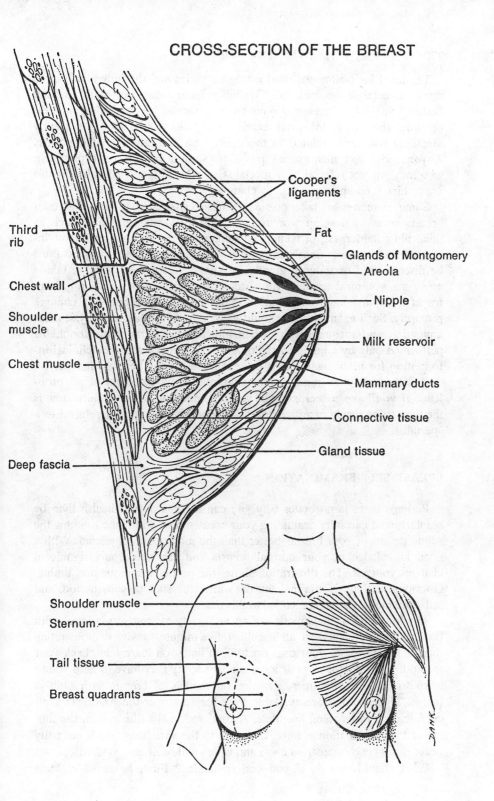

Cooper's ligaments

Fat

Glands of Montgomery

Areola

Nipple

Milk reservoir

Mammary ducts

Connective tissue

Gland tissue

Third rib

Chest wall

Shoulder muscle

Chest muscle

Deep fascia

Shoulder muscle

Sternum

Tail tissue

Breast quadrants

The need for postmenopausal estrogens varies and the individual's need must be carefully considered. Disability from symptoms such as "hot flashes," vaginal dryness, and bone changes should be weighed against the possible risk of endometrial carcinoma. This risk is not yet clearly identified but seems related to the dose given and duration of exposure. Anyone who has menopausal problems should consult their physician who may suggest referral to a specialist specifically knowledgeable in this area which is complex and rapidly changing.

Some women who take postmenopausal estrogen may find that their breasts seem to develop worrisome, relatively vague symptoms such as thickening, tenderness, or feelings of fullness. X-ray changes may show increased density more consistent with a younger age. Often estrogens must be discontinued or reduced greatly in dosage. Certainly if you are taking estrogens, you must examine your breasts regularly and see your physician for at least an annual examination. You should also report any changes promptly. Such examinations should include a careful history, physical examination and mammography when indicated. Mammograms should be performed only by a qualified radiologist who has access to the clinical information for interpretation. At present these are the best but not perfect diagnostic techniques, and do not guarantee early detection of all problems. If you have concerns about your examination or the results, now is the time to be firmly assertive and ask for another opinion or referral to a specialist.

BREAST SELF-EXAMINATION

Perhaps there is no better way you can safeguard your health than by regularly and carefully examining your breasts. You will come to know the subtle details of your breasts better than the most astute physician. With a good knowledge of your normal breasts you can detect any significant changes yourself. The illustration shows the proper technique and timing. Hormonal activity is minimal ten days after the start of your period, and self-examination is recommended at this time.

Any local unit of the American Cancer Society can put you in touch with further material, such as an excellent five-minute movie, demonstrating this technique. Also, your own doctor can help you learn and check your method. Your doctor or your local cancer society may have to help you to learn to find abnormalities. Practice on models of breasts with built-in lumps. These models are available from local units of the American Cancer Society and teaching hospitals. As outlined in the illustration, the timing of the examination is important, due to the variations which normally occur during each menstrual cycle and which will be discussed shortly.

What should you do if you find something? First, *be sensible!* Most problems are *not* cancer. Seek prompt attention from a competent physician. If you have found an early cancer, you have done yourself the biggest possible favor because these are highly curable. More will be said later regarding other problems you might discover.

EVERYDAY BREAST CARE

There are no mysteries regarding the care of your breasts. Good hygiene is important here as everywhere. The skin of the nipple and breast can be susceptible to dryness, particularly during the winter, and to allergic reactions to clothing. A cream or ointment that does not contain alcohol can relieve such dryness. Some women prefer to remove the few dark hairs around the areola by plucking them. Care should be taken not to cause infection by doing so. You should not "dig" them out; pluck gently as you would in shaping your eyebrows. Electrolysis may be helpful in some instances; however, it is suggested that you first consult your physician. It is not unusual to have occasional scaling of the nipple, but crusting or bleeding is another matter and must be checked by your doctor.

Women with large breasts can be plagued with rashes and dryness under the breast fold, especially in the summer. Often simple remedies such as baby powder are beneficial in relieving the condition.

Most women, particularly those with large breasts, wear a brassiere for both support and comfort. The most important thing about a brassiere is fit. One that is too loose, too small, or "uplifts" to the point of ridiculousness makes no more sense than the bygone custom of tight girdles and stays. Any good department store can help with fitting. Women whose breasts change a great deal with their menstrual cycles may require more than one size brassiere. Many women find that their brassiere size changes after pregnancy and after menopause. It is not necessary to spend a lot of money for a properly fitting brassiere. A brand name or other (admittedly desirable) features of decorations and material may enhance the cost, but not the support.

A well-fitted brassiere is especially important for most athletic activities. This topic is discussed in "Fitness," the chapter on exercise. In general little breast injury has been noted in women athletes.

When should a young girl obtain her "first" brassiere? Often this is a matter of local social custom. If everyone else is wearing a bra by a certain age or grade in school, there is no reason why a girl should not have one, even if she does not need one yet. At the other end of the spectrum is the more full-busted girl who probably needs a brassiere.

Some men and women feel that sexual attraction is often based on breast size. Sexual attraction has more to do with attitude, self-esteem, and personality characteristics than on any single physical characteristic. The American male while often joking about and overtly admiring breasts is

HOW TO EXAMINE YOUR BREASTS

When: Recommended time is ten days after period starts or same day every month for post-menopausal women

PART 1

After hot bath, sitting before a well-lighted mirror

Arms at sides — become familiar with superficial blood vessel patterns; look for any unusual swelling, dimpling or puckering of skin

Stretch arms high — observe any changes

Press hands firmly on hips to flex chest muscles

DANK.

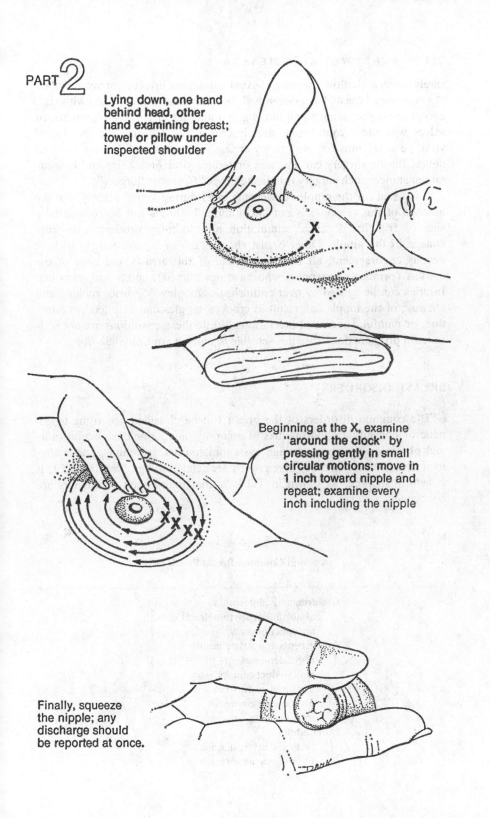

PART 2

Lying down, one hand behind head, other hand examining breast; towel or pillow under inspected shoulder

Beginning at the X, examine "around the clock" by pressing gently in small circular motions; move in 1 inch toward nipple and repeat; examine every inch including the nipple

Finally, squeeze the nipple; any discharge should be reported at once.

rarely such a shallow creature. Sexual attraction involves many nuances.

Once your breasts have developed, hormones have little to do with size, except during pregnancy and nursing. No amount of creams, ointments, or salves will affect your breast size. Exercises can only change the size of your pectoral muscles and rarely make a significant difference in your figure. Plastic surgery can increase or reduce your breast size and in some circumstances such surgery is indicated (see "Cosmetic Surgery").

It is usual for the nipples to become erect during sexual activity, but the absence of this response is not uncommon. It should not be considered a sign of frigidity if sexual stimulation and foreplay produce only little change in the nipple. Other breast changes during sexual activity include venous engorgement, an increase in size of the breasts and later of the areolas (primarily in women who have not nursed), and a pink mottling. Injuries can be caused by over enthusiastic sex play. Vigorous sucking and chewing of the nipple can result in cracked nipples that may lead to infection, or painful, superficial ulcerations. While these conditions are not serious, if a problem does arise it is sensible to consult your physician.

BREAST DISORDERS

The common disorders of the breast can be classified according to genetic or congenital abnormalities of anatomy, endocrine dysfunction, normal physiologic changes, benign cysts and tumors, infections, and malignant disease. Disorders in these groups are related to age (see Table 1). It is helpful to note, as shown in Table 2, that many adult complaints are not cancer.

TABLE 1.

Age and Common Breast Problems

Children and adolescents
    abnormal or asymmetrical growth
    fibroadenomas
Adolescents and young adults
    fibroadenomas
    benign duct tumors
    cysts and cystic disease
    physiologic changes
    infections
Older adults
    cysts and cystic disease
    physiologic abnormalities
    cancer

TABLE 2.

Breast Conditions—1,000 Women Seeking Medical Consultation

750	symptoms not requiring medical care
85	abnormal physiology, requiring medical care
80	benign, of physiologic origin, requiring medical care
30	tumors, not cancer, requiring medical care
55	cancer, requiring medical care
1,000	

SOURCE: C. D. Haagensen, *Diseases of the Breast,* rev. 2nd ed. Philadelphia: Saunders, 1974.

Anatomical Abnormalities and Endocrine Dysfunction

There are several relatively common congenital anatomical disorders which do not become apparent until puberty. Failure to develop *any* breast tissue due to anatomical abnormality is exceedingly rare. However, "extra" breasts or parts of a breast occur in 1 to 2 percent of Caucasians, and more frequently in Orientals. In all mammals the breasts develop from an embryonic milk-line which extends on both sides of the body from the axilla to the groin. Breast tissue, nipples, or areolas in any combination may be present along this line and may be unilateral or bilateral. The presence of axillary breast tissue is common and of no particular significance. This is rudimentary tissue with no physiologic function. Even if enlarged during pregnancy these incompletely formed breasts will usually regress. A fully formed additional breast, however, may function normally and even provide satisfactory nursing. These more complete breasts are subject to the diseases affecting normal breasts.

Another problem which appears at puberty is a difference in the size of one breast compared with the other. This is quite common and not considered abnormal in most instances. Only if the difference in size is great should plastic surgery be considered. However, even a modest difference in breast sizes may be disconcerting and give rise to some anxiety.

Like navels, some nipples are always "inners" rather than "outers." An inverted nipple which a woman has had all of her life is no cause for concern. It is when there is a change that you should have an examination.

Abnormalities in the breasts which are associated with abnormal endocrine gland development or dysfunction are usually not noted until adolescence, unless associated congenital abnormalities involving the genital system are evident at an earlier age. Failure of the breasts to develop at all due to endocrine dysfunction is rare. When it does occur, it may be associated with the absence of ovaries or adrenal glands. Delayed or minimal breast development may be associated with ovaries which are functioning abnormally. Complex relationships between the pituitary, thyroid, and adrenal glands can produce numerous variations of delayed or minimal development. Failure of development of breasts by age 15, with or without associated onset of menstruation, should be investigated. Modern methods of evaluating gland function can usually pinpoint the precise problem. Replacement hormone therapy can often help to stimulate development of the nonadult breast. It should be noted that very small breasts may be completely normal. It is the function of the endocrine glands, not size of the breast, which determines the need for hormonal stimulation in adolescents. It should also be pointed out that hormonal medication will not increase the size of the normal adult breast and should never be considered for that purpose.

In some cases breast development begins early. If it begins before age 8, it is called precocious puberty. It is common for the other secondary sex characteristics, especially pubic hair, growth of the labia, and menstruation, to develop somewhat later than the onset of breast development. In the past it was thought that most of the problems of precocious puberty were related to a tumor of the ovary which caused increasing production of hormones. Since bone maturation and precocious growth often coexist, it now appears that precocious puberty is related to other or more general endocrine problems. For example, tumors of the adrenal gland have been known to cause the condition. A careful and complete endocrine evaluation is necessary to find the source of the disorder.

Children who develop breasts between 8 and 12 are considered to have early puberty not precocious puberty. Development may be unilateral and may be noted first as a soft, flat, 1 to 2 inch circular mass beneath the nipple. Since the opposite breast will begin to develop in several months, excision of this "mass" is not wise as the entire normal breast may be removed. It is not until about age 13 or later that some other common disorders such as cysts or fibroadenomas begin to occur.

Normal Physiologic Changes

During late adolescence and adult life normal physiologic changes in the breasts occur with each menstrual cycle. These changes do not represent disorders and understanding them can relieve much unnecessary anxiety and concern. For three or four days before menstruation the breasts may become engorged, that is you may notice that your breasts are fuller and more sensitive. In some women there is quite a marked change. There may also be some increase in the nodularity or lumpiness of your breast. Less commonly, you may notice a more distinct lump or cystlike mass, which may be uncomfortable, but which disappears with menstruation. The breast may become very tender. Other more general symptoms related to menstruation are fluid retention, mood changes, and pelvic "cramps."

Variability in symptoms is great. Such changes and complaints may not always occur with every cycle because there are times when, although the menstrual cycle is quite regular, you do not ovulate. The woman whose ovaries are intact after a hysterectomy should remember that menstrual symptoms, including breast changes, may be present, even though vaginal bleeding is of course absent. Awareness of your own pattern of symptoms and careful self-appraisal in these circumstances can be quite helpful.

No specific therapy other than a good supporting brassiere and aspirin is indicated or generally beneficial for such premenstrual complaints. Some women require or use a diuretic to reduce premenstrual fluid retention. This fluid retention does contribute to breast complaints. Once anxiety is relieved by knowledge and understanding, most women have no serious disability from these cyclic changes. Education of young girls regarding menstruation should certainly include information about all the normal physiologic changes that accompany it. Changes normally associated with menstrual cycles are often attributed to cystic disease. To label such normal physiology as a "disease" is improper and produces unnecessary anxiety and concern. (True cystic disease is discussed later.)

Benign Cysts and Tumors

It is during young adulthood that problems of an enlarging mass or masses begin to occur. Most often these masses are cysts, cystic disease, or fibroadenomas. (See illustration.) Cysts and cystic disease are a common problem in the adult woman. They rarely make their initial appearance after menopause, and indeed, menopause frequently "cures" the problem.

There is much confusion regarding this group of benign diseases. It is helpful to think of cysts as larger and less numerous in occurrence than the smaller multiple nodularities that characterize cystic disease. Other terms frequently used to describe cystic disease include chronic cystic mastitis, fibrocystic disease, and fibroadenosis—a term used to describe some of the microscopic findings associated with cystic disease.

A cyst is a fluid-filled sac like a small balloon. The cause and significance of cysts and cystic disease is poorly understood and a source of controversy among medical experts. They are probably interrelated. At the present time no specific hormone imbalance has been identified, and the entire problem may be a "normal" result of the cyclic hormonal changes to which the breasts respond. The first general form of the problem is the presence of larger cysts containing fluid which can be withdrawn through a hollow needle. The second form is associated more often with nodularity and often the nodules are shown to be cysts only under microscopic magnification. There are other highly variable cellular changes noted under the

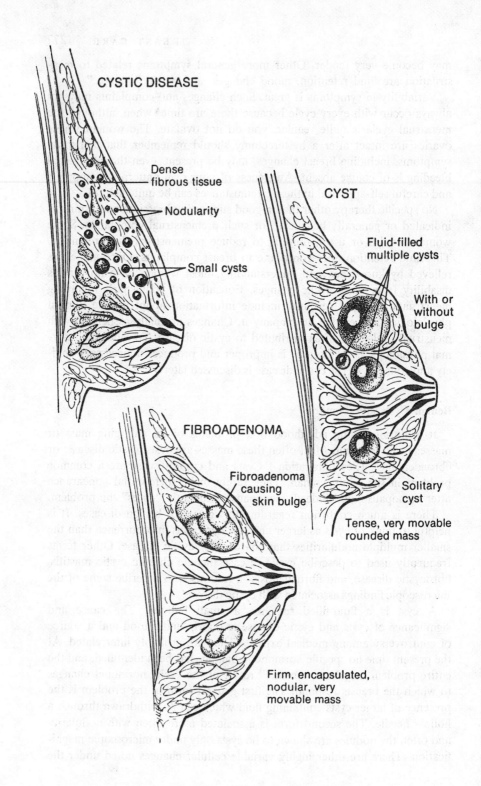

CYSTIC DISEASE

Dense fibrous tissue

Nodularity

Small cysts

CYST

Fluid-filled multiple cysts

With or without bulge

Solitary cyst

Tense, very movable rounded mass

FIBROADENOMA

Fibroadenoma causing skin bulge

Firm, encapsulated, nodular, very movable mass

microscope in both types of this disorder. Sometimes cysts and cystic disease follow the menstrual cycle. Occasionally a cyst may completely disappear as the menstrual cycle proceeds. In addition, it is common to have chronic and continuing difficulty with cysts or cystic disease. Whether or not there is an increased risk of cancer in a breast that has had cysts or cystic disease is unknown.

Continued monitoring by both you and your physician is indicated. No specific therapy is indicated. The influence of exogenous hormones, such as birth control pills, is not totally clear.

Another disorder of adult women is a form of benign tumor known as a fibroadenoma. Usually these appear in younger women than do cysts. Initial appearance after menopause is rare. Black adolescents seem more prone to develop fibroadenoma than white adolescents. This tumor, like a cyst, may produce a skin bulge. It is also movable and difficult to distinguish from a cyst. However, fibroadenomas are solid masses rather than fluid-filled, like cysts. In general, there is little influence upon these tumors by the menstrual cycle and they are seldom painful. Usually they grow very slowly, although in rare cases they grow rapidly during pregnancy. Equally rarely, they spontaneously disappear or get smaller, particularly with onset of menopause. There is no nipple discharge and usually no pain. In young women the diagnosis is often based upon personal history and physical examination. Women over 25 should have the diagnosis confirmed microscopically, which means either excisional biopsy (removal of the whole mass) or needle biopsy (withdrawal of tissue sample). If the mass is not producing symptoms and is not enlarging, there is no medical reason to remove it. However, if there is any doubt in the physician's mind regarding the diagnosis or if you wish, surgical removal can be readily done. There is no known relation between fibroadenoma and the development of subsequent cancer. The role of birth control pills and the natural history of fibroadenomas is not clear.

Less common in the young adult is another benign tumor, an intraductal papilloma. This is a growth of the cells lining the breast ducts, similar in some respects to a kind of wart. These growths can produce nipple discharge; the discharge is often dark and contains traces of blood. The discharge may come from a single or several duct openings in the nipple. You may become aware of it by a stain on your brassiere. Such symptoms, even without a palpable mass, require investigation by a physician. Intraductal papilloma has no known relationship with cancer, but can mimic the symptoms of some cancers. There is no known specific relation to the menstrual cycle.

Another benign lesion which can produce nipple discharge is breast duct ectasia. Duct ectasia is the dilatation of the ducts just beneath the nipple with changes in the tissue surrounding the ducts. These changes are variable, but can cause new nipple inversion. The lining cells of the ducts are thinned, rather than proliferating as in papillomas. Nipple discharge or discharge along with a slight suggestion of ropiness under the nipple may be the only symptom. Duct ectasia seems to be more common among women who have nursed for long periods of time. Duct ectasia is not malignant nor is there a known association with cancer. However, bloody nipple discharge and *new* nipple inversion are also signs associated with cancer. Usually, excision of the involved area is indicated for diagnostic purposes.

Copious nipple discharge that is clear or milky is called galactorrhea. Detailed endocrine studies can pinpoint the cause of this problem. Galactorrhea may be caused by antidepressant and antihypertensive drugs, as well as oral contraceptives. Rarely the cause is a tumor in the pituitary gland.

Sometimes, there is a mild, clear nipple discharge for which there is no satisfactory explanation. As age increases and menopause ensues, this problem seems to decline.

Another relatively common breast disorder which makes its appearance in the adult woman and has signs similar to cancer is fat necrosis. Injury to the breast, such as a significant bruise, can cause scarring and damage to the fatty tissue. It can distort the skin and the damaged area may feel like a hard knot (a sign often associated with cancer). Such symptoms, which may occur long after any recalled injury, require prompt evaluation and usually biopsy to determine the specific diagnosis.

Infections

The breast and its overlying skin are subject to inflammation, infection, and possible abscess formation. Most infections are related to nursing. Infection of the mammary glands is called mastitis, which may begin with oversecretion or retention of milk. A fissure in the nipple may cause infection, usually with staphylococci bacteria. Symptoms of infection include diffuse redness, swelling of the skin or nipple, a tender painful mass appearing like a boil, fever, and general weakness. Breast infections require appropriate antibiotics. If the infection is not controlled soon enough an abscess may develop which usually requires surgical drainage in addition to antibiotics.

Serious infections may cause residual thickening of the skin, scarring of breast tissue, and distortion of the nipple. However, most cases leave no residual change. Such infections are relatively infrequent today, except among women with diabetes, who are more prone to infections of all kinds.

It is rare, but possible, for a breast cancer to be associated with an infection, especially as age increases. Therefore, every effort must be made to investigate this possibility, particularly, in an older nonnursing woman who has a serious breast infection.

Malignant Disease

With increasing age the kinds of breast disorders change. Cysts and cystic disease, fibroadenoma, intraductal papilloma, and duct ectasia decrease and the frequency of cancer rises. Most breast cancers occur after the age of 40. For reasons not entirely clear, there are established risk factors in addition to age. These are listed in Table 3. Any woman over 40 or with any of these risk factors should certainly examine her breasts regularly.

TABLE 3.

Increased Risk of Breast Cancer

Over 40 years of age
Family history of breast cancer
First child after 34 years of age
No children
Previous breast cancer

Early detection of breast cancer is of the greatest importance for ultimate cure. In order to be most effective in detecting breast cancer at an early and curable stage, breast self-examination should be practiced faithfully each month. Important signs that require investigation include:

· *Nipple discharge.*
· *Any change* such as the nipple drawing inward or pointing in a different direction.
· Any chronic *scaling* or *bloody secretion of the nipple.*
· Any *change in the contour or the symmetry* of the breast.
· Any *lump or thickening* which persists through a menstrual cycle.
· Any *skin dimpling.*
· Any *new lumps.*

Generally, there is a lead-time during which a cancer may be quite small and quite localized. The enlargement and spread may take many months or years. Cancers of the breast usually arise in the cells lining the ducts and glands and then progress outside the ducts. (See illustration.) There are rare forms of cancer arising from other tissues of the breasts and even more rare cancers which arise from other parts of the body and spread to the breast. Thus, any suspicious abnormality noted by a woman

SIGNS OF BREAST CANCER

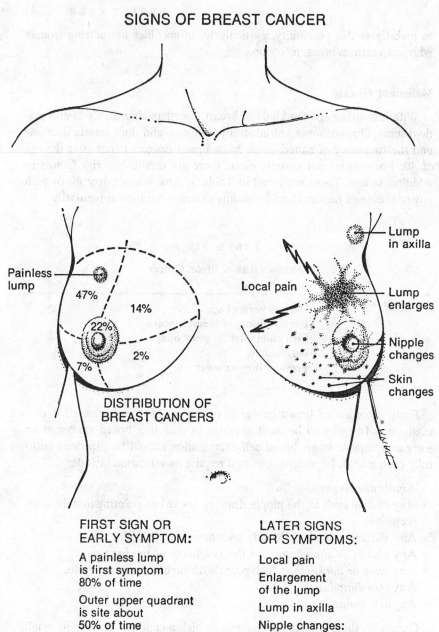

Painless lump

47%

14%

22%

7%

2%

DISTRIBUTION OF BREAST CANCERS

Lump in axilla

Local pain

Lump enlarges

Nipple changes

Skin changes

FIRST SIGN OR EARLY SYMPTOM:

A painless lump is first symptom 80% of time

Outer upper quadrant is site about 50% of time

LATER SIGNS OR SYMPTOMS:

Local pain

Enlargement of the lump

Lump in axilla

Nipple changes:
soreness
discharge
retraction
ulceration

Skin changes:
dimpling
puckering

GROWTH OF BREAST CANCER

GROWTH RATE OF BREAST CANCERS IS EXTREMELY VARIABLE

Cancer arising in mammary ducts

Normal ducts

Cancer invading surrounding tissues

Axillary nodes

Cancer spread to adjacent lymph nodes (primarily axillary)

or her physician requires diagnosis by examination of the area. Usually this is done with a biopsy. Having a breast biopsy, however, is not equivalent to having cancer. As shown in Table 4, many breast biopsies reveal nonmalignant conditions or tumors.

TABLE 4.

Breast Conditions Found in 5,604 Breast Operations

Breast Condition	Percent
Cystic disease	33.9
Fibroadenoma	18.5
Duct disease	10.0
Cancer	27.1
Other	10.5

SOURCE: Henry Patrick Leis, Jr., *The Diagnosis of Breast Cancer*. American Cancer Society, 1977.

Most often breast cancer does not spread until after it has grown outside of the duct. Once outside the duct, spread is frequently first to the lymph nodes (primarily in the axilla). Almost any other area of the body can then be involved as subsequent metastases occur. It must be stressed that early detection and treatment can usually prevent this distant spread. Survival is greatly enhanced if the cancer is confined to the breast itself. Even when it has spread to the lymph nodes, survival is good. Once, however, the cancer has spread beyond the breast and local lymph nodes, complete cure is not possible although there may be many months or years of fairly comfortable living.

DIAGNOSIS

The anxiety a woman feels when some abnormality of the breast is detected is heightened as she tries to gather her courage and visit her physician. Indeed sometimes a woman will delay seeking diagnosis partly because of her anxiety regarding the "routine" examinations and procedures with which she is not familiar. It should be helpful for you, therefore, to know what to expect when you visit your doctor for a breast examination and evaluation. It should also be helpful in allowing you to *judge for yourself if the evaluation of your problem is complete and reasonable.* The following are only guidelines and may vary according to the age of the patient and to the specifics of the individual problem.

Prompt evaluation is usually necessary. Telephone your physician immediately to describe your situation (age, Table 3 risk factors, time of your menstrual cycle, etc.). He or she will decide how soon you need to be seen. At the time of your visit a complete history will be taken. You should certainly bring along any medications that you are taking. Particular questions regarding your risk factors will also be asked. It is then that attention will be directed to your specific complaint and its relation to your menstrual cycle, duration, changes, and other associated symptoms.

Usually, you will be asked to dress in a half-sheet or shawl-like garment for your examination. The first part of the examination is careful inspection of your breasts and nipples. A palpation of your breasts and examination of the nipples will be performed, first while you are sitting and then while you are lying down. You will be asked to put your hands on your hips and squeeze to tighten your pectoral muscles and to raise your arms above your head perhaps several times. These movements allow the doctor to examine the contour and symmetry of your breasts as well as their movement as you exercise your pectoral muscles. Sometimes very subtle but important changes can be seen in the skin with these techniques. The axillae and the areas above your collar bone will be examined.

Do not be embarrassed or concerned if the physician has some difficulty finding the abnormality you have found. After all, you have been checking yourself regularly and this may be your first visit to the doctor. You may have to help the physician when such a problem arises. Sometimes, however, a cyst or nodularity that may have been related to your menstrual cycle will have disappeared.

Your doctor will ask you to describe in detail any complaint or history of nipple discharge and may examine your nipple using a magnifying glass. You might be asked to help obtain a sample of the discharge. This may involve some discomfort, but it is necessary. The discharge may be tested for blood or smeared on a glass slide for microscopic study.

The remainder of the examination varies greatly. You may be asked to have a mammogram, a specialized type of X-ray for detecting small tumors and other tissue changes of the breast. There are other techniques for examining your breast. Xerography is very similar to mammography. Both use X-rays to expose the film. Xerography film, developed by techniques similar to those of the Xerox copy machine, can better detect differences in the tissue of the breast. Thermography measures the heat radiating from the breasts. The newer CAT (computerized axial tomography) scanners are being modified and investigated for possible use in breast examinations. The use of ultra-sound (like sonar) is also being investigated. Questions about which of these techniques is best for you should be directed to the specialized radiologist who performs these kinds of examinations.

During mammography, each breast is placed on a small examination plate, and up to three different pictures made. Sometimes the radiologist may ask for other views or ask to examine your breasts. For nipple discharge complaints a tiny plastic tube may be inserted into the duct from which the discharge comes, and a small amount of special radiologic dye injected and additional mammograms taken.

There has been a great deal of controversy regarding who should have mammograms and how often they should have them. The following guidelines take all known risks into account:

- Women under 50 and women *without risk factors* and *without complaints* should *not* have annual screening.
- Women *over 50* and women *with risk factors* should have an annual checkup, including physical examination and mammography in addition to their own monthly self-examination.
- Women *with specific breast complaints at any age* may require a mammogram.

For the individual patient specific recommendations can best be made by your own physician. It should be noted that mammograms are not usually helpful in evaluation of disorders common in younger women, primarily because the density of young women's breast tissue gives an X-ray picture that is difficult to interpret. Occasionally, however, mammograms are obtained in the younger woman and again this is a judgment to be made in individual instances.

In addition to these techniques, the evaluation of a lump or mass in the breast quite often includes a needle aspiration. This aspiration is done using a small amount of local anesthetic in the skin so that a needle can be inserted into the mass. Sometimes several attempts may be needed to set the needle into a very movable mass. Fluid is removed, if there is any present, through the needle. Those masses which are true cysts will collapse when the fluid is removed and usually do not return. Normal breast cyst fluid varies in color from clear yellow to various shades of green or green-brown. As yet there is no known reason for these color differences. It is not always necessary to have normal appearing breast fluid examined since rarely are there any cell abnormalities noted. Abnormal fluid may be cloudy and/or contain blood or tiny tissue fragments. This fluid requires microscopic examination. Even if no fluid is obtained there may be enough cells in the needle for a pathologist to examine. The needle is rinsed with saline and the cells are sent for microscopic examination.

If the mass does not completely disappear with aspiration of the fluid, if a solid tumor is noted, or if a diagnosis cannot be made from the fluid or cells in the needle, a biopsy is indicated. The biopsy may be performed either with a much larger needle or through an incision. The choice is individualized. Such biopsies can frequently be performed in the office or clinic under a local anesthetic and have several advantages. They avoid the risk involved in general anesthesia. They do not require hospitalization, which is expensive, interrupts activities, and may be more anxiety-producing than outpatient treatment. There is no rush with pathological analysis as there is when the patient is under general anesthesia and the surgeon is waiting to proceed with treatment. If the results do indicate treatment is necessary, you and your physician have time to discuss all the therapeutic alternatives. There is no evidence that in the case of breast cancer (as in some other forms of cancer) proceeding in this manner will "spread the cancer."

After a needle aspiration, needle biopsy, or incisional biopsy there is some bruising. Sometimes after an incisional biopsy a small, thin rubber drain may be left in place for one or two days. Generally, there is modest discomfort that can be controlled by aspirin or other mild analgesics. It is very important to follow your doctor's instructions regarding activity and changing surgical dressings after such biopsies.

Hospitalization and a general anesthetic are indicated for the removal of intraductal papillomas, plastic surgery, and other more extensive breast surgery or biopsy. Fibroadenomas can usually be removed on an outpatient basis.

Any examination of fluid, tissues, or cells removed may take several days. A "frozen section" is faster, but not considered as final as a more detailed study requiring three to four days. The pathologist may have difficulty with some cases and require longer than several days for a specific diagnosis. The time it takes to do a careful examination of the tissue is time very well spent.

TREATMENT

Nonmalignant Disorders

Congenital anatomic abnormalities rarely require specific treatment. Some of the developmental disorders described earlier can, if related to hormone imbalance, be helped with hormone treatment. Developmental disorders also may be helped with specific surgery, particularly if there is a great discrepancy in size between the two breasts. Cyclic changes in the breast related to the menstrual cycles often require no specific therapy, especially when the woman understands their nature. Cysts large enough to be aspirated successfully and which then disappear completely usually do not require further surgery. Cystic disease of the smaller cyst variety and with more nodularity may require closer follow-up and also a biopsy to be certain of the diagnosis. Women with this type of "lumpy" breasts need most of all to perform careful regular self-examination in addition to the regular follow-up by their physician. No known medical therapy is at present indicated for cysts or cystic disease unless a specific hormonal imbalance can be identified and corrected. After menopause, most cystic disease regresses.

The benign masses such as fibroadenomas, papillomas, duct ectasia, and fat necrosis often require surgical excision either to confirm the diagnosis or to remove an annoying problem.

Breast Cancer

Rapidly accumulating data from national and international studies make it imperative that any woman who has a diagnosis of breast cancer discuss her treatment plan with her physician on an individual basis.

Surgery (mastectomy) is, and for many years has been, the cornerstone treatment of breast cancer that has not spread at all or at least has not spread beyond the axillary lymph nodes. If the cancer is found to have spread beyond the axillary nodes at the time of initial diagnosis, surgery will be of no or only limited benefit. The amount of tissue removed (type of mastectomy) depends on certain characteristics of the cancer such as its size and location, on the general health and age of the woman, and on her and her physician's personal preferences. There are eight surgical procedures used in the United States at the present time.

1. Supraradical or extended radical mastectomy. The breast, the pectoral muscles which cover the chest, and the axillary and substernal lymph nodes are removed. To remove the latter, some sections of the rib must also be removed. Some surgeons also remove the supraclavicular lymph nodes (where the neck joins the shoulders). This procedure is rarely done now.
2. Classical or standard mastectomy (also called a radical mastectomy or the Halsted procedure). The breast, all the axillary nodes, and the pectoral muscles are removed.
3. Modified radical mastectomy. This is like the classical procedure except that the pectoral muscles are not removed.
4. Extended simple or extended total mastectomy. The breast is removed and a few axillary lymph nodes are removed for microscopic analysis to see if the cancer has spread to them. The pectoral muscles are not removed.
5. Simple or total mastectomy. This is like the extended simple mastectomy except that no, or only one, lymph node is removed.
6. Partial mastectomy, segmental resection, or wedge resection. The tumor and a fairly large amount of surrounding breast tissue are removed. The breast is not removed, but will be smaller. If the axillary nodes are also removed, the procedure is called a partial radical mastectomy.
7. Lumpectomy, tylectomy, or local excision. The breast lump is removed

along with a small amount of surrounding tissue. The breast is not removed and may or may not be smaller.

8. Subcutaneous mastectomy. Breast tissue is removed but overlying skin is not. The axillary nodes may or may not be removed. The nipple may be removed or left in place depending upon the individual situation. The nipple may be temporarily grafted, usually in the groin.

It must be stressed that the specific type of surgery is tailored to the individual circumstances. Surgery is *local treatment* and the type of surgery performed is greatly influenced by the specifics of location, size, and microscopic type of the cancer as well as other medical conditions. Also it is now common to consult with other oncologists (cancer specialists) regarding the complete treatment plans of which surgery may be one part. Should you require surgery for breast cancer you should be certain you understand the proposed treatment.

Depending again upon your individual circumstances, treatment may include surgery, radiation therapy, endocrine (hormone) treatments, or chemotherapy. The presence of microscopic involvement of lymph nodes often indicates that such post-operative treatments are indicated.

Recent research has made a new test available based on the sensitivity of a breast cancer to hormone treatments. This test is called the estrogen receptor assay and must be done on a portion of the actual cancer tissue. Hormone treatments may be of several types. Depending upon the specific circumstances, hormones can be added, removed (such as removing the ovaries) or blocked in their actions. Such hormone treatments can be very effective.

Chemotherapy (drugs which poison cancer cells) is also used. Most chemotherapy is accompanied by side effects such as nausea and vomiting, hair loss, injury to the bone marrow, and generalized weakness. At present there are many drugs and combinations of drugs being used and no single regimen is clearly the best. If you need chemotherapy you should understand the benefits and risks.

Recent advances in the use of radiation therapy in the treatment of early breast cancer, as well as more advanced disease, are most encouraging. Usually these treatments are part of a plan which includes surgery and/or chemotherapy. Several studies are under way and have shown good local results, but it is too early to tell what the long-term influence on survival rates will be. Radiation treatment is often available in major medical centers throughout the country.

Immune treatment (immunotherapy) is also being studied. This treatment can stimulate your body's own defense mechanisms against cancer—much like a vaccine stimulates your defenses against polio and tetanus.

Other treatments are often discussed in medical literature, women's magazines, newspapers, television, and among friends. If you have any questions about their worth, you should consult your physician.

One further point must be made regarding breast cancer treatment. If, at the time of diagnosis, the cancer has spread to body parts beyond the lymph nodes, no form of mastectomy may be indicated. To determine this, you may be asked to undergo multiple tests. Some of these are blood tests, bone scans, liver scans, X-rays, and possibly biopsies of areas other than the breast.

Reconstruction of the breast following breast surgery is an important question which should be discussed with your surgeon before the operation and should, if indicated or desired, be part of the overall treatment program. Such surgery is performed by plastic surgeons. There is an excellent booklet available, *Breast Reconstruction Following Mastectomy for Cancer,* which answers many questions. It is often available from local American Cancer Society units, or write to the American Society of Plastic and Reconstructive Surgeons, 29 East Madison Street, Suite 800, Chicago, Illinois 60602. Please remember though, that the doctor's first concern, and hopefully yours, should be the best chance of saving your life. Reconstruction options *should not be the major deciding factor regarding the exact type of surgery performed.* As in any other circumstance, you have freedom of choice both in selecting your physicians and in decisions regarding your treatment. A little assertiveness in your approach to your physician can help elicit the understanding and concerned support you need.

There are many myths regarding the psycho-sexual aftermath of breast surgery (well discussed in the referenced articles by Mildred Witkin and Alan Wabreck). It is clear that the most important goal is building and maintaining a positive self image. The fears that others will be repulsed by the new you are more easily put to rest when you face reality. There are no physiologic or sexual capabilities lost when a breast is lost, except nursing. You are as fully capable of joyful sex and sexuality as you were prior to surgery. There are certainly severe stresses and multiple problems related to going home, back to work, and in relationships. These are not insolvable. The Reach for Recovery Program of the American Cancer Society can help. The women volunteers in this organization have had mastectomies and will visit you in the hospital and help you when you return home. They have been trained to help other patients and understand the anxieties, fears, and problems accompanying breast surgery. Your doctor or nurse can readily contact them. The volunteer will usually bring you a temporary breast prosthesis to wear home and can accompany you when it is time to obtain a permanent one.

Relationships with your family, husband, lover, and friends will be affected as they would by any other serious and difficult problem in life.

Seldom are sturdy relationships seriously harmed. Weak or difficult relationships are sometimes strengthened but can deteriorate. Unmarried or divorced women patients have told me that the true worth of a developing relationship with a man is strongly tested following breast surgery.

The human breast is a complex organ, and it is important to you in many ways. Psychological investments, however, should *never* keep you from prompt diagnosis and proper therapy. Even if the treatment involves removal of a breast you can live well and lead a full, loving life after such surgery. There is, after all, so much more to a woman than the mere presence of a bustline. The reassuring fact seems to be that love and communication—not breasts—are central to man-woman relationships.

Armed with more knowledge of the structure and function of your body, I urge you to be sensible regarding your breasts. Check your breasts once a month, tell your doctor about any changes, and insist on being fully and clearly informed about any suggested treatment.

REFERENCES

Breast Reconstruction Following Mastectomy for Cancer: Some Questions and Answers, Chicago: American Society of Plastic and Reconstructive Surgeons, 1979.

Foster, R. J., et al. "Breast Self-Examination Practices and Breast Cancer Stage." *New England Journal of Medicine* 299. (August 10, 1978): 265–270.

Gillette, J. V., and C. E. Haycock. "Women in Athletics." Eighteenth Conference on the Medical Aspects of Sports, American Medical Association, 1976.

Greenwald, P., et al. "Estimated Effect of Breast Self-Examination and Routine Physician Examinations on Breast Cancer Mortality." *New England Journal of Medicine* 299. (August 10, 1978): 271–273.

Haagensen, C. D. *Diseases of the Breast.* 2nd ed. Philadelphia: Saunders, 1971.

Henderson, C. I. and G. P. Canellos. "Cancer of the Breast: The Past Decade." *New England Journal of Medicine,* 1, no. 1, 2 (1980).

How to Examine Your Breasts. New York: American Cancer Society, 1975.

Leis, H. P., Jr. *The Diagnosis of Breast Cancer.* American Cancer Society, 1977.

Moskowitz, M. "Mammography in Medical Practice: A Rational Approach." *Journal of the American Medical Association* 240 (October 20, 1978): 1898–1899.

Peck, D., and R. Lowman. "Estrogen and the Postmenopausal Breast." *Journal of the American Medical Association* 240 (October 13, 1978): 1833–1835.

Seltzer, M. H. and M. S. Skiles. "Diseases of the Breast in Young Women." *Surgery, Gynecology, and Obstetrics* (1980): 360–362.

Wabreck, Alan J., et al. "Marital and Sexual Counseling After Mastectomy." *Human Sexuality.*

Witkin, Mildred. "Psychosexual Myths and Realities of Mastectomy." *Human Sexuality,* December, 1979.

FURTHER READING

Storch, M. and L. May. "The Complete Breast Book." *Good Housekeeping,* February, 1979, p. 75.

Cosmetic Surgery

KATHRYN STEPHENSON, M.D.
Santa Barbara Cottage Hospital, Santa Barbara, California

There is nothing new about the desire to improve one's appearance—to look younger or prettier, to uplift the breasts or pare down the hips, to refashion the nose or flatten the ears. Surgery to achieve these desires is not new either. What is a recent development is the fact that cosmetic surgery has come out of the closet. Operations once considered the hush-hush prerogative of the rich and famous are now freely discussed with news reporters, magazine writers, and friends. "New" looks are launched at "coming-out" parties; the old look is discarded—sometimes along with old jobs, old spouses, or psychiatrists.

Many factors account for the increasing popularity and democratization of cosmetic surgery. Contemporary culture in the United States is preoccupied with youth and with appearances. Women threatened with the loss of a job at the age of 45 because they look too old (they are likely to have a life expectancy of 30 more years) are more and more determined to compete not only on the basis of skills and experience, but on the basis of wrinkle-free faces. In the scale of values of many employers, years of experience and a mature sense of responsibility weigh less than the look of blooming good health associated with youth. Even though many young women are more conventional and conservative than some of their elders, a youthful appearance is usually associated with "a fresh point of view," "an active mind," and "up-to-the-minute attitudes."

Coupled with these factors are changing circumstances within the profession: more and more doctors are specializing in cosmetic surgery. Improvements in instruments and refinements in technique, particularly in the techniques of microsurgery, are constantly being made, and with the ongoing advances in medicine and anesthesia, operations can be undertaken with greater safety and more assurance of a successful result.

Where does the money come from for this surgery? Except for some ear alteration, breast reduction, and, increasingly, breast reconstruction after mastectomy, it is rarely paid for by any form of medical insurance; it is not covered by Medicare or Medicaid, although it is tax deductible. Secretaries, waitresses, executives, housewives, part-time parents who are reentering the job market are sufficiently motivated to make the necessary sacrifices in order to pay the bills. Some women forego vacations; others spend practically no money on clothes for years so that they can save up for the surgery. Some borrow money; others sell a valuable piece of jewelry. Girls in their teens are sometimes given the choice of money to spend on a nose job or on a sixteenth birthday party.

DECIDING TO UNDERGO COSMETIC SURGERY

Cosmetic surgery is a specialty within the larger field of plastic surgery. Plastic surgery concentrates on the repair of congenital defects (such as a cleft lip) and the restructuring of parts of the body damaged by disease (as in the case of breast cancer) or by injury (such as might be sustained in a fire, in war, or in an automobile accident). Cosmetic surgery is usually elective. Its purpose is to improve physical appearance by such procedures as nose alteration (rhinoplasty), face lift (rhytidoplasty), ear alteration (otoplasty), eyelid correction (blepharoplasty), and breast augmentation or reduction (mammaplasty).

Cosmetic surgery cannot perform miraculous changes in physical appearance or in basic personality defects such as self-rejection, incurable envy, the "if-only" syndrome, or hopelessly childish notions about "beauty and romance." Women with unrealistic expectations about results are almost sure to be disappointed. A woman with a specific and limited problem—whose livelihood is at stake because of premature wrinkles, whose husband has been urging her to have the bags under her eyes removed, who is self-conscious about being flat-chested, or who loathes her nose—is likely to be pleased with the solution cosmetic surgery can provide and go about the business of her life with a feeling of satisfaction.

While a face lift won't save a marriage that's on the rocks or guarantee a better job or a bigger salary, it can be helpful in building self-confidence and the assertiveness that can play a crucial role in many competitive situations. However, women whose obsession with looking young is profound and whose terror of aging is acute might benefit more from sustained soul-searching than from surgery. Any woman who wants to get the best return for a considerable investment of money and time should therefore be as honest with herself as possible about the motives that bring her to the surgeon's office.

Past or present therapy for unresolved emotional problems need not rule out the use of cosmetic surgery as one way (but never the only way) of dealing with psychological stress. The surgeon should be informed of the therapeutic situation and perhaps consult with the psychotherapist to evaluate the patient's suitability for the desired operation. Women who for many years have focused on some aspect of their appearance that is unsatisfactory to them as the reason for their sexual or professional inadequacies should be gently guided toward what may be painful introspection about major flaws in their behavior and away from obsessive inspection of minor flaws they see in the mirror.

Surgery should not be undertaken when the patient's emotional stability has been threatened by a shocking experience. There is no doubt that some women who have experienced an unusually stressful crisis, such as a divorce, a sudden death in the family, the unanticipated loss of a job, or the unexpected responsibility of taking care of an invalid child or parent, can benefit from the positive effects of a long-postponed improvement in appearance. But other factors must be taken into account. Psychic stress has an adverse effect on the physiology of the body and in many cases can slow down the healing processes.

Ideally, a person about to undergo elective surgery should be in top physical and mental condition, always taking into account the fact that if the surgery is to be extensive, it will inevitably produce some feelings of anxiety in the patient about the outcome. A reputable surgeon will also ask the prospective patient a long list of questions to find out if she has had a recent severe illness, if she is addicted to alcohol, smoking, or any drugs such as tranquilizers or sleeping pills, and if she is a chronic user of any medication such as aspirin and antihistamines. Surgery may have to be delayed until she has ceased using drugs or alcohol for sufficient time so that they no longer affect the body. Some medications, such as aspirin and antihistamines, reduce the body's blood clotting efficiency, thereby increasing the potential hazard of postoperative bleeding. A patient addicted to certain types of drugs may require dangerously high doses of sedatives for adequate relief from pain. Estrogen medications may affect pigmentation following certain procedures. A patient who has been taking cortisone presents special problems and needs more than the usual amount of monitoring by an internist and an anesthesiologist before, during, and after the operation.

Before any woman goes to a cosmetic surgeon, she should attempt an honest assessment of her appearance and precisely how she wishes it to be changed. Where exactly is the problem? Does the chin need strengthening? The nose shortening? Is it the set of the ears that should be corrected? If a particular body contour should be changed, take a good look at it with no clothes on. Perfect symmetry of either the face or the figure is usually out of the question; in fact, it is the slight asymmetry of facial bones that gives most faces an interest and individuality that is more attractive than classic "perfection."

Advice from friends and family about cosmetic surgery should generally be avoided. Conflicting opinions of friends can be extremely confusing. Close relatives may be offended at the idea that a physical trait shared by the family is offensive to one member; while they may be as tactful as possible, their feelings or ethnic pride may be severely wounded. One or the other parent may refuse to permit a daughter to have her nose changed. In other cases a teenager may not have strong feelings one way or the other—in fact, may feel that her nose is exactly like Barbra Streisand's—but her mother may want her to have her nose trimmed or straightened. With young people especially, if people close to the patient take a negative view of prospective surgery, their attitude is likely to persist after the operation, causing the patient to be unhappy about the result. When the decision for surgery is finally taken, it should be taken as independently as circumstances permit.

CONSULTATION WITH THE COSMETIC SURGEON

Once the decision is made, look for a properly accredited surgeon. To check a surgeon's credentials, write to the American Society of Plastic and Reconstructive Surgeons, 29 East Madison Street, Suite 807, Chicago, Illinois 60602. This organization has a listing of surgeons certified by the Board of Plastic Surgeons as well as detailed information about their training. Board certification indicates that the surgeon has completed the necessary years of training in general surgery and two or three years of special training in plastic surgery and that following an examination, qualifications for practicing this specialty have been established. Fellowship in the American College of Surgeons is further evidence of qualification. To have surgery undertaken by a physician who does not have the proper credentials not only adds to the risk of the surgery, but may also lead to irreversible mutilation. The surgeon who has received the most publicity is not necessarily the most skilled or the most conscientious, and while more and more cosmetic surgeons are creating minihospitals in their own offices to lessen costs due to hospitalization, it is important to check on their conventional hospital associations, too. While shopping around for a surgeon may cause a certain amount of confusion, it is essential that the patient find a specialist who is not only well qualified, but also congenial to her and makes her feel confident rather than apprehensive.

When making an appointment with a surgeon for a first visit, the prospective patient should ask how much the fee will be for the consultation.

The amount is collected at the time of the consultation and in some cases it may be deducted from the surgical fee. All questions relating to fees should be discussed in the greatest detail at the time of the first visit to avoid future misunderstandings. The patient would be well-advised to ask about and make written notes on the cost of the surgery, additional fees for anesthesia, X-rays, and laboratory procedures, and all other associated fees. If hospitalization is involved, the patient should consult her insurance policy to find out what her coverage will be. While it may come as something of a shock, most cosmetic surgeons expect to be paid in full in advance of an operation. The reason for this involves several practical considerations: unless the commitment to have the operation is made final by prepayment, cancellations and postponements can pile up to the point where the surgeon cannot maintain any kind of schedule. Also, when the work is paid for in advance, it is likely to be viewed with more satisfaction by the patient than if it is to be paid for postoperatively.

During the consultation the surgeon will question the patient about her medical history and her physical condition. The woman who is not entirely honest or is evasive in her answers is asking for trouble and being unfair to herself and to the doctor. Special problems associated with previous surgery should be described in detail. Any bleeding tendencies should be mentioned. Drug dependencies and the use of any medication must be discussed. A history of hypertension, diabetes, asthma, kidney or heart disease, allergy, or mental illness must be mentioned.

Not only is it important for the patient to speak openly to the surgeon, but the patient should expect to get certain specific information from the surgeon. During the consultation the prospective patient should be told about the following matters: problems ordinarily connected with the particular type of surgery requested; the patient's particular suitability or unsuitability for it; realistic limitations of the procedure and expectations in the results; potential complications; preparations essential before the surgery is performed; the actual technique by which the surgery is performed; the nature and length of postoperative recovery.

If after this discussion the patient wishes to proceed with the surgery and the surgeon feels she is a suitable candidate for it, photographs will be taken either during this first visit or during a visit following the first one. The surgeon evaluates the photographs with the patient at a subsequent visit prior to surgery. It is during this visit that the patient should feel free to ask any and all questions that remain unanswered in her own mind.

It must be especially emphasized that the patient should make a determined effort to hear what the surgeon says to her. If she doesn't trust her memory, she should write the responses down and have the accuracy of her transcription checked by the surgeon on the spot. Controlled studies of patients undergoing plastic surgery have shown that few patients remember postoperatively the statements made to them by the surgeon before the operation. The reason for this memory lapse appears to be the fact that in most instances patients have so firmly decided in advance to have the surgery that they are incapable of absorbing the information communicated to them by the surgeon. There are also those patients whose nervousness about the procedure or the presence of a physician prevents their hearing anything that is said to them. They simply do not listen to the surgeon's recounting of the limitations of the procedure, the possibility of having to undergo secondary surgery, the immediate and delayed anticipated results, the time necessary for recuperation, or the potential complications.

While complications are not common, they do occur. There is no operation that is risk free. Hemorrhage may occur at the time of surgery or immediately following it; adverse response to anesthesia may occur despite all precautions and impeccable techniques; postoperative infection may complicate and delay healing and recovery. Incisions, although designed and sutured by the surgeon to be as inconspicuous as possible, do result in scars. Some individuals form elevated red scars termed hypertrophic or keloidal. Some scars stretch regardless of the physician's technique. How conspicuous the scars will be varies with the area of the body involved and with the patient's type of scar formation.

In recent years it has become increasingly popular to introduce foreign materials into the body. All patients should be aware of the normal response of the body to such substances as metal, glass, ivory, paraffin, silicone, and other synthetic materials. To protect itself from damage, the body's normal response is to extrude or to wall off these substances by the formation of scar tissue. Countless breasts have been lost or maimed by the injection of silicone, and there has been discoloration and loss of tissue in other parts of the body due to these injections. The substance migrates and can cause death if blood vessels are invaded and circulation is blocked off.

All of these substances have been used in the past by both qualified surgeons and charlatans. However, qualified surgeons have discarded them all except for synthetic prosthesis and silicone-filled bags. All surgeons agree that the most satisfactory substitute for missing tissue is autogenous tissue, that is, similar tissue taken from the patient's body. For example, tissue needed for nasal reconstruction may be taken from a rib, ear, or septal cartilage.

Once expectations and complications have been considered, the patient is ready to schedule surgery.

SURGICAL PROCEDURES

Rhinoplasty

Rhinoplasty, alteration of the contour of the nose, is one of the most frequently requested cosmetic operations and one of the most difficult. It should not be done until after age 16, when bone development and cartilage growth are complete. The difficulty is due to the fact that the overlying soft tissue on the ridge of the nose is not sufficient to conceal even the slightest irregularity. The development of excess scar tissue beneath the skin may alter the result desired by both the surgeon and the patient.

A nose may protrude too much or not enough. It may be hooked or depressed. The tip may be bulbous or pinched; it may turn up or turn down too much for an attractive profile. The nostrils may be too wide and flaring or too narrow. The septum may deviate or it may be markedly crooked. The nose is rarely symmetrical; even the beauty queens of Hollywood constantly request that cameramen take their "best" side.

The patient who consults the surgeon about nose reconstruction often has many misconceptions about the problems involved. It is only after multiple photographs are taken from various angles, with the face in repose and smiling, that the problem can be analyzed and clarified. In a discussion that keeps referring back to the photographs, the limitations of the alteration should be made as clear as possible to the patient. If the nose is to be augmented, there may not be enough soft tissue available for covering the cartilage, bone, or silicone implant used by some surgeons. If the tip of the nose is to be reduced, there may be an excess of inelastic tissue that will not shrink adequately to drape over the reduced cartilaginous support. When this problem exists, it may be necessary to make an external incision which will result in a visible scar.

A reduction rhinoplasty, commonly called a "nose bob," is the most frequently requested correction. This surgery is usually done under local anesthesia: the nerves are blocked with injections of Xylocaine or procaine containing epinephrine, a synthetic hormone that limits bleeding. The surgeon can work without having his vision or his instruments obstructed by cumbersome anesthetic equipment. If general anesthesia is necessary, because of squeamishness or other reasons, endotracheal anesthesia is used; a breathing tube is inserted through the mouth into the trachea (the windpipe) to prevent the patient from getting blood into the lungs while unconscious. When general anesthesia is used, most surgeons also inject local anesthesia containing epinephrine to limit bleeding which obscures the operative field.

The surgery itself is performed through incisions within the nostrils unless the nostrils are to be decreased or otherwise reshaped. Through these

COSMETIC SURGERY OF THE NOSE

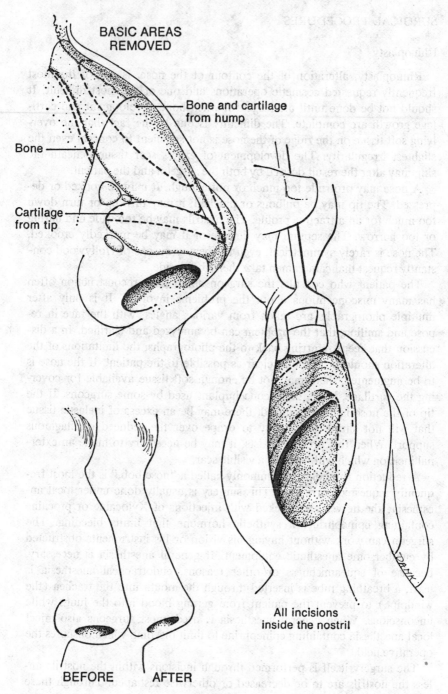

BASIC AREAS
REMOVED

Bone and cartilage
from hump

Bone

Cartilage
from tip

All incisions
inside the nostril

BEFORE   AFTER

incisions, the soft tissues are separated from the underlying bone and cartilage. The cartilages of the tip are modified, the undesirable bony hump is
removed by saw or chisel and filed for smoothness, and the lateral nasal
bones are fractured to re-create the pyramidal form of the upper portion of
the nose.

When the crookedness of the nose is caused by the deviation of the septum (the cartilage that separates the two nostrils), a modification or resection of the septum is indicated. This is usually done before reducing the
size of the nose. In many cases, only the upper portion or the tip needs to
be modified. If the width of the nostrils is to be altered, it is necessary to
make an incision at the margin of the ala (the wing of the nose) where it
joins the upper lip and cheek.

Following the completion of the surgery, nasal packs are inserted and
an external splint is applied to maintain the new position of the bones,
limit postoperative swelling, and protect the operated sites. The packs are
removed within a few days, but the external splint is likely to be retained
for about a week. The postoperative pain is negligible, but the eyelids may
become swollen and discolored, and while the nose is packed, mouth
breathing causes the nuisance of dryness of the mouth. Some oozing of
blood is common. The nose may feel stiff and numb. The numbness disappears gradually, and by the tenth day most of the swelling subsides. The
appearance of the nose gradually improves, and usually by the sixth month
the scar tissue has softened.

Following removal of the splint, the patient should not handle the nose,
sneezing should be avoided, and all violent exercise should be eliminated
for three weeks. Participation in contact sports should be discontinued for
six months.

The most common complications of this procedure are the following.
The formation of excessive scar tissue may result in distortion and a less
delicate contour than anticipated. Asymmetry or deviation may occur. A
flat arch and pinched nostrils or even partially occluded nostrils may present a postoperative problem. Profuse bleeding may occur with septal surgery. Following septal surgery, there may be a perforation of the septum
or a collapse of the bridge of the nose. While most of these complications
rarely occur, the patient embarking on a rhinoplasty should take these possible failures into account.

Rhytidoplasty

Rhytidoplasty, face lift, is a major surgical procedure. For the best possible results it is essential that in addition to being in good health the patient be at her lowest normal weight. Any planned dieting should be done
before rather than after surgery so that the skin is slack and a maximum
amount of tissue can be removed during the operation. The patient is usu-

ally advised to keep her hair long enough to cover the scars which will be pink immediately after the surgery. Most surgeons do not shave the hair. Prior to surgery the patient will be told to wash her hair with antiseptic soap.

The procedure may include a forehead lift, cheek lift (meloplasty), and neck lift. Whether these operations are undertaken at the same time as the face lift or are done subsequently as separate procedures depends on the appearance of the patient and her overall physical condition.

While the surgery can be accomplished under local anesthesia with adequate premedication, many surgeons prefer to use supplemental intravenous or inhalation anesthesia as well.

A face lift consists of the separation of the skin and subcutaneous fat from the underlying muscles and fascia (fibrous connective tissue) and the pulling back and cutting away of the excess tissue. The incision extends across the forehead, usually behind the hairline where the scar will eventually be concealed, and down into the area of the temples. Some surgeons prefer to make the incision below the hairline, and in an unusually high forehead this is preferable. The incision goes in front of the ear, around the lobe, upward on the back of the ear or in the crease where it joins the head, and then as far as necessary into the hair-bearing area. While the incision may encircle the entire head, it usually extends only as far back as necessary to allow for the removal of an adequate amount of tissue. Vertical incisions in the midline of the nape of the neck are sometimes used, but they are likely to produce unsightly scars. However, if such incisions are necessary, the scars can be partially hidden by wearing the hair longer in the back. Patients with a "turkey gobbler" neck may require an incision beneath the chin for the removal of excess fat.

After the incisions are made and the skin and fat are separated from the tissue beneath them, they are retracted (pulled up and back) and the excess is cut away. Some surgeons think that they accomplish a better correction if the fascia is also retracted, folded back on itself, and sutured down. An additional procedure consisting of partial excision of the neck muscles may be necessary to give optimal correction.

Many surgeons insert drains which are attached to suction to remove oozing blood and serum. The removal limits somewhat the extent of postoperative swelling and monitoring the drains can alert personnel supervising the patient's condition to the onset of undue bleeding. Other surgeons prefer to rely on the around-the-head pressure dressing.

For smoothing away fine lines in unoperated areas, usually just around the mouth but sometimes on the forehead, abrasion may be performed at the time of the face lift. Some surgeons advocate chemosurgery instead of abrasion (the two procedures are described later).

Postoperatively, there is surprisingly little discomfort or pain, although some patients become agitated by the comprehensive dressing that covers a large portion of the head, face, and neck. When there *is* pain, it should alert the surgeon to investigate the wound. Swelling and ecchymosis (black

COSMETIC SURGERY OF THE FACE

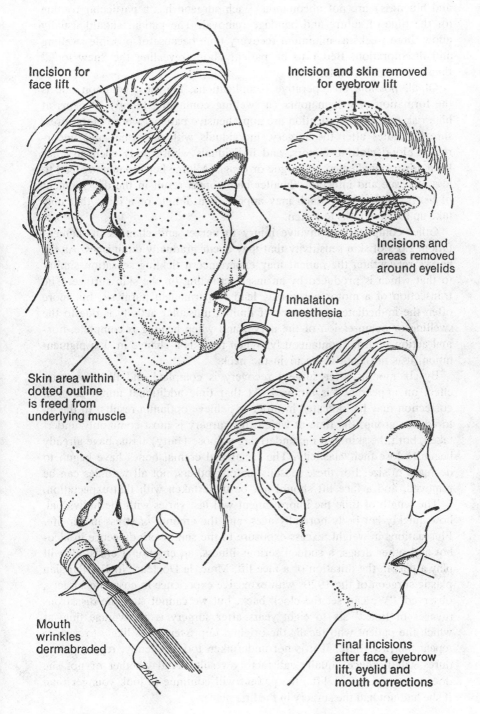

Incision for
face lift

Incision and skin removed
for eyebrow lift

Incisions and
areas removed
around eyelids

Inhalation
anesthesia

Skin area within
dotted outline
is freed from
underlying muscle

Mouth
wrinkles
dermabraded

Final incisions
after face, eyebrow
lift, eyelid and
mouth corrections

and blueness) are not uncommon. Each surgeon has a particular routine for the time of suture and bandage removal. The patient should usually allow three weeks as minimum recovery time because of possible swelling and discoloration. Better to be patient about revealing the "new look" than to present it prematurely.

Of all possible postoperative complications, the most common one is the formation of a hematoma (a swelling containing blood). Persons at high risk for this complication are apprehensive patients whose blood pressure fluctuates after the surgery, individuals with abnormal and uncorrected blood clotting factors, and individuals whose body chemistry has been adversely affected by fatigue or drugs. A large hematoma may lead to loss of tissue and infection. Smaller hematomas result in the development of heavier scar tissue which may appear as a dimple or a lump that may take up to six months to soften.

Other complications involve injury to nerves and changes in pigmentation. Loss of skin sensitivity that may occur gradually diminishes. As the nerves regenerate, the patient may experience a tickling sensation similar to that which is produced by an insect crawling on the skin surface. The transection of a motor nerve may lead to permanent paralysis, but more often the immediate appearance of limited muscular activity is due to the swelling or compression of the nerve, and when healing is complete, normal action returns spontaneously. When there is a change in skin pigmentation, it is most apt to occur in the neck.

By six months after surgery recovery is complete and the maximum effect on appearance is attained. At that time additional minor surgical correction may be indicated in order to achieve optimum results. In the 40 to 45 age group, the time at which this surgery is most commonly undertaken, both the skin and the underlying adipose (fatty) tissue have already begun to lose their elasticity. The facial and cranial bones have begun to decrease in size. For these reasons, among others, not all wrinkles can be removed, and a face lift should not be undertaken with that expectation.

The length of time the improvement will last varies with the individual, how quickly her body normally ages, and the amount of stress in her life. Fluctuations in weight, excess exposure to the sun, overindulgence in alcohol and other drugs, a sudden serious illness, an emotional crisis, all will play a part in the duration of a face lift. Mme. le Docteur Noel, a Parisian plastic surgeon of the 1920s with extensive experience in cosmetic surgery, observed, "We can set the clock back, but we cannot stop the disastrous ravages of time." Six to eight years after surgery is an average time at which the patient who recalls the original improvement is likely to wish to repeat the procedure. If it is not undertaken too frequently, repeat procedures will produce equally satisfactory results. And whether or not she does have repeat face lifts, the patient will continue to look younger than if she had not had the surgery in the first place.

I know of no procedure that produces such a high degree of euphoria in such a large number of patients. Some of this sense of well-being may be due to the character of the women who seek the improvement; usually they are energetic, determined to cope with life's more unpleasant realities, and eager to participate in the activities of the world around them.

Abrasion, Chemosurgery, and Collagen Injection

Abrasion (or dermabrasion) is the removal of outer layers of the skin. Scars due to acne can be improved by beveling the edges of the scars if they are not the deep pitted "ice pick" type, although the abrasion may have to be repeated several times to achieve a skin surface that approaches the normal in appearance. Abrasion may also be done to smooth fine wrinkles. Because elevated levels of estrogen affect the pigmentation of the skin, the procedure should not be done on a woman who takes estrogens as replacement therapy or as contraception. It should not be done on a woman who has a history of chloasma of pregnancy (pigmentary changes of the skin, primarily of the cheeks) or on a pregnant woman due to her altered endocrine function.

The procedure can be done under local anesthesia or by topical refrigeration (spraying on a solution that freezes the skin surface), but since dermabrasion takes a long time, many patients elect to have a general anesthetic or supplementary intravenous anesthesia. Most surgeons prefer to work on the entire face at one time in order to blend or feather out the margins at the hairline and beneath the jawline to get results as close as possible to the texture of the normal skin. At one time, sandpaper was used to remove the outer skin layers. Now most surgeons use a rotary diamond fraise, a revolving cylinder in which diamond dust is embedded. A rotary wire brush is also used by some surgeons.

Immediately following the surgery the face swells, as it would after a second-degree burn, and the swelling continues for at least two days more. Pain is not acute after the first six hours, but the patient does suffer from a most disagreeable appearance caused by the accumulation of plasma that forms a crust. The crusting usually falls off within ten days, exposing rosy-colored tissue beneath. This color gradually fades and the skin takes on its normal coloration. It is absolutely essential that for six weeks the patient totally avoid any exposure to the sun and that for six months she protect her skin against the sun by wearing a large-brimmed hat and using a sun-blocking skin cream. If the face is exposed earlier, spotty pigmentation will occur. In individuals with darker skin the exposed abraded area is usually darker than the unabraded area; in fair-skinned individuals it is usually lighter.

Occasionally there may be a difference in pigmentation even though the patient is not taking estrogens and was not exposed prematurely to the sun. Sometimes there is a formation of milia (white papules due to the retention of sebum). More rarely the procedure may result in red and elevated (hypertrophic) scarring.

Chemosurgery (or "chemical peel"), the removal of the outer layer of skin by the application of chemicals, is preferred to abrasion by some surgeons treating fine wrinkles due to aging. It is not as satisfactory as surgical abrasion for acne and scars. Because the solution used contains phenol, individuals with kidney disease are not considered candidates for this procedure. The application of the chemical solution must be performed with extreme care to control the depth of penetration.

The patient's face is carefully cleaned and then the patient is heavily premedicated. As the surgeon applies the phenol solution with an applicator, the patient experiences a stinging sensation. The face is then blotted and a tape mask is applied unless the individual has very thin skin. The mask is left in place for 24 to 48 hours. During this time and for an additional 24 to 48 hours the face swells as following any burn and often the pain requires narcotics. Following the removal of the tape, thymol iodide powder is applied to dry the weeping surface. In ten days to two weeks this powder is removed and cosmetics may be applied to the bright pink skin. This coloration gradually fades.

Complications following this procedure are similar to those following abrasion, but are more apt to occur. The patient must protect her face from exposure to the sun for six months. The texture of the skin is more altered and hypo/or hyperpigmentation of the skin or a blotchy discoloration may occur. Although the improvement may be more prolonged following chemosurgery, some surgeons do not perform it because of the increased likelihood of complications.

Collagen is a purified derivative of the dermis of the skin. It forms a mass at body temperature, but has recently been made soluble so that it can be injected into the skin and subcutaneous tissue to elevate depressed areas and wrinkles. Following the injection of collagen, swelling and redness last for about 48 to 72 hours and then gradually disappear. An occasional individual develops a hyperpigmentation in the area, and infection is a possibility as with any injection. Although still in the investigative phase and not yet approved by the FDA, collagen is a biological substance and does hold promise of not eliciting the adverse reactions associated with the injection of a foreign substance such as silicone.

Maxilloplasty, Mandibuloplasty, Mentoplasty, and Malarplasty

The premaxillary portion of the facial bones (the upper jaw) just below the nose may protrude or recede too much for an attractive appearance. While some correction can be obtained from orthodontia, if the malocclusion is severe, maxilloplasty, the surgical recession or advancement of the bone itself, may be advisable. This is a major surgery that demands careful preoperative study, hospitalization, and longer postoperative care than most cosmetic surgery procedures. While it does in fact improve the patient's appearance, a maxilloplasty does not generally come under the heading of cosmetic surgery, but rather is considered reconstructive surgery since function, namely, proper occlusion, is always involved.

Severe malocclusion may also be corrected by mandibuloplasty, the resecting or advancing of the mandibular (lower jaw) bone. Frequently, the addition of bone, cartilage, or some type of silicone implant is used to bring the chin forward to achieve better facial balance. This surgery is often performed in conjunction with a rhinoplasty, making possible the use of the bone and cartilage removed from the nose for the reconstruction of the chin. As an additional procedure accompanying a face lift, it is especially valuable to the individual whose chin has receded excessively because of the premature loss of the lower teeth.

Chin surgery (mentoplasty) is undertaken under local anesthesia unless it is necessary to obtain bone from some other part of the body. The incision is made either inside the mouth or just beneath the chin, where the scar will be inconspicuous. The chin incision is used for the removal of excess bone to reduce an excessively long or prominent chin. After the operation the patient is limited to a soft diet for about ten days. While complications are rare, a nerve may be damaged, producing numbness and lack of mobility of the lower lip either temporarily or in rare instances permanently. Another postoperative complication may be the deviation (separation or slippage) of the material inserted. This is corrected by a secondary adjustment.

The appearance of some women is enhanced by malarplasty, the augmentation of the malar eminence or cheekbone. Bone or silicone is inserted to achieve greater prominence of the cheekbone. The incision may be made in the mouth, through the lower eyelid, or behind the hairline in the area above the ear. A pocket for the insertion of the bone or silicone is created by separating the overlying tissue from the bone beneath. The inserted material may angulate slightly, be asymmetrical, or in the very thin patient be slightly apparent on close inspection, but aside from complications that may accompany any surgery, this operation presents no special problems.

Blepharoplasty

Blepharoplasty is the correction of puffy or wrinkled eyelids. Fullness or puffiness of the eyelids may occur even in young women, and it is usually a familial characteristic. In this condition the orbital fat that cushions the globe of the eye weakens the orbital muscle and a pseudo-hernia develops. The resulting puffiness sometimes characterizes patients with periodic or chronic edema and may be the symptom of a kidney disorder. After a period of time the puffiness becomes conspicuously wrinkled. In older women the wrinkling may occur without the puffiness. In some cases the overhang of the upper lid interferes with peripheral vision.

Surgery for the correction of this defect can be performed under local anesthesia, but since most patients are nervous about surgery close to the eye, supplemental intravenous or inhalation anesthesia may be advisable. The additional anesthesia relaxes the patient who may suffer some pain when the fat is being removed. Vision is checked before the operation. The surgeon also makes an estimate of the amount of tissue to be removed and usually draws an outline on the eyelid with a colored solution. The incision on the upper eyelid is ordinarily made in the fold of the lid where the eyeball meets the orbital bone. The scar is thus concealed when the patient's eye is open. The incision on the lower lid is usually made just beneath its edge, where it will be hidden by the lashes. The excess skin is removed, the muscles separated, and the fat gently extracted. Following the suturing of the skin, ice may be applied to limit swelling and discoloration. The sutures are removed by the fifth day following surgery. After the first week it is safe to stroke the eye horizontally, but not until the third week should it be rubbed vertically. By the tenth day after surgery, the patient generally is presentable without dark glasses.

In some cases excessive swelling may turn the eyelid out, or the lid may droop in a "hound dog" effect. These postoperative conditions almost always disappear with time. The eyelid tissue heals with practically no visible evidence of surgery. When scarring does occur, it is usually in the lateral area where the incision may have extended beyond the eyelid tissue and into the area of the "crow's feet." The patient should not anticipate the removal of all wrinkles. There is the occasional patient who may develop a persistent darker pigmentation of the lower eyelid. In others, if too much skin is removed, the lower eyelid may droop to the extent that the ability to close the eyes completely is lost. When this complication occurs, it has to be corrected by subsequent surgery. The muscular action of the upper eyelid is rarely damaged. While interference with the drainage of tears through the tear duct can occur, it rarely does. A few rare cases of blindness in one or both eyes, both temporary and permanent, have been reported.

Eyebrow Lift

There are some women whose eyebrows are so low that rather than perform an operation on the upper lid, the surgeon may suggest the excision of tissue above the eyebrow so that it can be repositioned. This improves the upper lid droop. While incisions in this area are likely to result in more conspicuous scars than those in eyelid tissue, the general total effect is likely to be more pleasing than before the eyebrows were elevated.

Otoplasty

Cosmetic surgery for the alteration of ear contour may involve reducing the size or form of the entire ear, the lobe, or the rim, but the most common operation is the correction of protruding ears. The protrusion results when the midportion of the ear (the concha) is too deep or the upper portion of the ear (the auricle) does not have such well-developed or acutely angulated folds as the normal ear. Making ears lie closer to the head can be accomplished only by surgery.

The surgery can be undertaken any time after the age of 6 when the ear has reached almost full development in most children. It should be done before the child has suffered psychological damage from taunts by thoughtless classmates and equally thoughtless relatives, but it can be done on adults.

The surgery is usually done in the doctor's office or on an outpatient basis in a hospital. With proper medication and a quiet reassuring environment, the operation can be performed on most children and adults under local anesthesia, although a restless or apprehensive child may require a general anesthetic. Most frequently the incision is made in the crease that separates the ear from the head. If the surgeon prefers to perform the operation from the front side, the incision is made just inside the rim. The soft tissue is elevated, and then the ear cartilage is revised either by cutting the cartilage, excising an ellipse, or thinning it by abrasion or crosshatching. The tissue is sutured into the desired position. After the muscles and the skin are sutured, a bandage is applied around the head to splint the ear in the new position and protect it.

The first dressing is often left in place for one week unless there is bleeding or the patient complains of pain. Pain may be caused by a bandage that is too tight or some other reason that should be investigated. In most cases after the first day little medication is required since there is practically no pain. A head band may be substituted later and worn for about three weeks while the fractured cartilage is healing. The postoperative numbness or insensitivity of the ears usually disappears within a few months.

Complications are minimal compared to those of the far more complex rhinoplasty. The cartilage of the revised ear may not become reunited. If the cartilage does not reunite spontaneously, it may be necessary to resuture it. The gentle anterior curve may be too angular and necessitate a minor corrective procedure. While the possibility of bleeding and infection can never be ruled out entirely, they occur rarely.

Mammaplasty

AUGMENTATION MAMMAPLASTY

When augmentation mammaplasty was first done breasts were increased in size by the transplantation of fat. In later operations fat and the dermal portion of the skin taken from the hip or abdominal area were used. Later still, glass balls and many synthetic prostheses of various materials were manufactured for the purpose of insertion. Then came the injection of silicone fluid. A silicone fluid or gel injected directly into the body migrates not only into the soft tissues in various parts of the body, but into the lymphatics and small blood vessels and thus can be transported to the liver, kidneys, lungs, heart, and brain. The use of this substance in mammaplasty resulted in the destruction and loss of otherwise healthy breast tissue and in some cases death caused by silicone embolism. At present, to prevent such disasters, the breast is augmented by the insertion of a silicone bag filled with silicone gel or fluid. Instillation of cortisone has been explored, but there is at present no sure way to control the complications of rejection by the body.

Before augmentation is undertaken, preoperative mammograms are recommended to ascertain whether there is an unsuspected malignancy. As in all breast surgery, the patient is usually advised to use an antiseptic soap to wash her upper torso for several days before the operation. The surgery may be performed under local anesthesia, general anesthesia, or a combination of local and intravenous anesthetics. Many surgeons do this operation in their office or in the outpatient facilities of a hospital.

The size and shape of the prosthesis is determined before the operation to be appropriate to the patient's thorax, the estimated recipient cavity, and the amount of tissue the patient has to cover it. The surgeon shows a sample prosthesis of the anticipated size to the patient. The surgeon may take two sizes to surgery to allow for variation in the actual cavity. The incision for the prosthesis may be below (submammary), at the armpit (axilla), or at the junction of the areola with the skin. The areolar and axillary incisions leave less conspicuous scars than the submammary incisions. The surgeon separates the overlying breast tissue between two layers of fascia. When the submammary approach is used, there is less likelihood of transecting the breast tissue.

Although bleeding at the time of surgery is minimal, later oozing or bleeding from a large vessel may occur and result in hematoma. This in turn can lead to necrosis (death) of the overlying skin or disruption of the wound. Visible scars can occur, but since the incision is small, they are a minor problem unless the patient forms keloids (raised red scars). Asymmetry is always a possibility, especially if the chest wall is asymmetrical.

The most common complications result from the body's rejection of the

COSMETIC SURGERY OF THE BREAST
REDUCTION MAMMAPLASTY

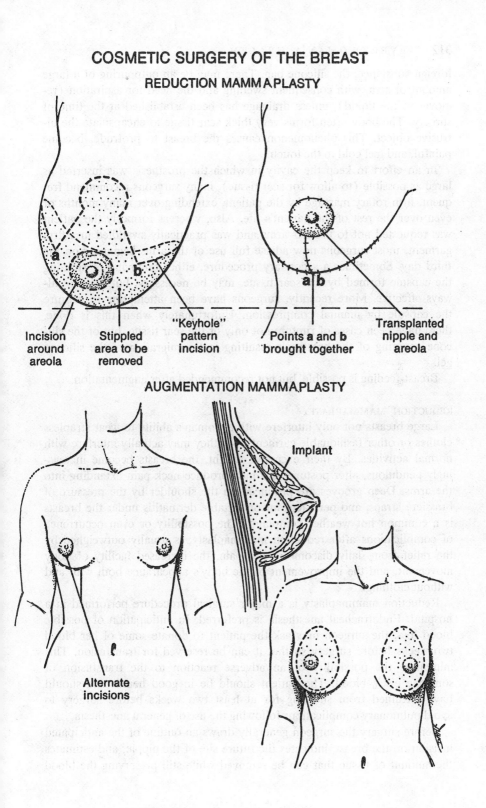

Incision around areola

Stippled area to be removed

"Keyhole" pattern incision

Points a and b brought together

Transplanted nipple and areola

AUGMENTATION MAMMAPLASTY

Implant

Alternate incisions

foreign substance, the silicone bag. There may be an outpouring of a large amount of sera, with consequent swelling and the need for aspiration (removal of the liquid), unless drainage has been established at the time of surgery. The body often forms very thick scar tissue to encapsulate the intrusive object. This phenomenon causes the breast to protrude, become painful, and feel cold to the touch.

In an effort to keep the cavity in which the prosthesis was inserted as large as possible (to allow for scar tissue), many surgeons recommend frequent, firm rotary massage by the patient, extending over many months or even over the rest of the patient's life. Also, whereas formerly the patient was requested not to use her arms and was practically swaddled in a firm garment, most surgeons now advise full use of the arms beginning on the third day. Sometimes a secondary procedure, either removing or splitting the capsule formed by the scar tissue, may be necessary, but it is not always effective. More recently, surgeons have been attempting to rupture the capsule by manual compression. Unfortunately when this is done, there have been cases of rupture not only of the scar tissue, but of the silicone covering of the prosthesis resulting in the migration of the silicone gel.

Breast-feeding is possible, but not recommended after augmentation.

REDUCTION MAMMAPLASTY

Large breasts not only interfere with a woman's ability to wear strapless clothes or other fashionable garments, but they may actually interfere with normal activities. By their excessive weight, the breasts become increasingly pendulous, alter posture, and may produce neck pain extending into the arms. Deep grooves are produced on the shoulder by the pressure of brassiere straps, and persistent uncomfortable dermatitis under the breasts is a common hot weather complaint. The possibility or even occurrence of complications after reduction mammaplasty, is usually outweighed by the relief from daily discomfort and pain, the increased facility of body movement, and the improvement of the body's appearance both with and without clothing.

Reduction mammaplasty is a major surgical procedure performed in a hospital. Endotracheal anesthesia is preferred. In anticipation of possible blood loss, the surgeon may ask the patient to donate some of her blood two weeks before surgery so that it can be reserved for transfusion. This minimizes the possibility of an adverse reaction to the transfusion of someone else's blood. The patient should be in good health and should have refrained from smoking for at least two weeks before surgery to avoid pulmonary complications following the use of general anesthesia.

Before surgery the surgeon generally draws an outline of the anticipated incision on the breast, indicates the future site of the nipple, and estimates the amount of tissue that can be removed while still preserving the blood supply to the areola and the nipple. The incisions are usually made around the pigmented areola and extended either laterally or in the midline to the submammary area, where they are further extended horizontally. The skin, fat, excess breast tissue, and usually some of the oversized areola, are all excised. The remaining breast tissue and fat are then fitted into the "skin brassiere" and the nipple is secured in its higher location. In some very oversized breasts it is necessary to separate the areola and nipple from the underlying tissue. After the tailoring of the breast tissue has been completed, the areola and nipple tissue are then applied as a free graft. Many surgeons insert drains attached to suctions for the removal of blood, sera, or liquified fat that might accumulate postoperatively and jeopardize the final results.

After the operation the patient wears a bandage around the chest or a special brassiere for approximately three weeks. During this postoperative period physical activities involving the use of the upper arms are strictly limited.

The complications that can occur after this operation are bleeding, infection, prolonged drainage, loss of tissue, inversion of the nipple, and unsightly scars. Because of the large amount of fat in oversized breasts, there is a greater chance of infection than in most other cosmetic surgery procedures. Tissue loss may occur because the blood supply is inadequate to the retained skin or areola and nipple complex, or the loss may result from infection or pressure. When such complications occur, a secondary procedure may be necessary. Follow-up surgery may also be necessary to correct asymmetry or depressed nipples. While the scars following breast reduction operations are more apparent than those resulting from other plastic surgery, they can usually be modified. Noticeable scarring is most likely to occur and to recur even after modification in the submammary area.

The nipple may be hypersensitive for a period of time, and there may be some permanent decrease in sensitivity and erectility. With the passage of time the breasts will gradually become more pendulous than they were in the immediate postoperative period. Following a transposition procedure in which the nipple is secured into a higher position, a woman may breast-feed a baby, but she is not encouraged to do so. Future breast-feeding is impossible when the operation involves a free grafting of the nipple.

MASTOPEXY

Breasts naturally sag (ptosis) with the passage of time even when they are not abnormally large. The elevation of the ptotic breast is a much less complicated operation than the correction of oversized, dependent breasts. The designs of the incisions and the surgical procedure for lifting the sagging breast are similar to those of a reduction mammaplasty, but because the procedure is simpler and quicker, the attendant risks are fewer and the scars are less conspicuous.

PLASTIC SURGERY PROCEDURES FOLLOWING MASTECTOMY

After a simple mastectomy or a modified radical mastectomy, if enough subcutaneous fat remains, the form of the breast can be re-created by the insertion of a prosthesis as in augmentation mammaplasty. Many surgeons believe that a more attractive breast contour can be created by inserting the prosthesis under the pectoral muscles. If an areola and nipple have been removed, a portion of each from the remaining breast may be used as a free graft. If both breasts have been removed, it may be necessary to use tissue from the labia minora to simulate the areola and the nipple. Sometimes, during the mastectomy procedure, the nipple and the areola are preserved for later transplantation by temporarily transplanting them to the groin to keep the tissue viable.

After a radical mastectomy, if extension of the cancer or of metastisis appears to be unlikely, consideration can be given to breast reconstruction. When the radical mastectomy has necessitated a skin graft or coverage, it is necessary to transplant an adequate amount of fat and skin in order to obtain enough coverage for the prosthesis. This "flap" is taken from some adjacent part of the body and rotated into position. The procedure is done under general anesthesia in a hospital, and several operations may be scheduled, separated by an interval of three weeks. The nipple and the areola can be simulated as they are in a modified mastectomy.

The particular postoperative routine is determined by the surgeon and must be followed meticulously in order not to jeopardize the blood supply to the transplanted tissue. In addition to the possible complications outlined in other breast surgery, the patient must take into account various other factors: prolonged hospitalization, inevitable scarring at the site of the body from which the tissue was taken for grafting, and the question of money and whether coverage for breast reconstruction has been included in her medical insurance. The decision to embark on breast reconstruction is also affected by many unconscious factors, especially the degree to which a woman equates her breasts with her femininity.

Lipectomy

ABDOMINAL LIPECTOMY

Abdominal lipectomy was originally undertaken to correct extreme cases of obesity by removing some of the skin and subcutaneous tissue of a grotesquely pendulous lower abdomen. Today this surgery is also performed for the correction of the excessive flaccidity of the skin that may result from pregnancy or weight loss and for the improvement of the striae (stretch marks) caused by pregnancy. Often a lax, obese abdomen is associated with weakened or separated central abdominal muscles, and to obtain a good result in such cases, it is necessary that the fascia surrounding these muscles be plicated across the midline (folded back on themselves) to pull the muscles together.

The patient should be in excellent health before the surgery is scheduled since this is a major procedure performed under general anesthesia. The patient is usually requested to bathe with antiseptic soap for several days before entering the hospital. Preceding surgery, the pubic hair is shaved. The incision is usually made just above the pubic area and extends laterally across the area that would be covered by the lower part of a bikini. If there is an old midline scar, if improvement of the waistline is to be accomplished, or if the surgeon decides it would be more advantageous, a midline incision may be made instead of a horizontal incision. In some cases both incisions are made. The skin and subcutaneous tissue are separated from the underlying fascia as far up as the rib margin and sternum. The patient is placed in a flexed position, with knees and upper torso elevated so that the maximum amount of tissue can be removed. The excess is cut away, and the navel is relocated in a new opening made for this purpose. Blood loss is minimal. However, drains attached to suction are inserted as there may be some postoperative ooze and liquefaction of fat as in a reduction mammaplasty. The flexed position is maintained as the wound is dressed. Various types of dressings are used, but most of them are designed to exert pressure and are similar to a panty girdle. The wearing of a supportive girdle for six weeks after the surgery is recommended. Ambulation usually begins on the third day and gradually increases as healing proceeds, and the patient gradually becomes more upright in position.

Postoperative bleeding may occur and drainage may be excessive. Because the area is one of fatty tissue with a relatively small blood supply, infection may occur, but this is rare. Loss of tissue can occur because of a hematoma, excessive tension, or inadequate blood supply. When tissue loss does occur, a second procedure may be required for correction. Scars may be conspicuous. Rarely are all stretch marks removed. Those that were located in the excised skin are, of course, gone, but those in other areas remain. However, since the skin is more taut, the remaining striae are less conspicuous.

THIGH, HIP, AND ARM LIPECTOMY

Excessive flabbiness of skin or excessive fat or both can also be removed from hips, thighs, and arms. The preoperative preparation and procedure are fundamentally similar to those required by the abdominal lipectomy, and potential complications are the same in all. The excision of arm tissue is the simplest.

The incision for the removal of excess tissue from the hip is usually made in the gluteal fold where the buttocks join the upper thigh. If the problem exists over the lateral portion of the upper thigh (trochanteric) area, the incision may extend around three-quarters of the thigh or at a slightly higher level where the scar will be hidden by a bikini.

For the removal of excess skin from the inner thigh, a modified T incision is made extending vertically at the midline of the inner thigh and extending forward and backward for a limited distance at the groin.

To remove the excess skin and subcutaneous tissue of the upper arm, a modified T incision is made, with the vertical portion of the cut placed along the least visible portion of the arm and the horizontal cut extending into the armpit. The scar will be visible when the arm is raised. In deciding whether to have this surgery, the patient must choose between flabby arms and a visible scar.

For all these procedures three weeks of disuse should be anticipated. After three weeks scars may increase in width but they also become paler and less conspicuous.

Spider Hemangioma and Capillary Varicosities

Spider hemangiomas, which appear on the face or the body as little red spots with tiny radiating blood vessels, and capillary varicosities, which usually appear on the thighs and legs, can be eliminated. This is accomplished by the injection of air and a chemically irritating (sclerosing) solution into the blood vessel through a very small needle. More than one visit to the physician may be required. It is imperative that the solution be injected directly into the vein so that it does not come in contact with adjacent skin. Contact with the skin may cause an alteration in pigment or even loss of the affected tissue. Some surgeons prefer to treat the little vascular lesions by touching them with an electric needle.

In this chapter I have presented a nontechnical survey of current procedures in cosmetic surgery. It is neither comprehensive nor definitive, but it is an attempt to explain what is involved in various operations as an aid to the woman considering them.

During a consultation, the patient should be told exactly what will take place before, during, and after the operation. All doubts and possible misunderstandings should be resolved before the operation. If the doubts remain, it is best not to schedule the surgery. To obtain the best results, the surgeon's instructions should be followed as closely as possible. Many a good result at the time of surgery has become a disaster because of the patient's lack of cooperation.

The criterion for the ultimate success of cosmetic surgery is the patient's greater pleasure in her appearance. Unfortunately, an operation that may be considered successful by the surgeon in terms of physical and esthetic results may not be viewed with the same enthusiasm by the patient. For those few women whose dreams of rejuvenation are so unrealistic as to be totally beyond the possibility of accomplishment, no improvement will ever be good enough. However, in spite of the limitations and the problems that must be taken into account, the vast majority of patients who have had surgery for the improvement of their appearance were the happier for having done so.

FURTHER READING

Englebardt, Stanley L. "What You Should Know About Cosmetic Surgery." *Reader's Digest*, April 1979.

Goin, John M., and Marcia K. Goin. *Changing the Body: Psychological Effects of Plastic Surgery*. Baltimore: Williams and Wilkins, 1981.

Rosenthal, Sylvia. *Cosmetic Surgery: A Consumer's Guide*. Philadelphia: Lippincott, 1977.

Drugs, Alcohol, and Tobacco— Their Use and Abuse

ADELE HOFMANN, M.D.

Associate Professor of Pediatrics,
Director of Adolescent Medical Unit, New York University
Medical Center–Bellevue Hospital, New York City

What peps us up? What turns us on? What calms us down? What puts us to sleep? What drugs keep us going?

ALCOHOL	DOM (or STP)	METHADONE	PSYLOCYBIN
AMYL NITRATE	DORIDEN	METHAQUALONE	QUAALUDE
AMYTAL	EQUANIL	METHEDRINE	SCOPOLAMINE
ATROPINE	HALDOL	MILTOWN	SECONAL
BENZEDRINE	HASHISH	MORPHINE	SOPOR
CAFFEINE	HERBAL TEA	NEMBUTAL	STELAZINE
COCAINE	HEROIN	NICOTINE	TALWIN
CODEINE	ISOBUTYL NITRITE	OPIUM	THC
DALMANE	LIBRIUM	PCP	THORAZINE
DARVON	LSD	PERCODAN	VALIUM
DEMEROL	MARIJUANA	PEYOTE	
DEXEDRINE	MELLARIL	PHENOBARBITAL	
DMT	MESCALINE	PRELUDIN	

DEFINITIONS

Drug For purposes of this chapter, any chemical substance, legal or illegal, including alcohol, which is used to achieve the effects listed below under drug use. Drugs can be found in legitimate medicines, in plants, and on the street.

Drug use The voluntary, self-controlled administration of a chemical substance to achieve a desired psychological (psychotropic) effect or physical sensation. This may be anything from the relief of moderate tension or mild aches and pains, to promoting relaxation and social intercourse at a party, to easing the passage to sleep, to seeking spiritual perception and a vision of eternal truth, to heightening self-awareness. There are many uses to which a drug may be put. Some are beneficial, others do outright harm, and there is a middle ground in which we simply do not yet know whether dangers do or do not exist.

Drug abuse   The excessive, indiscriminate use of a drug such that it sometimes passes beyond self-control and interferes with normal function. Abuse is one step away from compulsive emotional need or habituation.

Habituation   *Psychological* dependence upon a drug; the user's compulsive emotional need for its effects in order to function or get through the day. All drugs cited in this chapter are potentially habituating, depending on the individual's psychological predisposition. Habituation can be just as compelling as addiction.

Addiction   *Physical* dependence upon a drug; adaption of the body to the presence of a drug so that its continued use is required by the user just to feel well and to continue to function physiologically. Addiction occurs only with narcotics and depressants and only if taken regularly on a daily basis. Whether or not stimulants are addicting remains uncertain. After a number of days without a drug, addiction is lost.

Tolerance   The body's gradual adaptation, with regular, daily intake over one or two weeks or longer, to the presence of a particular amount of a drug so that that dosage produces a diminishing effect. In order to achieve the desired effect, larger and larger amounts of the drug are required. Susceptibility to overdosage decreases, and the user is able to take amounts which would be lethal to anyone else. Tolerance regularly occurs with the use of narcotics, stimulants, and, to a lesser degree, with barbiturates and alcohol. It also occurs with marijuana. Tolerance is lost rapidly, within a few days or weeks, upon abstinence.

Cross-Tolerance   The capacity of one drug to substitute for another in meeting the habituated person's need, in relieving withdrawal symptoms, or in satisfying an addict. Such drugs are also additive in their effects. Cross-tolerance generally exists between all members of a class of drugs, for example between alcohol and Valium (depressants), cocaine and Dexedrine (stimulants), heroin and morphine (narcotics). The term is unrelated to tolerance as defined above.

THE UNIVERSALITY OF DRUG USE

Drug use has been and continues to be part of human history, in ancient and modern societies, in sophisticated and primitive cultures, and in Eastern and Western civilizations. Opium poppy capsules decorate the base of an early Greek vase and the headdress of an ancient terra cotta head unearthed in Crete. Marijuana was used in China over four thousand years ago. Mushrooms and cacti with hallucinogenic properties have been essential elements in the religious ceremonies of South and Central American Indians. As for the uses of alcohol, the *Rubaiyat* of Omar Khayyam makes this comment:

> I drink Wine not for Pleasure, nor for Profligacy,
> nor to renege Religion and good Morals;
> but solely to escape a Moment from myself.
>
> *Quatrain 63*

In our own lives drugs are found at every turn, to be used as an escape from physical pain or emotional distress or as a quick way of dealing with daily pressures. Most women are at one time or another faced with the choice of whether to have an alcoholic drink at a business lunch or dinner party, whether to take something stronger than aspirin after a tooth extraction, whether to smoke a cigarette or light up a marijuana joint as a way of relaxing after a family quarrel, whether to gulp a cola drink or a cup of coffee as a pick-me-up, whether to experiment with over-the-counter sedatives, or whether to try a tranquilizer prescribed by the doctor.

Many of us have the opportunity to explore still other drugs, yet the decisions we make about whether or not to do so are often made not rationally and on the basis of available facts, but rather in response to social pressure or a momentary impulse. Many of us will have to deal with drug use by a family member or a close friend. We may have to consider the effects of regular use of "diet" pills or "pep" pills or "sleeping" pills on a teenage daughter. We may have to weigh the effects of caffeine and alcohol on an unborn child.

KNOW YOUR FACTS

Facts and figures are difficult to come by, and the truth is sometimes distorted for the sake of a sensational news story, to increase commercial profits, or to bolster an emotional, unscientific point of view. The indiscriminate use of the term "addiction" may create a picture much blacker than the reality. Scarcely any of us can be immune from the pervasive hard sell of advertising and the images that bombard us from the media in the interest of greater profits for the drug manufacturers, alcoholic beverage companies, the cigarette industry, the "health and beauty" business. It's macho, mature, sexy to smoke. Beer makes the party; wine makes dinner for two more romantic. Have you got a headache? Suffering from a stuffed nose? Can't sleep? Got a backache? Is bad breath a problem? Want to weigh a few pounds less? Someone out there has just the pill, the cream, the medication to make you feel better, look better, and live happily ever after.

The federal government has not always been a reliable source of unprejudiced facts either. Although false information is rare today, as recently as the 1930s, marijuana was presented as a substance that inevitably resulted in madness, insatiable sexual appetite, and uncontrollable violence.

How can you assess the material presented in print, on the radio, and on television? Pay attention to the statistics and try to understand what they mean in relation to the total picture. Use your common sense. Remember that the initial reports of a new drug or an old one used in a new way appear before the public without sufficient regard for an accumulation of facts over a considerable period, especially about such matters as side effects, cumulative effects over a long period, reactions when combined with other medications. Material in the media may raise your awareness about drugs, but it may give only a one-sided picture, to extol therapeutic values or to condemn negative aspects. Take the time to inform yourself by reading balanced articles and books by reputable authorities. Discuss your uncertainties with your doctor. What does he or she think about the drug? Its safety? Its benefits?

WOMEN AND DRUGS TODAY

How many women have a drug problem? This question cannot be answered unless there is some agreement about the definition of "problem." A strict teetotaler might think that anyone who has a glass of wine with dinner every evening is heading for trouble, and at the same time view with equanimity a woman who "needs" six Valium a day or who can never get to sleep without a sedative. As a physician, I would feel that the pill-taker had the problem.

But even if we were to agree on a definition of "problem," it would be difficult to get at all the facts since the consumption of drugs is often clandestine. Take the question of women and alcohol abuse. Current estimates suggest that over 40 percent of the approximately 10 million alcoholics in the United States are women, that is, over 4 million women are suffering from the disease of alcoholism according to the generally agreed upon criteria established by experts in this area. It is difficult to say how many are addicted to sleeping pills or tranquilizers. Estimates by the National Institute on Drug Abuse suggest that there are about 20 million women in the United States with a drug abuse or alcohol problem, more than twice the number of men. Some 200 million or more prescriptions are written each year for mind-altering substances, and two out of every three of these prescriptions are for women. Twice as many women as men have used amphetamines at least once, 72 percent more take tranquilizers, 45 percent more use sedatives. Women are also more susceptible than men to mixed patterns of abuse, to self-medication, and to "borrowing" pills from friends. Yet 60 percent of all patients have little idea what these medicines really are. Ignorance can lead to disaster for the pill-popper when certain substances are combined. The mix of alcohol and sedatives can be deadly; the mix of tranquilizers and antihistamines can lead to dozing while driving—a dangerous circumstance indeed.

While the most frequently abused substances are alcohol and depressants, a significant number of women get involved with stimulants as a way of losing weight. Obesity has long been treated with this category of drugs because they are known to curb the appetite temporarily. Among the more widely used are Dexedrine, Methedrine, and Preludin, as well as other related compounds. At the same time that they restrain the desire to overindulge in chocolate cake, they provide a pick-me-up, a relief from depression and chronic fatigue. Many women are caught up in unwitting habituation to these drugs. Nowadays, most responsible physicians recognize this hazard and refrain from prescribing these drugs except under limited and special circumstances. Even those doctors who are running profitable weight-reduction mills have become increasingly careful in how they prescribe amphetamines, thanks to a crackdown by the federal government on the frequency of such prescriptions.

It is not uncommon for women to become addicted to narcotics. While heroin is characteristically a problem of both sexes in inner city ghettos, women in all walks of life who are in chronic pain serious enough to be immobilizing may find that the Demerol or Percodan prescribed by their doctors provides something more than physical relief and will continue the use of the drug beyond its original purpose. Or they may become addicted during proper medical use when taking the drug as a pain-killer and find it difficult to stop on pain's surcease. It is estimated that at the turn of the century, about 20 percent of the female population was addicted to one or another derivative of opium, usually laudanum or morphine, in the form of "nerve medicine" or an "elixir for monthly discomfort." Nowadays, the physician is legally permitted to prescribe narcotics to the point of addiction and to maintain the patient's habit only for the alleviation of the intractable pain that may accompany terminal cancer or some similar fatal disease.

Female habituation to tobacco is increasing despite continued warnings by the government and other health authorities. Indeed, the rising incidence of lung cancer and heart disease among women is attributed to this cause. It also appears more difficult for women to give up smoking than for men; "stop smoking" programs are generally more successful for the male.

While marijuana use is widespread among young women, it does not appear to be associated with habituation to a marked degree. Those with susceptible personalities may get "strung out" and need more than one or two joints a day in order to face the world, but this is not common (less than 1 to 2 percent of all users).

Fads for drugs that produce "highs" come and go, but the depressant drugs—alcohol, tranquilizers, and sleeping pills—have always led the list of habituating substances and probably will continue to do so. It is this class that should therefore be subjected to the closest scrutiny.

WHAT YOU SHOULD KNOW ABOUT DRUGS IN GENERAL

Before considering particular drugs, you should know certain facts that apply to drugs in general.

How Drugs Are Taken

The way in which a drug enters the body has a significant effect upon the user's experience. When the substance is swallowed and absorbed through the digestive tract, it tends to produce a reaction which is slower in onset and less intense than other methods of use, but the reaction lasts longer. The rate of absorption is also affected by previous food intake: more rapid if the stomach is empty, slower if the stomach is full, and slower still if the recently ingested meal was particularly fatty.

In intravenous use, or "mainlining," the drug is dissolved in a liquid, usually water, and taken up in a syringe. It is then injected into a surface vein, usually in the arm or hand. This method produces the most rapid onset and the most intense effect (known as a "rush" and stated to be similar to a sexual orgasm) and, because of the rapidity and intensity, may produce sensations that cannot be achieved by taking the drug in other ways. But the experience is relatively short-lived. Quick results can also be attained through injection under the skin, or "skin popping," although the effects are somewhat slower in onset and less intense than in mainlining. Injection carries with it the risk of infection from contaminated needles, syringes, or drug.

The mucous membranes of the mouth and nose readily absorb many drugs. Dissolving a tablet under the tongue or sniffing a powder can achieve an effect as rapid as the effect achieved by skin popping. Cocaine is characteristically used in this way; so is LSD on occasion. Limitations are imposed by the irritant properties the drug may have; sneezing and a runny nose are not particularly desirable consequences.

Smoking and inhaling are highly effective ways of getting a drug into the body. Absorption through the lungs is rapid, about on a par with the mucous membrane or subcutaneous route. Marijuana, hashish, angel dust

(PCP), isobutyl nitrite ("poppers"), glues, and various solvents are regularly used in this way. Irritant factors, especially associated coughing, may preclude this method.

Frequency, Strength, and Purity of Contents

It is obvious that the strength of a drug dose and the frequency with which it is taken will significantly vary the achieved effect and its duration. Frequency is generally under the control of the user; the amount not always. While alcohol and medically prescribed pills are consistent in their strength, drugs obtained on the illegal market may be quite a different matter. Such substances often are highly variable in the amount of the active chemical they contain, and this variability is often unknown to the seller or user. What other substances they contain in addition to the desired drug also may be unknown. Thus the user may end up with a substance that has no effect whatever, one that produces the usual effect, or one so strong as to cause a fatal overdose.

While alcohol or drugs purchased at licensed stores or pharmacies are pretty much guaranteed as to the strength, purity, and safety of their contents (except where a label indicates a warning to be observed), this reliability is often questionable when drugs are procured illegally. Heroin and cocaine are regularly "cut" or diluted with anything from quinine to talcum powder to even house dust. Also, since they are far from sterile, they may contain disease-producing bacteria or viruses. Hepatitis is the most notorious example, but tetanus and infections of the heart or bones also may occur. Hallucinogens are especially notorious for being something other than claimed. Chemical analyses of samples of LSD, for instance, have revealed that 13 percent either contained other drugs in addition, were an entirely different drug, or contained no active material at all. Pills sold as mescaline have been found to be as "advertised" in only 10 percent; those purported to be psilicybin were so in only 13 percent. Both were far more likely to contain LSD or PCP. Indeed, of all drugs commonly subject to abuse, only marijuana actually was marijuana in more than 90 percent of the tested samples. Even marijuana is increasingly found to be adulterated with PCP.

Experience and Environment

Drugs taken by experienced users in a congenial setting are more likely to produce optimal pleasurable results than those taken by novices under threatening circumstances. Both the experience of the user and the environment may alter the quality, intensity, and duration of the drug effect. A novice's anxiety or false expectations may limit effects or produce undesirable sensations. For example, novice smokers of marijuana regularly report little more than dizziness and nausea. Convivial settings are said to enhance the desired effects of LSD, while uncongenial ones sometimes result in unpleasant experiences, or "bad trips." However, attitude and environment are only contributing factors to effects, not the determining one. Anyone will experience some kind of effect if the drug is taken in sufficiently large doses, no matter what the time, place, or mental attitude. Even a congenial and/or supportive environment is no guarantee against having a bad trip, overdosing, or becoming addicted.

Individual Vulnerability to Drug Abuse

Not all drug users succumb to abuse, and not all drug abusers become habituated or addicted. Indeed, the majority of individuals can take alcohol and sedatives, smoke marijuana, or even experiment with other drugs with relative impunity. We do not understand all the factors that contribute to a particular person's vulnerability to drug abuse, but certain characteristics seem to be shared by those who develop a drug problem, regardless of the nature of the drug in question. These characteristics invariably include personal adjustment difficulties, low self-esteem, few apparent options or choices in dealing with life's problems, increasing feelings of helplessness and hopelessness, inadequate communication with others, or a family history of heavy drug abuse. Additional specific risk factors are typically associated with alcoholism.

It is not yet clear whether physiological or genetic predisposition exists. Certain individuals do seem to be on the road to alcoholism after a single drink, although for the majority the disease develops only after prolonged and excessive intake. Studies of drug abuse among adolescents and young adults generally confirm the conclusion that use becomes abuse primarily in those who are psychologically vulnerable. But in a few instances even the most seemingly well-adjusted youths have succumbed to narcotic addiction or to psychotic reactions after taking LSD.

Effect of Availability, Popularity, and Acceptance of Drug Use

The ease with which a drug can be obtained has a significant impact upon whether it is used or not. Alcohol, Valium, and sleeping pills are all easily available from the corner liquor store or from physicians who treat symptoms rather than underlying problems. When police efforts against narcotic traffic in New York City's inner-city made street heroin hard to get and exceedingly weak, addicts and abusers felt that it was hardly worth their effort and turned to methadone instead, easily available through illegal diversion from legitimate treatment centers.

Some of the more exotic or newer drugs become popular through rumors about a new and great high. Such rumors are especially apt to arise among the experimenting young or jaded poly-drug users. Often the substances in question are relatively easy to manufacture by underground chemists, who themselves promote the drugs through the grapevine in expectation of making large profits. The current popularity of the hallucinogen PCP is a case in point. DOM (desoxymethylamphetamine), a hallucinogen, entered the drug scene in this way several years ago. Its popularity was brief, because although it had a stupendous effect, its action lasted for days rather than hours, and since it was associated with an exceedingly high incidence of bad trips, it soon fell into disrepute.

Drugs that receive the overt or covert acceptance of society certainly are more likely to be used than those that are rigorously proscribed. Alcohol, cigarettes, marijuana and the full range of tranquilizers, pep pills, and sedatives are examples. The approval of a particular substance by a subcultural group, even if not by society at large, is also influential. (The recent taking up of cocaine sniffing by the disco set is an example of trendiness in drug use.) And the converse is also true: alcohol consumption may be less popular in a strict teetotaling community.

In many respects the medical profession has to take part of the responsibility for widespread drug use and abuse. Health care in the United States has evolved along lines that suggest that medicines cure all, and the view that medicine is magic has been capitalized upon by the pharmaceutical industry. Drug manufacturers profit not only from prescriptions written by doctors, but also from the promotion and advertisement of drugs that can be bought without a prescription: over-the-counter medicines to induce sleep, to maintain alertness, to reduce pain, to ease stress, or to relieve a nagging headache. A complex, tension-producing world coupled with a medical system that treats the patient's symptoms with pills or shots certainly creates the impression that self-medication, even with illicit drugs, need not be all bad. The frequency with which physicians prescribe tranquilizers and sedatives to relieve physical and emotional distress, without further investigation of the underlying cause and without consideration of alternative treatment, encourages patients to seek immediate relief from any discomfort, instills the habit of pill-taking, and provides some with the opportunity to accumulate large numbers of prescriptions for Valium or Demerol by visiting one doctor after another.

The Institute of Medicine of the National Academy of Sciences has recently recommended that current medical practices in relation to the prescription of depressants, particularly those intended to treat insomnia, be further curtailed and that doctors limit the number of pills prescribed at one time as well as how many times and at what interval the prescription may be refilled.

Women must recognize their rights and obligations to assume greater responsibility for their own well-being and to avoid the seductive message conveyed by advertising, trendy friends, and some doctors that pill taking is the best method of dealing with the normal stress of daily living on mind and body. Every woman should know specifically what medication she is taking, its intended action, its possible hazards and side effects, and what combinations with other substances can be harmful if not lethal. This personal responsibility extends to prescription medicines as well as to those purchased over the counter. She should question her doctor about prescriptions, read the labels on nonprescription substances, and never take prescription medication from friends or offer them any of her own.

DRUGS IN COMMON USE TODAY

Most substances on the drug scene today can be divided into four broad categories or classes according to their dominant effect. It is helpful to view drugs in this way since the effects of any member of a given class are generally representative of all. Among depressants, for example, what we know about alcohol bears much similarity to what we can expect from sleeping pills and tranquilizers. Among narcotics, heroin, morphine, Demerol, and methadone are very much alike.

- Depressants cause sedation, ease anxiety, and promote sleep.
- Stimulants promote alertness, diminish fatigue, and heighten mental processes.
- Hallucinogens distort perceptions, giving rise to visions and heightened sensations. They can closely mimic such serious illnesses as schizophrenia and paranoia in their effect.
- Narcotics have a depressant effect and also produce euphoria and alleviate pain.

A few drugs that are used less frequently do not fit into these categories and are mentioned separately.

These broad classes and their subgroups are described below in terms of their effects and medical complications for the user. Possible complications for the fetus resulting from use during pregnancy are discussed in the section following the description of drugs in use.

Depressants

This class is comprised of three major subgroups: (1) tranquilizers and sedatives, (2) alcohol, and (3) volatile solvents, gasoline, and aerosol propellant gases. All of these substances decrease anxiety, diminish inhibitions, and promote sleep. While they depress brain function as do narcotics, they do not produce euphoria or a dreamlike state, a rush sensation does not follow injection and none are effective in the medical treatment of pain. Depressants are colloquially called "downers."

Tranquilizers, sedatives, and alcohol have remarkably similar pharmacologic effects and could be considered collectively as a single group. Since they possess cross-tolerance, they directly supplement each other in the level of intoxication achieved. Sleeping pills do not counteract the effects of alcohol; rather, by increasing the inebriated state, they increase the likelihood of overdose. The division of these substances into the two subgroups is based on substantial differences in patterns of use and medical complications. The pharmacologic effects of solvent and aerosol sniffing more closely resemble the effects produced by the inhalation of certain anesthetics used in surgery. The drugs involved will therefore be considered to comprise a subgroup of their own.

TRANQUILIZERS AND SEDATIVES

Characteristics and medical use. Since most members of this group are generally legitimately manufactured and therefore chemically controlled, they are relatively pure whether obtained on the street or through prescription. They have the capacity to calm anxiety, decrease nervousness, and induce sleep. Sedatives are more effective in inducing sleep, while tranquilizers more selectively reduce anxiety. Sedatives also have a major role in the treatment of convulsions and epilepsy. Strong tranquilizers such as Thorazine, Stelazine, or Haldol are of particular benefit in the treatment of serious emotional disorders and mental illness.

Drugs commonly abused. The sedatives most widely used and most commonly abused are: Nembutal, Seconal, phenobarbital, Amytal, Quaalude (Sopor or methaqualone), and Talwin. The tranquilizers are: Doriden, Librium, Valium, and Miltown (Equanil). Dalmane, the most frequently prescribed sleeping pill today, is a close chemical relative of Valium and Librium.

In street terminology specific downers are likely to be called by names deriving from the color of their capsules: "blues" or "bluebirds" for Amytal; "yellows" or "yellow jackets" for Nembutal, and "reds" or "red devils" for Seconal.

Appearance and method of administration. Sedatives and tranquilizers are generally sold in capsule or pill form and are taken orally. On occasion, intravenous administration may be resorted to.

Effects. Anyone who has been intoxicated with alcohol can readily predict what the effects of tranquilizers and sedatives will be. Low doses produce a pleasant sensation of diminished tension and relaxation; slightly larger amounts result in the decrease of inhibitions. Sometimes this is perceived as a "stimulant" effect, especially when the drug causes the user to become livelier and more talkative. What has in fact occurred is the depression of customary emotional restraint, permitting a freer, less guarded, and more impulsive self to emerge. Large doses of either sedatives or tranquilizers produce marked drowsiness and sleep. Even larger doses suppress bodily functions to the point of coma and, if emergency measures are not taken, can result in death.

Just what constitutes a low, moderate, or large dose is difficult to define due to all the variable factors described before. One to two drinks or tranquilizer pills would constitute a low to moderate dose for the average individual. Four to six drinks or pills would probably induce sleep. It is extremely difficult to consume a fatal dose of alcohol before passing out. The fatal amount of sedatives or tranquilizers is variable depending on their overall strength.

All depressants interfere with muscular control. Initially, fine motor coordination is lost. Greater degrees of intoxication result in gross impairment, leading to a staggering gait and general clumsiness. Speech becomes slurred to the point of incoherence. Sexual impulses may be aroused and acted upon in the early stages of intoxication because of the reduction in inhibitions. With higher levels of drug intake, however, physiologic mechanisms of the sexual response are depressed to the point where the male becomes incapable of erection.

Sedatives and tranquilizers (and alcohol) are all addicting. But unlike addiction to narcotics, the problem does not occur with sedatives and tranquilizers unless a certain "threshold" dose is exceeded on a daily basis. Seconal requires daily intake of more than four 100-milligram capsules (red) and Valium more than twelve 5-milligram tablets (yellow).

Tolerance develops, but only partially. Heavy users or abusers find they do require somewhat larger doses over time in order to achieve the desired physical effect, but ultimately the dose stabilizes without further increase.

Withdrawal. If an *addicted* (not simply habituated) individual abruptly stops taking any depressant, the result may be fatal. Detoxification from alcohol, tranquilizers, or sleeping pill addiction must be carried out in a hospital under strict medical control. Withdrawal symptoms are directly related to the amount of daily intake. Mild signs include jitteriness, tremors, increased anxiety, restlessness, and insomnia. More severe withdrawal symptoms include disorientation, confusion, and hallucinations, usually of an unpleasant, even terrifying sort. (In alcoholism these latter signs are referred to collectively as the DTs or delirium tremens.) In its most acute form, withdrawal may lead to convulsions, physical collapse, heart failure, coma, and death.

Medically supervised withdrawal from sedatives is carried out in the same way as it is for narcotics: Phenobarbital or Nembutal is substituted for the addictive drug in amounts sufficient to relieve the acute symptoms, and then gradually the doses are diminished to the vanishing point by the end of a week or ten days. By this time the patient will be drug-free and physically comfortable, although the underlying psychological problems leading to the addiction in the first place may leave the individual emotionally distressed.

Overdose. All sedatives and tranquilizers, as well as alcohol, produce loss of consciousness and slowed breathing if taken in large enough amounts. As previously noted, when alcohol is combined with sedatives or tranquilizers, the effect is additive; thus what would not comprise a lethal dose if either were taken alone may be fatal when both are combined.

Medical complications. When users of sedatives and tranquilizers inject them intravenously, they become vulnerable to problems of contamination and infection. When taken by mouth, they cause fewer complications. Some persons may develop skin reactions to barbiturates on rare occasions. Liver cirrhosis and permanent brain damage are not prominent dangers as they may be with alcoholism. Transient side effects of the strong tranquilizers, such as Thorazine and Stelazine may include blurred vision and drooling. On rare occasions prolonged use of very high doses may result in tremors, a condition called tardive dyskinesia. Also, rarely, some individuals have an inherited defect of liver enzymes which shows up only with the use of Thorazine and the appearance of jaundice.

Self-injury may occur because of the decrease of muscle control and the impairment of judgment. When under the influence of depressants, it is not unusual for an individual to stagger and fall, sustaining cuts, fractures, contusions, and even concussion. Drivers intoxicated with sedatives or tranquilizers are just as likely to have accidents as drivers who are drunk. Since the effects of these drugs may last considerably longer than the effects of alcohol, they may pose an even greater danger.

ALCOHOL

Alcohol ingestion results in many of the same effects as the foregoing drugs. Here, attention will be focused primarily on those aspects that are different and on the syndrome of alcoholism.

Metabolism. Alcohol is readily absorbed through both the stomach and intestinal walls. Effective blood levels are achieved quickly on an empty stomach, more slowly on a full one, particularly if the meal has contained fatty material. When alcohol enters the bloodstream, it is acted upon by the liver and converted to a substance that enters the body's energy cycle to be burned as cell fuel. Only small amounts are exhaled in the breath or excreted in the urine. Alcohol is not converted to body fats, and it will not put on weight per se. But because it metabolizes so quickly, it is preferentially used by the body for energy instead of the sugars, starches, and fats that are part of the intake of food. Thus when the calories in alcohol and the calories in food add up to an excess of the daily requirement, the food is deposited as stored fat, and the net effect is weight gain.

Alcohol is metabolized or burned at an even and constant rate regardless of the amount consumed. In the average adult this rate is approximately 10 milliliters (2 teaspoons) of 100 proof whiskey per hour. Full clearance from the body of 4 ounces of whiskey or 1¼ quarts of beer takes from five to six hours. The constancy of this rate is an important factor, since the level and duration of intoxication increase in proportion to the amount consumed in excess of this metabolic rate.

Patterns of use. Alcohol differs from other members of this class in being the only drug generally considered part of socially accepted activity rather than a form of medication. It is in this sense not identified by most users as a drug and is subject to no medical regulation and only limited legal regulation. Because of its ubiquitous presence, it is the one drug of all those discussed in this chapter that is most likely to be abused. More people become disabled from drinking alcohol than from any other substance.

Most people can have a few drinks on an occasional evening without serious consequences provided they don't drive. But caution needs to be exercised by that one individual out of ten who feels emotional discomfort if it is impossible to have the evening cocktail; whose intermittent social drinking becomes a regular routine; who cannot limit the number of drinks after having one, even if that one is taken only from time to time; or whose few drinks sometimes turn into a "binge" affair. When any of these patterns develop, it is time to ask whether drinking is confined to pleasurable and relaxing occasions, whether it is still under the user's control, or whether it is a compulsion.

Effects. The effects of alcohol are the same as those of other drugs in the depressant class. In addition, heavy drinkers are more likely to "pass out" and to have what are called "blackouts" or episodes of amnesia, even though consciousness has not been lost. The blackout is a critical danger signal that the individual is losing control over alcoholic intake and may already be suffering from the disease of alcoholism.

Alcoholism. According to the World Health Organization, alcoholism is a medical disease characterized by compulsive drinking to a degree that persistently or intermittently interferes with effective functioning in the home and family, on the job, and in the community. About 10 percent of all social drinkers ultimately become alcoholics in variable degrees; of this number, up to 40 percent are women. The precise cause is unknown. Some authorities feel that there is a physiological or genetic predisposition, with an as yet unidentified chemical deficiency rendering the drinker vulnerable. Others claim that the disease is essentially psychological. Whatever the answer may be, the National Council on Alcoholism has identified the following factors as increasing a person's risk.

1. A family history of alcoholism, including parents, siblings, grandparents, uncles, and aunts.
2. A history of strict, moralistic teetotalism in the family, coupled with a change in the individual's social environment where drinking is encouraged or required.

3. A history of alcoholism or teetotalism in the marital partner or the marital partner's family.
4. Coming from a broken home or a home with much parental discord, particularly one in which the father was rejecting or absent, but not necessarily physically abusive.
5. Being the youngest child or among the youngest members of a large family.
6. Being of Irish or Scandinavian ancestry, two cultures in which alcohol has an enhanced role.
7. Having female relatives of more than one generation who have had a high incidence of recurrent depression.
8. Heavy smoking.

Once an individual has begun to drink, the following danger signs indicate potential or actual abuse. While it does not follow that abusers are or will become alcoholics, singly or in combination these signs are a cause for alarm.

1. Frequent drinking as a teenager.
2. Drinking to the point of heavy intoxication at social gatherings on a regular basis.
3. Drinking more than the other members of one's social group.
4. Drinking to relieve tensions and anxiety or to achieve intoxication, rather than as a social relaxant.
5. Drinking alone.
6. Drinking at inappropriate times of the day, in the morning, during daytime working hours, or at school.
7. Recurrent episodes of passing out.
8. Recurrent blackouts.

The fullblown syndrome of alcoholism appears to take about six to eight years to develop, during which drinking gradually escalates. Once established, the disease may vary in its effect on functioning from mild to severe and may proceed with many ups and downs. The only constant factors are that alcoholism is progressive; if untreated, it may be fatal; and even when treated, it renders the individual vulnerable to recurrence for the rest of his or her life, that is to say, an alcoholic who has successfully stopped drinking can never drink again with impunity.

The following are some of the more important characteristics of the disease, although all need not be present in every case of alcoholism.

1. Physiological dependence or addiction as manifested by withdrawal symptoms somewhere between the first and third day of abstinence.
2. Evidence of tolerance. Some alcoholics appear to defy pharmacologic expectations of the effects of depressant drugs and are capable of drinking unusually large amounts with little apparent physiological impair-

ment. The daily consumption of a fifth of whiskey (or its alcoholic equivalent in wine or beer) for two or more days without visible signs of intoxication is in and of itself an indication of alcoholism.

3. Blackouts.
4. Continued drinking despite strong social consequences, such as loss of a job, disruption of a marriage, or uncontrolled abuse of children and spouse.
5. Continued drinking despite compelling medical contraindications.
6. The presence of one or more medical conditions associated with heavy drinking, such as liver disease, chronic stomach inflammation, anemia, brain dysfunction, malnutrition, vitamin deficiency diseases, diseases of the nerves, increased frequency of infections, and problems with the muscles of the heart and limbs.
7. Feelings that self-control over alcohol consumption no longer exists.
8. Behavior patterns such as the following: gulping drinks; surreptitious drinking; morning drinking; repeated attempts at abstinence; frequent absence from work for spurious medical reasons; loss of interest in activities not associated directly with drinking; frequent automobile accidents; emotional instability marked by outbursts of rage, self-pity, resentment, jealousy, and paranoid attitudes sometimes resulting in unprovoked physical attack of others.
9. Blatant indiscriminate use of alcohol, skid row or equivalent social displacement, or psychological manifestations of permanent brain damage.

VOLATILE SOLVENTS, GASOLINE, AND AEROSOL PROPELLANT GASES

The solvent chemicals found in plastic model glues, cleaning fluids, nail polish remover, lighter fluid, and paint and lacquer thinners; gasoline; and some of the propellant gases (Freon and nitrous oxide) in aerosol spray cans all have similar effects. While their mode of action is predominantly that of other depressants, they will cause some users to experience hallucinations, delusions, and disorientation. One of the manifestations of these altered states of perception is the belief that one can fly, a delusion that has caused the death of a number of youngsters. Inhaling leaded gasoline can cause lead poisoning; sniffing Freon in aerosol containers can be fatal because of their effect on the heart. Solvent sniffing, an activity with special appeal for the very young, has fortunately declined in popularity, but parents should continue to be alert to this type of drug abuse. Recently, nitrous oxide sniffing (once known as laughing gas) has enjoyed popularity among some adults and young people.

Stimulants

Stimulants can be divided into three subgroups: (1) amphetamines, or "uppers," (2) cocaine, and (3) caffeine. These drugs produce effects opposite to those of depressants: sensations of heightened alertness, well-being, and energy. As in the case of other classes of drugs, the subgroups are distinguished by relative strength and patterns of use, rather than by pharmacologic differences. In the material that follows, amphetamines are the prototype. Consideration of cocaine and caffeine is limited to differential aspects.

AMPHETAMINES

Characteristics and medical use. Amphetamines have had their widest medical application in the treatment of obesity because of their ability to depress the appetite and act as a stimulant at the same time. Their use for weight control has been increasingly discredited in recent years, because achieved weight loss has rarely been maintained and a significant number of patients have become habituated to the drug. Amphetamines have also been used for the treatment of depression and bedwetting, although better medications for both conditions are now available. Currently they have an unqualified medical role only in the treatment of certain carefully selected children with abnormally hyperactive (hyperkinetic) behavior, of the sleep disorder called narcolepsy, and of some special instances of depressive illness.

Drugs commonly abused. Benzedrine, Dexedrine, Methedrine, Preludin, collectively referred to as "uppers," are the most frequently used. The most commonly abused is Methedrine, variably known as "speed," "meth," "crystal," or "crank." Benzedrine is the particular favorite among those who have to stay awake for long stretches, and it has been the traditional drug of choice on college campuses at exam time. Benzedrine tablets may be referred to as "cartwheels" or "bennies."

Appearance and method of administration. Amphetamines may be obtained in the form of a white powder, pill, or capsule. Since a major source is illegal diversion from legitimate manufacture, amphetamines are usually quite pure. Stimulants may be inhaled, or "snorted," in the powder form, dissolved in water and injected intravenously, or taken orally. "Speed freaks" (regular and heavy users) tend to prefer the intravenous route because it is associated with a marked rush. Serial injections are common and provide an intense, cumulative effect which can be prolonged for hours or even for days.

Effects. The first effect of stimulants is a sense of well-being, alertness, increased energy, and enhanced powers of concentration. If the drugs are mainlined, these feelings are introduced by a rush likened to a sexual orgasm. Appetite and fatigue are reduced, and the user feels filled with unusual energy and very talkative. Amphetamines are said to enhance sexual powers.

Higher concentrations of the drugs produce feelings of omnipotence, unlimited inner energy, and sensations of extraordinary mental and physical powers. Since sociability is greatly enhanced, "speeding" is often a communal affair. While the user feels incredibly alert, logical, and perceptive, the observer usually sees a restless, garrulous, and emotionally erratic individual who makes little sense.

Associated physical effects include a rise in blood pressure and pulse rate, dilation of the pupils, increased sweating, and decreased appetite. Later on the user will "crash," that is, experience a feeling of exhaustion leading to deep sleep. The post-intoxicated state is marked by a voracious appetite on waking, followed by extended periods of lassitude and depression during which strong suicidal impulses may be present.

Stimulants are not physically addicting. Abusers can take large amounts for prolonged periods of time and experience no adverse physical effects upon cessation. Some do consider the crash experience and extended lassitude a form of withdrawal syndrome; others see these effects as a manifestation of physical exhaustion which would be a normal consequence of any type of hyperactivity no matter how achieved.

Tolerance develops readily, with the user requiring ever larger amounts to achieve a high. Tolerance begins to appear early, with low daily doses of one or two diet pills spiraling upward rapidly to ten or more pills per day. This is a major drawback in medical use. But tolerance can be completely lost after five to ten days of abstinence. Cross-tolerance is a property of all members of the stimulant class; thus one drug can readily be substituted for another.

Overdose. Very large and sustained intake will cause a toxic paranoid psychosis similar to that of schizophrenia. The precise amount required to produce this effect is dependent on individual susceptibility, but is rarely seen unless repeatedly taken by injection over a period of several days. Victims lose touch with reality and rationality. They may perceive others as enemies, hear voices, and think that people are saying evil things about them. Typical behavior includes restlessness and agitation, abusive language, and attempts at physical assault. Hospitalization and containment may be necessary for the person's own safety or for that of others. A physician unaware that drugs were taken may make a mistaken diagnosis of a mental breakdown, rather than a toxic drug effect.

The abnormal state induced by drug toxicity usually clears within a few days, but in a significant number of cases, the individual remains in a prolonged or persistent psychotic state. Whether this is directly due to drug effect or whether an underlying psychological vulnerability has been triggered into psychosis remains unclear. Most authorities favor the latter view.

Medical complications. Several reports appeared in the 1970s giving evidence of serious inflammation of the blood vessels in "speed freaks." Subsequent studies have not confirmed this finding, nor is there any documented evidence of harm to body organs resulting from the use of amphetamines per se. However, when any drug is administered by injection, it can introduce contaminants or disease-producing organisms into the body. The major dangers that arise directly from the drug use are the potential for self-injury or the injury of others during the intoxicated state and the real possibility of a toxic psychosis.

COCAINE

Cocaine is a natural substance derived from the leaves of *Erythroxylon coca*, a shrub growing high in the Andes Mountains. For centuries it has been used as an essential element in the culture of the Indians of the area, and it is currently grown for commercial purposes as well. An extract from the plant, which is sold as a flavoring for cola drinks, did at one time contain cocaine, but this ingredient has long since been removed.

Appearance and method of administration. Cocaine is a white crystalline powder usually snorted or sniffed into the nose through a straw or other hollow tube. Absorption occurs fairly rapidly through the nasal lining. Intravenous injection is also a common method of use.

Effects. Because it is similar in appearance to heroin and because it is often distributed through the same illegal channels, cocaine is assumed by many people to be a narcotic. This is a total myth. Cocaine has the same properties and produces the same effects as Methedrine and Benzedrine, with one difference: it produces numbness and constriction of local blood vessels when applied to the mucous membranes or injected under the skin. These properties once led to its widespread use in medical practice as a local anesthetic, particularly in the nose. It has since been replaced by more effective substances.

Cocaine has a considerably shorter period of action than amphetamines. Since it is rapidly inactivated in the body, its effect lasts for no more than 20 to 30 minutes. Frequent or repetitive snorting or injection is therefore common. Dilution through cutting further reduces the intensity and duration of the drug effect. Because of these factors, toxic psychoses are extremely rare.

Medical complications. The destruction of nasal tissues and perforation of the bony septum due to the constriction of local blood vessels and resultant injury is a classic consequence of snorting cocaine frequently. Few other complications occur unless contaminants are introduced when mainlined.

CAFFEINE

Caffeine and caffeinelike substances are present in coffee, tea, cocoa, cola drinks, and many medicines, both over-the-counter drugs (pain-killers such as Anacin, Excedrin, Midol; many cold preparations; stimulants such as NoDoz) and prescription drugs (Migral, Cafergot, Fiorinal, Darvon compound). While the predominant effects of caffeine and chemically related substances are mildly stimulant in nature, they may also increase the flow of urine and constrict the blood vessels of the brain. They are considerably weaker in their effects than other members of this class.

Medical complications. While the amount of caffeine in 6 ounces of any of the beverages listed above is small, drinking several cups of coffee at once, having two cups of strongly brewed tea on an empty stomach, or drinking cola beverages throughout the day and evening, or drinking the beverages during the same period in which caffeine-containing medications are taken may have adverse effects in some individuals. This may include fine tremors, jitteriness, increased blood pressure, irritability, and insomnia. Heavy caffeine consumers should not mistake these feelings for the symptoms of anxiety and incorrectly treat them with a tranquilizer. Persons with hypertension should carefully assess the effects of caffeine-containing substances upon their blood pressure; avoidance would seem prudent. There is also a growing recognition of association between heavy caffeine intake and nighttime leg cramps.

Hallucinogens

The hallucinogenic (or psychotropic) class includes all those substances which can produce altered sensory perceptions: visions, distortions of reality, or delusions. These substances are capable of producing reactions that mimic serious mental illnesses, especially psychotic states such as schizophrenia. For the most part the drug experience is limited in time, and the user returns to normalcy after a few hours. A few individuals, however, have remained in seriously disturbed states for weeks or months. Some have never recovered. Whether the irreversibility of the psychotic state was caused by the drug itself or because the drug triggered an underlying predisposition is unknown. With the exception of marijuana, and probably of hashish as well, the use of hallucinogenic substances is accompanied by risks of major proportions.

Four sub-groups comprise this overall class: (1) LSD, mushrooms, and cacti, (2) PCP or angel dust, (3) marijuana, hashish, and THC, and (4) atropinic drugs (atropine and scopolamine). While the inclusion of marijuana in this class may be questionable, the fact of the matter is that sufficient amounts of the psychoactive substance (tetrahydrocannabinol or THC) can produce an experience identical with that of LSD.

Other than atropinic drugs, none have a fully established place in conventional medical practice. However, scientific research has suggested that LSD may be helpful in understanding the cause of true schizophrenia and in treating some mental disorders. Marijuana has been found to be singularly effective in controlling the severe nausea associated with the chemotherapy of cancer and in reducing pressure in the eyes of glaucoma patients, and it is legally available for the treatment of these conditions in many states. PCP was originally introduced as an anesthetic, but it was soon abandoned because of its disconcerting psychological effects.

LSD AND RELATED COMPOUNDS

Drugs used. LSD (lysergic acid diethylamide), peyote (the dried cactus *Lophophora williamsii*), mescaline (a purified form of peyote), psilocybin (derived from mushrooms of the genera *Conocybe, Stropharia,* and *Psilocybe*), DOM (desoxymethylamphetamine) and DMT (dimethyltriptamine, derived from plants of the genera *Mimosa, Virola,* and *Piptadenia*) are the major drugs of this group.

Appearance and method of administration. Hallucinogens generally are manufactured illegally and may appear in almost any form, color, and shape depending on the whims and imagination of the underground chemist. Pills are either dissolved in the mouth and absorbed through the oral mucous membranes, or they are swallowed, with absorption through the digestive tract. Powder or liquid forms (sometimes several drops on a sugar cube or a blotter) are ingested either directly or added to food and drink. Some users saturate cigarette papers with LSD and achieve intoxication by inhaling the chemical when smoking marijuana or ordinary tobacco. Peyote and psilocybin may be sold in the form of the dried cactus (peyote button) or mushroom or as a pill or powder purported to be the purified drug. However, in more than 85 percent of tested samples, these allegations of purity prove to be false, and the psychoactive material is likely to be LSD or PCP when psychoactive material of any kind is present at all.

Effects. The onset of the hallucinogenic effect occurs 30 to 40 minutes after ingestion and somewhat sooner if smoked or dissolved under the tongue. With LSD the peak effect is reached in about one to three hours, and the total duration of the "trip" is about eight to twelve hours. This time frame varies to some degree with other drugs in this class. Feelings of depersonalization and disorientation are characteristic. The user feels detached from both self and environment and has the sensation of observing things from a distance. Everything appears distorted in size, shape, and form. Colors assume unusual vibrancy. Sensory cross-overs occur, with the user "smelling" colors and "seeing" sounds. Mental processes are fluid and introspective. Thoughts assume a mystical quality, and new "truths" are discovered about the meaning of life. Some users may experience delusions and believe themselves capable of flying or holding back an oncoming car.

Usually these sensations are perceived as highly pleasurable and mind-expanding. Even though intoxicated, users are aware that they are in a drug-induced state and in most cases can reestablish contact with reality with relative ease. Sometimes, however, the experience is accompanied by terrifying hallucinations, a fear of loss of control, or mental disintegration. The user may become frightened when the ability to retain perception of what is real is lost. Such an individual is said to be on a "bad trip." While any user may unpredictably experience a "bad trip" regardless of other factors, new users and those who take the drug in an unfavorable environment or mood seem to be more prone to adverse effects.

In addition to its hallucinogenic aspects LSD is also a moderate stimulant to which the body responds as it does to amphetamines or cocaine. The heart rate and blood pressure are elevated, and the pupils are mildly dilated. An unsteady gait is also common. Psilocybin and mescaline have similar, but greatly reduced effects.

The evidence for either physical addiction or tolerance is meager since users tend to take these drugs intermittently. Even among heavy abusers, neither withdrawal symptoms nor the need for increasing doses to achieve an effect has been verified, although some investigators do believe tolerance does exist.

Medical complications. The serious problem of persistent psychotic states and the phenomenon of "bad trips" have been mentioned. Persons may also subject themselves to injurious or even fatal circumstances when they are delusional. Another complication is the "flashback," in which someone who has previously used LSD, even if only once, will suddenly and unaccountably relive some aspect of the original drug experience. The onset can occur days or weeks after the drug was taken. While such experiences usually taper off and disappear after a few weeks or months, some persons may have them over a longer period of time. Novice users may be more vulnerable, but any user may experience "flashbacks" at any time. The precise nature of "flashbacks" is highly variable. They may last for seconds or minutes; they may occur as a single episode or recur intermittently throughout a day. They may recapitulate pleasant or unpleasant aspects, they may occur spontaneously under the most unlikely circumstances, or they may be precipitated by the use of another drug, usually marijuana.

Controversy also surrounds the issue of possible permanent chemical alterations of mental processes. Many heavy users of hallucinogens and other drugs do have certain personality traits in common. They care little about achievement, are rarely goal-oriented, are passive and pacifistic in nature, and often have a deep interest in meditational religions and alternative communal life styles. While these traits have been termed the "amotivational syndrome," it is valid to ask just who determines what appropriate motivation should be and whether the search for alternatives to a highly competitive and stressful culture necessarily reflects a crippled psyche. In any event, it is hard to say whether hallucinogen abuse directly causes amotivation or whether amotivation is simply consistent with an individual's life style and counterculture values.

PCP (PHENCYCLIDINE)

PCP was first developed as an anesthetic for human use, but it was abandoned quickly because of its undesirable side effects. It is still used in veterinary medicine, and some street supplies are diverted from this source. Since PCP can be made even in the most primitive underground laboratory, illicit supplies easily reach the street from makeshift setups in basements and garages. Because it is cheap and readily available as compared to some of the more esoteric drugs, PCP is often substituted for other hallucinogens marketed as "pure" THC, mescaline, or psilocybin.

Known as "angel dust," "hog," "dust," "crystal," "peace," "weed," "rocket fuel," "cyclone," "elephant trank," and a host of other names, PCP appears on the street as a pill of any size, color, or shape, as a powder, or dried on cigarette papers. Since it is sometimes mixed with marijuana, serious hallucinogenic experiences attributed to marijuana may actually have been caused by PCP.

Effects. PCP appears to have a specific effect on the brain quite different from that of other hallucinogens in that it blocks the processing and integration of sensory stimuli and the organization of response. It thus produces an inability to perceive, register, and interpret sensations normally and accurately. The user's inability to test and relate to reality leads to the dissolution of personal boundaries and intellectual and emotional disorganization bordering on internal chaos. Since amnesia is a characteristic effect of the drug, the user may have no recollection of having taken PCP and thus lose the sense of control provided by awareness of being in a drug-induced state.

The specific sensations experienced are highly variable and relate both to dose and to individual reactions. In contrast to other street drugs because it was subjected to testing prior to marketing for human use as an anesthetic, we have some idea as to the relation between dose and response. A low dose of PCP (1 to 5 milligrams) tends to produce a floating sense of euphoria sometimes associated with numbness, a release of inhibitions, and emotional instability. Increased amounts (5 to 10 milligrams) produce an excited, confused state in which the body is perceived in distorted form, sensations of touch and of pain are markedly reduced, verbal communication is impaired, and the individual feels isolated from all external sensations and is preoccupied with inner turmoil.

At the level of 10 milligrams and above even more serious mental disturbances emerge. Schizophrenia may be mimicked to the point where the most skilled diagnostician cannot tell the difference. This breakdown of personality is manifested in stupor, grimacing, bizarre posturing, and a refusal (or temporary inability) to talk. Other manifestations include agitation, incoherent speech, unpredictable destructiveness, or assaultive behavior. Some users enter into a paranoid state: they hear voices, exhibit delusions of grandeur, suspect others of hostile intentions, and are unable to perceive what is and what is not real. These individuals are potentially very dangerous. Acute uncontrolled panic, suicidal depression, and feelings of total isolation and sheer nothingness have also been described.

The duration of this toxic effect is considerably more prolonged than that of other drugs. The minimum time for return to a normal state ranges from four to five days, but it is by no means unusual for the disturbed state to last for weeks or even months. In those who are vulnerable to schizophrenia, this illness may be triggered into an active form.

The physical effects on the body are similar to those of LSD. Additional signs following high doses are fever, drooling, rapid uncontrolled eye movements, slurred speech, and staggering gait.

Neither addiction nor tolerance has been identified with PCP, but definitive studies have yet to be carried out. The prolonged effect of the drug makes it difficult to discern whether abstinence symptoms occur or not. However, in the light of the dire and direct effects possible from a single dose of the drug, the question of tolerance or addiction is scarcely relevant.

Overdose. In addition to the previously described toxic psychoses, the high dosage may produce a comatose state resembling strychnine poisoning; the individual is rigid with an arched back rather than limp. If emergency measures are not taken, death can result.

Medical complications. As already noted, serious physical injury to self or to others may occur in the toxic state. Coma and death may follow overdose. Some users remain in a prolonged schizophrenic state, but permanent physical damage to specific body organs has not been identified.

MARIJUANA, HASHISH, AND THC

Marijuana and hashish are simply different forms of THC (tetrahydrocannabinol) and related chemical compounds found in the resin produced by the flowering tops of the marijuana plant *Cannabis sativa*. Marijuana and hashish differ from each other only in strength and appearance. Marijuana is a mixture of the dried upper leaves of the plant and the resin which has dripped down from the flowers above. Known as "pot," "Mary Jane," "grass," or "weed," marijuana appears as a brownish, sweetish smelling leafy material, often mixed with stems and seeds. It usually is smoked as a cigarette, or "joint," or in a pipe. It can also be mixed with and baked in foods. Hashish, or "hash," is the pure resin scraped off the leaves and formed into little brown cakes from which flakes are chipped and smoked in a pipe. This, obviously, is the stronger form. Pure THC is a brown, viscous liquid. It is difficult to make and rarely makes its way to the street. Pills or powders alleged to be THC are not since this chemical exists in liquid form only. Marijuana is the weakest of all three and THC the strongest, but any form is highly variable in potency depending on the conditions under which the plant is grown. Climate, rainfall, sunlight, and soil significantly influence both the amount of resin and of THC in the resin. Semitropical conditions produce stronger marijuana than temperate climates. A particularly good batch of "grass" or "hash" may be known by its place of origin, for example, "Aztec gold."

In some circles it is common to smoke marijuana and drink alcohol at the same time. The effects are additive, heightening the general level of intoxication.

Effects. First-time users of marijuana rarely report any psychotropic effect. Instead of experiencing the anticipated altered sense of awareness, they feel dizzy, lightheaded, and nauseated. Those with more practice regularly become "high" on the same dose. Some have termed this phenomenon "reverse tolerance," but it may in fact be due to the potentiating effects of expectancy rather than to any shift in the drug effect per se.

Mild effects include a sense of relaxation, a feeling of social ease, and a heightening of sensory experiences. Objects are brighter and more sharply defined; sound and rhythm have more subtlety and nuance; touch, taste, and smell are enhanced. Things which ordinarily do not provoke laughter become uproariously funny: pot smoking is often accompanied by much silliness and giggling. Time perception slows down to a marked degree, limbs feel lighter, and the general mood is one of mild euphoria and well-being.

Muscle control, muscular coordination, and mental performance deteriorate with increasing intoxication. Verbal output, counting, color discrimination, and short-term memory all become impaired after several marijuana cigarettes. To the degree that different categories of drugs can be compared in their effect, one marijuana cigarette has an intoxicating potential roughly equivalent to that of three bottles of beer or 3 ounces of 100 proof whiskey. Marijuana intoxication slows down a driver's response to a braking situation as well as recovery from nighttime headlight glare and users should exercise the same restraint in not driving while high as with alcohol.

With larger doses (whether obtained from heavy marijuana smoking, hashish, or the use of THC in pure form) heightened perceptivity gives way to distortions, delusions, and hallucinations and may approximate an LSD experience.

Physiological effects are an increased heart rate, dilation of the blood vessels, causing flushing of the skin and a characteristic redness of the eyes. Effects on other body organs are mild or nonexistent.

Addiction does not occur, but tolerance has been demonstrated conclusively. Cross-tolerance exists not only between members of this specific group, but also with LSD, mescaline, and, surprisingly, with morphine as well.

Overdose. Overdosage with marijuana and even hashish is exceedingly rare, and signs of acute physical toxicity are minimal, even with large amounts. (Coma, with full recovery, has been reported in the case of one individual who smoked ten large pipefuls of hashish.)

Medical complications. The most common adverse effects are dizziness, nausea, and vomiting. "Flashbacks" and "bad trips" are encountered on rare occasions.

Long-term heavy users experience irritation of the respiratory tract. Severe bronchitis and damage to the blood vessels has been found among heavy users in Eastern countries. Recent studies have demonstrated impairment of lung function. In addition, long term use may be carcinogenic.

A study in England in the early 1970s reporting atrophy of the brain among several young heavy marijuana smokers has not been substantiated by other studies conducted elsewhere. More recent animal research implicating marijuana with interference with the body's disease defense system has rather tenuous application for the human; there is no clinical indication that marijuana users experience more infections or other diseases related to compromised immunity than anyone else. The most significant deleterious effect relates to the finding of reduced levels of testosterone (the male sex hormone) and sperm count in men who are heavy marijuana smokers, but these functions return quickly to the normal range after cessation. Occasional anecdotal reports exist of gynecomastia (breast enlargement) in males and galactorrhea (milk from the breasts unassociated with pregnancy) in both males and females. While intoxication may temporarily diminish the sex urge, there is no evidence of permanently reduced libido, impotence, or infertility.

All in all, the evidence to date for significant, persistent medical risk is highly inconclusive as yet. However, while serious dangers have not been documented, additional studies are required, particularly over a long period, before all the facts about "pot" are in. It should be kept in mind that it took years for medical science to make the unequivocal connection between tobacco smoking, lung cancer, and heart disease.

ATROPINIC DRUGS

This group contains two drugs, atropine and scopolamine, that occur naturally in a number of plants, including deadly nightshade and jimson weed. The latter grows throughout the Southwest in the United States and has been ingested both deliberately and unknowingly. The purified drugs have been used medically to dry up secretions in the respiratory tract during surgical anesthesia, to induce what is called twilight sleep in women during labor, to soothe irritable stomachs and colons, and to alleviate asthma. More effective medicines for asthma are usually used today, and adverse side effects of twilight sleep have discouraged its use as anesthesia in labor.

Drugs for self-administration are acquired through the diversion of pills from legitimate sources of manufacture or by the ingestion or smoking of active plant materials. Scopolamine is sometimes mixed with marijuana to achieve an enhanced effect. Intoxication produces drowsiness, euphoria, giddiness, and hallucinations. Both members of this group also produce distinctly uncomfortable side effects: dry mouth, fever, blurred vision, severe headache, restlessness, and disorientation. Because of these consequences, neither atropine nor scopolamine has enjoyed wide use.

Overdose can produce heart failure, depressed breathing, coma, and, rarely, death; this is more common in children than adults. Toxic delirium, which can also occur, may mimic alcoholic DTs or acute schizophrenia.

Narcotics

Characteristics and medical use. Whether naturally derived from the opium poppy or chemically manufactured, members of this class are characterized by their ability to alleviate pain, calm anxiety, and induce sleep. Associated effects are constipation and the suppression of coughing. Strong narcotics are used in medicine for the treatment of severe pain; weaker ones are prescribed for a persistent cough, diarrhea, and lesser pain unresponsive to aspirin.

Drugs commonly abused. The stronger narcotics are opium, heroin, Demerol, morphine, methadone, Percodan; the weaker ones are codeine, Darvon, Talwin. When heroin was introduced in the 1930s in Germany, it was thought to be a nonaddictive painkilling agent which might serve as a substitute for addictive morphine. Only after its introduction were its narcotic properties recognized. Methadone was always recognized as a narcotic and was introduced in treatment to substitute for heroin addiction in a controlled manner.

Heroin, known as "H," "smack," "horse," "dope," or "Harry," is the most frequently used street drug. More recently, methadone has gained in popularity. All of the drugs listed have been tried on the street. Young adults and adolescents are especially apt to experiment with the weaker forms, since these are more easily available. While usually taken in such low doses as to have only modest effects, Darvon used intravenously has been the cause of several deaths. Physicians, nurses, and other health professionals, as well as patients who have required prolonged use of narcotics for pain relief, are at somewhat greater risk of addiction because of the easy availability of the drugs. In these cases of addiction the substances most often involved are morphine and Demerol.

Appearance and method of administration. Heroin is usually sold as a white powder in small glassine bags similar to those used by coin and stamp dealers. A single bag is known as a "fix"; it may also be referred to by its price, for example, $5.00 worth is called a "nickel bag." The amount of heroin contained in a fix is highly variable. It is usually cut or diluted with a nonactive material such as quinine which gives the drug its reputed bitter taste. Methadone appears as a pill or liquid, depending on the form in which it is used in the local treatment center. Codeine is available as a pill or as an ingredient in cough syrup. Until the 1960's such cough mixtures were available over-the-counter, but now can no longer be bought without a prescription. Demerol appears as a pill or injectable liquid, Darvon as a pink capsule, and Talwin as a pill.

Narcotics may be administered through any route. Intravenous injection is preferred. Subcutaneous injection is also common. While opium smoking is still popular in some Asian countries, it has not enjoyed widespread use in the United States, nor has swallowing or sniffing been employed with any frequency.

While all narcotics can be administered by needle without residual marks if the drug is chemically pure and the equipment is sterile, the contaminants of street forms do cause tissue damage. Mainliners may develop needle tracks, that is, darkly pigmented scars over the injected veins, while skin poppers may develop sores at the injection site. Such sores heal into pale round depressions of a quarter to three-quarters of an inch in diameter.

Effects. Narcotics produce a sense of euphoria and well-being, surcease from anxiety, and a dreamlike state. Sedation also occurs, and the intoxicated individual appears remote, withdrawn, and uninterested in his environment. When used intravenously, the drugs in this category produce an immediate rush. There is no impairment of time and place orientation, nor are hallucinations part of the experience. There is little danger to others from an addict who is high. Associated crime stems from the addict's need for money for the next "fix," rather than from any violent tendencies produced by the drug experience as such.

Dominant effects on the body include depression in the breathing rate, constriction of the iris of the eye (the telltale sign of pinpoint pupils), constipation, and a decrease in sexual interest.

All narcotics are addicting, and they produce tolerance when taken regularly. Early signs of addiction can appear following even small amounts taken over only four or five days, although few addicts initiate their habit this quickly. Addiction results in three stages of response: a "high" that lasts for an hour or two after administration, a "straight" sensation of sobriety unaccompanied by any physical discomfort and lasting for an additional hour or so, and a "sick" response with physical symptoms of withdrawal setting in when all the effects of the drug have gone. The cycle begins again when the next dose is taken. Addicts may require anything from three to ten or more "nickel" bags a day, depending on the strength of the drug itself and the user's tolerance level.

Since tolerance develops rapidly, even with relatively small amounts, in a brief time the user needs to increase the amount to achieve any effect. This is an ever-escalating situation, and an addict therefore faces serious economic problems in having to procure more and more drugs to support the habit. However, both tolerance and addiction will disappear within about a week or ten days after stopping.

Withdrawal. Any drug capable of producing addiction will also produce a genuine illness or withdrawal syndrome upon cessation of use. Narcotic withdrawal or detoxification is characterized by flu-like symptoms: general malaise, muscle aches, sweating, running eyes and nose, intestinal cramps, and diarrhea. The severity of these symptoms is directly proportionate to the degree of addiction and the total daily consumption of the drug. But no one ever dies in narcotic withdrawal, although many have wished that they would.

Withdrawal without any medical support is referred to as "cold turkey." When medically supervised, usually in a hospital, the addict commonly is given methadone in amounts sufficient to counteract the distress of the withdrawal symptoms. This amount is then gradually decreased as tolerated to zero over a five- to seven-day period. By this process the patient is kept comfortable and physical dependence eliminated. Habituation or psychological dependence remains; this is a much more complicated issue and the emotional craving for the drug's effect usually persists unchanged unless help geared to this problem is obtained.

Overdose. Particularly large doses of a narcotic produce marked sedation, depressed breathing, and mental confusion. Loss of consciousness and even death are not uncommon. When an especially pure batch of heroin makes its way to the street, overdose reactions and deaths tend to occur with greater frequency because of the user's miscalculation. Users who have just completed withdrawal may also miscalculate their drug needs. Methadone tends to produce more overdose reactions because it is considerably stronger than heroin, even in street form. There are cases of methadone poisoning among small children who sampled their addicted parent's supply of the drug which was kept at home during participation in a treatment program. Such an occurrence is a grave medical emergency requiring prompt treatment.

Medical complications. Complications other than the problems associated with overdosage and withdrawal confront those who administer their drug via needle and syringe. First, the presence of solid, particulate matter in the drug that is being injected may cause the blockage of small blood vessels and the formation of microscopic scars throughout the organs of the body, especially in the lungs. While most users try to filter out foreign material by drawing up the dissolved heroin powder or the crushed pill into the syringe through a wad of cotton, this method is rarely wholly effective. Addicts may develop chronic lung problems over time.

An even greater hazard is posed by the possible introduction of disease-producing organisms into the body through the use of improperly sterilized needles or contaminated drugs. Hepatitis is the most common disease contracted in this way, but tetanus (lockjaw), brain abscesses, and infections of the heart, blood, or bones are also likely.

Pure narcotics as used in medicine are not known to cause any permanent damage to body organs, even when used in large amounts in the treatment of patients suffering from serious and prolonged pain.

Tobacco

The three major components of tobacco smoking that cause medical concern are tars, nicotine, and carbon monoxide. Tars are not absorbed by the body, but since they are deposited in the cells lining the respiratory tract and lung air spaces, they may act as cell irritants. Research studies have shown that such irritation can produce cancer in animals, and it is now felt that this may occur in humans, although human cancer may not develop unless there is a combinant effect by both tars and various environmental factors.

Nicotine is absorbed into the bloodstream and has a variety of sometimes paradoxical effects. It may either increase or slow the heart rate; it may increase the breathing rate, raise blood pressure, and stimulate the body through the release of adrenalin, yet inhibit muscle activity to the point of paralysis. (It is this latter effect that makes nicotine useful as a garden insecticide.) Nicotine is also a brain stimulant and in high doses can produce tremors and convulsions. Vomiting, intestinal cramps, and diarrhea may also occur. Obviously this is an extremely toxic drug, and while ordinary smoking is not associated with many of the above symptoms, subtle forms of intoxication are inevitable. Nicotine can also be fatal: death would result if the average adult were to swallow the contents of two high-tar cigarettes all at once. The lethal dose is in the range of 60 milligrams, and some brands contain 30 milligrams each. Cigarette smoke, however, contains 25 to 30 percent of this total amount. Chronic exposure to nicotine results in tolerance and habituation.

Appreciable amounts of carbon monoxide are also present in smoke. This gas is readily absorbed into the blood, where it combines with red blood cells and prevents them from performing their essential function of transporting oxygen from the lungs to the body's tissues. In regular smokers anywhere from 5 to 10 percent of the red blood cells are immobilized in this way. The immobilization produces a condition similar to anemia, even though the smoker appears to have sufficient red blood cells.

This consequence may have particular implications for athletes, for individuals with heart impairment, and for pregnant women.

Medical complications. The major medical risk associated with smoking is an increased likelihood of heart attack. There is also an increased risk of chronic lung disease, including bronchitis, emphysema, and asthma, and of cancer of the lung and other organs (mouth, larynx, esophagus, pancreas, and bladder). The probability of developing any of these conditions is closely related to the number and strength of cigarettes consumed each day and the number of years of such intake. Cigarette smoking presents a considerably higher risk of medical complications than pipe or cigar smoking, because the latter two habits are not usually associated with inhaling.

While smoking is a significant and even dominant factor in the development of heart disease, it does not appear to be solely responsible; other concomitant factors, chiefly obesity, hypertension, high blood fat levels, physical inactivity, and stress, greatly increase the vulnerability of the cigarette smoker to a heart attack. Lung cancer may also be influenced by other factors, but these have not yet been as clearly identified, except for the role played by high levels of environmental air pollutants.

Women smokers are subject to additional sex-related risks. Those who are over 35 and take estrogen medication as oral contraception or replacement therapy following menopause, are more than 11 times likelier to have a heart attack than nonsmokers. If a woman cannot give up smoking, she would be wise to stay away from estrogens after the age of 35 unless they are absolutely necessary; if they are necessary, they should be taken for no more than a year or two.

Discontinuation of smoking at any time significantly reduces the risk of disease and disease-related deaths. This risk gradually decreases over time and approximates that of nonsmokers after 10 to 14 years of abstinence. Switching to a low-tar nicotine brand or cutting back to less than one pack a day can reduce the greater likelihood of illness and premature death, but it will not eliminate the higher risk altogether.

It is difficult to cite the precise statistics that compare various illnesses as they appear in smokers and nonsmokers or respective mortality figures. While various studies are consistent in establishing that the increased risk exists, the magnitude of the risk has not been quantified for all smoking-related illnesses. However, even though many variables are involved, overall figures clearly indicate that the death rate among smokers aged 45 to 65 years is 70 percent higher than for nonsmokers in the same age category. Another way of stating this fact is that a woman who smokes two packs a day at age 23 and who continues to smoke can expect to die 8.3 years sooner than her nonsmoking counterpart.

Miscellaneous Drugs

ISOBUTYL NITRITE

This drug is closely related to amyl nitrite, used medically to treat anginal heart pain. Indeed, abuse of amyl nitrite preceded that of isobutyl nitrite until federal control restricted its availability. Sometimes touted as the "poor man's cocaine," isobutyl nitrite (also known as "poppers") is legally manufactured as a room deodorizer, but illicitly sold for abusive purposes under such trade names as "Rush" and "Bolt." It is marketed as a liquid in small bottles or in glass ampules surrounded by absorbent cloth. The user sniffs directly from the bottle of liquid or breaks the ampule and inhales the resultant vapor.

Almost instantly, all blood vessels are dilated; the user experiences a rush and sensation of giddiness. The quick high may also be accompanied by a pounding heart, dizziness, persistent severe headache, and nausea. In many respects the feelings are similar to fainting, and sudden movement from sitting to standing may cause the user to pass out. Relatively little danger exists for the healthy person, but someone with heart disease may not be so fortunate and can sustain a serious or even fatal heart attack.

"HERBAL" TEAS

Beverages brewed from various mixtures of dried plant materials are enjoying increasing popularity. Those who buy such ingredients at local "health food" stores should be aware that herbal teas contain a wide variety of biologically active materials. Catnip, juniper, hydrangea, lobelia, jimson weed, wormwood, indian tobacco, nutmeg, and mandrake all have euphoric, stimulant, or hallucinogenic effects, albeit very mild ones in most instances. Ginseng is not only both sedative and stimulant, it also contains hormones reported, in at least one instance, to cause painful and swollen breasts. Other herbal teas may increase urinary flow, cause diarrhea, affect the heart, or contain general body toxins. For many people the use of such teas is pleasant, relaxing, and sometimes beneficial. This section is not intended to condemn the use of such teas, but simply to make the reader aware that not everything sold in a health food store is harmless and that discrimination and common sense are in order.

DRUGS AND PREGNANCY

Many drugs are potentially capable of adversely affecting the growth and development of the fetus during pregnancy. Complications include intrauterine addiction and withdrawal symptoms after birth, low birth weight, brain damage, and spontaneous abortion.

Sedatives and Tranquilizers

Regular daily intake of sedatives and tranquilizers, at least during the last few months of pregnancy, may cause the newborn baby to be addicted and to suffer withdrawal symptoms. Intermittent or low doses is not likely to have an addictive effect on the fetus. Symptoms are similar to the withdrawal syndrome experienced by addicted adults; extreme restlessness and convulsions are typical.

One particular tranquilizer, Thalidomide, became notorious for its direct association with serious deformities of the baby's arms and legs. Thalidomide has been discontinued from medical use. No similar consequences have been traced to the use of any other tranquilizers now available. However, it is a wise precaution to abstain from all drugs during pregnancy, particularly in the first three months, unless medically essential.

Alcohol

The fetal alcohol syndrome is a specific disorder of babies born to mothers who drink excessively. These infants are permanently brain damaged and grow up retarded. They often have certain peculiar facial characteristics: small eyes, thin upper lip, receding upper jaw, and unusually short pug nose. A variety of other birth defects may also occur, including hare lip, eye problems, heart malformations, and kidney abnormalities.

The precise amount of alcohol intake required to produce these consequences has not been determined. Clear risk is associated with the consumption of six hard drinks or more per day. An even more recent discovery is that even 1 ounce of whiskey slows the fetal heart rate to a significant degree for several hours. The implications are unknown, but this slowdown could compromise the flow of blood to developing organs. Taking everything into consideration, current recommendations suggest that pregnant women should limit their alcohol intake to no more than two drinks once or twice a month, if they must drink at all.

Stimulants

No particular syndrome or increase in birth defects has been associated with amphetamines or cocaine. Nonetheless, these substances do cross the placenta and make their way into the fetal blood stream with the potential for marked pharmacologic effects. It is difficult to conclude that the infant would not be adversely affected by frequent maternal use, but this is more hypothetical than proven.

Caffeine use has been the subject of recent debate. A 1982 study found that coffee drinking has no detectable ill effects on the fetus. Avoidance of heavy caffeine intake during pregnancy, however, would be wise.

Hallucinogens

Laboratory studies indicate that all members of this category, including marijuana, have the capacity to damage chromosomes and genes, although the damage appears to be no more than temporary, similar to that encountered with many virus illnesses. There is no compelling evidence as yet that any defect that affects the reproductive cells could be passed on, since sperm and egg cells that are damaged become incapable of reproduction. Nor have users or their offspring shown any evidence of diseases or conditions traceable to genetic mutation. Some reports suggest that children born to women who used LSD during pregnancy have a somewhat higher occurrence of birth defects than infants not similarly exposed. Other studies report that this is not true, and the issue of fetal damage by hallucinogens therefore remains controversial. Insufficient time has passed for assessment of their long range effects or their effects on subsequent generations. The absence of clear evidence of damage, however, does not justify the use of hallucinogens or, indeed, of any other drug, during pregnancy.

Narcotics

Babies of heroin addicts are prone to low birth weight. They also may be born addicted and suffer many of the same symptoms of withdrawal as does the addicted adult. Some infants may experience convulsions as well. In the course of time, these children develop more slowly and perform less well intellectually than the offspring of nonaddicted mothers.

A choice with less adversity for pregnant women who cannot abstain from heroin has been to place them on methadone treatment. While the problem of fetal addiction remains with this drug as well, prenatal care is likely to be more responsibly carried out. While infants born under these circumstances do tend to weigh less than the norm, the disparity is less pronounced and withdrawal is less acute than it would be if the mother were using heroin. Most of these youngsters seem to develop normally, without significant long-term negative effects. Little experience with mothers addicted to other narcotics has been reported, but it can be conjectured that it would be similar to that of heroin addicts.

Tobacco

Particular problems are engendered by pregnant women who smoke. The baby faces a significantly greater probability of low birth weight and has a greater likelihood of being stillborn or of dying early in infancy than the offspring of nonsmokers. There is further evidence of some increase in physical and intellectual impairment as these children develop. Some researchers believe that these disabilities are the result of fetal poisoning by carbon monoxide.

Babies of nursing mothers may also encounter problems when nicotine is present in breast milk in significant amounts. Nausea, vomiting, diarrhea, and rapid heart rate in the infant have been observed. There is enough compelling evidence to suggest that pregnant women and nursing mothers should not smoke for the sake of their babies, if not for themselves.

SIGNS OF TROUBLE

Many patterns of drug use exist, running the gamut from a single exposure to heavy compulsive daily use. Casual social use may be viewed with tolerance, but justifiable alarm sets in when self-control goes. The vast majority of those who use drugs do so in moderation, with only a small percent succumbing to abuse. While 40 percent of all high school students in the United States have used marijuana and 80 percent alcohol even to the point of modest intoxication, only a small number will become "pot heads" or alcoholics. Use per se is insufficient cause for pushing the panic button indiscriminately. We need to be able to identify specific danger signals that inevitably accompany the transition between use and abuse or that suggest special vulnerability. The following characteristics and behavior patterns are subjective and objective indicators that either trouble is at hand or just ahead.

1. A vulnerable personality structure characterized by an inability to deal effectively with stress and anxiety. Feelings of isolation, frustration, low self-esteem, and helplessness are dominant. This may be a lifelong pattern or it may emerge in connection with situational crises: working people arriving at the realization that their dreams of glory will never be fulfilled; mothers faced with the need to find a new identity when their children grow up; adolescents struggling to achieve independence and take on responsibility for their own behavior.

2. Signs of poor adjustment and a deterioration of effective functioning, whether at home, school, or work; increasing emotional instability, with

rapid mood swings from high spirits to rage; evidence of increasing depression, with longer periods of time spent in bed; persistent fatigue even after many hours of sleep; decreasing appetite and weight loss; increasing inattention to personal hygiene and dress and a general aura of sadness.

3. Highly secretive behavior; improbable excuses for absences from commitments; unexplained and prolonged periods of time away from home; studied efforts at self-control; general evasiveness.

4. Recurrent episodes of intoxicated behavior, particularly when associated with vigorous denial that such episodes occurred. Such behavior would include slurred speech, unsteady gait, and other signs of drunkenness; unusual drowsiness or remoteness; withdrawal from reality; flights of grandiose ideas and philosophical musings lacking in coherence; agitation, restlessness, and unusual energy levels; inappropriate laughter or silliness.

5. Presence of drug paraphernalia (needles and syringe) or drugs, pills, empty liquor bottles, tubes of glue hidden in profusion.

6. Sudden acquisition of unusual amounts of money from unexplained sources (resulting from selling drugs); disappearance of money or valuable objects from the home.

Motivation for Help

Drug abuse is a difficult problem to pinpoint through physical symptoms since physical indications may be minimal. In the absence of intoxication doctors can rarely tell whether or not a person has used drugs by a physical examination alone. Blood and urine can be tested, but these will show positive results only if the drugs were used within the previous few days. Few laboratories are equipped to test for the hallucinogens.

Even when unmistakable signs of drug abuse do exist, it is one of the most difficult emotional problems to deal with. It is hard for someone who finds easy relief from problems to give up drugs for the alternative of physical and emotional pain. The period between cessation of drug use and ultimate rehabilitation is long and difficult. Even when confronted with incontrovertible proof, the habituated or addicted individual may still deny drug abuse or shrug off the notion that a problem exists. In many cases serious "bottoming out" experiences and overwhelming fear or guilt must occur before motivation to seek help becomes strong enough. Such experiences may be the loss of a job, a serious overdose reaction, the death of a friend from overdose, the breakup of a marriage, causing physical harm to a loved one, being picked up by the police, or experiencing a humiliating situation. Even when help is sought, periodic failure and reversion to drug habituation are common.

Ideally, the drug abuser should seek help as soon as there is an awareness that volitional control is being lost. But since denial is a common aspect of abuse, family members may have to take the initiative for getting help. They should not succumb to denial themselves and continue to cover up for the abuser. Early intervention increases the probability of successful treatment since it is much more difficult to deal with the problem when abuse patterns are of long duration.

Family members should make every effort to talk over their concerns openly and honestly without delay. It is to be hoped that the concerns will be discussed in an atmosphere of supportive and loving care rather than in anger and vituperation. Unfortunately, communication is likely to be least effective in precisely those families where tensions were cause for escape into drug use in the first place. The entreaties of spouse or parent have probably been angry and frustrated over a long period, suggestions about seeking help falling on deaf ears. In these instances family members will simply have to take the initiative and make independent inquiries about treatment options.

Family physicians, local drug treatment facilities, Alcoholics Anonymous, Alanon, social workers in hospital clinics and mental health centers, and the police are all sources of help. In recent years many large companies have begun to provide on-the-job alcohol and drug treatment services. Group health insurance is also likely to provide coverage for hospitalization when detoxification is indicated.

Treatment

Since drug and alcohol abuse have proved to be resistant to traditional one-to-one psychiatric techniques, specialized programs are usually required. The following are options that exist in many communities:

ALCOHOL

Initial detoxification or "drying out" is best achieved over a period of several weeks in a special hospital setting. The alcoholic then needs a continuing support system and must remain abstinent. Alcoholics Anonymous is the major nationwide (and international) organization established for this purpose. Regional and local chapters exist in most cities and towns and are listed in the telephone directory. Support groups for family members are also offered: Alanon for spouses, close relatives, and concerned friends, and Alateen for adolescents. These support groups have proved extremely helpful even if the alcoholic individual refuses to be involved in his own treatment. AA can often be helpful in identifying treatment programs for other drug problems as well.

Another alternative for the alcoholic is the taking of Antabuse, a medicine which causes acute gastrointestinal upset and vomiting if it is followed by alcohol consumption. Doctors and some treatment programs may recommend it, but its success as a deterrent to drinking depends on the willing compliance of the patient to take it every day, and this discipline can be difficult for some.

NARCOTICS

Initial detoxification is best carried out in a hospital during a stay of several weeks. State and city health or mental health departments can make the proper referrals if there is an unwillingness to consult the family doctor who may also be a personal friend. Inquiries are confidential, and the addict need not fear that criminal prosecution will be a consequence of seeking help.

There are several alternatives for long-term treatment after detoxification. The first option is a drug-free residential center. Rehabilitation consists of a combination of behavior modification and encounter therapy in a program of graduating levels of responsibility, self-determination, and reengagement with society. None of these programs has locked doors, and the resident is free to leave the center at any time. The turnover rate is very high, but if the individual is able to make it through the first few months, the outlook for successful rehabilitation is vastly improved. The treatment process takes from one and a half to two years. Most of these residential centers are geared to handle individuals with multiple drug problems. Among the nationally known centers are Odyssey House and Daytop Village.

Some drug-free programs are organized for outpatient rather than for residential care. Since individuals attend only during waking hours but go home to sleep, the major drawback to successful therapy is the patient's continued exposure to all the environmental tensions and drug availability that created the problem in the first place.

Narcotic addicts who cannot cope with a drug-free program have another alternative in methadone maintenance treatment centers. Methadone, also a narcotic, is substituted for heroin and given in daily doses large enough to produce a level of tolerance which renders any street heroin ineffective. At the same time methadone is maintained at a level that keeps the addict "straight" and produces neither intoxication nor withdrawal symptoms. While many addicts have done very well with methadone maintenance, others have moved on to abuse alcohol and sedatives.

A third alternative is a program based on treatment with nalloxone, nalline, or a similar narcotic antagonist that directly neutralizes the effects of heroin, rendering any amount taken incapable of producing intoxication. This differs from methadone maintenance in that the medication involved has no psychotropic effects and is not addicting. These programs have not been well received, as the addict must have a high level of motivation; if he stops taking the medication even for a brief period, he can experience a heroin "high" again.

BARBITURATES

Any individual addicted to this group of drugs must be detoxified in a hospital and given continuing psychological treatment. Facilities suitable for narcotic addicts or alcoholics (excluding drug replacement programs) often will treat the barbiturate addict as well.

OTHER DRUGS

Individuals abusing any of the other substances discussed in this chapter, whether singly or in combination, are usually welcome in residential or day treatment programs. Regular mental hospitals and mental health clinics, medical programs for adolescents, free clinics, and other health facilities may also have drug treatment programs. A number of youth community programs and schools also have special groups to help adolescents who are involved with drugs.

Sources of Information

- Alcoholics Anonymous
- Regional "hot lines"
- State and city departments of health, mental health, and social service
- Local general and mental hospitals
- County medical societies
- Family physicians
- School guidance offices
- Boys and girls clubs and other youth programs
- Community mental health centers
- Juvenile and family court probation officers
- Any local drug treatment program

DRUG ABUSE EMERGENCIES

Drug abuse emergencies generally result as a consequence of overdose, commonly referred to as OD by drug users and doctors alike. The specific physiological and psychological reactions to each class of chemicals have been given in the previous discussion. When an emergency arises, the wisest thing to do is call an ambulance *at once*. Questions of pride and shame must be set aside and lifesaving measures given top priority.

Overdose reactions generally fall into two classes: (1) stupor or coma and (2) a psychotic, schizophrenic-like state. If breathing has stopped (and be sure that it in fact has and is not simply shallow and slow), cardiopulmonary resuscitation should be instituted at once while awaiting an ambulance. However, this should be attempted only by those who have had instruction in CPR. In the absence of CPR training, insure that the victim has no obstruction in the nose or mouth, loosen any tight clothing, place him on his back, and keep him warm.

With persons experiencing a psychotic reaction, it is important that those in attendance be as calm and reassuring as possible; this is no time for panic. The victim should be kept in a quiet, softly lighted room. Someone he knows well should stay with him and communicate by both words and touch that everything is "OK" and help is on the way.

In those who are extremely agitated or violent it may be necessary to use physical restraint as a last resort to avert the danger of self-harm or harm to others. Less drastic methods are preferable while waiting for professional help, but these are not options when serious harm is likely to occur.

The attending physician should be given as much information as possible about what drug may have been taken. Any pills, powders, liquids, or empty bottles found in the victim's possession or the immediate surroundings (including the medicine cabinet) should be taken to the hospital. Persons present when the drug might have been administered should be questioned at once for detailed information not only about what the substance might have been, but also about what is currently popular and available on the street. When an emergency patient turns up in a psychotic state, it is particularly important that doctors be aware of the possibility of drug ingestion. The possibility of PCP ingestion in particular definitely needs to be considered as the cause of a schizophrenic-like reaction to avoid a mistaken diagnosis and improper treatment.

PERSONAL DECISIONS ABOUT DRUGS

While it might be easy to recommend that all drugs be avoided under all circumstances, this is not a realistic approach. The use of mind-altering substances for recreation, relaxation, and celebration is an immutable fact with long historical precedent. Since everyone is exposed to the availability of drugs, the decision of whether to use them or not should be based on sound factual knowledge about the drug under consideration and knowledge of personal vulnerability to addiction. To act out of impulse, social pressure, or ignorant curiosity is to do ourselves harm. Any reader should look to the following points before she acts.

Alcohol has a definite place in human socialization. The choice of whether to drink or not is a personal one. The average drinker's primary responsibility rests in not placing oneself or others in jeopardy while intoxicated. Persons with a high percentage of factors predisposing to a risk of alcoholism should be particularly careful about how much and how often they drink or whether they should drink at all. If you decide to drink alcohol, you probably desire only its pleasures and wish to avoid its dangers. Here are some guidelines.

- Eat both before you drink and with your drinks, preferably fats which slow absorption.
- Sip your drink and pace yourself—one drink of whiskey or equivalent per hour. Limit yourself to two or three drinks an evening. Keep your own count and don't let your half-empty glass get filled up.
- If possible, pour your own drinks and dilute them well.
- Be sensitive to your personal signs of "too much"—a fuzzy feeling, a feeling of warmth in ears or face, trouble getting your tongue to perform properly, a little unsteadiness when you walk—and change to a soft drink.

Women who are under considerable emotional stress of more than a temporary nature, feel a sense of futility and frustration, and find it particularly difficult to cope with life are most vulnerable to abusing drugs. The seeking of professional help is a far better alternative.

When drug or alcohol consumption begins to be necessary to get through a day, when being high is preferable to being straight, and when drugs are taken regularly in amounts exceeding what a doctor would recommend, the user is in trouble and should seek professional help.

Cigarette smoking now has established long-term risk factors for women as well as men. It can significantly reduce life expectancy and increase the likelihood of heart attacks, lung disease, and cancer. There can be no rational justification for smoking cigarettes.

However, many women do smoke and most begin in their teens, presumably to appear sophisticated or to achieve early adulthood. They quickly become habituated, probably more to the "mechanics" of lighting up and the association of smoking with various activities—reading, talking, cooking, driving, playing cards—than to tobacco itself. Smoking becomes a conditioned reflex, a bad habit. That's really the reason it's so hard for many people who desire to do so to stop. They are unable to modify their behavior. Help in stopping requires either a tremendous amount of self-discipline or professional psychological help.

The facts on marijuana are not all in and further study needs to be done, particularly on the effects of long-term use. But no serious side effects or deleterious consequences from occasional recreational use have yet been confirmed. Legal aspects of marijuana are in flux. While selling continues to bear significant criminal liability, simple possession of small amounts for personal use is increasingly being regarded as just a misdemeanor. This varies from state to state.

Many substances, although bearing minimal risks for the user, may have adverse effects upon a fetus. All drugs, including caffeinated beverages, should be avoided during pregnancy and alcohol consumption eliminated or at least reduced to minimal amounts.

Know the action of the substance you are thinking of taking. Read about it; ask knowledgeable people; think about it first. Do not act on rumor and hearsay or out of impulse.

Be sure you are getting what you think you are. Do not take substances whose purity or content is in question. More times than not you will be getting something other than what the seller alleges. Psilocybin and mescaline are particularly notorious in this regard and usually contain LSD or PCP instead.

LSD, PCP, and other strong hallucinogens should be strictly avoided. Their results are highly unpredictable even with a single dose. They may cause permanent mental illness or cause the user to perform dangerous and reckless acts.

Neither can the illegal or unprescribed use of stimulants, narcotics, sedatives, or tranquilizers be condoned, although it is true that a single dose of any of these drugs is not associated with the same degree of harm as are strong hallucinogens. They each have their own particular hazards, and illegal possession bears risk of criminal prosecution.

Many of the drugs subject to abuse also have a legitimate place in the treatment of disease under medical supervision. You have the right and need to be informed about the nature of the medication prescribed, its effects, and possible risks. You have the power to control your own life, to make reasoned rather than impulsive choice. Be aware of yourself, know your strengths and vulnerabilities, and be informed; these are the two cornerstones upon which the rational and appropriate use of drugs is based and their abuse avoided.

FURTHER READING

Books

Brecher, Edward M., and the Editors of Consumer Reports. *Licit and Illicit Drugs.* Boston: Little, Brown, 1972 (hardcover); Mount Vernon, N.Y.: Consumers Union, 1972 (paperback).

Drug Literature Review. Washington, D.C.: National Coordinating Council on Drug Education, 1979.

Hornik, Edith. *The Drinking Woman.* New York: Association Press, 1977.

Lingeman, Richard R. *Drugs from A to Z: A Dictionary.* New York: McGraw-Hill, 1969.

Mann, George A. *Recovery of Reality: Overcoming Chemical Dependency.* New York: Harper & Row, 1979.

Marijuana and Health, a Report to the Congress from the Secretary, Department of Health, Education and Welfare. Washington, D.C.: Department of Health, Education and Welfare, 1976 (rev. 1979).

Marin, Peter, and Allen Y. Cohen, *Understanding Drug Use: An Adult's Guide to Drugs and the Young.* New York: Harper & Row, 1971.

Musto, David F., M.D. *The American Disease: Origins of Narcotics Control.* New Haven: Yale University Press, 1973.

Pamphlets

Federal government publications available from National Clearinghouse for Drug Abuse Information, 5600 Fishers Lane, Rockville, Md. 20852:
  Alcohol: Some Questions and Answers
  Cigarette Smoking: Some Questions and Answers
  Drug Abuse: Some Questions and Answers
  Federal Source Book, Answers to the Most Frequently Asked Questions About Drug Abuse
  Marijuana: Some Questions and Answers
  Sedatives: Some Questions and Answers
  Stimulants: Some Questions and Answers
  Terms and Symptoms of Drug Abuse
  Volatile Substances: Some Questions and Answers
  Youthful Drug Use

Barbiturates: Important Facts for Your Survival. DO-IT-NOW Foundation, P.O. Box 5115, Phoenix, Ariz. 85010.

The Conscientious Guide to Drug Abuse. DO-IT-NOW Foundation, P.O. Box 5115, Phoenix, Ariz. 85010. (Aimed at people who are using drugs.)

Drug IQ Test. DO-IT-NOW Foundation, P.O. Box 5115, Phoenix, Ariz. 85010.

Drugs of Abuse: An Introduction to Their Actions and Potential Hazards. Student Association for the Study of Hallucinogens (STASH), 638 Pleasant Street, Beloit, Wis. 53511.

The Facts About Drinking and Accidents. Available from the National Safety Council, 425 North Michigan Avenue, Chicago, Ill. 60611.

"Major Drugs: Their Uses and Effects" (3-page multicolored chart by Dr. Joel Fort). Playboy Enterprises, Inc., 919 North Michigan Avenue, Chicago, Ill. 60611.

Drug Education and Treatment Resources

National Clearinghouse for Drug Abuse Information, 5600 Fishers Lane, Rockville, Md. 20852.

The clearinghouse is operated by the National Institute on Drug Abuse and serves as a distributor of federal information on drug abuse. Single copies of some publications and posters are provided free upon request. In addition, the clearinghouse refers specialized and technical inquiries to federal, state, local, and private information resources.

National Coordinating Council on Drug Education, 1200 Connecticut Avenue, NW, Suite 212, Washington, D.C. 20036.

The council is the largest national, private, nonprofit drug education network. It is aimed at organizing effective community action programs, evaluating drug education programs, campaigns, and materials, and disseminating factual information about drugs.

A wide variety of local and state programs exist for drug and alcohol prevention and treatment. Each state has a State Drug Abuse Coordinator. Check with this individual, local drug treatment agencies, Alcoholics Anonymous, and others to identify specific resources to meet your needs.

Rape and Spouse Abuse— Two Crimes of Violence

DOROTHY HICKS, M.D.

Professor of Obstetrics and Gynecology, University of Miami
School of Medicine, Director, Rape Treatment Center,
Jackson Memorial Hospital, Miami, Florida

The increasing violence in our society is reflected in the growing incidence of sexual assault and spouse battering. Professionals working in these fields have come to understand that these crimes are the result of anger and hostility culminating in violence. It is now our goal to see that the general public is educated so that they can understand the basic emotions behind these crimes and so that they know where to turn for help if they are the victims. This education can be accomplished through many media— books such as this, other publications, and plays and documentaries on television, in the theater, in the schools.

The various sections in this chapter deal with the individual crimes and their victims, but the underlying theme which connects them all is violence.

SEXUAL ASSAULT: FORCIBLE RAPE

Forcible rape is a violent crime, not an act done for sexual reasons, and it precipitates a crisis situation in the victim. The degree of the stress involved may become more understandable if you think of rape as a crime against your person. This places it in the same category as other aggressive crimes such as robbery, assault, and the ultimate act of aggression, murder. In fact, as far as damage to the innermost self is concerned, rape is the most traumatic act short of murder.

The word "rape" comes from the Latin *rapere*, "to take by force."

Other meanings are to plunder, to destroy, to seize and carry away by force. The traditional legal definition of rape is carnal knowledge (vaginal penetration) of a female through the use of force or the threat of force, without her consent.

Although present laws vary from state to state, most states have changed or are in the process of changing their old rape laws so that they now speak of "sexual assault" or "involuntary sexual battery" and have degrees and penalties similar to those found in the laws for murder. Oral, rectal, and vaginal contact, as well as penetration, are grounds for conviction. A witness to the crime is no longer necessary. There is a range of penalties for the offender. These newer statutes are far more realistic in terms of the nature of the crime and the effect on the victim. Women and girls can be damaged psychologically as much from an attempted rape as they are from an actual rape. Penetration of the oral and rectal cavities are often more humiliating than vaginal penetration and the effects more serious. Since sexual assault is usually a one-on-one crime, requiring a witness was ridiculous. The key word is "consent" to the sexual activity.

During the 1970s the feminist movement began to publicize the problems of rape victims, and the pressure to change the old laws has been felt at all levels of government and in many areas of the world. In 1978 a rapist was arrested in Paris for the first time in history. In Egypt the prime minister asked the legislature for a law making rape a crime. The state of Oregon passed a law making it illegal for a husband to rape his wife. In September 1979 in Massachusetts a man was convicted of raping his wife; the couple were in the process of getting a divorce and were living apart, but the divorce was not final. Times are changing, and some day women may have equal rights and protection under the law in every country on earth. Unfortunately, in many countries women are still considered to be inferior to men and are treated as chattel.

The United States government has recognized the scope and urgency of the problem. The National Center for the Prevention and Control of Rape has been established in Washington, D.C. Programs are being developed and legislation is being written to compensate the victims of rape and other violent crimes. Courses are being held at criminal justice training centers and at police academies to educate and sensitize law enforcement personnel working with the victims of sexual assault.

Efforts are being made to educate the public so that they realize that sexual assault is a crime and not "hanky-panky" as it has been thought to be for centuries. Even when the victims were abused physically, people often felt the woman had "asked for it." Women's groups have organized crisis centers, hotlines have been established, colleges and universities have sponsored seminars to educate the students and personnel, public information and education programs have been presented by radio, television, newspapers, and magazines. Remember that in our court system the juries are made up of citizens and if they are to come to a correct verdict, they must comprehend the nature of the crime that has been committed. The public must be made to realize that sexual assault is a crime.

History

The threat of rape has been a fear of women from prehistoric times to the present. It is interesting to research ancient laws and historical practice to see how they approached the problems posed by rape.

In ancient times, the Babylonian Code of Hammurabi and Mosaic laws allowed capture by force of women from outside the tribe. Such women were considered to be prizes of warfare. Acquisition of women within the tribe required payment of goods or money to the family. Perhaps this was a basis for the concept of criminal rape: to take the virginity of a maiden was equivalent to destroying property or stealing the goods and money she would have brought to the family.

Under the Code of Hammurabi a female had no independent status. She lived as a virgin daughter in the house of her father or as a wife in the house of her husband. A married woman who was raped shared the blame with her attacker and both were bound and thrown into the river, although her husband was permitted to rescue her if he so chose. A virgin who was defiled was held innocent and the rapist slain.

Hebrew laws were similar. The "offending" wife and her attacker were stoned to death. A virgin raped within the city walls was considered guilty because she could have screamed for help, but a maiden raped in the fields was considered guiltless, the rapist paid the girl's father a fine, and the two were forced to marry. If the virgin had been betrothed before the incident, the rapist was stoned to death.

Tales of rape and similar stories are found in the Bible and in the folklore of all peoples. Variations on the story of Potiphar's wife, the woman who unjustly accused Joseph of rape, are found in Moslem, Christian, and Hebrew folklore as well as in the myths of the Celts and the Egyptians as far back as 1300 B.C. The moral of the story is that a woman can cause a man a lot of problems by falsely crying rape.

The practice of forcible seizure of women for mates was for centuries considered acceptable. One way to obtain property in the Middle Ages was to abduct an heiress and marry her; it was not until the fifteenth century that this was considered to be a felony. Arranging marriages was a common method of acquiring property during these times, and in some forms this practice continues today.

In Europe in the eighteenth century an assault was not considered rape if a woman conceived, because it was believed that if she did not consent, she could not have conceived. The law was very vague about the rape of women who were not virgins. There are few records; apparently these victims were not taken seriously and the accusations quashed.

In the United States during the days of slavery it was accepted practice to use slave women as the owner desired, and it was common for them to be raped by the men in charge. There was no attempt to maintain a slave family, but instead the women were considered to be "breeders" and were valued as such.

During wars and occupations of the conquered countries women have always been considered a part of the spoils of war and were ravished by invading troops. The primary basis for the assaults was not sexual gratification, but rather the acts were part of the psychology of conquest—the right of the conqueror to overwhelm and humiliate his victims.

These attitudes about what was considered acceptable behavior and the old laws concerning rape seem to reflect the need to preserve social stability and to protect property more than any concept of protection of the woman as an individual against a criminal act.

The Startling Facts: Current Statistics

Rape is the fastest growing of the violent crimes; since 1960 the reported number of forcible rapes has increased almost 200 percent. In 1977 there were 63,200 forcible rapes reported to the Federal Bureau of Investigation, and even the most conservative observers believe that only one in four rapes is reported to the authorities. The FBI estimates that in 1977 in the United States one forcible rape occurred every two minutes, although the reported rate was one rape every eight minutes.

It is unfortunate that we have no clear picture of the actual numbers of rapes and sexual assaults, but this is impossible to determine because of many factors. Statistics of law enforcement agencies may be misleading. The way in which the crimes are categorized is one reason. A rape is classified in one of three ways: forcible rape, which includes attempted rape but does not include statutory rape or homosexual rape; child molestation; or rape-homicide. On the national average 15 percent of the rapes reported to the police are dismissed as unfounded, that is, the police establish to their satisfaction that neither forcible rape nor the attempt to rape occurred. Still another reason for the lack of accurate figures is that many accusations of rape are reduced via plea bargaining to a lesser charge, such as breaking and entering or aggravated assault, and thus are included in the figures for those crimes instead of being counted as rapes.

Victims also contribute to the inaccuracies in the known number of rapes. Most of the assaults are unreported because of the stigma attached to being a victim of sexual assault. Many people still have the attitude that the woman is responsible for tempting or teasing the attacker and is therefore at least partially to blame for the rape. Failure to report the assault is especially true in the case of the child victim. Parents are afraid of the re-actions of family and friends and want to protect the child from any addi-tional psychological trauma. Even in such cases the victim, the child, may be accused of being seductive and therefore responsible for the attack. We must educate people that rape is not a sex act, but a crime of violence; the victim is no more to blame than if she were mugged and robbed.

The statistics from a rape treatment center in a typical metropolitan area are more comprehensive than those kept by law enforcement agen-cies. One large center in Dade County, Florida, serving approximately 1 million people, reports that it has cared for 4,700 victims since January 1974. In 1978 32 percent of the patients were under the age of 16; 5 per-cent of the victims were males; the youngest patient was a 2-month-old girl and the oldest a 93-year-old woman. These last two cases alone should make everyone realize that rape is not committed for sexual reasons.

Contrary to what most people expect, the rapes reported at the center were usually not interracial. In most cases whites were attacked by whites and blacks by blacks; there was very little cross-over. Victims were 45 per-cent black, 49 percent white, and 4 percent Hispanic. Dade County is one-third Latin, one-third black, and one-third other; the incidence of rape in the Hispanic community is assumed to be higher than reported, but Latins seem to be least likely to report rape to the authorities.

Weapons were used in 26 percent of all cases; in cases in which victims were 16 or over, this percentage increased to 37 percent. A knife was used in 24 percent of the cases and a gun in 13 percent. At the Jackson Memo-rial Hospital Rape Treatment Center, the number of cases in which a weapon is used has been increasing, and the violence is increasing. More victims have physical injuries.

Thirty-one percent of the assaults took place in the home of the victim, 19 percent in the home of the offender, and 25 percent outdoors.

The offenders were known to the victims in 45 percent of the cases.

In this group of patients, 89 percent reported the crime to the police, al-though some of these did not prosecute the case. Most of the others agreed to submit an anonymous report to the authorities; in such a report all the details of the crime are given except the name and address of the victim.

In general, past statistics for rape and sexual assault do not give an ac-curate picture of the frequency of the crime itself. Only recently have women been able to come forward and identify themselves without jeopardizing their reputations and relationships.

Myths About Rape

Many myths have persisted throughout the ages about the crime of rape, and they must be corrected if we are to make progress in dealing with this problem. Although we cannot deal with them all, here are some of the most prevalent.

1. *The rapist acts to satisfy sexual desires.* From the work that has been done with convicted sex offenders, it is well known now that sexual gratification is not the reason for sexual assault. The need of the attacker is to overpower, degrade, and humiliate. Violence, not sex, is expressed by the attack. The majority of rapists have a sexual partner with whom they identify and have a relationship and many have children.

2. *A woman cannot be raped if she doesn't want to be.* This is absolutely untrue. The primary reaction of a woman to a rapist is fear, fear that she will be killed or maimed. In addition, weapons are used in about 37 percent of the assaults, and anyone who argues with a knife or gun is foolish.

3. *If women did not wear sexy clothes and act in a provocative manner, they would not get raped.* Since violence and not sexual gratification is the motive for the attack, what the woman wears and how she acts have nothing to do with it. Many of the victims are at home asleep in their own beds. Most of the victims are fully clothed in conservative attire. A woman becomes the victim because she was in the wrong place at the wrong time.

4. *Rape is part of the sexual fantasies of women, or all women want to be raped.* It may be true that some women have sexual fantasies in which varying degrees of force play a part and that some women at some time and for a variety of reasons want to take a submissive role in sexual relations. However, these thoughts are completely different from and are unrelated to fantasizing rape in the sense of wanting to be the unwilling victim of a violent, nonsexual criminal act.

5. *Most rapes are reported to the police.* As we have pointed out, even the most optimistic observers feel that at best one in four attacks is reported to authorities; some think it is only one in ten.

6. *Only young attractive women get raped.* Statistically this is not true. All females regardless of age, race, socioeconomic status, and attractiveness are potential victims for the rapist. Most vulnerable is the woman alone at any time of day or night. One reason the majority of victims is between 16 and 29 is that this group is the most active and mobile. Vulnerability, not appearance, is the quality that attracts the attacker. Rapists look at their victims as objects or things rather than as people and often cannot identify the victim after the attack.

7. *White women are being raped by black men.* As we have said, there is very little racial cross-over between rapist and victim. About 80 percent of the time the victim is the same race and class as the attacker.

8. *You can tell a rapist by looking at him.* Rapists come in all shapes and sizes and from all socioeconomic and educational levels. Most rapists are physically attractive males and have no problem finding female companions. At least 50 percent have a steady partner, married or unmarried,

and the partners have no idea that their man is a sex offender. The average rapist attacks about once a week and many as often as two or three times a week. Each rapist follows a method of operation, and often can be identified by this pattern even though his name is not known.

Protecting Yourself

What can you do to prevent being raped? Most important is to recognize that you are a potential victim. Every female is vulnerable to attack regardless of her age. Sexual assaults occur in broad daylight as well as in darkness, in suburbs as well as in the downtown areas and ghettos, in homes as well as in alleys and automobiles.

Your home should be protected as well as possible. Use initials rather than your first name on the mailbox and in the telephone directory. If you live alone, add a fictitious name on your door, so that the fact that you are alone is not apparent. Install good quality locks and dead-bolts. When you move into a new house or apartment, change or rekey the locks on the exterior doors so that the old keys will no longer work. Do not keep an extra key in the mailbox, under the door mat, or over the door; these are the first places an intruder will look. Instead, give a key to a close friend or a trusted neighbor. Lock the door whenever you leave, even if you will be gone for only a moment; all a rapist needs is an opportunity.

Never open the door to strangers. The front door should be fitted with a peephole with a 180° angle so that you may see who is there without being seen yourself. A peephole is essential because a chain on the door may not be strong enough to prevent forced entry. If there is any doubt, do not let the person in. Ask for identification from utility men, repairmen, etc., and if there is any doubt, call the company to verify the identification. If a stranger wants to use the telephone because of an emergency, offer to make the call and ask him to wait outside.

Be alert to suspicious telephone calls. Never let the caller know you are alone and never give personal information about yourself, your family, or your neighbors. If you receive calls that are obscene or those in which the caller is silent or hangs up, notify the telephone company immediately. The police should be notified if threats are made.

Walking or jogging alone, especially after dark, can be hazardous. Rapists look for women who are vulnerable. Walk with a purpose and be aware. Do not stop to give directions to a stranger unless you are far enough away to avoid being grabbed and forced to go with the questioner. If you think you are being followed, check by crossing the street and reversing your direction. If there is any doubt, find a populated area and call the police.

Follow the same precautions when using public transportation. In addition, be suspicious of transit stops if only one person is in the area. Try

A Woman's Body

STRUCTURE AND FUNCTIONS IN FULL COLOR

Illustrated by Leonard D. Dank

SKELETAL SYSTEM

VOLUNTARY MUSCULAR SYSTEM · CIRCULATORY SYSTEM

ENDOCRINE SYSTEM · RESPIRATORY SYSTEM

DIGESTIVE SYSTEM

NERVOUS SYSTEM · URINARY SYSTEM

REPRODUCTIVE SYSTEM

THE BREAST

EMOTIONS AND THE BODY

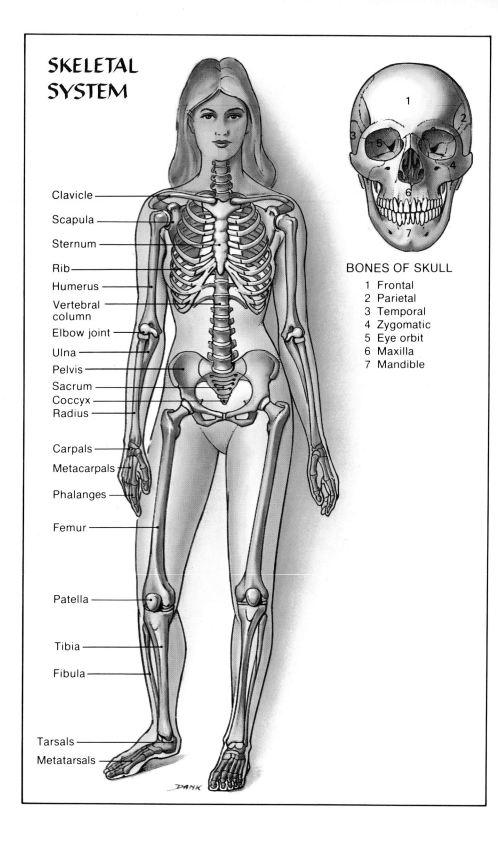

SKELETAL SYSTEM

Clavicle

Scapula

Sternum

Rib

Humerus

Vertebral column

Elbow joint

Ulna

Pelvis

Sacrum

Coccyx

Radius

Carpals

Metacarpals

Phalanges

Femur

Patella

Tibia

Fibula

Tarsals

Metatarsals

BONES OF SKULL

1 Frontal
2 Parietal
3 Temporal
4 Zygomatic
5 Eye orbit
6 Maxilla
7 Mandible

DANK

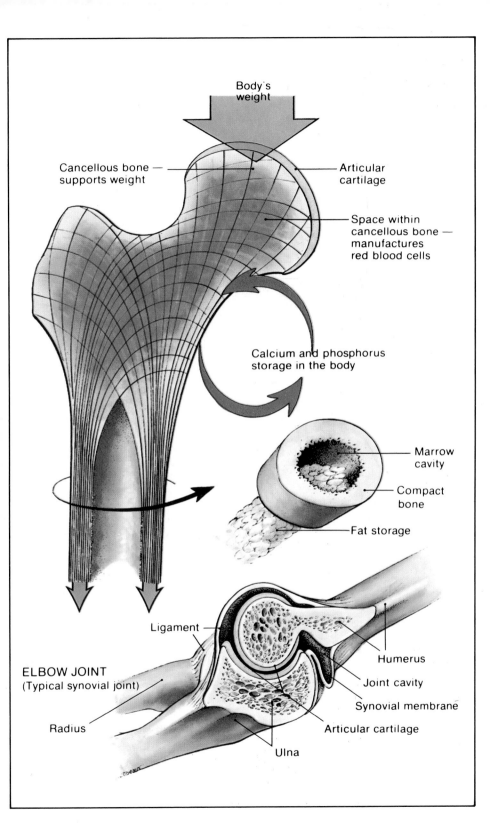

Body's weight

Cancellous bone — supports weight

Articular cartilage

Space within cancellous bone — manufactures red blood cells

Calcium and phosphorus storage in the body

Marrow cavity

Compact bone

Fat storage

ELBOW JOINT
(Typical synovial joint)

Ligament

Radius

Humerus

Joint cavity

Synovial membrane

Articular cartilage

Ulna

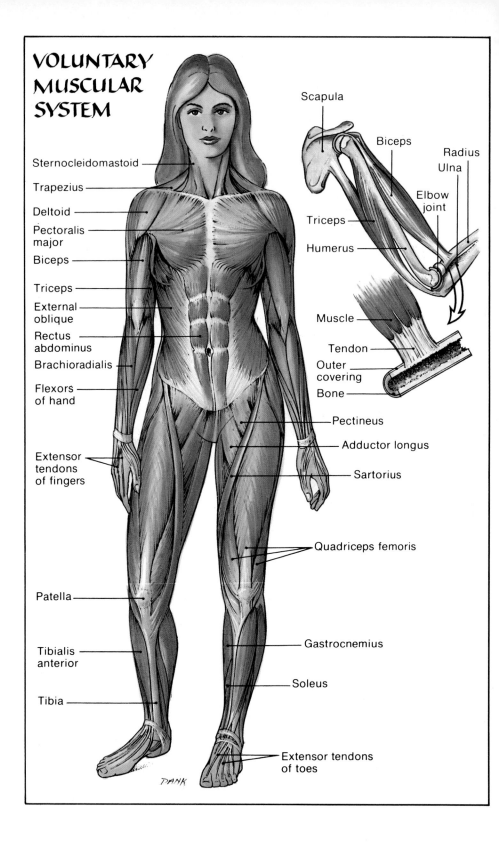

VOLUNTARY MUSCULAR SYSTEM

Sternocleidomastoid

Trapezius

Deltoid

Pectoralis major

Biceps

Triceps

External oblique

Rectus abdominus

Brachioradialis

Flexors of hand

Extensor tendons of fingers

Patella

Tibialis anterior

Tibia

Scapula

Biceps

Radius

Ulna

Triceps

Elbow joint

Humerus

Muscle

Tendon

Outer covering

Bone

Pectineus

Adductor longus

Sartorius

Quadriceps femoris

Gastrocnemius

Soleus

Extensor tendons of toes

DANK

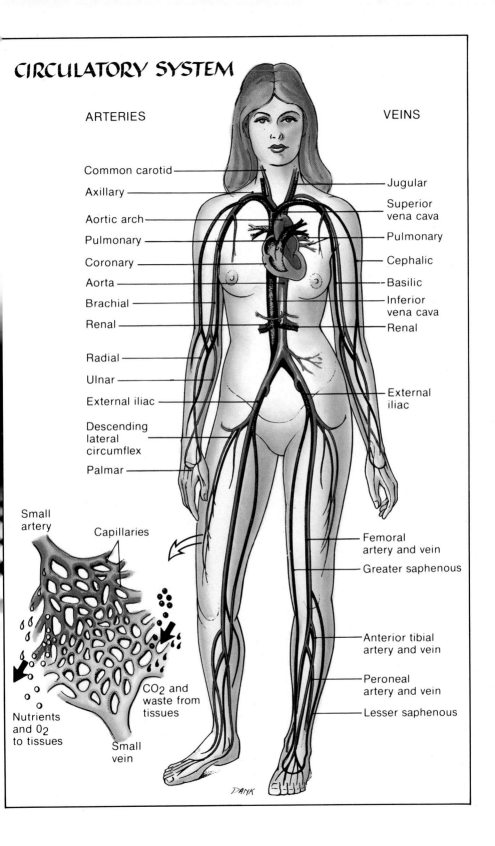

CIRCULATORY SYSTEM

ARTERIES

VEINS

Common carotid

Axillary

Aortic arch

Pulmonary

Coronary

Aorta

Brachial

Renal

Radial

Ulnar

External iliac

Descending
lateral
circumflex

Palmar

Jugular

Superior
vena cava

Pulmonary

Cephalic

Basilic

Inferior
vena cava

Renal

External
iliac

Femoral
artery and vein

Greater saphenous

Anterior tibial
artery and vein

Peroneal
artery and vein

Lesser saphenous

Small
artery

Capillaries

CO_2 and
waste from
tissues

Nutrients
and O_2
to tissues

Small
vein

DANK

ENDOCRINE SYSTEM

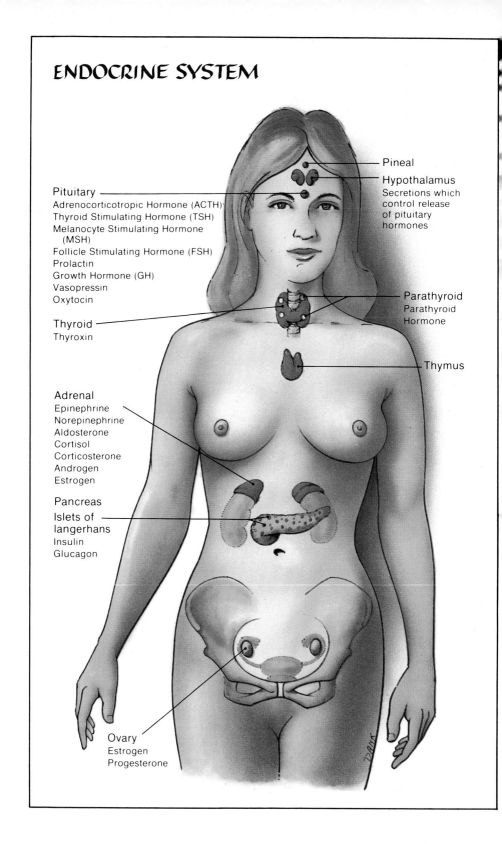

Pineal

Hypothalamus
Secretions which
control release
of pituitary
hormones

Pituitary
Adrenocorticotropic Hormone (ACTH)
Thyroid Stimulating Hormone (TSH)
Melanocyte Stimulating Hormone
 (MSH)
Follicle Stimulating Hormone (FSH)
Prolactin
Growth Hormone (GH)
Vasopressin
Oxytocin

Parathyroid
Parathyroid
Hormone

Thyroid
Thyroxin

Thymus

Adrenal
Epinephrine
Norepinephrine
Aldosterone
Cortisol
Corticosterone
Androgen
Estrogen

Pancreas
Islets of
langerhans
Insulin
Glucagon

Ovary
Estrogen
Progesterone

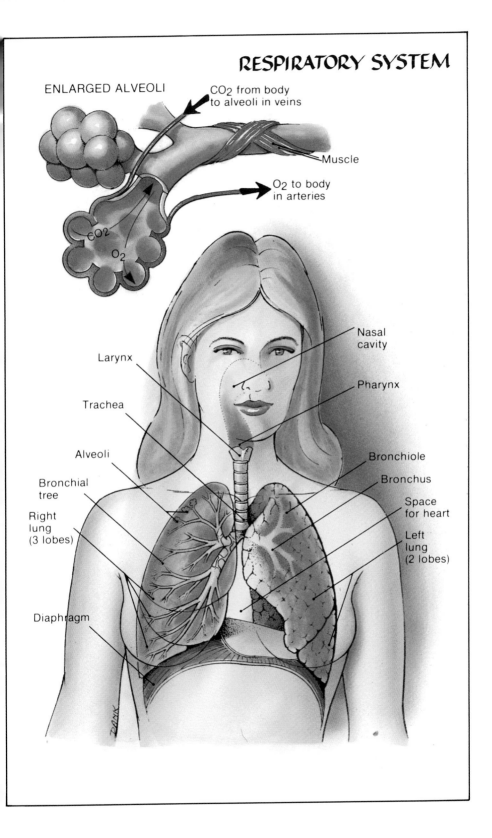

RESPIRATORY SYSTEM

ENLARGED ALVEOLI

CO_2 from body
to alveoli in veins

Muscle

O_2 to body
in arteries

CO_2

O_2

Nasal
cavity

Larynx

Pharynx

Trachea

Alveoli

Bronchiole

Bronchus

Bronchial
tree

Space
for heart

Right
lung
(3 lobes)

Left
lung
(2 lobes)

Diaphragm

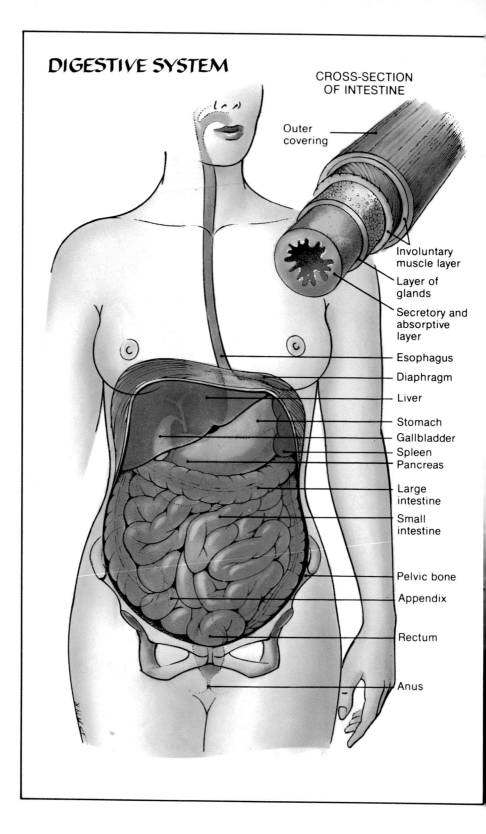

DIGESTIVE SYSTEM

CROSS-SECTION
OF INTESTINE

Outer
covering

Involuntary
muscle layer

Layer of
glands

Secretory and
absorptive
layer

Esophagus

Diaphragm

Liver

Stomach

Gallbladder

Spleen

Pancreas

Large
intestine

Small
intestine

Pelvic bone

Appendix

Rectum

Anus

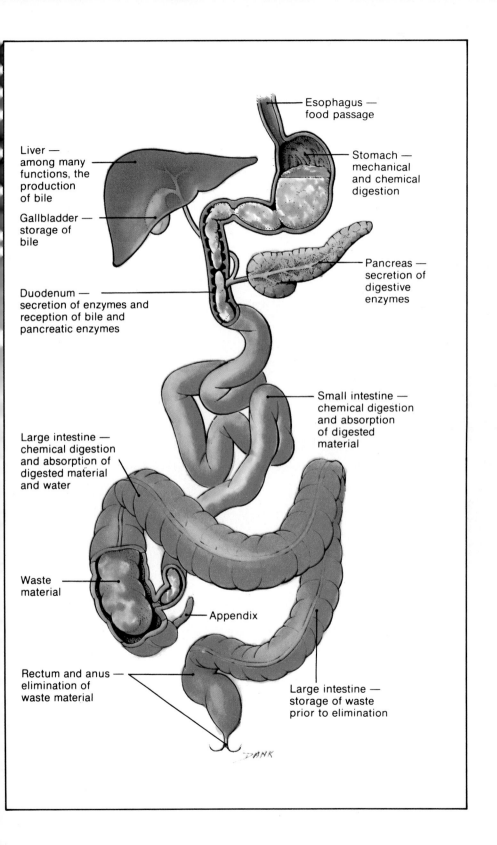

Esophagus —
food passage

Liver —
among many
functions, the
production
of bile

Stomach —
mechanical
and chemical
digestion

Gallbladder —
storage of
bile

Pancreas —
secretion of
digestive
enzymes

Duodenum —
secretion of enzymes and
reception of bile and
pancreatic enzymes

Small intestine —
chemical digestion
and absorption
of digested
material

Large intestine —
chemical digestion
and absorption of
digested material
and water

Waste
material

Appendix

Rectum and anus —
elimination of
waste material

Large intestine —
storage of waste
prior to elimination

DANK

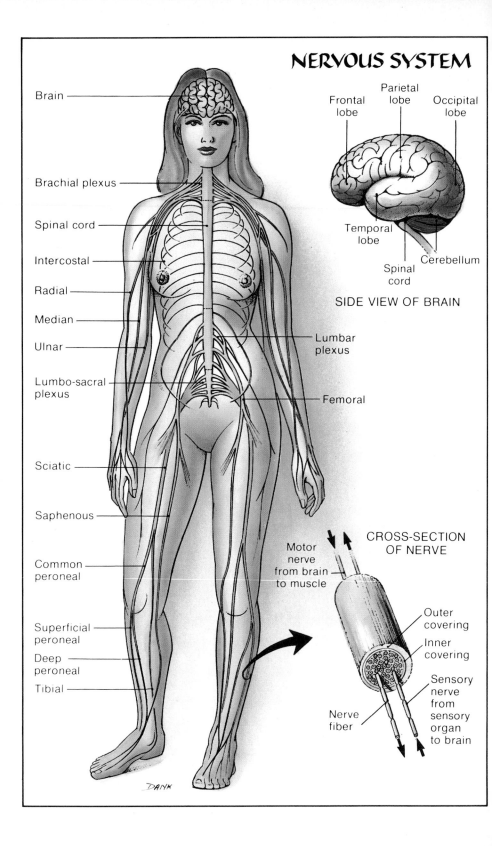

NERVOUS SYSTEM

Brain

Brachial plexus

Spinal cord

Intercostal

Radial

Median

Ulnar

Lumbo-sacral plexus

Sciatic

Saphenous

Common peroneal

Superficial peroneal

Deep peroneal

Tibial

Lumbar plexus

Femoral

Frontal lobe

Parietal lobe

Occipital lobe

Temporal lobe

Cerebellum

Spinal cord

SIDE VIEW OF BRAIN

CROSS-SECTION OF NERVE

Motor nerve from brain to muscle

Outer covering

Inner covering

Sensory nerve from sensory organ to brain

Nerve fiber

DANK

URINARY SYSTEM

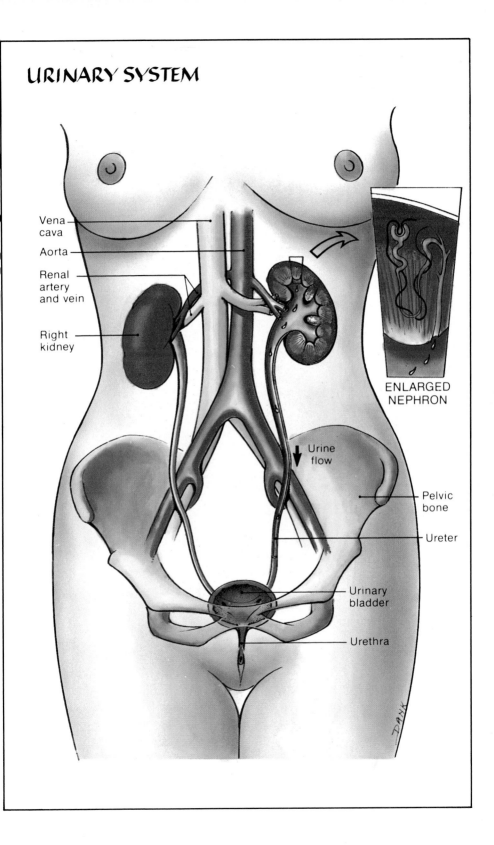

Vena cava

Aorta

Renal artery and vein

Right kidney

ENLARGED NEPHRON

Urine flow

Pelvic bone

Ureter

Urinary bladder

Urethra

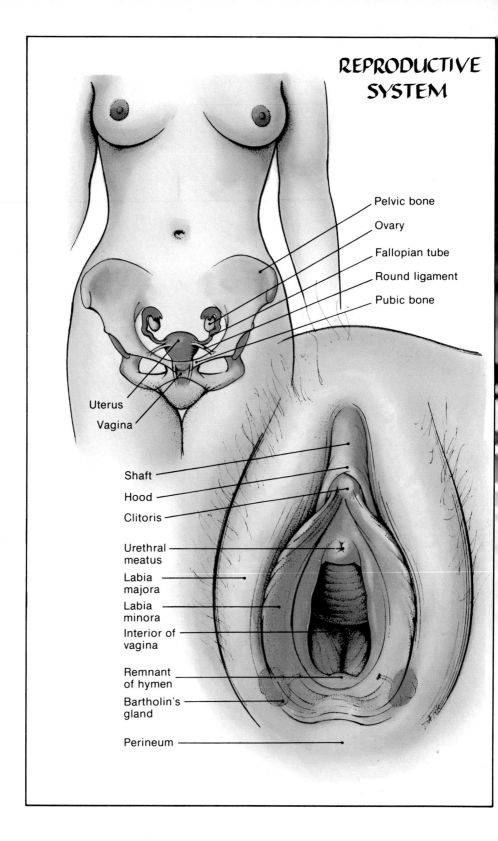

REPRODUCTIVE SYSTEM

Pelvic bone

Ovary

Fallopian tube

Round ligament

Pubic bone

Uterus

Vagina

Shaft

Hood

Clitoris

Urethral meatus

Labia majora

Labia minora

Interior of vagina

Remnant of hymen

Bartholin's gland

Perineum

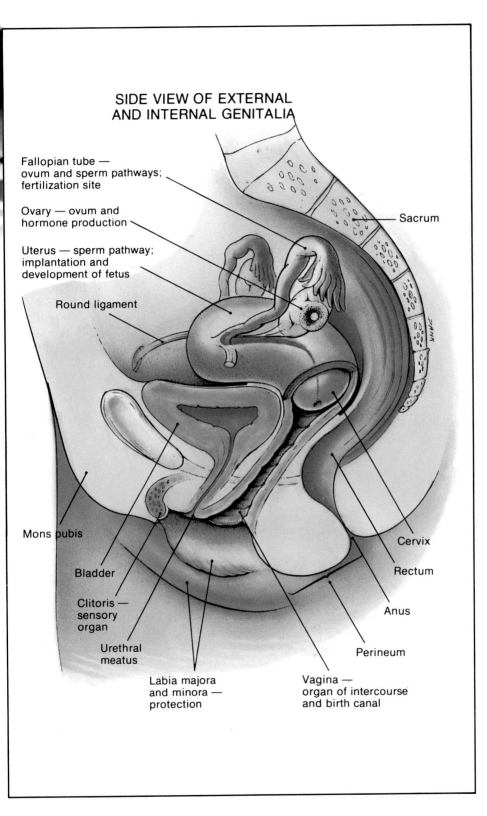

SIDE VIEW OF EXTERNAL AND INTERNAL GENITALIA

Fallopian tube — ovum and sperm pathways; fertilization site

Ovary — ovum and hormone production

Uterus — sperm pathway; implantation and development of fetus

Round ligament

Sacrum

Mons pubis

Bladder

Clitoris — sensory organ

Urethral meatus

Labia majora and minora — protection

Cervix

Rectum

Anus

Perineum

Vagina — organ of intercourse and birth canal

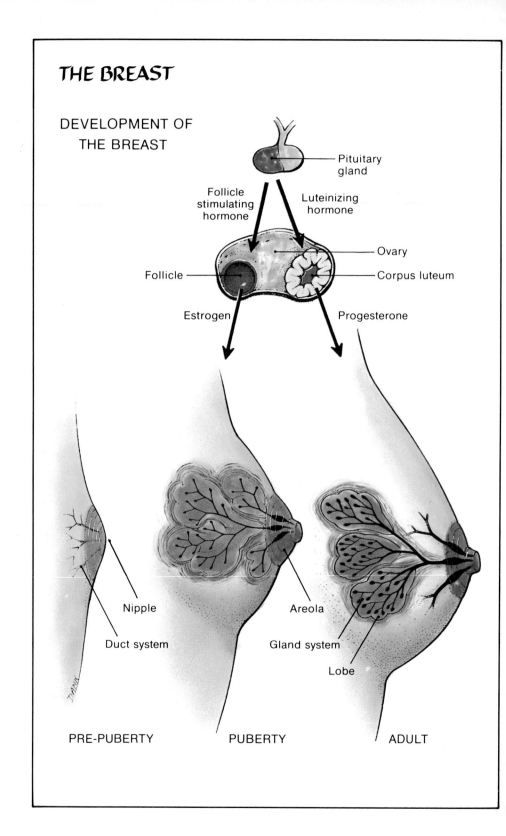

THE BREAST

DEVELOPMENT OF
THE BREAST

Pituitary gland

Follicle stimulating hormone

Luteinizing hormone

Ovary

Follicle

Corpus luteum

Estrogen

Progesterone

Nipple

Areola

Duct system

Gland system

Lobe

PRE-PUBERTY

PUBERTY

ADULT

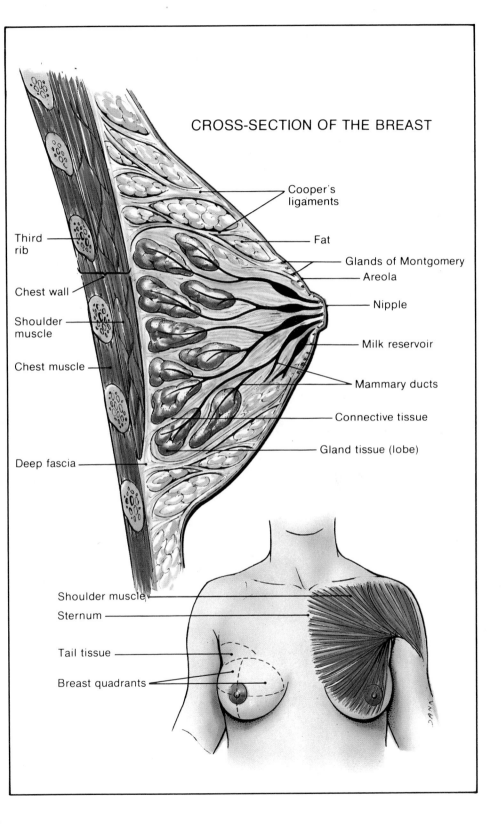

CROSS-SECTION OF THE BREAST

Cooper's ligaments

Fat

Glands of Montgomery

Areola

Nipple

Milk reservoir

Mammary ducts

Connective tissue

Gland tissue (lobe)

Third rib

Chest wall

Shoulder muscle

Chest muscle

Deep fascia

Shoulder muscle

Sternum

Tail tissue

Breast quadrants

EMOTIONS AND THE BODY

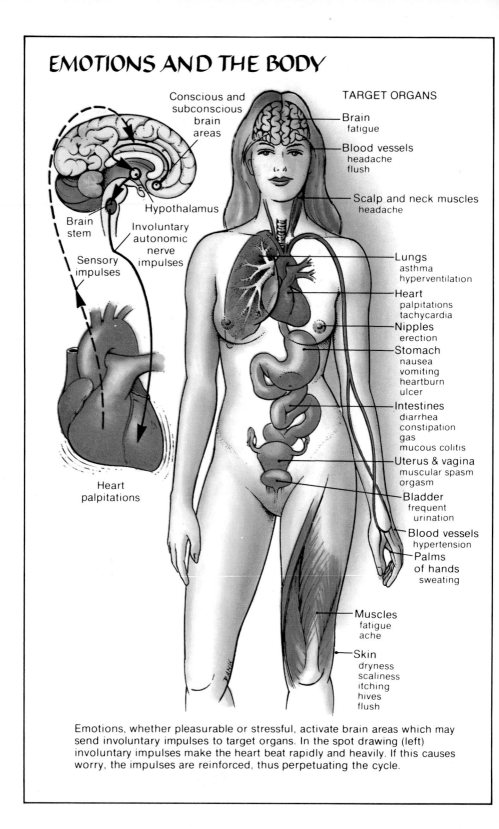

Conscious and subconscious brain areas

Hypothalamus

Brain stem

Sensory impulses

Involuntary autonomic nerve impulses

Heart palpitations

TARGET ORGANS

Brain
fatigue

Blood vessels
headache
flush

Scalp and neck muscles
headache

Lungs
asthma
hyperventilation

Heart
palpitations
tachycardia

Nipples
erection

Stomach
nausea
vomiting
heartburn
ulcer

Intestines
diarrhea
constipation
gas
mucous colitis

Uterus & vagina
muscular spasm
orgasm

Bladder
frequent
urination

Blood vessels
hypertension

Palms
of hands
sweating

Muscles
fatigue
ache

Skin
dryness
scaliness
itching
hives
flush

Emotions, whether pleasurable or stressful, activate brain areas which may send involuntary impulses to target organs. In the spot drawing (left) involuntary impulses make the heart beat rapidly and heavily. If this causes worry, the impulses are reinforced, thus perpetuating the cycle.

never to travel alone at night and take well traveled routes whenever possible.

When driving an automobile, be sure there is enough fuel to make the trip without stopping in a strange area. The car should be locked at all times and should always be parked in as safe a place as possible. Have your key ready in your hand when you walk to the car. Look in the back seat before getting into the automobile. Once inside, lock the doors. Never pick up hitchhikers. Never stop for an accident or a disabled vehicle; instead drive to the nearest safe telephone and call the police. If your car is disabled, raise the hood and wait inside the car with the doors locked and windows up until the police arrive to help. If someone offers to help, unless you know him, simply ask him to call the police. Rapists have been known to let the air out of an automobile tire and then offer to change the tire.

These are some of the measures you can take to avoid becoming a victim. Above all, however, is the necessity to realize that you can be assaulted even though you do nothing to encourage the offender.

What You Should Do If Attacked

No one knows how she will react when actually confronted by an attacker. Age, physical condition, previous experience and training, religious convictions, and basic personality traits, all come into play in a crisis situation.

In general, rape victims can be divided into two types. The first group is more afraid of being seriously injured than being sexually assaulted. The second group cannot bear the thought of being raped and will risk serious injury, even if the attacker has a weapon, to avoid the "fate worse than death." The response of the victim will depend upon the group to which she belongs as well as the circumstances under which the rape occurs.

One thing you must keep uppermost in your mind, however, is the fact that rape is a violent crime, and that the need to humiliate and overpower, not sexual gratification, is the motivation for the attack. This will help you to prevent panic and to think clearly and make the best decisions possible.

Some of the following tactics may be used to try to avoid the attack. A loud noise such as that made by a police whistle or a Freon horn may be enough to frighten off the attacker. Sometimes screaming will do the trick. Yell "call the police" or "fire." Do not yell "help"; no one wants to help, but almost everyone wants to see a fire. Try to be sure there is someone near enough to hear the noise or your scream. This tactic may infuriate the attacker, and if no one is there to respond, the problem may be intensified.

Stalling is another tactic that may help. Several ploys have proven to be useful. Among these is feigning a fainting attack or a convulsion. Pretending to have severe pains in the abdomen or chest may be effective. Vomiting or urinating on the attacker are other tricks that have aborted an attack.

Running to a safe place may be a successful tactic if the circumstances are favorable. However, you must be able to run fast and have a safe place to run to, one that is within a reasonable distance. If you are in an isolated area, any attempt to flee may make the situation worse by angering the rapist.

If it is impossible to avoid the attack, try not to do anything that will threaten the attacker. If you stay calm and do not antagonize him, it is usually possible to defuse his anger and should prevent any serious physical injury.

Talking may be the best way to abort an attack if it is impossible to frighten him away or escape. It is necessary to talk calmly "with" him, not "to" him. Enhance his ego. Never cry, plead, moralize, or make small talk; this may be just what he is looking for and expects to hear. Each rapist has planned the rape carefully in detail and operates within his fantasy. Therefore, if the victim can talk with him and make him see her as a person rather than as an object and himself as a worthwhile individual instead of some kind of monster, he may come to his senses and stop; the attack is over. Some women have talked about their families, religion, plans for the future; try anything to break his fantasy.

Fighting is the last tactic to use. All rapists are potentially violent and are capable of inflicting serious physical harm. If he has a weapon, he will not hesitate to use it. Many victims have been sprayed with their own mace or shot with their own guns, and several "fighters" have had broken bones and other severe physical injuries in addition to genital trauma. Fighting is not the method of choice unless you have been well trained. Surprise and speed of reaction are necessary if you are to be successful. You must be able and willing to overpower and disable the attacker because the struggle itself may enrage him and increase his violence. The risk of serious injury is definitely increased when the victim responds with physical force. Remember the emotional stimulus for rape is anger and hostility, not sex.

If an attack is inevitable, try to get it over with as easily and as quickly as possible. Submit and try to show no emotion. Although it is not necessary to cooperate, do not resist unless he is going to beat or maim you. Be alert to anything that may help to identify the man: height, weight, skin color, eye color, hair type and color, scars, language, odors, clothing. You can help the police immeasurably if you are alert and do not panic.

Remember rape is a crime and there is no more reason for you to feel embarrassed or ashamed than if you had been the victim of any other crime. You will need help because the psychological trauma of the attack, even if physical rape was not completed, can be destructive to you and others close to you. Some studies report that 50 percent of the victims are separated from the man in their life within two years after the rape.

The police should be called. (Unfortunately, because of persistent attitudes toward rape, there may be personal reasons for not wanting to call the police. For example, in one case a woman involved in a custody battle felt her husband might use the attack as evidence of her promiscuity.) Rapists are repeaters, and the police may be able to identify the attacker just from your story. It is not necessary to prosecute just because the crime is reported. The police will usually take the victim to a hospital or rape treatment facility for skilled care and will provide transportation in any case.

It is important to go "as is." No shower, bath, or douche should be taken, and the same clothes should be worn. Bed sheets, towels, and so forth should not be disturbed if the police are to be involved. The "scene" should be preserved, and all physical evidence of the attack saved.

If you do not want to call the police, call a rape crisis counselor or someone knowledgeable in crisis counseling. They will recommend a physician who will examine you and give any medical treatment that is indicated. Either the counselor or the doctor will give you the psychological support and care you need. Do not underestimate the psychic trauma of sexual assault. Rape victims have special needs. Seek help from people who have been trained to help rape victims. This skilled care is necessary if you are to survive the attack successfully and have no permanent emotional damage.

Treatment

All victims of sexual attack need care and counseling. If the problem is not dealt with properly at the time, the effects may surface weeks, months, or even years after the attack and may take longer to resolve than if it had been taken care of at the time of the incident. (Special treatment needed by children is discussed on pages 376–79.)

Comprehensive care, both medical and psychological, should be available to every victim of sexual assault. No one who does not understand the problems of these victims should be involved in their treatment. These personnel must have empathy, not sympathy, for the patient. Understanding is essential; sympathy is degrading. Rape is a legal not a medical diagnosis; therefore, no judgments should be made by the medical team.

Today most areas have some kind of treatment facility available to the rape victim. Large cities have crisis centers, and many smaller communities have volunteers who are ready to counsel victims of sexual assault. This is especially true in university towns and those cities in which the women's groups are well organized. In Miami, the Rape Treatment Center is at Jackson Memorial Hospital and a floating team concept is used to insure expertise at all hours. The team consists of a gynecologist, a nurse, and a social worker, all of whom have been trained in crisis counseling and caring for the specific needs of the victim of sexual assault.

It is absolutely necessary that the victim regain control of her life as soon as possible after the attack. She has just been through an ordeal over which she had no control. One way to accomplish this quickly is by allowing her to make any decisions that are necessary. It is essential to explain to her that even if she does not wish to report the crime, she needs a medical examination and may need medication to prevent venereal disease and pregnancy, and that she and others close to her will need some counseling if they are to handle this crisis properly and go on with their lives. However, it should be her decision whenever possible how much is to be done to and for her. Usually victims are quite willing to cooperate if this plan is followed, and they understand the reasons for the examinations and treatment.

The examination of the patient should be done with only the physician and the nurse in the room unless the patient requests the presence of

---

RAPE TREATMENT CENTER
JACKSON MEMORIAL HOSPITAL   UNIVERSITY OF MIAMI SCHOOL OF MEDICINE

ADDRESS _____   BIRTHDATE _____ RACE _____ M S W D SEP

PLACE OF EXAM _____ TIME _____   POLICE DEPT. _____ CASE # _____

PERSONAL HISTORY   OFFICER _____

PARA ___ ___ ___ ___ GR. _____   GENERAL EXAM: (bruises, trauma, lacerations, marks)

LMP: DATE _____ NORMAL ABNORMAL   NO HISTORY

LAST COITUS: DATE _____ TIME: _____

CONTRACEPTION: YES NO TYPE: _____

DOUCHE BATH DEFECATE VOID SINCE ASSAULT

VENEREAL DISEASE: YES NO TYPE_____RX_____

HEPATITIS: YES NO WHEN _____ RX _____

HISTORY OF ASSAULT _____

DATE:_____TIME:_____

LOCATION: _____

NO. OF ASSAILANTS _____ RACE: B W L O UNK   PELVIC EXAM: (include signs of trauma, bleeding, foreign bodies)

ATTACKER: KNOWN _____ UNK _____ RELATIVE _____   VULVA _____

THREATS: YES NO TYPE_____   HYMEN _____

RESTRAINTS: YES NO TYPE _____   VAGINA _____

WEAPON: YES NO TYPE _____   CERVIX _____

　　　　　ORAL ANAL VAGINAL DIGITAL FOR. BODY   FUNDUS _____

TYPE OF SEX: ___ ___ ___ ___ ___   ADNEXAE _____

PENETRATION: ___ ___ ___ ___ ___   RECTAL _____

EJACULATION: ___ ___ ___ ___ ___

COMMENTS:_____

PAGE 1 | SEXUAL BATTERY FORM

someone else. The police should never be in the room, even if they are involved.

The medical examination varies depending on the history of the attack. It is not only unnecessary, but cruel to do procedures not indicated by the history. All examinations, however, should include careful documentation of injuries, tests for gonorrhea and syphilis, and tests to see if semen is present in the vaginal canal. If the police have been called into the case, specimens such as vaginal fluid, foreign bodies, pubic hair, venous blood, and saliva, are collected as evidence. Photographs of any injuries are essential because most bruises and abrasions are healed by the time the case goes to court; the patient has no visual evidence of the attack. Severe injuries should, of course, be treated before the routine examinations are done. In several instances in our experience the specimens to be used as evidence were collected in the operating room while the patient was under anesthesia.

Prophylactic medication should be offered for sexually transmissible dis-

---

RAPE TREATMENT CENTER
MIAMI, FLORIDA
JACKSON MEMORIAL HOSPITAL   UNIVERSITY OF MIAMI SCHOOL OF MEDICINE

PHYSICIAN _____ NURSE _____ COUNSELOR _____

TESTS	TREATMENT
GC CULTURE: ORAL ANAL CERVICAL OTHER_____	V.D. PROPHYLAXIS: YES NO TYPE_____
VDRL: YES NO (5cc venous blood—red top)	PREGNANCY PROPHYLAXIS: YES NO TYPE_____
PAP TEST: YES NO	TETANUS: YES NO OTHER MEDS: _____

EVIDENTIAL SPECIMENS, TESTING AND RECEIPT

RESULTS OF PRELIMINARY TESTS: A.P.: NEGATIVE WEAK MODERATE STRONG
SPERM: NONE 1-5 6-10 10+ MOTILE NON-MOTILE

SPECIMENS OBTAINED:		GIVEN TO POLICE	OTHER TREATMENT
10 cc VENOUS BLOOD (red top) _____			X-RAY _____
FINGER NAIL SCRAPINGS _____			SURGICAL CONSULT._____
PUBIC HAIR COMBINGS_____			PSYCH. CONSULT._____
VAGINAL	{ SMEAR / SWAB _____		OTHER: (Explain) _____
CERVICAL	{ SMEAR / SWAB _____		
VAGINAL ASPIRATE _____			
RECTAL	{ SMEAR / SWAB _____		
ORAL	{ SMEAR / SWAB _____		
SALIVA SPECIMEN _____			GIVEN TO POLICE
CLOTHING (number) _____	{ TYPE / CONDITION_____		
FOREIGN BODIES (number)_____	{ TYPE / LOCATION _____		
OTHER SPECIMENS _____		PHOTOGRAPHS: YES NO TAKEN BY_____	
TOTAL NUMBER SPECIMENS _____		TOTAL TO POLICE _____	

RECEIPT OF EVIDENCE: THE ABOVE EVIDENCE HAS BEEN RECEIVED BY ME ON (DATE) _____ AT_____

(TIME) _____ (OFFICER'S SIGNATURE) _____

PHYSICIAN'S SIGNATURE: _____

WITNESS SIGNATURE _____

PAGE 2 | SEXUAL BATTERY FORM

ease (STD), and the patient should be encouraged to take it. Although the reported incidence of gonorrhea following rape is only 3 percent and of syphilis 0.1 percent, proper medical attention can ensure that neither is contracted because of a rape. If there has been abrasion of the skin, tetanus prevention may be indicated.

The incidence of pregnancy following a rape is reported as 1 percent. Despite this low risk, medication to prevent conception should be offered unless the victim is already pregnant or on a method of family planning or the assault occurred more than 72 hours before the examination. Pregnancy secondary to rape is not a pleasant prospect, and prevention is less traumatic than menstrual extraction or interruption of the pregnancy after conception has occurred. Several contraceptive methods may be offered, but the one most often used is the morning-after pill (diethylstilbestrol, or DES) or another form of estrogen. Insertion of an intrauterine device has been suggested, but this is questionable. Placing such a device is not always a simple procedure in women who have not been pregnant; in addition, any unnecessary manipulation in the vaginal area only adds to the trauma of the rape victim.

If the patient was treated with prophylactic or contraceptive medication, she should be reexamined and retested six weeks after the initial examination to be sure that she has not contracted STD or become pregnant in spite of the medication. If no antibiotics were given, the patient should be reexamined for gonorrhea two weeks after the attack.

The psychological assessment and counseling of the patient should begin as soon as the patient reaches a treatment center, although the formal counseling usually occurs after the physical examination. The doctor, nurse, and counselor evaluate the victim's mental state and her ability to cope with the situation as they talk with her.

The rape experience precipitates a crisis, and the trauma fits within the framework of the general crisis theory. A crisis is an event that produces stress and comes with suddenness; there is no opportunity to prepare for the emergency. The reaction of the rape victim is similar to that seen when one deals with grief. However, in addition to the deep sense of loss that the rape victim experiences, she must also deal with the emotions resulting from the threats to her safety and the invasion of her body. The loss of self-esteem and the threats to her relationships with others close to her only add to her difficulties. An inability to develop or recapture her sense of self-worth and realize that she is a worthwhile person is one of the long-term problems of a rape victim that can jeopardize her future success.

It is reassuring when the victim can talk with a counselor and find that the emotions and reactions that she is having are the same as those of other women who have been sexually assaulted and that she is not the only victim who has felt that way.

In the post-rape syndrome described by several investigators, the victim goes through three stages of recovery: the acute stage, the outward adjustment stage, and the integration stage. The length of time needed to pass through these stages may vary with the basic personality and previous experiences of the victim, but all rape victims go through these steps.

During the acute stage the woman experiences a gamut of emotions including shock, anger, fear, hostility, disbelief that it could happen to her, and often denial that it did happen. It is essential that she receive practical help as well as medical and psychological support during this time.

Some of the practical problems that must be dealt with are whether she will tell her family or friends, where she will stay, if she needs money, whether she will report it to the police. All these things must be dealt with almost immediately after the attack.

She may have many physical complaints that will persist for weeks after the attack. Some of these are headaches due to the tension, inability to sleep, nightmares, abdominal pains, loss of appetite, and even nausea. Usually all these somatic complaints are the result of the psychological trauma she has experienced. It is important to make her realize that she is not to blame for the attack and that the offender is a criminal to be caught and punished.

It is during this first phase that it is so important that family and friends provide adequate support and that, if there is a special man in her life, he be understanding and realize the sexual fears she may have. If no one is available to understand and support her during this early phase, the victim may become disorganized, that is, be unable to regain a healthy self-image and thus be unable to function or relate to others as she did before the attack.

The outward adjustment stage is the period during which the patient seems to be doing well, sometimes too well. She resumes her life, returns to work or school, and is apparently adjusting to and coping with the trauma. It is common during this phase for the patient to suppress her feelings, and she may be depressed. She may try to forget that the assault ever happened, and unless she is forced to, she may not face the problem and may stay in limbo for weeks. The longer this phase persists, the more difficult it is for the patient to begin the reorganization process.

Once the patient has faced the problem, she begins the integration stage. This is the period during which resolution of the rape experience takes place, and it may be several months or even years before this phase is completed. It is common for a patient to change her residence and telephone number in an effort to prevent the attacker from finding her and perhaps doing it again. She may seldom go out alone even during the daylight hours. The support of friends and family is again essential. The counselor encourages the victim to seek support, but at the same time expresses confidence that she will again be able to function at least as well as she did before the assault.

During this period the woman is willing to discuss her experience and can talk about it without becoming distraught. She may even be angry and be eager to punish the offender. However she reacts, she is ready to face her anxieties and verbalize her fears; she is ready to recover and return to her world.

If the woman decides to prosecute the offender, she will need ongoing support from her family and from the police and prosecutors. The court procedures are not easy, and it is difficult to win rape cases if the victim is young and pretty and has not had serious physical injuries. The police investigation is often long and tedious. The actual trial does not take place until months after the attack. It is impossible for the victim to resolve the experience and get on with her life until the trial is over. However, many victims, once they realize that the rapist is a criminal and repeats his crime over and over, are quite willing to prosecute and try to send him to jail "so he can't do this to another woman."

Women who decide to prosecute the rapist should look at themselves as trail blazers. Five years ago the case would not have gone to court; ten years ago no one would have listened to them at all.

Sexual Abuse of Children

Sexual molestation of children under the age of 16 is something about which we know very little. Until recently the literature has been sparse, and much of the information remains entwined with myth and error. Molestation may involve a range of sexual contact from touching to intercourse. Although physical force may be used, the attack may also be accomplished because of the child's lack of comprehension of the act and habits of obedience to and trust of older individuals.

It is estimated that at least 350,000 cases of child sexual abuse occur in the United States each year. Only a few are reported. Some authors feel that about 80 percent of the attacks known to the parents are never reported to the authorities unless there has been physical injury. Parents are loath to report because of their desire to save the child and the family from the stigma that sexual assault and rape still carry. Again, sexual assault is violence, not a sex act per se, and no one need be ashamed of being a victim of this crime.

In most instances the offender is known to the child. There is some indication that in cases involving the very young (under the age of 4), at least 90 percent of the offenders are known to the child. This percentage decreases as the age of the child increases, but at any age the attacker is most often a member of the family (incest), a friend, or someone in a supervisory capacity. Again, the numbers are based on limited information because cases are not reported to the police and parents do not always seek medical help. In small children there seldom is physical trauma because fondling is the chief method used by the child molester. Even if there has been physical trauma to the child, many parents do not take the child to a hospital or doctor, in order to keep the assault secret. Families that do go to the hospital tend to be limited to lower socioeconomic classes.

Once the problem has been uncovered, the medical examination is one of the main concerns of the family and the authorities. The parents are anxious to know whether or not their son or daughter has been violated. The police are looking for physical evidence of an assault.

The examination can be frightening for the child unless it is done with care. It should never be hurried, and the approach varies with the age of the child. The smaller child will behave much better if the mother is in the room and, if the procedures are explained, will cooperate so that the necessary things can be done. Speculum examinations are usually not necessary in the case of small children, and cotton swabs can be used to collect evidence from the vulvar and vaginal areas. If any extensive, detailed examination is needed to see if there has been severe trauma, the child should be examined under an anesthetic. Restraining her is the same as raping her. As in the adult, prophylactic medication should be given for STD and tetanus when indicated.

The adolescent must also be treated carefully. Victims in this age group are often resistant to examination and may refuse to answer any questions about the assault. It is necessary to gain their confidence if they are to be helped. Adolescents generally behave much better if the parent is not in the room. The examination is similar to the one done on the adult, including prophylactic and contraceptive medication.

Skilled counseling is essential in all cases of sexual assault, but it is absolutely essential in those cases dealing with children because the entire family needs help. Both parents and child need help to cope with this crisis in their lives. It is important to develop communication and understanding among the family members or there may be irreparable damage.

The rape trauma syndrome, with its short-term and long-term phases, is similar in children and adults. If there has been no physical injury, the younger child will usually recover and be relatively problem free. The parents of a younger child will need the counseling. However, the older child will need counseling even if there has been no physical damage. The behavior of all child victims must be monitored for a long period of time because a child's reactions to stress are usually nonverbal, for example, bed wetting, nausea and vomiting, anxieties, embarrassment, withdrawal. Any behavioral changes should be investigated by skilled personnel.

The reactions of parents to the sexual assault of their child varies greatly. The crisis may precipitate problems within the family that were marginally controlled before the assault. Adults are often unable to cope with the problem of rape because they have never been able to handle any issues related to sexuality.

Many become irrational and act as though the child is "soiled" or "damaged goods"; some parents have actually used those terms in front of the child. Many tend to blame the child for allowing the assault to occur, and if the incidents have continued over a period of time, they accuse the child of encouraging the molester. While it is true that some children seem to exhibit seductive behavior, the child is not responsible because he or she has no real comprehension of the act and its significance to the adult mind. If anything, the child is looking for love and favors.

Often parents blame each other because there is a need to blame someone during the acute phase of the reaction. They are angry and feel guilty because they were unable to protect the child at all times. They may be overprotective because of their guilt and concern or they may discipline the child unfairly. A common reaction is "I don't believe you," which to the child means "I won't help you," and the child feels betrayed and psychologically abandoned. The parents should be reassured that permanent scars are unnecessary if the situation is handled intelligently. Best results are obtained when the parents trust and believe the child until proven otherwise. Children seldom lie about this situation. The parents then should be able to discuss the incident with the child and try to prevent a recurrence of the experience.

Incest may be narrowly defined as coitus between close blood relatives, although in our society it is extended to include as well any form of sexual contact between members of a family, including relatives such as stepchild and stepparent. The problems consequent to molestation by a stranger or friend are compounded and made more intense by the interfamily relationship.

It is accepted fact that there are invariably three people involved in incest situations. The mother, for example, is almost always aware of the situation but refuses to believe that such a thing could be happening in her family and makes no conscious effort to stop the assaults. There is more guilt on the part of the child in incest situations because the interfamily relationships have been upset. The mother often blames the child for seducing the father and often forces the child to leave home. If the father is arrested, the economic level of the family is usually lowered. The mother may have to get a job or the family may be forced to go on welfare. Other members and siblings may blame the victim for causing these changes in their standard of living. Therefore, it is necessary to look at all the aspects of the situation before any plans can be made to manage these cases.

Prosecution is difficult in child molestation cases because there is seldom any physical evidence, and the child is often considered to be a poor witness. When cases do come to trial, the courts try to protect the child as much as possible. Sometimes the cases are heard in the judge's chambers or the courtroom may be cleared of visitors when the child is testifying.

The parents should prepare the child for the court appearance because it can terrify a youngster. Family support is the key if the child is to have no permanent damage from the experience.

SPOUSE ABUSE

Spouse abuse is a subject that has received attention only recently. Although it is not a new phenomenon, it has usually been ignored except as a source of humor for cartoonists and comedians. Because this type of violence occurs within the home, it is generally considered a matter of private, rather than public concern.

Although wife beating has received more publicity, husband beating is just as serious a problem. In *The Violent Home: A Study of Physical Aggression Between Husbands and Wives* (Beverly Hills, Calif.: Sage, 1974), Richard J. Gelles' study of 80 families, he found that 22 percent of spouses were assaulted on a regular basis; 47 percent of husbands had hit their wives at least once, and 11 percent hit them regularly; 32 percent of the wives had hit their husbands at least once, and 11 percent hit them regularly. In most of the families, wives who realized that if they persisted in an argument they were going to be physically abused, kept arguing anyway. Most husbands and wives felt that they hit their spouse only when she or he deserved it, and in most instances both parties considered their actions to be well within the realm of normal behavior for married couples.

There is little doubt that the pattern of family violence is learned in childhood and that it is reinforced by the outside world through stereotyped imagery in mass media and social interaction. The stereotyped masculine hero uses physical violence to achieve his objectives and is successful. Therefore, violence is not only acceptable, but to be admired.

The data supports the theory that family violence is a learned response. Almost all the husbands came from homes in which there had been physical abuse between their father and mother. Although the connection was not as common in the case of the wives, many of them did come from violent homes. Both husbands and wives in this group came from families in which physical punishment was used regularly to discipline the children. Since parents serve as powerful role models, this behavior teaches their children not only that violence is a useful and effective way to accomplish desired behavior, but also that it is morally correct.

Another thing that the child learns from violence within the immediate family is that males are stronger than females and that if a battle is lost verbally, it may be won through the use of physical force. The male child learns from watching his mother's reaction that she is afraid of the father, even if they do not fight physically. He may apply this knowledge in adulthood by using violence or the threat of violence to maintain superiority over family members whose traditional rank is subordinate to his and to control those who challenge his authority.

Although the middle class tends to identify family violence with lower income status and ethnic minorities, family violence is not limited by economic class or social status. In one study at least 20 percent of the people questioned approved of slapping one's spouse if the occasion were appropriate, and approval of this type of behavior increased as the income and educational levels increased. Perhaps violence within the family seems more common among the poor because more of these cases become police matters; the affluent are better able to keep the incident from becoming public knowledge.

Family violence does not appear to be related to early adjustment problems during a marriage, but instead seems to result from problems that occur during the relationship over a period of time. The group having the greatest amount of violence was from 41 to 50 years of age and married for several years. There was an inverse relationship between the husband's educational level and the amount of violence; the opposite was true for women.

The relationship between alcohol and abuse is not clear. Some studies by law enforcement agencies show that alcohol was the primary cause in only 14 percent of the cases, and the police felt that in some cases alcohol may have a calming effect to reduce the incidence of violence in a family quarrel.

Throughout the years the wife has been considered to be the "property" of the husband and this has led society to allow husbands the right to physically punish their wives. The woman has been trapped in the violent relationship because of the sexist orientation of our culture. She has been largely responsible for child-rearing and has been unable to leave the home without jeopardizing her right to economic support because she "deserted the bed and board." Since ours is largely a "couples" society, she also loses her social status. Groups no longer include her because she is a "single." Clubs do not carry her on their roster because the membership is in her husband's name.

Next to acceptance of the learned response of violence, economic survival is perhaps the most important reason that the battered wife does not leave home. Many women have been conditioned since childhood to have no expectation for a career and therefore are not trained for employment. A woman still has fewer job opportunities than a man and often earns less holding a similar job. Since she is usually responsible for an unequal portion of the childcare, her time is more limited and therefore her earning further restricted.

Even a court award of child support to the woman with children who does leave is no guarantee of economic stability. Fewer than half the husbands comply even during the first year, and efforts to make the fathers contribute are not only expensive but often futile. She, therefore, feels bound to stay for the economic good of the children. Wives who are fully dependent upon their husbands for financial support often feel they can not even call for help. They need some kind of job and strong psychological support before they can find the courage to break away.

However, if she stays, the children's psychological well-being and her own suffer, for no one thrives in a violent home environment. Most individuals involved develop multiple complaints; headaches, gastrointestinal disturbances, and chronic fatigue are common. The wives often have nightmares and are almost always depressed. The children usually have emotional problems which may manifest themselves as "illnesses" or sleep problems; aggressive behavior is common, especially in the boys.

Shelters for battered women and programs to give them and their children emotional support and financial aid are now functioning in some areas of our nation. The office on Domestic Violence, an agency in the Department of Health and Human Services, serves as an information center for sources of federal aid available to such programs. Unfortunately, this help is limited to larger cities and areas which have received some sort of grant money and is usually available only for the short-term period of the crisis. What is needed is funding for long-term counseling and adequate monetary assistance so that the mother and her children can stay together and survive until she can make arrangements. The entire family will need counseling and in some cases psychotherapy may be indicated if the family is ever to live as an intact unit again. Any mental health therapy is costly and long-term.

Spouse abuse and especially wife beating is a hidden crime in our society. Few women will admit that their husbands beat them and almost no husbands will acknowledge that this physical violence is an issue in their marriages. Until family violence is recognized to be a common occurrence in our culture and until the people realize that this abuse results in long-term disabilities and extensive socioeconomic problems for all involved parties including the children, no significant effort will be made to solve the problem.

CONCLUSION

The sources of the increasing violence throughout our society are frustration, anger, and hostility. If we realize this and learn to recognize the developing tensions, we may be able to manage them before they overwhelm the individuals and erupt in the violent crime and problems discussed here.

Until that day comes, however, it is essential that men and women understand the underlying reasons for sexual assault, child abuse, and spouse abuse. We all must learn that these are crimes, and the victims will need skilled counseling in addition to any necessary medical treatment if they are to return to their normal activities and function in an efficient and organized manner. Only understanding will enable individuals to protect themselves against these offenders, and only understanding the problem will produce juries which will reach proper and just conclusions when offenders are brought to trial.

FURTHER READING

Bard, M., and D. Sangrey. *The Crime Victim's Book.* New York: Basic Books, 1979.

Brownmiller, S. *Against Our Will: Men, Women and Rape.* New York: Simon and Schuster, 1975.

Burgess, A. W. and L. L. Holmstrom. *Rape: Victims of Crisis.* Bowie, Md.: Bradys, 1974.

Halpern, S., D. J. Hicks, and T. Crenshaw. *Rape: Helping the Victim.* Oradel, N.J.: Medical Economics Book Co., 1978.

Hicks, D. J. "Rape: Sexual Assault," *Obstetrics & Gynecology Annual* 4 (1978): 447–465.

Hicks, D. J. "Rape: A Crime of Violence," *Contemporary OB/GYN* 11 (1978): 67–78.

Hilberman, E. *The Rape Victim.* New York: Basic Books, 1976.

Hirschowitz, R. G. "Crisis Theory: A Formulation," *Psychiatric Annals* 3 (1973): 36–47.

Sutherland, S., and D. J. Scherl. "Patterns of Response Among Victims of Rape," *American Journal of Orthopsychiatry* 40 (1970): 503–510.

"Uniform Crime Reports: Crime in the United States." Washington, D.C.: Federal Bureau of Investigation, 1977.

Viano, Emilio, ed. "Spouse Abuse." *Victimology: An International Journal* 2, no. 3/4 (1977–1978).

Viano, Emilio, ed. "Child Abuse and Neglect." *Victimology: An International Journal* 2, no. 2 (1977).

Your Mind and Feelings— Mental and Emotional Health

JOAN J. ZILBACH, M.D.
Associate Clinical Professor of Psychiatry,
Tufts University School of Medicine, Boston, Massachusetts
Co-Director, Family Therapy and Research Program,
Judge Baker Guidance Center, Harvard Medical School,
Boston, Massachusetts

I could barely heave myself out of bed this morning. I was furious when Tommy couldn't find his shoes when he was getting ready for school, and I just snapped at a colleague in the office. Now I have a headache. I wonder if I have the flu. No, I know I don't. I wonder if I'm falling apart.

Should I do something about how I feel? How do I feel? What should I do?

Do I need help?

Every woman at some time feels this way. Most often she will dismiss the vague concern about her feelings, but sometimes she may try to answer the questions raised by these feelings. She is, in effect, trying to determine the state of her mental health.

We all learn to deal quite directly with our body's responses to physical injury or common illnesses. After you have bumped into the corner of a table, the sight of the bruise is expected and not disturbing. If you've dug out a garden bed or spent a day handling a crisis in the office, you are not concerned about feeling tired at night. You may have been miserably uncomfortable with your last cold, but you knew you didn't have a serious illness.

Understanding what is happening to you, knowledge of physical reactions, past experience with similar situations, and realistic expectations of how your body will feel in such situations allows you to evaluate the state of your physical health. You are able to recognize healthy body reactions and temporary reactions to unusual situations. You can distinguish these reactions from signs of illness which may require treatment beyond the normal self-corrective mechanisms of the body.

A similar understanding of how the healthy mind functions and how it responds to different conditions is necessary to assess the state of your mental health. Unfortunately, much of what we learn about emotions and feelings dwells on mental illness rather than on mental health. The source of much of what is known about emotions is the study of cases in which something has gone awry. We may learn that certain behaviors or responses accompany certain types of disturbances or that certain conditions contributed to their development. However, it is not always made clear that the presence of similar responses or conditions does not mean that the disturbance is necessarily present. For example, it has been observed that children suffering from certain types of emotional problems do not like to fingerpaint; it does not follow that any child who does not fingerpaint is suffering from these problems.

Emotional health is more difficult to describe than physical health because it is harder to identify the causes of emotional responses than of physical responses. They are rarely as clearcut as the blow to your leg or the cold virus. Also, the responses are highly variable. A particular event may trigger a strong response in one person and almost none at all in another; for one person the same event in different circumstances or at different stages of life may produce different responses.

Added to these difficulties are the current popular psychologies and sales pitches that promise to make you happy, anxiety free, aggressive, and successful, implying that these are the signs of mental health, and that if you do not display these signs, something is wrong with you and you had better get help. Quick and easy help is then offered in the form of the purchase of a new book, a new self-development program, or a new therapeutic technique.

We cannot here explore questions of the nature of the mind or the complexity of its functioning. We can, however, attempt to define a state of mental health, describe some normal processes of the healthy mind, indicate some signs of illness, and provide a guide to sources of help.

DEFINITION OF MENTAL HEALTH

Mental or emotional health can be defined as the ability to handle the stresses, tensions, and anxieties of daily life with sufficient equilibrium to maintain daily activities and to participate in relationships. A complementary definition is the ability to love, work, and play.

Stress in its most general sense means a force which exerts pressure (presses on) or which strains (pulls on) an object and by such force tends to deform the object, that is, tends to change its shape. So we can think of stress as a force which changes the body from its normal state. For example, the corner of the table exerts pressure on the tissue of your leg, and the physical exertion of gardening makes your heart and other organs function at a rate greater than they do at rest. In emotional terms, too, stress can be understood to mean the presence of an event or condition which elicits an extraordinary response from the individual, which makes her feel or behave in a way different from her established patterns of response. Conflict is the opposition between these established patterns and the pressure to deviate from them.

Stress may arise from obvious events in the individual's environment, for example, loss of a job or death of a spouse. It may also arise from psychological or physiological processes. Although external events may be easier to identify than internal processes, the two categories cannot really be separated. In most cases the external event, stressful in itself, triggers the internal processes as well. For example, the loss of a job represents obvious cause for concern in practical matters, but it may also involve diminished self-esteem, threats to the self-image, arousal of unresolved hostility toward authority figures, and so forth. Each person's temperament and history determine which events will be stressful and the degree of response they will elicit. (In this chapter we talk about how the individual handles stress rather than the psychological process by which a particular event comes to be stressful for that individual.)

Tension is response to stress. It may be expressed emotionally as a feeling of striving or fear and is most often expressed physically as feeling restless or "knotted up." The response may range from positive feelings, such as heightened energy, to negative feelings, such as distress or pain resulting from a sense of danger or need.

Anxiety is that form of tension in which the condition creating stress is not fully known, a feeling of danger or threat in which the danger cannot be clearly identified. Fear is the response to an explicit, known danger— either external (a car swerving into your path) or internal (a phobia).

It is important to emphasize that our definition of mental health does *not* imply an absence of stress. Stress in one form or another is inevitable in every area and at every stage of life. Nor does the definition imply an absence of response to stress, that is, an absence of tension or anxiety. Sufficient equilibrium does not mean an absence of conflict, but the ability either to resolve conflict or to function in the presence of unresolved conflict. Mental health includes the ability to continue activities and relationships in the presence of tension and anxiety.

Normal Tension and Anxiety

Within this definition levels of tension which do not interfere with functioning can be seen as a normal reaction to stress, not a sign of emotional malfunction. Returning to the physical analogy, the rush of blood to the site of the bruise is part of the healing process; fatigue after exertion allows the body to regain its strength and prevents overexertion. We know that a voluntary muscle that is never tensed atrophies; we have learned that the strength and stamina of the heart are improved by periodic subjection to stress.

If stress is a force that creates change or demands a new or different response, tension then can be interpreted as a sign of resistance to that change. By this response the healthy mind can maintain its integrity. If there were no resistance, we would simply be at the mercy of any pressure. At the other extreme of response is the inability to make any adjustment, even if the change might be beneficial. Tension is the means by which the mind maintains its balance in the face of opposing forces until the conflict between them is resolved.

Of course, we are not saying that it is healthful to live in a constant state of tension. We are simply trying to defuse the word, to point out a positive function it might serve, so that the presence of tension does not in itself become a cause for anxiety, and so that you can accept in yourself a normal level of tension and distinguish it from a serious disturbance.

The signs of tension are familiar to all of us. Emotional and physiological signs are so closely interconnected that it is impossible to separate them. At a low level of stress, a low-level response of increased heart and respiration rates may be experienced as a mild energetic feeling, while in a fear reaction or anxiety attack these same responses are intensified and are clearly observed as palpitations and rapid or difficult breathing. Certain parts of the body are particularly susceptible to these effects. The most common physiological reactions to tension include "queasiness" in the stomach, diarrhea or constipation as the intestines are affected, stiff neck from tightness of muscles in the neck and upper back, and headache from the constriction and subsequent dilation of blood vessels.

Another common sign of tension is a depressed feeling, the "blues." Just as the sensation of fatigue helps to prevent muscle strain, so perhaps the feeling of "not wanting to do anything" may be a way of slowing us down to keep the effects of stress under control. A day of sleep, a "good cry," a period of withdrawal from involvement, although experienced as an unpleasant "down" feeling, can still be interpreted as part of the spectrum of normal response to stress.

The current tendency to "pop a pill"—a tranquilizer, an antidepressant, or the latest psychological "help" movement—rests on the assumption that any anxiety is a sign of illness and that somehow we are never supposed to be uncomfortable or "unhappy." But we do experience stress, and under the influence of this kind of thinking, the normal, appropriate, and healthy reactions involved in the maintenance of equilibrium come to be perceived by us as illness. Recurrent or persistent severe physical symptoms or prolonged periods of depression are symptoms which should be investigated, but an occasional tension headache or "blue" day can certainly be accepted as within the range of expected responses to stress.

Universal Stresses—Individual and Family Life Cycles

In our definition of mental health we use the term "stresses of daily life." These include not only random events and stresses peculiar to each individual, but also stresses which accompany different stages in the human life cycle. Once we begin to think of stress and tension in terms of pressure to change and response to that pressure, it becomes clear that transitions from one stage of life to the next are necessarily periods of increased stress for everyone.

These transition points within the life cycle of an individual have been called "developmental crises" and "critical steps" to emphasize the inevitable and universal stress that accompanies them.

1. Birth—transition into life outside the uterus.
2. Infancy—acquisition of skills of physical survival, learning to eat, to walk, and so forth.
3. Toddler—first experiences of autonomy and steps away from mother.
4. Childhood—movement from the home into the larger community through school.
5. Adolescence—identification of self as separate from family, efforts toward competence and independence.
6. Young adulthood—establishment of one's own household or family; search for life's work.
7. Middle adulthood—time of reappraisal in the light of a perception of limited time left for the rest of one's life.
8. Old adulthood—adaptation to altered physical and social conditions.

The family also goes through a series of stages.

1. Coming together as a couple.
2. Forming a household.
3. New member joins the family (child, in-law, etc.).
4. Movement of family members (child, in-law, etc.) into larger community.
5. Departure of family members.

6. Smaller family unit—or possible extended family (grandparenthood).
7. Death of spouse; end of family unit.

The transition of the entire family through these stages produces inevitable stress on all family members, while at the same time each member is experiencing his or her own individual life cycle transitions.

In this chapter we want only to identify the major points of transition and emphasize their universality. (Some of the physiological, psychological, and social complexities involved are described in the next three chapters and in sources listed under Further Reading at the end of this chapter.) Being aware that these are difficult periods for everyone can help you to handle tensions in yourself and to understand the problems of others, particularly family members, as they pass through individual and family life cycles.

MECHANISMS TO MAINTAIN EQUILIBRIUM

Defense and coping mechanisms are the mind's way of dealing with conflict. Defense mechanisms are internal processes for handling stress and anxiety. Their operation within the conscious and subconscious mind is complex, but we can here mention some of the types of processes involved: denial, refusal to admit that the stressful situation or tension relating to it exists; sublimation, transformation of responses into a more acceptable form; projection, attribution of one's own feelings to others; reaction-formation, development of an opposite reaction to an impulse; intellectualization, attempt to give rational form to responses to minimize intense feelings associated with them; counterphobic reaction, deliberate involvement in a fear- or anxiety-producing situation.

Coping mechanisms are methods of dealing directly with the stressful situation and actions taken to relieve tension. Techniques of coping with stress include changing position in relation to the stress situation, information gathering, maintaining flexible attitudes, and redirecting energies.

Changing one's position is often the most easily accomplished. If you are afraid of living over a seismic fault, moving to another location will relieve that tension; if you don't get along with your boss, a new job will remove that source of stress. However, if the source of the stress has not been accurately identified, the geographical cure (moving from California), the new husband, or the new job will turn out to be ineffective.

Information gathering—location, clarification, and verification—is a more effective approach. Can you locate the source of the stress (is it your job or an unrelated anxiety)? Can you clarify the situation (does the boss make the job unpleasant or is the job not satisfying)? Can you verify the appropriateness of your response (is your boss really impossible to work with, for you and for others, or have you misread her or him or contributed to the conflict)?

A most important aspect of handling stress is flexibility, or the ability to respond or change your response in terms of good information gathering. Many people have rigid, automatic reactions to some kinds of situations; after an initial perception of possible conflict or danger, they do not pause to observe the situation or to examine their reactions. For example, upon hearing a stranger say that her husband's employer was about to fire a few men, Mrs. X immediately became tense, assumed her husband would lose his job, and became totally absorbed in worry that he would not be able to get another. Her automatic reaction precluded information gathering and the intensity of her reaction made it impossible for her to view the situation realistically, to consider alternatives, and to anticipate options. Anticipation allows one to plan and thereby lessen the impact of inevitable stress.

In the course of dealing with stress everyone develops techniques to allay tension through a redirection of energy. For example, some women work their way out of a depression by putting more effort into a current office project, by writing or painting, by digging in the garden, by going shopping, or by taking naps. These actions may or may not be related directly to the stressful situation or to an anxious response, but they do serve to reduce the tension, certainly have none of the possible adverse effects of taking unnecessary medication, and may in fact have productive results which are beneficial to self-esteem.

Most people are not able to cope with stress entirely on their own throughout their lives. The ability to turn to others for support is another important aspect of maintaining equilibrium. Talking about a problem is likely to be much more helpful than taking a pill. The pill may make the feeling go away temporarily, but talking may provide not only relief from tension, but also needed support and an opportunity to gather information that can help you cope with distress. Trying to think your way through some of these problems by yourself can be difficult or even self-defeating if automatic reactions limit your view. It's easy in isolation to begin to think that others seem to cope better and to function better and that you are somehow at fault. In an exchange with a friend you may both find out that what you think of as your particular problem is actually quite common (neither of you has produced the world's first 2½-year-old monster; they're all like that); that others experience their own form of tension in similar situations (either you're not so sick or at least you're as normal as everyone else). You can provide verification for each other and confirmation that it is rational to be concerned about a particular problem. Thus, in turning to another for support, you may find that at the same time you can also give support.

It is encouraging to notice that our definition of mental health turns out to be somewhat circular, the means and the goals tend to blur in the process of functioning. If you turn to a friend for support to maintain equilibrium, you have begun to participate in relationships. If you relieve some of your tension in work, you are remaining active. Every person develops individual mechanisms and techniques for dealing with conflict. If yours work to keep you functioning with equilibrium, then you have found a way to deal healthily with stress. It is only when a mechanism doesn't work or when it becomes the only means to maintain equilibrium and replaces or interferes with the activities and relationships it is designed to support that the question of impaired mental health arises.

IMPAIRED MENTAL HEALTH

Stress Overload

Even though normally you may deal quite effectively with tension and a temporary feeling of imbalance, there are times when your ability to handle stress seems to diminish and there is a restriction of daily activities and relationships. You accept the presence of a bruise as a normal body reaction, but you also know that extreme pain or a failure of the tissue after a reasonable time to return to its normal state is a sign of some disorder. The slowness of healing may be due to an inadequacy of the self-corrective mechanisms of the body or to the severity of the blow. So, too, emotional disequilibrium can result from a failure to develop effective mechanisms to handle daily stress or from a situation of extraordinary stress.

A single, traumatic event beyond the limits of normal daily stress, such as rape, the death of a child, or mastectomy, in itself may be expected to create an equilibrium disturbance. Or, an overload may result from the coincidence of several stressful events at once. For example, a woman who might be able to handle her transition from young to middle adulthood with minimum disruption may arrive at that point in her life at the same time her family moves into a crisis stage, other family members approach individual crises, and an elderly parent has a serious illness. Too many such crises at once are likely to upset anyone's equilibrium.

No one can predict the point at which an overload will occur for herself or others. As we have said, we cannot anticipate which events will be stressful or the strength of our response to them. Just as each individual has a threshold of physical pain which may change under different physiological and psychological circumstances, so each individual has a threshold of psychic pain.

Effects of Overload—Signs of Imbalance

What are some of the signs of overload? Perhaps you begin to notice that minor events seem to elicit a more intense response compared to your previous responses to similar situations, that you do not seem to get over things as quickly as you used to, that you seem to be less effective in your activities. The point of overload is the point at which you feel overwhelmed by events, because you cannot discharge the tension they create, and you begin to experience serious psychic pain.

DEPRESSION

The word depression has a wide range of meanings from the brief "down" feeling we have described to a form of severe mental illness. To distinguish it from ordinary "blues," we can describe a depressive state as profound feelings of sadness, discouragement, or self-deprecation. The depression may express itself in crying spells, sleeplessness, agitation, expressions of anxiety, fear of being left alone, and severe loss of appetite. Or it may take the almost opposite form of withdrawal into extreme fatigue, long hours of sleep, unwillingness to talk to anyone, and serious overeating. It may also be masked by excessive activity or by excessive consumption of alcohol or other drugs.

There is a difference between a depressive episode and depressive illness. An episode of depression quite frequently follows an extraordinarily stressful event which involves a significant loss to the individual—the loss of a loved one, as in the death of a spouse, or the loss of self-definition, as in a debilitating illness. Almost anyone is likely to go through such a state if the stresses are sufficiently acute. If an individual's mechanisms to maintain equilibrium are generally effective, she may need extra support and guidance for a while, but she will usually recover from the episode with time.

A depressive illness is a condition of continuing disequilibrium in which a person may not be able to recover from the depression induced by a severe stress or may experience frequent and persistent periods of depression with no identifiable cause. The seriousness of the illness is related to the degree to which the symptoms interfere with daily activities and the intensity of feelings experienced in the depressive state.

PSYCHOSOMATIC ILLNESS

We have already given examples of some physiological responses to states of tension. When tension continues unabated for considerable periods of time, physiological responses which were mild and transitory may become more severe and chronic, may cause more long-lasting malfunctions, and may eventually damage the body.

EMOTIONS AND THE BODY

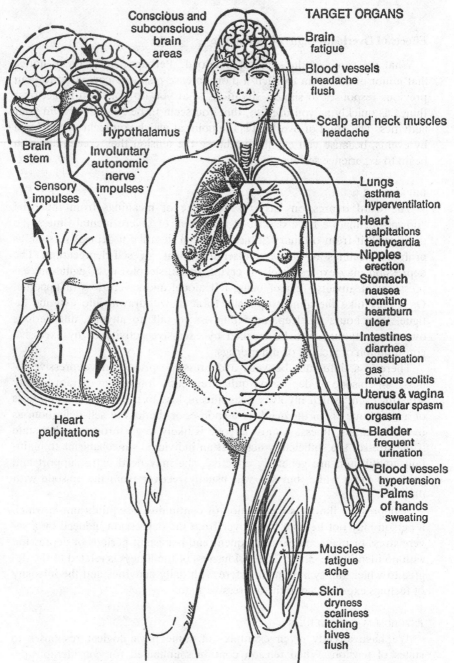

Emotions, whether pleasurable or stressful, activate brain areas which may send involuntary impulses to target organs. In the spot drawing (left) involuntary impulses make the heart beat rapidly and heavily. If this causes worry, the impulses are reinforced, thus perpetuating the cycle.

The term psychosomatic (from *psyche,* "mind," and *soma,* "body") refers to the interaction between emotional states and the condition of the body. Although the exact electrochemical mechanism is not fully understood, it seems to be clear that emotional states activate areas of the brain, thus stimulating the autonomic nervous system to "send" nerve impulses to susceptible parts of the body. For example, the stimulation of the stomach, which produces the "queasy" feeling, over a long period may begin to produce malfunctions such as hyperacidity (heartburn) or recurrent nausea and vomiting. Continued and increased stimulation may lead to actual tissue damage, ulceration of the stomach lining. Resulting pain and concern about the malfunction causes additional tension which further increases the involuntary impulses. (Effects on other organs are shown in the illustration.)

The susceptibility of an organ to the effects of tension is determined by a number of psychic and nonpsychic factors, most of which are still unknown. Some of the factors may be congenital, some may possibly be genetic, but most seem to reflect psychic conditioning, mainly during childhood and adolescence, and thus may be described as familial. For example, someone brought up in a family that is very concerned about bowel function may develop chronic constipation or recurrent diarrhea. Whatever the origin of these disorders, the effects and symptoms are similar and thus the treatment of the symptoms is generally the same. However, to enhance the treatment and to prevent recurrences of the symptoms, the primary cause should be identified if possible and treated appropriately. Therefore, when the problem is psychosomatic, psychological investigation and treatment of the emotional disequilibrium are essential.

Neurosis

Neurosis is another term with a wide range of meaning. In popular use it may be applied to any activity considered unusual, while a neurologist might specify its meaning as a functional nervous disorder with no physical lesion. Every school of psychology probably has its own variation of meaning. In relation to our definition of mental health we can see neurosis as a disorder of the mind resulting from unresolved internal conflicts and ineffective mechanisms to maintain equilibrium. A neurosis may affect or impair the individual's activities, relationships to others, and relationship to self, but it is generally not accompanied by a total inability to participate or by a loss of contact with reality.

In discussing mental health the question of degree should be considered. For example, in our list of defense mechanisms we mentioned reaction-formation. A case of such a mechanism is the development of a compulsion to neatness and cleanliness as a means to avoid anxiety. A woman who finds she "feels better" after she has collected the debris left around by her children has perhaps found a healthful technique to relieve tension. A woman who in a moment of heightened tension stops other activities to clean house may be displaying an incident of neurotic behavior. However, the woman who cannot stand to have anything out of place or who is fastidious beyond a rational standard of cleanliness to the degree that it interferes with daily activities can be said to have a neurosis. The tendency to display neurotic behavior increases as internal and external stresses increase, while neurosis has a continuing effect on all behavior because it is the expression of a continuing high level of internal stress.

Severe Mental Illness and Psychosis

"Nervous breakdown" is a popular, nonspecific term used to label anything from a moderate emotional disturbance to insanity. Most generally, it is used to indicate any failure of normal mental processes to a point where an individual can no longer function in her environment. But this description still encompasses a wide range of disorders from extreme neurotic symptoms to psychosis.

Serious mental disorder is present when the signs of disequilibrium are so severe as to disrupt almost totally the maintenance of daily activities and participation in relationships. Psychosomatic illness may be debilitating or life-threatening; an individual may become absorbed in depressed thoughts; compulsive behavior may severely limit participation in other activities.

A psychosis is a specific mental illness characterized by loss of contact with reality and disintegration of personality; a disconnection between the inner person and the real world is expressed in bizarre and antisocial feelings and behavior. It is this disconnection that distinguishes psychoses ("insanity") from other forms of mental disorders. The term psychotic is used to describe the behavior of a person who has a psychosis; sometimes the term is given a more general application to indicate a disorder which totally interrupts functioning for a period of time. For example, in what is termed psychotic depression the expression of the illness—withdrawal, agitation, or other symptoms—replaces almost all other activities.

There are specific clinical definitions of the different types of psychoses. The most common are manic-depressive psychosis and schizophrenia. Manic-depressive psychosis is characterized by mood swings from high elation and delusions of grandeur to brooding depression, feelings of persecution, and often a distorted sense of body appearance. The definition of schizophrenia is not as clear and is the subject of some controversy. In a general sense it is an escape from reality in the form of serious regression (hebephrenia), long periods of stupor (catatonia), or hallucinations and delusions of persecution (paranoia). The literal meaning of the word, *schizo,* "split," and *phrenia,* "mind," does not refer to split personality as is commonly thought, but rather refers to the separation of self from reality. The appearance of two or more distinct personalities within one individual is more properly called multiple personality.

The genesis of psychosis is not clearly understood. Heredity appears to play some part. Physiological factors, such as chemical processes in the brain, are being explored. Environmental influences appear to play a major role in precipitating the onset of psychosis if other predisposing factors are present. Any person under severe stress may experience some distortion of reality or some interruption of normal thought patterns in the form of strange ideas, bizarre feelings, or eccentric behavior, but the onset of true psychosis appears to depend on the presence of these not yet understood predisposing factors.

The Need for Help

We have described some signs of mental problems ranging from minor disturbance to serious illness. Clearly, treatment and perhaps hospitalization are required for psychotic illness, neurotic behavior which interrupts functioning, and psychosomatic illness. It is at lesser levels of disequilibrium that the decision to seek help is more complicated. At what point is help necessary? When is it perhaps not necessary for your survival, but still desirable to increase your ability to love, work, and play?

If you can learn to recognize and accept processes that are normal for you, you can then begin to recognize mechanisms that are not functioning as well as they might or stresses which are beyond your capacity at the moment. You can think about the state of your emotional health with the same kind of knowledge, expectations, and sense of proportion you use when thinking about your physical state: "The bruise still looks and feels awful today, but I know it will be healed in a few days" or "I had better see a doctor because the pain is increasing and the skin doesn't look the way it usually does when it is healing."

You know that sometimes you are better able than a person struggling with a problem to recognize signs of disequilibrium in that person. The same is true for you, and friends may be able to help you assess your mental health. But, it is you who must answer the questions: Do I feel ineffective in my activities and relationships? Do I feel overwhelmed by my feelings? Am I in pain? If the answer is yes to any of these questions, then you might consider calling on someone who is trained to evaluate the seriousness of your problems, to give support, or to begin to look for underlying causes.

TYPES OF HELP

There are now many medical and nonmedical professionals who specialize in giving advice, support, and treatment for the wide range of emotional disturbances we have described. Although they are all concerned
with some aspect of psychotherapy, the treatment of mental disorder, they
vary in extent and scope of treatment, training, form and method of treatment, and theoretical basis of approach. Some focus on relief of symptoms, while others concentrate on the underlying cause of the disturbance.
Treatment may range from short-term counseling in time of crisis, to attempts to modify behavior, to long-term exploration of the operation and
origin of internal processes.

There is no sure way to know in advance exactly which approach or
which particular practitioner would be best for you. It will take some
research, investigation, and experimentation to find the help you feel you
need. The best advice at this stage is to ask questions and read; find out as
much as you can from your physician, friends, clergyman, local mental
health center, and any other source of information.

A consultation with a well-recommended practitioner may clarify your
needs. A consultation is not a commitment to a course of treatment, but a
means of investigating your problem and alternative therapies. The practitioner may be able to help you evaluate the seriousness and nature of your
problem, describe some treatment approaches, make his or her own approach clear, and perhaps make recommendations as to which approach
might be most beneficial for you. One or two sessions may very well
relieve your anxiety about your problems so that you decide you need no
further help. You certainly will begin to get some feeling for the type of
person you would feel best working with.

We cannot here explain the theoretical bases of the many therapeutic
approaches. We can, however, briefly describe four major areas of help:
psychotherapy (types of practitioners and approaches to therapy), drug
therapy, hospitalization, and self-help groups.

Psychotherapy

PRACTITIONERS

Among the types of mental health practitioners are the following.

1. *Psychiatrist.* A psychiatrist is a physician who has had at least five or
six years of postgraduate training in psychiatry, the specialized branch of
medicine that deals with mental, emotional or behavioral disorders.

2. *Psychologist.* A psychologist has an advanced degree (usually a

Ph.D.) granted after four to ten years of postgraduate training in psychology. Not all psychologists are therapists. They may concentrate on academic, research, or educational applications of the field of psychology. The education of a therapist includes not only general academic study of psychology and research, but also includes clinical psychology, that is, study and training in specific kinds of psychotherapy and an internship to gain clinical experience. This category is confusing because there are therapists with degrees other than a Ph.D. with training similar to that in clinical psychology programs. The Psy.D. is a doctorate in psychology in which the counseling aspects of psychology are emphasized. The Ed.D. is a doctor in education in which the study of psychology may be included, but the research is in the field of education.

3. *Social worker.* A social worker has two years of postgraduate training in social work leading to a master's degree in social work (M.S.W.). The training includes academic study, clinical work, and training placement. There are some advanced programs in social work leading to a doctorate in social work (D.S.W.).

4. *Counselor.* There are a number of counseling fields which involve undergraduate programs and specialized advanced training leading to a degree or other form of certification. For example, a degree in pastoral counseling is granted after specialized training within a divinity school.

5. *Other therapists.* Specializing training programs in particular therapeutic methods—art therapy, occupational therapy, etc.—are offered at undergraduate and graduate levels.

6. *Psychoanalyst.* To add to the complexities, psychiatrists, psychologists, and other therapists may, in addition to the above, become psychoanalysts. This means that in addition to the training previously described, they enter a psychoanalytic training institute and do additional academic and theoretical work in psychoanalysis plus supervised work in psychoanalytic treatment. There are a number of schools of psychoanalysis, including those based on the work of Freud, Jung, William Alanson White, and Karen Horney. Most psychoanalysts are M.D.s, but some training institutions do admit clinicians from other fields. These people may be referred to as "lay analysts."

APPROACHES TO TREATMENT

There are a variety of approaches to treatment that all or some of the mental health practitioners may recommend or practice.

1. *Individual psychotherapy.* This is commonly called "one-to-one treatment" in which you and a therapist talk about your troubles and feelings. Again, there are a variety of schools which determine the theoretical orientation of the therapist. Psychoanalysis is one form of individual psychotherapy.

2. *Group psychotherapy.* In this method several patients discuss their

problems under the guidance of a trained leader. Interaction among the patients is used to bring to light and consider each individual's and common group problems.

3. *Marital counseling.* In this approach the therapist concentrates on problems and interactions which affect the relationship of the couple. The couple has sessions together and also may have separate sessions.

4. *Family therapy.* In this approach all members of the family are involved in the therapeutic process. The family meets the therapist together, and in addition one or more members may have sessions with the therapist.

5. *Assorted therapies.* There are a rapidly growing number of other approaches such as psychodrama, encounter therapy, psychomotor, meditation, and others. Be sure to check on the training of the therapist and to find out exactly what the program involves.

6. *Activity therapies.* There are well-established forms of treatment that include methods other than the primarily verbal methods just described. In these forms, such as dance therapy, art therapy, and occupational therapy, therapists use body activities to promote self-understanding and symptom relief.

Drug Therapy

Medication with or without psychotherapy is a form of treatment frequently used today. Psychotropic drugs, that is, medications which act on the mind, are used primarily for the purpose of symptom relief. These drugs can be divided into three categories: antipsychotic, antianxiety, and antidepressant. Note that the categories represent effect on particular emotional states rather than chemical effects on the nervous system. Thus, a sedative such as phenobarbital or a depressant such as maprobomate would be categorized as antianxiety drugs in terms of their similar mood-changing effect. (See "Drugs, Alcohol, and Tobacco" for a description of the effects of various drugs on the nervous system). When you or a family member is given medication be sure to find out what kind it is, what effect it is supposed to produce, and what its side effects may be.

The antipsychotic drugs are sometimes called the major tranquilizers. In 1954 reserpine was the first drug used to treat mental illness. Because of side effects and with the increasing research in this area, reserpine was supplanted by other drugs. Chlorpromazine (brand name Thorazine) is the most frequently used. Antianxiety drugs—generally sedatives and the minor tranquilizers—include diazepam (Valium), meprobamate (Miltown), chlordiazepoxide (Librium), phenobarbital, and others. Antidepressants such as imipramine (Tofranil) and amitriptyline (Elavil) are frequently used in order to alleviate symptoms of depression. Lithium is used in the treatment of manic-depressive psychosis.

There is no doubt that drugs are overprescribed and overused. There is also little question that, when properly used, psychotropic drugs can be invaluable. The use of antipsychotic medication to bring about relief of psychotic symptoms often shortens the duration of hospitalization. But too often when a woman has vague complaints, she receives a pill rather than a sympathetic or understanding ear. It may be easier to take a pill than to endure strong feelings and think about unresolved inner problems and tensions. But a pill will only bring temporary relief and not aid the process of the problem-solving. If your doctor or therapist writes a prescription quickly and without discussion, ask questions. If questions and discussion are discouraged, another source of information should be requested. Referrals for a second opinion are often more useful than the prescription for sedatives and tranquilizers.

Hospitalization for Mental Illness

The decision to seek psychotherapy is in most cases a personal one. You feel you need help and look for it. However, in the case of serious mental illness a person may be too disorganized or too separated from reality to make this kind of decision. Family members or friends who recognize the signs of illness, such as bizarre behavior, antisocial acts, or serious bodily symptoms, should seek evaluation by a psychiatrist. At times the recommendation for evaluation may be made by a family physician or by a member of a community agency, such as church, police, or social worker.

At the time of the evaluation hospitalization may be discussed. The idea of hospitalization for physical illness is vaguely frightening to most people because it is associated with serious or even life-threatening conditions. The thought of hospitalization for mental illness is even more frightening because of its association with ideas about the "lunatic asylum," "bedlam," the "cuckoo's nest." If hospitalization is suggested, it is important to remember that the main reason for this is that the professional feels that the person needs intensive treatment and care. The patient may need around-the-clock care, supervised medication, or more intensive treatment than can be provided in an office, clinic, or other outpatient setting. First and foremost, the psychiatric hospital is a place for treatment.

To minimize the effects of this fear, it is important for the patient and the patient's family to ask many questions and perhaps even to visit the place that is being suggested. The hospitalization of one of its members will be a crisis for the whole family. Adult members may be too afraid to ask questions clearly. Children too young to understand exactly what is happening or to ask questions will often show reactions in their bodies and in their behavior. Their sleep may be disturbed; they may become discipline problems or, in contrast, too well-behaved for their age. It is important to encourage discussion and questions about the hospitalization of a family member. Both adults and children may feel considerable guilt about the hospitalization. The spouse and children of the patient are likely to feel that they are to blame for the patient's serious emotional disturbance. Also, children often feel that the parent has gone away forever and need strong and frequent reassurance. The time perspective of children is different from the adult's and to say "Mommy will be gone only for a month" may mean "forever" to the child. It is important to be open and flexible to whatever questions arise, including, "Did I do it to her?" Yet, in practice, flexibility and open discussion within the family may be very difficult to achieve. This is another time when help may be needed. The mother may have to take the major role in recognizing that the sleepless child whose father has been hospitalized may be crying "help" in his or her own young way.

The hospital recommended may be a private hospital or a government hospital. The decision may be made on the basis of the family's economic situation and estimates of the length of hospitalization. Insurance coverage and fees vary.

Self-Help and Support Groups

A growing number of self-help organizations are being formed today. Individuals facing the same problem may meet to discuss their experiences and to provide support for one another. Many such groups remain temporary and informal, but an increasing number are expanding to become clearinghouses for information.

The movement toward self-help was stimulated by the women's movement when it formed groups to focus attention on women's social problems and then on the inadequacy of education about their bodies and the medical care they receive.

An outgrowth of the consciousness-raising and body awareness groups has been the development and growing use of "support groups." These support groups are usually focused on physical concerns, such as childbirth, breast-feeding, mastectomy, weight issues, sexuality, and others. Other groups have been formed to help the families of alcoholics; even within professional institutions, such as psychiatric hospitals, support groups have been started by the staff as part of the overall treatment program. The groups are a form of self-help group therapy. Members form discussion groups in which they talk to each other about their concerns and also learn new facts. Often professional consultation is available in the early stages of support group formation. They may be started by a professional and then go on to become self-run and apparently leaderless.

It is clear in these groups that physical concerns and those of the mind cannot be separated. Emotional issues are involved and enter into the discussions. However, the old and ever-present dichotomy between body and mind is one which deserves some consideration. Self-help has centered on the body and political issues of "consciousness-raising." In the coming years it is likely that the self-help movement will move more directly into areas that may be classified as mind or mental health. It seems appropriate to encourage the development of mental health groups that, for example, discuss the stresses and strains of everyday life without necessarily being centered around illness. Clarification, demystification, and increasing centeredness of self will be aided by more direct consideration of the mind and its processes.

FURTHER READING

Mental Health, Psychology, Life Cycle

Erikson, Erik H. *Childhood and Society,* rev. ed. New York: Norton, 1964.

Erikson, Erik H. *Identity: Youth and Crisis.* New York: Norton, 1968.

Freud, Anna. *Psychoanalysis for Teachers and Parents.* New York: Norton, 1935.

Freud, S. *Five Lectures on Psychoanalysis* (1909). New York: Norton. (Also in Standard Edition of *Complete Psychological Works of Sigmund Freud.*)

Freud, S. *The Complete Introductory Lectures on Psychoanalysis* (*1916–1917*). New York: Norton, 1966. (Also in Standard Edition of *Complete Psychological Works of Sigmund Freud.*)

Jones, Ernest. *The Life and Works of Sigmund Freud,* edited and abridged by L. Trilling and S. Marcus. New York: Basic Books, 1961.

Jung, C. J. *The Portable Jung,* ed. Joseph Campbell. New York: Viking, 1971.

Infancy and Childhood

Brazelton, T. Berry. *Infants and Mothers.* New York: Delacorte Press/Seymour Lawrence, 1969.

Brazelton, T. Berry. *Toddlers and Parents.* New York: Delacorte Press/Seymour Lawrence, 1976.

Brazelton, T. Berry. *Doctor and Child.* New York: Delacorte Press/Seymour Lawrence, 1976.

Gesell, A., and F. L. Ilg. *Child Development: An Introduction to the Study of Human Infants.* New York: Harper & Row, 1970.

Fraiberg, S. *The Magic Years.* New York: Scribner, 1959.

Adolescence

Blos, P. *The Young Adolescent.* New York: Free Press, 1970.

Adulthood

Levinson, D. J. *The Seasons of a Man's Life.* New York: Knopf, 1970.
Rubin, Lillian. *Women of a Certain Age: The Mid Life Search for Self.* New York: Harper & Row, 1979.
Sheehy, Gail. *Passages.* New York: Bantam, 1976.

Self-Help

Boston Women's Health Book Collective. *Our Bodies, Ourselves.* New York: Simon and Schuster, 1971.
Heide, Wilma Scott. "Feminism: Making the Difference in Our Health." In Malkah Notman and Carol C. Nadelson, eds., *The Woman Patient.* New York: Plenum Press, 1978.
Marieskind, Helen. "The Women's Health Movement: Past Roots." In Claudia Dreyfus, ed., *Seizing Our Bodies: The Politics of Women's Health.* New York: Vintage, 1977.
Miller, J. B. *Toward a New Psychology of Women.* Boston: Beacon Press, 1976.
Notman, M. and C. Nadelson. *The Woman Patient* (Vol. I.) New York: Plenum Press, 1978.

Changing Roles—
Women from 18 to 40

CAROL NADELSON, M.D.

Professor of Psychiatry, Tufts University School of Medicine
Vice Chairman, Department of Psychiatry,
Tufts—New England Medical Center, Boston, Massachusetts

As a young woman enters her adulthood and begins to plan her future, what choices are open to her and what roles will she be expected to fulfill? Accepted behavior is determined by society for all of its members, and traditional expectations are slow to change. However, changing social and economic conditions have forced us, both men and women, to consider the limitations of traditional roles and the possibilities for change. The women's movement in particular has focused on the consequences to the individual of restrictive, and now perhaps outmoded, attitudes. For many women society has not yet changed enough to allow for alternatives to existing roles; for others, new choices and opportunities do exist. We shall look at some of these new choices and the problems they create, mainly in terms of their effect on family structure. What is the impact of the pressure toward career? What has happened to marriages? How are children affected? Is the status of the single woman changing? Where do women see themselves going?

RIGIDITY OF ROLE EXPECTATIONS

Throughout most of human history average life expectancy was short, serious disease was rampant, there was no real possibility of fertility control, many children failed to survive to adulthood, and the world population was small and expanding slowly. Even at the beginning of this century general health care was poor, occupational risks were high, and there was considerable pressure to increase the population.

Average life expectancy for women now is more than 70 years and most children survive to adulthood. Since, if current growth rates continue, the world population will double in 33 years, decreasing the rate of population growth has become a major concern and control of fertility is not only possible, but desired. This has enormous impact on how women view themselves and plan their lives.

A young woman in our culture is torn by contradicting values and priorities. She is encouraged to have a small family and to develop her own personal life goals apart from her role as a wife and mother, but often she is still led to believe that if she chooses motherhood, she must do it full-time to avoid profoundly damaging her children. Despite the focus on individuality in today's culture, young women's attempts to develop that individuality create an enormous burden of guilt and anxiety.

While an increasing number of women with children do work, many feel that their work is secondary to their role as mother. The working mother carries the full responsibility for being the caretaker of her children regardless of what else she does. She finds herself in a double bind: her longer life span and better education provide the opportunity and capability to function outside the family structure, but she often cannot compete in a career or pursue other goals because the definition of her role as wife and mother has not changed. Her private expectations are simply added to her traditional family function.

The woman has a narrow range of options because, regardless of what else she does, she is expected to become a "good" wife and mother, and "good" is rigidly defined. We do not define and measure husbandhood or fatherhood in the same way. The man is expected to succeed at work, to provide economic support for the family, but he is encouraged to explore and choose areas of work commensurate with his skills and talents. Thus his pursuit of personal life goals is taken as his fulfillment of his responsibility as husband and father with only a limited additional obligation to share in household burdens and child care.

Rigidity of role expectations clearly limits the options of both men and women. In our culture we are as uncomfortable about a man who is ambivalent about work or his traditional role, as we are about a woman who is ambivalent about maternity or marriage. The strong, silent model of masculinity inhibits the development of sensitivities in men, just as the helpless, dependent model of femininity inhibits the expression of activity and independence in women. There is evidence suggesting that when children are pressured to assume culturally defined sex-appropriate roles too early, they may pay a price in the development of their capacity for flexibility and self-expression. The process of socialization appears to expand the options of the little boy, who is encouraged to be competent and active in tasks. However, many boys may be handicapped intellectually because the kind of physical activity which is encouraged may make it difficult for them to develop the ability to concentrate on intellectual tasks. The effects of socialization on girls are not as positive in relation to competence, because the development of independence, autonomy, or an orientation toward achievement is discouraged.

It seems likely that the tendency to define sex roles and expect sex-appropriate behavior in young children has negative consequences for both boys and girls for their maturation and development. We tend to behave as if we are certain that sex roles are biologically determined and that they are thus unchangeable and fixed, despite the lack of supporting evidence for this view. Thus, expectations are imposed on children on the basis of how they "should" be, rather than on the basis of individual personality and skills.

If girls have been exposed since childhood to the idea that women are not as serious or committed to developing and pursuing their goals as men are, they may underestimate themselves or limit their progress. A girl may find it difficult to allow herself to be competitive or successful. She may worry about her femininity and attractiveness if she actively pursues areas of competence, especially if she chooses a "masculine" field such as a career in engineering or management. She may instead capitulate and do what is expected, often with regret, but at least with less guilt or anxiety about being a "good girl." Even those women who succeed often have negative feelings about their abilities despite obvious successes.

In the early 1960s Matina Horner, now the President of Radcliffe College, found that women tend to avoid success more than men do. They were fearful that success would bring adverse consequences, especially socially. When the same research was repeated six years later at the same school, men were as likely as women to show evidence of a motive to avoid success. While the underlying reasons for this motive in men may be different from what it is in women, the finding does appear to reflect a change in men's orientations. Many women in the past gave their husband's career precedence over theirs, in part because they felt it was a more intrinsic part of his self-concept and in part because they saw it as an expected and acceptable position to take.

CHANGING ATTITUDES, VALUES, AND BEHAVIORS

The 18-year-old woman of today is different from her 40-year-old mother and even from the women in the middle of that age range. In the past few years there have been changes in our attitudes about careers and families for both men and women, especially among young people. Marjorie Lozoff recently found some striking differences from the students of only a few years earlier. When considering the number of children they desired, about 67 percent of a 1965 group (male and female) wanted three or more; later only 16 percent wanted three or more, and 10 percent wanted no children at all. In the area of career 50 percent of women students in 1967 stated that having a career was important in addition to being a wife and mother; later this figure had risen to 81 percent. In addition, contrary to prevailing mythology, 91 percent of male students expressed interest in a wife with a career, 60 percent of male and female students thought that fathers and mothers should spend equal time with children, 44 percent of males felt that men and women should share household responsibility, and 70 percent of females and 40 percent of males felt that both male and female should contribute equally to family financing. The discrepancy in opinion on financing may represent either a realistic evaluation of the present differences between male and female earning power or a reluctance to relinquish the privileges accompanying the role of the major "breadwinner." In another recent study, 75 percent of college men said that they expected to spend as much time as their wives in bringing up children.

Marital patterns also appear to be changing. More people are now marrying later—or not marrying at all—than a decade ago. More choose to live together rather than marry. The divorce rate continues to rise. People are having fewer children, and more are choosing to remain childless. The change in marital patterns is reflected in a striking increase in the number of adults who live alone. To the elderly—primarily widows—are added those who choose not to marry, those who remained unmarried in their young adulthood, and divorced men and women.

Another important change has been in the number of women in the work force. Currently, more than 50 percent of all women 16 years or older are in the work force or actively seeking employment. Fifty-three percent of all women in intact families are in paid employment, and 41 percent of these families have children under 18 years. Furthermore, 31 percent of all children under 6 have working mothers. The number of women in the work force has increased by 60 percent in the past decade.

At this time only 6 percent of American families fit the traditional model of two parents with husband working and wife caring for children. Even if we accept this model as traditional, in statistical terms, families which follow it can be considered deviant, while dual worker families are the norm. However, the pattern we call traditional actually evolved as an adjustment to modern industrialization and affluence and has in reality existed only for one or two generations of white, middle-class Americans. It has never included minority people or the poor. The idea of the full-time, lifetime mother is a relatively new concept which evolved for middle-class women in the past half century. In the more distant past women had always filled many roles and shared the burden of work in order to sustain their families.

Until recently the fact that a woman was employed did not change the basic role expectations within the marital situation. However, new patterns, such as a dual career marriage, job sharing, and the commuting family, are emerging. Dual career marriage is a relationship in which both partners are in high commitment activities with responsibilities extending beyond the work day. This situation implies that modification in roles, decision making, and tasks must be made. For example, a husband cannot assume that his wife will take off from work when a child is ill or a repairman must come; and likewise a wife cannot count on her husband to be available to escort her to a social engagement or to repair the car when it breaks down.

This kind of relationship is relatively recent, and couples work out varying strategies to cope with both the ordinary and special aspects of a life in which neither partner functions as the "wife," that is, the partner who tackles the chores, arranges child care, schedules social activities, and buffers the other partner from the demands of daily life.

Some couples continue the traditional sex role division of labor model, others choose a nontraditional reversal of roles, and still others opt for equality. Equality implies that the couple make decisions together about the best options for each of them and for them as a unit. Decisions, such as whether they will move when one is offered a job, are not made by one partner deciding what is best for the family or couple.

Joint interaction may produce some strain, especially when one or both partners have been raised in more traditional families. The husband who was brought up to believe that housework is women's work may, while espousing egalitarian views, be resentful of the demands of this life style on his time, or he may even experience anxiety because of his perceived failure to live up to what he believes is a masculine role. He may also find that colleagues at work are unsupportive when he takes time off to take a child to the dentist or to attend a parents' meeting. He may even find family and friends openly hostile or belittling. The wife in this situation may experience similar conflicts and anxieties, despite her commitment to equal sharing.

Furthermore, children exposed to a more traditionally oriented environment at school, in the community, and via the media may expect and even demand more traditional behavior. They may be reluctant to invite friends to their house because neither parent is home or find it difficult to be the child who may not have a parent who can volunteer to chaperone a school dance.

Job sharing, where two people divide one job, has been successfully carried out by some companies and organizations, although the only formal study with husbands and wives was reported by a Norwegian group.

While the project was an experimental one, the couples who participated found this to be a satisfying solution both for them and for their children. This alternative may not work for many kinds of careers; it is, however, important as a possibility for the future.

In the commuting family, partners live apart on work days, because of job commitments in locations too far apart for daily commutings, but live together on weekends or non–work days. This alternative has not been well studied, but obviously involves difficulties if there are young children in the family.

How widespread these changes in life style patterns will become is not yet known. Also, their impact on social structure and individual attitudes is yet to be understood and evaluated. Social systems and internalized values take time to shift.

THE SINGLE WOMAN

Today, more women are choosing to remain single, either temporarily or permanently, for a variety of reasons including their desire to remain childless, their experience of marital unhappiness or divorce, or their belief that marriage is restrictive or unfulfilling. However, since the majority of people in our society eventually marry, the single woman, while she has freedom and autonomy, may find that she is increasingly excluded from social activities which are oriented around couples or families, especially as she grows older.

Friendships become an important source of support and sustenance to ease the isolation of being alone. Sometimes, intense relationships, either heterosexual or homosexual, may help develop a sense of community or family. Many single women live together or with their parents or families for emotional and economic support.

There continue to be differences between the life experiences of single men and women. Research indicates that unmarried women have better physical and psychological health than unmarried men. It is not clear why this is true, although people have speculated that, given the fact that it is generally easier for a man than a woman to find a relationship if he chooses to, men who do not marry may have more serious physical or emotional problems than women who do not marry. Single women often find themselves more frustrated than single men in obtaining intimacy and relationships. Since a relationship with a younger partner is less accepted for women than for men, as time passes the number of potential male partners decreases for women. Since women have tended to marry up (that is, marry men of higher social status) while men tend to marry down, the higher the woman's status, the fewer potential partners. Furthermore, since there are more available women than men, it has in the past been more important for women than for men to be physically attractive and have agreeable personality traits in order to find a partner.

There have been few studies which have examined the reasons for remaining single or the consequences of remaining single for a lifetime. There has been even less information on women who remain single because they choose lesbian relationships, since most research on homosexuals focuses on males. Lesbians tend to have long-term stable love relationships. Some lesbians also desire to be parents and may achieve that either by adopting or bearing children. There has been increasing interest in lesbian mothers and the effects of their sexual preferences on their children. Although there is little long-term data available, it appears that the children of lesbians, including those who live in lesbian households, grow up with the same range of sexual interests and preferences as do other children.

THE MARRIED WOMAN

Individuals marry for a number of complex reasons, including societal and family pressures, fantasies about a "perfect" life, concerns about loneliness, and needs for intimacy. Specific choices are made on the basis of romantic expectations and wishes as well as on more practical considerations such as similarity of life goals or the ability to work out problems together.

Marriage presents a paradox. The marriage ceremony states that the two shall become one: "For this cause shall a man leave father and mother and shall cleave to his wife and they twain shall be one flesh." Yet within the relationship the task of developing and maintaining a separate identity is important.

Marriage can foster development in a number of important ways. The close, sexual relationship offers the partners, perhaps for the first time, the opportunity to relate reciprocally with another individual, without regard to age or status, as in a parent-child or teacher-student interaction.

If each partner is perceived as separate and autonomous, they may support each other. In the ideal two person relationship, each partner is seen by the other as a separate individual with his or her own desires and needs. Within the relationship each partner attempts to fulfill both his or her own needs and those of the partner, without resorting to regressive behavior. It is also important for both to understand that even with individuals capable of true mutuality, it is not likely that this kind of interaction is attained consistently and predictably.

Together they may be able to work through unresolved conflicts from the past, relieve rivalries and repressed sexual feelings, and fulfill frustrated longings, allowing new opportunities for self-realization. Ultimately, however, for the success of the marriage each partner must face the reality of who his or her spouse is and often each must face some disappointment.

While people do consider a number of factors, including the compatibility of ideas, values, expectations, desires, family background, age, education, financial success, and future goals, most often romance starts a relationship and, while it may persist and even expand, the realities of building a life with another person often present problems which were not initially expected. Incompatibilities disregarded for romantic reasons may eventually be a source of conflict. Unconscious issues related to past experiences and conflicts remain with the individual after marriage and may not be resolved even in a supportive relationship. Future events and feelings may have unpredictable consequences despite attempts at working out the complexities of a relationship.

The level of psychological readiness to make a commitment to a marriage as an intense relationship is an important factor in the success of a marriage. Some individuals are prepared to cope with the tasks of marriage, but others may be burdened by excessive dependency needs, unrealistic expectations, or psychological deficits which make the resolution of marital tasks more difficult. While some individuals who enter a marriage when they are less mature can grow toward maturity within the marriage, others who either cannot cope or cannot resolve past conflicts are vulnerable to disturbance.

Recent work in adult development has indicated that important emotional shifts occur at different stages in the individual life cycle. Marital life also proceeds through a cycle. Conflicts can result if the partners are at different stages in their lives or if either's stage is not compatible with demands at particular times in the marriage cycle, such as shifts in tasks, the birth of children, changes in careers, relationships with relatives and friends, and the physical environment. Since complementary shifts may not occur in both partners, the balance of the relationship may be disturbed.

From the perspective of mental health, marriage appears to be more stressful for women than for men for a variety of reasons. The woman who marries modifies her life more than her husband does and risks more loss of autonomy. Although this pattern is changing and there are increasing numbers of dual career and commuting families, these patterns are by no means problem free for either partner.

For women who marry, there is a tendency toward lack of role differentiation and diversity which may lead to decreased self-esteem. The fact that the housewife role is an ascribed rather than an achieved role and that it is expected that women perform well in it without opportunity for diversification implies that all women must succeed. In fact, women who do not succeed in this role are often seen as life failures.

A loss of status may occur for a woman who has had an active career and then gives it up to marry. She often finds her role as housewife and woman devalued, although lip service is paid to its importance. While women without children are less likely to give up work, many women alter their career or work patterns and take positions with more flexibility, time, and fewer demands in order to spend more time at home or to be available to travel or entertain.

THE DECISION TO HAVE CHILDREN

More and more couples today are choosing not to have children. Many decide to postpone childbearing temporarily or indefinitely because of career goals, dislike of children, anticipated problems or desire for more freedom. Some of these people seek sterilization; others rely on birth control. This is a major social change; it is the first time in human history that the choice of childlessness has been safe and possible. The impact of this change is not yet clear. Certainly the stigma of childlessness has diminished.

Many people who make the initial decision to remain childless later change their minds. This is evidenced by the increasing number of women past 35 bearing their first child who state that they had decided not to have children earlier in their lives, and by the increasing number of people who have requested reversals of sterilization procedures as those techniques have become available.

The decision to bear children is a complex one. Motivations include the feeling that children will offer a more complete and full life, that it is "natural" to have children, that children will create a family atmosphere, that children will please a partner or parents, and that children will create a kind of immortality. In addition, people also love and want to care for children, and because they love each other, they want to consummate that love in the creation of a new family. At times people want children because they are insecure, dependent, or seek love and approval which they believe will come from a child. Sometimes it is a way of seeking normality, approval, or reaffirmation of their sexuality. There are positive and negative factors in everyone's decision.

While there is evidence that women who marry but remain childless are more successful in their careers, the higher a woman's educational level, the less likely she is to stop her career when she has children. The stresses of motherhood are high because of beliefs and attitudes about child-rearing which place higher demands on mothers than on fathers. Pregnancy and childbearing involve mothers more, and they continue to remain the major rearers of children.

Women who are single parents suffer significant economic problems. Women with children who are without men are increasingly likely to be poor. In 1974 one-eighth of all families in the United States were headed by women, and one-third of these had incomes below the poverty level. This rising figure includes women who were formerly considered middle class.

Little long-term data is available concerning women who have chosen to remain childless. Couples who are childless do report greater marital satisfaction than those with young children, during the early years of marriage. Over the course of their adult lives, however, women with children have been reported to have greater overall life satisfaction than childless women.

THE CAREER-FAMILY DILEMMA

Until the late nineteenth century women, married or single, worked almost exclusively in the house (either their own or as domestics in other peoples' homes) or as unpaid labor in family enterprises. As rapid industrialization created a greater demand for labor, single women began to be allowed by their families to take jobs outside of the home, and work for the single woman until she married became an accepted pattern.

The idea of women working after marriage still has not been universally accepted. During the labor shortage of World War II married women began to work when their children were in school or if they were poor. In the 1960s and 1970s economic necessity caused a rapid increase in the number of working women with preschool or school age children, and many married women began work because of their desire for self-fulfillment and independence.

Work has presented a dilemma for women since, as noted, they add the work roles to their traditional ones, resulting in work overload and considerable strain. Little adaptation has been made either by the work environment or the family to address this issue. While the family has been seen as a passive institution which adapts to the needs of the man-breadwinner, the new working woman has not been incorporated into the picture. With rigid, traditional division of labor, family functions cannot continue if the woman works. If the wife is at work, for example, no dinner will be cooked until she arrives.

The resolution of the career-family dilemma cannot be evaluated without considering the entire family structure, including the husband's orientation to his family and career and his resolution of conflicts between these areas. In our society it is assumed that every man will spend a major portion of his energy and time on his work regardless of his degree of commitment and satisfaction.

Most women who work, however, often think of their work as an extension of their nurturant maternal role rather than as an independent activity about which they may have some choice and in which they obtain personal gratification. They often prefer to work part-time or to limit the scope of their commitments. This presents problems with regard to job or career advancement and generally results in the view that they are not so serious about their work as men are. Furthermore, for the same jobs, women generally earn 60 percent of what men earn.

However, if we look at total life patterns, it appears that childbearing and rearing occupy only a small portion of the life of today's middle-class married woman. If she prepares only for a role as a mother and caretaker of small children, she may not be prepared for what will be a major part of her life. The statistics make the picture vividly clear. According to Alice Rossi, the average woman of 22 marries a man of 24, has two children two years apart, and dies at 74, nine years after her husband's death at 67. Of her years of adulthood starting at age 18

23 percent (13 years) are without a husband.
41 percent (23 years) are with a husband but no children under 18.
36 percent (20 years) are with a husband and at least one child under 18.
12 percent (7 years) are with a husband and preschool children.

Therefore, today's married woman will spend almost twice as many years with neither husband nor dependent children than she will caring for pre-school children (23 vs. 12 percent) and will spend almost two-thirds of her adult years either alone or living with a husband but no children under 18. In view of the rising divorce rate, it is also possible that she will be alone for even a longer time.

If we examine the actual time housewives spend on various activities, we find that they spend less than two hours a day in adult conversation. The remainder of their time is devoted to household chores. Interestingly, a look at household work with the advent of labor-saving devices reveals that more time is spent on these activities than in the past. Considerations of household responsibilities fail to include husbands and other family members as participants. Women are asked about their priorities and conflicts as if they existed alone. While participation in doing household chores may not be substantially affected by the fact that a woman works, many studies have found that the husbands of working women are more actively involved in the care of their children. Other studies show that this active involvement of the father has a positive effect on both male and female children.

Whether she works outside the home by her own choice or of necessity, guilt plays a prominent part in women's lives. They are rarely free of it, particularly if they have a career which involves a significant commitment of time and energy outside the home. This is even more of a problem for women with children. Old attitudes change slowly, and the persistent argu-ment that maternal work has negative consequences for children supports the guilt that so many working women feel. The working mother of young children continues to be seen as a less than good mother or even as an inadequate mother. Working women whose children develop physical or emotional problems are usually quick to be blamed and to blame themselves for causing the problems, although the relationship between cause and result may not be at all clear. The same criticisms are not leveled against women who spend equal time away from home in noncareer oriented activities, such as volunteer work, helping their husbands, or simply social engagements, because their home is seen as their primary commitment.

Those who oppose work for mothers are quick to generalize from studies showing that infants reared in inadequate day care institutions, without any stable one-to-one relationships with an adult, suffer serious emotional and learning deficits. While the importance of early attachments is clear, many day care centers are healthy alternatives. Research suggests that putting a small number of babies with an attentive and caring person avoids many of the adverse effects of institutional care. Often the increased stimulation found in such an environment is a benefit. Day care and alternative care can be warm, attend to the needs of children of different ages, and can provide the support necessary for children.

There is a growing body of evidence from many sources to support the idea that there are significant benefits for mothers, children, and families when the mother works, especially if her work is out of desire rather than necessity. The mothers express more positive feelings, use less coercive discipline, and feel less hostility and more empathy toward their children. However, working mothers who like their work often do feel guilty and overcompensate. For example, children are asked to help less around the house than children of the nonworking mothers.

Most of the information available in this area comes from middle- and upper-class families. In these families there is considerable evidence that having a working mother has a positive effect, particularly on girls. The daughters of working mothers have been reported to be more likely to choose their mothers as models and as the people they most admired. Adolescent daughters of working mothers, particularly in the middle and upper socioeconomic groups, were found to be active, autonomous girls who admired their mothers, but were not unusually tied to them. These girls usually approved of maternal employment and planned to work when they grew up and became mothers.

At all ages daughters of working mothers saw the role as less restricted and with a wider range of activities and independence than did daughters of nonworking mothers. The daughters of working mothers, unlike those of nonworking mothers, did not assume that women were less competent than men. Furthermore, the fact that the husbands of professional women also are more likely to respect competence and achievement in women is an important factor in the development of a positive self-image in their daughters.

Studies of nonworking women indicate that achievement frustrations are not great when children are young, but do increase with time. After about twelve years of marriage the nonworking woman often finds that her need for achievement rises, her self-esteem is low, her feeling of self-sacrifice is high, she is prone to depression, she worries about her competence in general and particularly as a mother, she is anxious about her children, and she feels guilty about occasional losses of her self-control. Despite her eagerness for her children to achieve, she is more likely to be ambivalent about their growing independence than the working woman. At this time many women do begin to plan for the future. Some go back to school, others consider retraining in a new field, and still others begin to work, often part-time initially, until they have found what they want and they have the time to devote themselves to full-time work.

As we look to the future, we find an increase in the percentage of women planning to combine careers and motherhood. These younger women who will pursue careers may be quite different from one another in values, self-concepts, and expectations. However, in view of changing attitudes they may very likely marry the kind of man for whom personal achievement and career goals may be less central to his life than the man they might have married in the past. The sharing of household tasks, child care, and career commitment by a husband and wife may well become a possibility. And if career-oriented women do become mothers, styles of mothering may also change. Child care centers may be more available and more acceptable. The pattern of women interrupting and dropping their careers may diminish, and parenting may attain priority as a primary commitment for both parents.

DIVORCE

One of the manifestations of problems resulting from social change can perhaps be seen in the divorce rate. While it clearly is not a good measure of success, happiness, or adjustment, since many people remain in unsatisfactory marriages, it does provide one kind of indication of "failure," whether caused by impatience, unrealized expectations, or other factors.

The divorce rate has increased considerably in the past decades. From 1920 to 1940 it was 10 per 1000 marriages. By the mid 1940s the number had risen to 24 per 1000. It fell in the 1950s, and then in the 1970s rose to a high of 26 per 1000. The number of divorces is estimated at about 10 percent of all marriages per year. The highest rate appears to be for those aged 25 to 39, but since the rate of marriage in this group is lower, the rate of divorce may be difficult to assess accurately.

People considering divorce often do not see themselves as vulnerable to the stress which occurs particularly in the period shortly after the divorce. They may be unprepared for the loneliness, the isolation, and the emptiness they often feel. While separation may initially be a relief if a marriage has been filled with tension and conflict, those who divorce usually do experience profound feelings about the loss at some point. In addition, the demands as well as the anger and anxiety of children may be draining and difficult. Parents often feel guilty about the distress they see in their children, and they may be oversensitive to criticism or disappointment. Even normal problems of growing up can be seen as related to the marital failure. Self-blame and anger at the partner frequently increase the burden for the children.

On the other hand, when a marriage has been extremely stressful or conflict-filled, the outcome of a divorce can benefit all of those involved. It offers an opportunity for maturation and growth. When there are children, divorce should be seen as representing a change in the structure and function of a family, rather than a dissolution of the family itself, since the children continue to have their original family. When bitterness is contained, and the best possible decisions are made, adaptation can be easier.

Divorce necessarily creates significant changes in family structure. This includes the reconstituted families created when a divorced parent remarries, and the increased number of single parents. Some parents seek remarriage to provide a home or to make up for an absent parent, only to find that new problems emerge. Children may reject the new partner because they had hoped for the reunion of their parents, they may see the new "parent" as a competitor, or they may not like the new partner. It is important to recognize that the new partner is in fact a step-parent and not a replacement. A relationship must develop over time. It is a new relationship with unclear definition for all members of a family. Because a marriage has taken place and the parent and new partner view themselves as a couple does not mean the children see it the same way.

Women often find themselves with fewer life options and many burdens after divorce. The single mother may have difficulty supporting herself and her family. She may not be able to work if there are no resources to help with child care, or she may not be able to earn enough if she has no experience or training for employment.

The price of divorce may be a high one for many women, although the gains may be well worth this price. It would seem that the myth of living happily ever after must give way to reality. This implies that women must see themselves realistically and plan for a potential future alone. They should acquire the education and training necessary to take care of themselves rather than limit their development in the expectation that they will be cared for by a husband.

NONTRADITIONAL LIFE STYLES

There is increasing interest in nontraditional choice in relationships, and a number of alternatives have emerged. Many more couples are making decisions to live together without marriage. The number of such couples has increased 117 percent since 1970. People may enter this kind of relationship for many reasons, including loneliness, the superficiality of the dating game, the search for intimacy, the emotional satisfaction of living and sleeping with someone who cares, the desire to try out a relationship before marriage, as well as doubts about marriage as a workable institution. Some couples feel committed to each other and see their relationship as akin to marriage, others are transiently attached, and still others merely find it convenient to share living quarters and household activities.

For some it works well and is a source of growth. The intimacy of the relationship may foster maturation. For others it is confusing and a source of anxiety. It may interfere with exploration and with the development of sexual identity. The lack of institutional definition of the relationship may create many fantasied expectations and the possibility of disappointment, if the couple do not establish clearly the nature of the relationship.

Most people who enter a nonmarital living situation do say that they eventually plan to marry. Their concept of marriage includes a high degree of intimacy and mutual sharing which they expect can evolve early, before they make the decision to marry. Available evidence indicates that most patterns of living together are monogamous. They are not casual, and sexual relationships with others is not a prominent feature. Also, both partners usually work and share financial responsibilities.

Communes as an alternative style gained popularity in the 1960s and many continue to exist. They consist of a group of people who decide to live together to share certain or all aspects of their lives, such as housing, a joint work enterprise, child-rearing, combinations of these, or an all-encompassing philosophic conviction. Many communes have evolved into self-contained communities and have been in existence for ten or more years, whereas others last only as long as the members remain in similar positions in life.

Most often the commune members maintain monogamous life styles within the structure of the community. Group marriages, that is, polygamous situations in which sexual exchange occurs and women may have children fathered by any man of the group, have tended to be unsatisfactory to the participants because of the difficulty most people have in sharing all aspects of their lives.

Another alternative, the open marriage, is a formal marriage with a degree of freedom within that relationship defined by the couple. For some it implies total freedom of life style, including the possibility of multiple sexual partners. For others, freedom is limited to nonsexual friendships and activities.

There have been few careful evaluations of the successes or problems of these alternatives because they are relatively recent. While there are distinct advantages to sharing goals, values, and property or granting new freedoms within old institutions, many of these alternative living situations fail because the participants have not yet been able to internalize the new values they represent. Jealousy, competitiveness, anxiety, and communication problems may ultimately disrupt the group or couple. In this situation, as well as in traditional marriages, the fairy tale concept of living happily ever after does not necessarily pertain. It is clear that changes and experiments will continue and that there are many reasons for seeking other sources of support, companionship, and intimacy.

THE FUTURE

A woman now has the opportunity to look objectively at her "traditional place" and to consider her alternatives as part of a changing society. She can consider various aspects of personality; does she choose to be dependent or independent, active or passive, helpless or competent, competitive or "feminine"? It is clear that although the anatomic destiny of a female may be to bear children, there is no valid reason to limit additional or other choices. The current atmosphere of feminism has fostered choice and flexibility. It is clear that in order to pursue alternatives, changes will be necessary in a number of areas. These may include living and working arrangements, priorities and expectations with regard to job and family, and definition of responsibilities of partners in child care, finances, and social status.

REFERENCES

Bailyn, L. "Family Constraints on Women's Work." *Annals of the New York Academy of Sciences,* 208 (1973): 82–90.

Birnbaum, J. "Life Patterns and Self-Esteem In Family Oriented and Career Committed Women" in Mednick, M., Tangri, S., Hoffman, L. (eds.) *Women and Achievement: Social and Motivational Analysis,* New York: Wiley, 1975.

Block, J. "Conceptions of Sex Role: Some Cross-Cultural and Longitudinal Perspectives." *American Psychologist,* 28 (1973): 512–525.

Campbell, A., and P. Converse. "The Human Meaning of Social Change." New York: Russell Sage Foundation, 1972.

Hoffman, L. "Early Childhood Experiences and Women's Achievement Motives." *Social Issues,* 28 (1973): 129–155.

Horner, M. "Sex Differences in Achievement Motivation and Performance in Competitive and Noncompetitive Situations." Doctoral dissertation, University of Michigan, 1968.

Howell, M. "Effects of Maternal Employment on the Child." *Pediatrics,* 52, no. 3 (1973): 327–343.

Howell, M. "Employed Mothers and Their Families." *Pediatrics,* 52, no. 2 (1973): 252–263.

Johnson, F., and C. Johnson. "Role Strain in High Commitment Career Women." *Journal of the American Academy of Psychoanalysis,* 4, no. 1 (1976): 13–36.

Katz, J. "Past and Future of the Undergraduate Woman." Paper presented at Radcliffe College, Cambridge, Mass., April 1978.

Lozoff, M. "Changing Lifestyles and Role Perceptions of Men and Women Students." Paper presented at Women: Resources for a Changing World at Radcliffe College, Cambridge, Mass., April 1972.

Moroni, R. "Note from the Editor." *Urban and Social Change Review,* 11 (1978): 2.

Murray, A. "Maternal Employment Reconsidered: Effect on Infants." *American Journal of Orthopsychiatry,* 45, no. 5 (1975): 773–790.

Nadelson, C. "Adjustment: New Approaches to Women's Mental Health." In *The American Woman: Who Will She Be?* Beverly Hills, Calif.: Glencoe Press, 1974.

Nadelson, C. "Current Impact of Women's Rights." *Basic Handbook of Child Psychiatry.* In press.

Nadelson, C., and M. Notman. "Medicine, A Career Conflict for Women." *American Journal of Psychiatry,* 130, no. 10 (1973): 1123–1127.

Nadelson, C., and M. Notman. "The Woman Patient" in *The Woman Patient: Medical and Psychological Interfaces.* New York: Plenum, 1978.

Nadelson, C., and M. Notman. "Women and Work: Impact of Social Change." Presented at Annual Meeting of the American Psychiatric Association, Chicago, Ill., 1979.

Nye, F., and L. Hoffman. *The Employed Mother in America.* Chicago: Rand McNally, 1963.

Pearce, D. "The Feminization of Poverty: Women, Work, and Welfare." *Urban and Social Change Review,* 11 (1978): 28–36.

Pifer, A. "Women and Working: Toward a New Society." *Urban and Social Change Review,* 11 (1978): 3–11.

Rossi, A. "Family Development in a Changing World." *American Journal of Psychiatry,* 128, no. 9 (1972): 1057–1066.

FURTHER READING

Bardwick, J. M. *Psychology of Women: A Study of Biocultural Conflicts.* New York: Harper & Row, 1971.

Bernard, J. *The Future of Marriage.* New York: Bantam, 1973.

Bernard, J. *Women, Wives, Mothers: Values and Options*. Chicago: Aldine, 1975.

Frieze, I., J. Parsons, P. Johnson, D. Ruble, and G. Zellman. *Women and Sex Roles: Social Psychological Perspective*. New York: Norton, 1978.

Grunebaum, H. and J. Christ, eds. *Contemporary Marriage: Structure, Dynamics and Therapy*. Boston: Little, Brown, 1976.

Holmstrom, L. *The Two Career Family*. Cambridge, Mass.: Schenkman, 1972.

Maccoby, E. E., and C. N. Jacklin. *The Psychology of Sex Differences*. Stanford, Calif.: Stanford University Press, 1974.

Miller, J. B. *Toward a New Psychology of Women*. Boston: Beacon, 1976.

Notman, M., and C. Nadelson, eds. *The Woman Patient: Medical and Psychological Interfaces*. New York: Plenum, 1978.

Paolino, T., and B. McCrady, eds. *Marriage and Marital Therapy: Psychoanalytic, Behavioral and Systems Theory Perspectives*. New York: Brunner/Mazel, 1978.

Rapoport, Robert, and Rhona Rapoport. *Dual Career Families*. Baltimore: Penguin Books, 1971.

Rapoport, Robert, and Rhona Rapoport. *Dual Career Families Reexamined*. Rev. ed. New York: Harper & Row, 1977.

Rapoport, Robert, and Rhona Rapoport, eds. *Working Couples*. New York: Harper & Row, 1978.

Visher, E., and J. Visher. *Stepfamilies*. New York: Brunner/Mazel, 1979.

Weiss, R. S. *Marital Separation*. New York: Basic Books, 1975.

Williams, J. *Psychology of Women: Behavior in a Biosocial Context*. New York: Norton, 1977.

Williams, J. *Psychology of Women: Selected Readings*. New York: Norton, 1979.

Midlife Transitions

MALKAH NOTMAN, M.D.

Associate Clinical Professor of Psychiatry,
Harvard Medical School, Boston, Massachusetts

After many years of neglect middle age is coming into its own. "Adulthood" has become recognized as a time of development rather than as a static period or a transitional stage on the way toward aging and death. This in part reflects a changed world. Longer life spans and changes in patterns of work have extended the midlife stage for all people. Changes in patterns of family life, control of fertility, and smaller families have extended the post-parental period and have helped identify the middle years as a distinct phase of life. The potential for development and growth during this period becomes apparent once it is viewed as more than a period of providing for children's needs and waiting for them to become independent.

To some extent new concepts of adulthood have emerged, with a change in definitions of sex roles as well as age roles. With middle age there is a further shift in the characteristics which are traditionally defined as "masculine" and "feminine." Some researchers find that men change in ways which make them more feminine in traditional terms, that is, they value relationships more and achievement less. Women change in the other direction, perhaps as their child-rearing tasks diminish and opportunity for achievement in more traditionally masculine terms increases. Biological differences between men and women and their apparent consequences in determining masculine and feminine personality characteristics appear to be less influential than was thought. When they reach middle age individuals may work out more personal and flexible adaptations in their lives than earlier stereotyped patterns.

WHAT IS MIDDLE AGE?

Defining middle age is not easy. Chronological age has often seemed to be the obvious criterion. The age of 40 is used as a basis by some people, others feel that 35 is the important transition age, and others choose 30 as the significant birthday that marks the end of "youth." For women middle age is linked with the menopause all too frequently.

But chronological age does not accurately represent the important experiences of this period. Not every individual is at the same place in life at the same age. The idea of using age to indicate life phases is derived from work with children where physical and psychological development is related more closely to actual age. This approach is not necessarily appropriate for adults whose lives diverge in more varied ways, and development in one or another area may occur at one point for one individual and another point for someone else.

The problem of arriving at a definition of middle age is further complicated by the fact that there are important differences in the life phases for men and women, in midlife as well as other periods. Most studies in psychology have been based on populations of men, for whom development tends to proceed through a series of predictable stages. For women this pattern is much less uniform. To some extent, becoming independent, establishing one's own identity, and developing some autonomy normally take place in early adulthood for everyone. However, for women dependency has been socially supported; some women move from being dependent on their parents to being dependent on their husbands and do not experience growth toward independence until much later than men of the same age. The adolescent and early adult development of independence, in the sense of being on one's own, may be temporarily replaced or accompanied by the development of interrelatedness, attachment, and responsiveness to the needs of others in the important experiences of motherhood and the formation of one's own family. Issues of independence may not be returned to until later in the course of life events or until some disruption, such as when children leave, a husband dies, or other circumstances, makes it important for a woman to think of what she wants for *her* life. If at that time she considers expanding her life beyond the home, for example, by returning to school or work, she may then have to face the old problems of adolescence, such as dealing with competitive feelings toward others, or anxiety about taking a stand on issues, or learning to do things on one's own without dependence on and guidance from others. For instance, some women never travel alone until some point in their middle years and find it both frightening and liberating.

In addition to the basic differences in life cycle patterns between men and women, a further source of variability comes from the current period of social change which has created even greater variation in the sequences of peoples' lives. Many women are waiting to establish themselves financially or in their careers before they marry or have children. Women may occupy different role patterns at different times, with combinations of children, work, and marriage. At a given age, therefore, it is not so clear what a woman can expect to have accomplished or what point in her life she feels she should have reached. Her husband may have established himself in work, trying out his place in the adult world, while she has been taking care of children. When the woman is ready to go "into the world," her partner may be ready for something else—a more quiet life, a change of career, or even retirement—which is quite out of keeping with her needs. The meshing of these different phases is very important in working out the eventual success of a marriage.

A study done by Bernice Neugarten illustrates a number of these points. She interviewed a sample of 100 successful men and women between 40 and 60 about their awareness of middle age and what they felt was important for them about this period. They described "a heightened sensitivity to one's position within a complex social environment and a clear sense of differentiation from both the older and younger generations."

The theme of reassessment of the self was found to be important, as was the changing time perspective in which "life is restructured in terms of time left to live rather than time since birth." Men and women both felt the growing awareness of the "rest of one's life" as an important characteristic of middle age. The infinity of time stretching ahead diminishes and disappears. A "lifetime guaranty" of a watch or a fountain pen no longer carries the same connotation of a rich and indefinite future. Chronological age for these middle-aged people was a less important marker than for young or old people. This is understandable in part because there are legal events which mark early adulthood and late adulthood; the young reach the age of legal driving, attain their majority, become eligible to vote, while the old reach the age of retirement, become eligible for pensions and medicare. There are no such legal events for midlife.

The Neugarten study confirmed that men and women see their life phases in relation to different experiences. Women in the study defined their age status in terms of timing of events within the family cycle. For married women middle age was closely tied to the launching of children into the adult world. An interesting additional finding was that even unmarried and childless career women often discussed middle age in terms of the family they might have had when assessing their lives' possibilities.

In contrast, men perceived a closer relationship between their stage of life and their career or work and particularly their assessment of the position they had reached. This difference is supported by the work of Daniel Levinson and his colleagues in their studies of men in which central importance is placed on the role of work in establishing one's self in the world. Although the importance of family relationships for the adult man is acknowledged, they are not the organizing theme of his life. Family concerns may be very significant for some individuals, but not in as central a way in defining their lives as seems to be true for women. In Levinson's attempts to define the important phases of adult development for men, he placed the separation from parents more centrally than the birth of the first child.

WOMEN, MIDDLE AGE, AND CHILDREN

Women's lives often have been described as influenced more strongly by biological variables and "natural forces" than men's lives, and for women reproductive function plays a more critical role in determining the phases of development than it does for men. It is important to understand this relationship without at the same time automatically concluding that women are "closer to nature" or that the biological events are inevitably the central ones. Such a view leaves out the critically important function of roles and the social context in which they occur, not to speak of individual experiences. An example of the different effect of the same events can be seen by comparing two women with different life patterns. One woman marries young, has children early, her children follow a similar pattern, and she is a grandmother at 40. Another woman pursues work and educational goals, marries late, and then decides to have "a child or two, before it's too late" at 40. Both women are the same age, yet they now face vastly different life experiences involving different attitudes toward commitment, independence, the need for stability as compared to their wishes for freedom, and what they need and expect from their husbands and families. Neither is likely, at 40, to be menopausal. Nor is either likely to think of herself as "young."

Women's lives have been closely bound up with children. Whether or not she chooses to have them, an important component of a woman's self-concept is her capacity to create children. Although there has been increasing involvement of fathers in the care of their children, women bear them, are the primary caretakers, and stop being able to become pregnant at a particular point.

So it is not surprising that men's and women's life phases and their sense of middle age as well are based on different criteria. The finiteness of time, which we have seen as an important characteristic of middle age for both, is for women closely related to their family roles and to the issue of having children. In fact, in a woman's psychological development the first pregnancy has been thought by many to be important in the development of her autonomy and separation from parents.

The social definition of a particular life stage is highly important.

Whether age is valued or demeaned in a particular society will affect a person's view of a particular life phase. In a society where women's sexual attractiveness is associated with youth and that attractiveness is considered an important part of life, women feel devalued as they age. In our society, for instance, women lose status with age more than men do, and to consider oneself middle aged is usually a negative view.

To consider the relationship to children as a reliable marker of middle age, although true in a wider sense, brings about some paradoxes, particularly in the current social climate. Conventionally, sociologists have considered middle age as beginning with children's independence, with the end of the parental role, "with launching children into the adult world," or similar events. However, these marking points of traditional definitions may not now be as applicable as they were, if indeed they ever were. The usefulness of these marking points has always been limited by the fact that children are born over such a wide range of maternal years that there has always been a wide variation in parental age when the children leave. Now that effective birth control and abortion allow women to delay childbearing and to reserve the period of early adulthood for other pursuits, there are an increasing number of families in which children do not leave home until well past the time at which parents regard themselves as having reached middle age and well past the mother's menopause, a conventional biological marker of middle age.

Another paradox is that now the decision to have a child may in itself be part of a midlife phenomenon. In reassessing herself from the midlife perspective of "time left to live," the childless woman may decide she does after all want to have a child and be a parent.

It is important to distinguish a woman's concerns about her reproductive potential from the concept that fulfillment and self-realization for women is automatically obtained from her children, is limited to childbearing, or is dominated by children. Many women have not found their children or their role as mother predominantly gratifying. Child-rearing may be draining, stressful, and conflict-producing. However, the finite years during which pregnancy is possible make the decision to have a child, or a second child, an issue which cannot be avoided in the process of midlife reassessment.

These decisions usually come well before the actual menopause, which has long been stereotyped as dominating women's midlife phase, and seem to be most critical between the ages of 35 and 40. Childbearing after the age of 40 has been approached with caution since it has been associated with increased risk of obstetrical complications and genetic abnormalities, particularly Down's syndrome (mongolism). In the past, medical advice encouraged early childbearing, and the optimal time was thought to be the early twenties. However, under current conditions of physical health and medical care, obstetrical complications in older women who are in good health are less frequent, less severe, and more easily controlled. Also, new data based on reexamination of current statistics raise some questions about the absolute connection between the mother's age and genetic abnormalities, since younger women also have babies with mongolism, although this is less likely. The technique of amniocentesis reveals the presence of this problem and thus provides an opportunity for aborting a defective fetus.

The midlife decision to have a child does not automatically satisfy reproductive concerns. When after years of postponement a couple is ready to have children, they may encounter infertility problems they did not know existed. There often is a great deal of stress associated with these problems, particularly if the couple feels very strongly the pressure of time running out.

Although more women now do marry late and have babies after 40, most see the way their lives are going earlier and before they reach 40 either have children or come to terms with not having one or not having another before their menopause. There may be sadness and depression and some mourning associated with this decision; however, some women are relieved that they no longer have to consider a choice which arouses internal conflict.

Once a woman has children, the stage of family development becomes an important determinant of the stage of life in which she is or feels herself to be. The ages of children, whether or not they are living at home or have left for school or other reasons, their development level, their activities, the interests of their peers, and the ages of their friends' parents all have important, if sometimes subtle effects on whether a woman feels young or middle aged. An older woman whose children are young often finds herself sharing time and activities with younger women whose children are her children's friends. Even if she works or is involved in other activities outside the home where she is more likely to be able to associate with her own peers, she may experience strong feelings of isolation. Consider the case of a woman who had her first child, a boy, at age 25 and did not conceive again until 15 years later. She and her husband were uncertain about what to do, but then felt they really did want a second child. When a daughter was born, they were delighted. Her son went to college two years later, and she returned to work as a nurse. Each day when she came home to a demanding toddler she felt stressed and often irritable. She found she could not make conversation with the other play group and day care mothers. All her friends were free of young children and she felt unable to muster the enthusiasm for all the developmental milestones of her daughter, experiences which she remembered having enjoyed with her son, but had "put away" as her son grew out of childhood. She felt the demands of work, the demands of her child, and the demands of her husband left her with no time for herself. The support she had found from friends who were going through the same experiences when her son was little was not available. She tried to turn to her husband for these needs. He was also feeling stressed, having less time from his wife for his own needs and never having been very communicative. When she found herself crying at work and losing her temper with her daughter, she sought counseling. It was helpful to be able to talk over her feelings, feel less guilty about her irritability, find ways to involve her husband more both with herself and her daughter, and also arrange for free time to spend with old friends who shared many of her current interests. She also became more aware of how much she missed the son who had left home. Her depression lifted and with this change her tolerance also increased.

For some women the experience of having their first child relatively late, perhaps in their late thirties, presents a very positive discovery of their sense of identity as women and a commonality of feelings and experiences with other women which they might not have predicted. One woman said, "I never really thought of myself as a mother—that would have meant like my mother, who never 'did' anything important. I felt like a professional. I discovered when my baby was born that I had so much to talk about with other women, things that I had ignored or that had never seemed to matter. It felt so good that that part of life was available to me too."

There have been many social changes in the past ten years which have profoundly affected women's lives. The increasing percentage of women in the labor force includes mothers of young children, but also includes women who will choose never to have children or to marry. Many of these are primarily involved in their work, some reflect changing social values which do not stigmatize an unmarried woman as much as previously, and others make a homosexual adjustment, temporarily or on a more permanent basis. The increasing options for women—and men—will bring some changes in life patterns and produce situations which require new adaptations.

MENOPAUSE

Turning to the later period of adult development brings us to a consideration of the menopause, stereotyped as the dominant factor in the midlife phase for women. Actually, there is a good deal of ignorance about menopause, even among physicians, and research has been neither plentiful nor careful. There have been problems in arriving at a consistent definition of the menopausal period and thus in agreeing on what is being studied. There is a tendency to ascribe all symptoms occurring during the menopausal period to the biological menopause. The more reliable studies show that psychosomatic and psychological complaints are not expressed more frequently by menopausal women than by younger women and that many of the symptoms attributed to menopause are not due to the actual physical and hormonal changes of this period at all.

Menopause is defined as the cessation of the menses for one year and therefore is a diagnosis which is made retrospectively. A more inclusive term to describe this part of life is perimenopause. During the several years that this occurs, there is a gradual diminution of ovarian function and a gradual change in endocrine status.

After the menarche the part of the brain called the hypothalamus, which has a regulatory effect on the pituitary gland, produces "releasing" substances which influence the pituitary to produce and release its gonadotrophic (stimulating to the ovaries) hormones (FSH and LH). Through feedback mechanisms a sufficient blood level of ovarian hormones inhibits the production of the stimulating hormones; a drop in the ovarian hormones is accompanied by increase in stimulating hormones by the hypothalamus and pituitary. This cyclic activity continues for years until the menopausal period approaches.

During perimenopause the ovary gradually diminishes its estrogen production. Progesterone, produced as a result of ovulation, also stops when ovulation ends. So for a time the ovarian estrogens decline while the pituitary and hypothalamus are still producing high levels of their stimulating hormones and there is thus an imbalance. The ovary does not stop all at once or smoothly, and the menstrual irregularities which are manifestations of menopause are a reflection of this variability. Although it is the uterus which shows the effects via the menses, it is the ovary which causes them. The actual pattern varies. Some women notice a shortening of the menstrual period and an increase in the interval between periods until they stop. Less frequently women describe periods which continue regularly until they stop abruptly. Sometimes bleeding is irregular with clots, profuse, or minimal. These patterns are thought to be a reflection of the hormonal imbalance, although some gynecological abnormalities may also contribute to them.

The understanding of these phenomena is complicated by the great complexity of hormonal pathways and the diverse sources of creation and release of hormones. Sometimes one substance is transformed into another within the body. For example, even after the ovaries have completely stopped secreting estrogen, it continues to be produced by the adrenals directly or is converted from adrenal androgens.

Age at menopause varies from the late thirties to the middle or even late fifties. This variation supports the tendency to assign a variety of symptoms occurring in these years to a woman's presumed menopausal status. McKinley, Jeffreys, and Thompson found that "the median age at menopause in industrial societies now occurs at about fifty and there is no firm evidence that this age has increased at least in the last century, nor any indication of any close relationships between the age at menopause and the age at menarche or socioeconomic status."

Menopause has been labeled a "deficiency state" by some because of the decreased ovarian production of estrogen and diminished circulating estrogen levels. The logical consequence of this concept is to remedy the "deficiency" by supplying estrogen. This is a subject of considerable controversy which we will discuss later. However, the concept of deficiency state for a normal developmental process brings up an interesting issue. One might see this as an example of the way in which adherence to a male model of development has affected thinking about women's bodies. For women it is normal to enter a postmenopausal phase where ovulation stops and hormonal levels decline. It is normal to end the childbearing years. For men there is no parallel experience which is as dramatic and definite, and male fertility usually continues well into old age.

What are the symptoms directly attributable to the menopause? Endocrinological and social-psychological data indicate that many misconceptions exist about the nature and extent of the menopausal symptoms. In a review of endocrinological data, Perlmutter states, "There are multiple disorders that have been ascribed to the changing hormonal balance and are equated with menopause. In reality, not all the changes that are noted are due to hormonal imbalances; some are the consequences of aging and others have a basis in psychological factors and life patterns."

In a review of symptoms of women aged 45 to 54 in the London area, McKinley and Jeffreys found that hot flashes and night sweats are "clearly associated with the onset of a natural menopause and that they occur in a majority of women." The other symptoms which they investigated, namely, "headaches, dizzy spells, palpitations, sleeplessness, depressions, and weight increase, showed no direct relationship to the menopause, but tended to occur together." Other symptoms sometimes attributed to menopause are irritability, diminished sexual interest, and mood swings.

Vasomotor instability, causing "hot flashes" or flushes (episodes of perspiration during the day or at night), has been one of the consistent symptoms accompanying menopause, with up to 75 percent of women reporting it.

The length of time a woman experiences hot flashes is variable. They may originate several years before actual menopause, signaling waning estrogen levels, reach a peak at about the time of the actual cessation of the menses, and persist as long as five years.

The cause of the vasomotor instability is unclear and appears to be related to the hormonal imbalance rather than to simple estrogen deficit. There are some conditions, such as anorexia nervosa, in which estrogen levels are less, but are not associated with hot flashes.

Psychological factors, such as anger, anxiety, and excitement, are considered important in precipitating flashes in susceptible women, as are activities giving rise to excessive heat production or retention, such as a warm environment, muscular work, and eating hot food. However, the symptoms may arise without any clear psychological or heat-stimulating mechanism.

Women are often worried about whether their flashes are visible. It is reassuring to know that most of the time no one can tell, although some women do break out in visible perspiration or find they need to take off a jacket or sweater. Generally the sensations and behavior are much more noticeable to the woman herself than to those around her. The concern and embarrassment result from her inability to control their occurrence and from the feeling that the flashes expose to public knowledge her menopausal state. The desire to conceal the state is a reaction to society's tendency to depreciate and ridicule the menopausal or postmenopausal woman as an aging person who has lost her sexual attractiveness.

Some of the symptoms considered part of the perimenopause do not occur consistently, may be unrelated to hormone changes, and in fact may be depressive symptoms or indications of anxiety in response to the stresses of the transitions of this period. Neugarten and her co-workers studied 100 women aged 43 to 53 using menstrual histories as an index of whether or not a woman was actually in the period of her menopause. They found little relationship between a variety of personality measures and the state of menopause and also little relationship between personality as a category and the severity of physical symptoms. However, women who previously had psychological difficulties, such as low self-esteem and low life satisfaction, were likely to have difficulties with menopause. This leads to recognition that menopause, as one of the most important experiences for women, may be best understood in the context of their entire lives.

Women's reactions to turning points in their lives, such as menarche and pregnancy, are usually consistent with their reactions to menopause. Two early psychoanalytic writers on the psychology of women, Therese Benedek and Helene Deutsch, observed from their clinical experience that a woman's reaction to menopause was similar to her reactions to puberty. Experiences which were milestones in her life as a woman would draw upon similar fundamental psychological responses. They predicted that a girl who felt puberty was a disaster and became depressed to have to acknowledge that she was a girl, might show strong reactions to her first period, expressed in psychological or perhaps physical symptoms. She would then be likely to have some strong response to the other transitions in her reproductive life, such as pregnancy and menopause.

Deutsch and Benedek also predicted that childless women would have more intense reactions at menopause, but studies by others and studies from other cultures contradict this idea. Women who have not had children do not necessarily have the most difficulties at menopause. Many of them have had to come to terms with their childlessness earlier than the biological menopause and have found other ways of organizing their lives. The biological menopause then represents a less critical event for these women. Having remained childless may have been the result of underlying reservations and hesitations about motherhood, attitudes more readily expressed in contemporary society than they used to be and also more possible to act on with better contraception and available abortions. Although the menopause does really mark the end of an important option for childless women, it is women who have invested heavily in childbearing and rearing who are most likely to experience intense reactions. It represents to them the loss of a personally and socially valued role and position.

Depression has been linked with menopause, but recent reviews emphasize that there is no clear connection between depression and female endocrine status. There is also good statistical evidence that the menopause is not a factor which increases rates of depression. Depression as a response to the loss of reproductive capacity and to aging seems to be more clearly associated with the individual's established psychological responses. It is also associated with cultural factors which determine the importance of menstruating, childrearing, and mothering in the self-esteem and status of women at a given time and place.

Estrogen Replacement Therapy

Treatment of menopausal symptoms with estrogen is a long-established practice. The symptoms for which women are treated are irregular uterine bleeding, hot flashes, various psychological symptoms, dryness and painfulness of the vagina, burning with urination, and osteoporosis, the postmenopausal loss of structural bone material which is a problem for many women, particularly women over 60.

Although clinical experience has shown that estrogens are effective in relation to some of these symptoms and are questionable in regard to others, the assessment is hampered by the lack of adequate research on the postmenopausal period. Recent statistics suggest that of the 75 to 85 percent of women who have some symptoms referable to estrogen deprivation only 10 to 15 percent seek medical consultation and then obtain treatment.

Questions of effectiveness have been further complicated by the implication of estrogen in one form of uterine cancer, and although the incidence is not high, the relationship now seems well established. This does not affect women who have had a hysterectomy, of course. The doses of estrogen necessary to treat menopausal symptoms do not seem to be involved in other cancer or in a clear way in other problems, but further study is needed.

The general agreement at this time is that estrogens are effective in treating vasomotor symptoms, which occur most severely at the time of the drop in estrogen function. These symptoms seem to be related to the change in function rather than to a low estrogen level, and they diminish naturally after the initial drop. However, for women who suffer severely, some gynecologists feel that low-dose estrogen treatment may be offered for a short time. The patient should be made fully aware of the potential risk; the therapy should be discontinued at intervals to see if it is still necessary; and an examination of the uterus to detect precancerous or cancerous changes should be repeated at intervals as long as therapy continues. Other gynecologists hold that other forms of therapy are preferable and that estrogens should not be used. This is still an area of controversy and needs further study.

Estrogens are also effective in overcoming the effects of the changes in the vagina which occur postmenopausally and seem to be associated with estrogen lack. These hormonal changes may cause dryness, itchiness, and pain on intercourse. Estrogen for this problem can be used in the form of a cream applied locally. Although the estrogen is absorbed by the body and enters the general circulation and thus is also potentially of concern, the doses tend to be much lower and the treatment can be intermittent.

Osteoporosis, or bone loss, does seem to be retarded if estrogen is given around the time of the menopause. However, as soon as estrogen is stopped, the process of bone loss can resume, and estrogen is not effective in restoring bone which has already been lost. There are some indications that other approaches, such as maintaining good nutrition, particularly with adequate amounts of calcium and vitamin D, and engaging in regular physical exercise, are also effective in warding off bone loss.

Estrogen does not seem to have a direct relationship to the relief of other symptoms which have been attributed to menopausal effects. Clearly, this is an area in which a great deal of research is in progress, and at present it seems to be a decision a woman must make as an informed choice, together with her physician. Any woman who does take estrogen should promptly report unusual vaginal bleeding or other symptoms and remain in close contact with her doctor.

MIDLIFE FAMILY ISSUES

As we have indicated before, family experiences during this period are important. The midlife transition for men, often the husbands of menopausal women, brings new stresses. This period for men is often accompanied by sexual problems sometimes leading to their having affairs, with consequent marital disruption and the abandonment of the women. In any event marital stress is frequent. Adolescent children may be sexually and aggressively provocative, as well as challenging or at times disappointing.

Children leave home for school or marriage, thus changing the family balance.

Although it is often assumed that the departure of children will always be felt as a loss, some women view it as an extension or expansion of parenting and find they begin to widen their own lives to include the wider interests and location of their children. In some marriages satisfactions increase as children leave the home. The "empty nest syndrome" appears not to be universal, and many studies now report that it is fathers who miss the departed children more than mothers. Women find their relationships with husbands changed. In some cases relationships become closer; in others the absence of children confronts husband and wife with the problems in their own relationships and new adaptations need to be made.

Departure of Children

Separation is an important developmental task at this time. The departure of children may revive the memory of earlier separations in the woman's own past and cause difficulty if these separations are still unresolved. She then may interfere in covert or overt ways with the development of independence in family members. The following example illustrates this problem.

Mrs. N is a 45-year-old married woman who would have been considered successful and fulfilled had her life been assessed two years before she sought help. She came from a small town and had extended family who were close and whose relationships were stable. She met and married her husband there. They then moved some distance away in search of better opportunities for both of them. She had two daughters, eleven months apart, who were in their mid-twenties at the time of the referral. When the children first entered school, she herself returned to school, went on to graduate training, and worked as an accountant. Her husband was an engineer.

Although she has never liked the area they moved to and missed her family, her husband loved it. They lived in the suburbs, had a large house, and from the very beginning raised their children to be successful and achievement oriented, an important value to both parents. The older daughter entered law school. Two years later the younger was accepted at business school. The parents were pleased at the achievement, but ambivalent about the shrinking of the family.

After both children left, Mrs. N and her husband became closer. They started "dating" again. Although her husband had been somewhat uncommunicative through the earlier years of marriage, their communication improved and so did their sexual relations. They made plans to travel and remodel the house. She kept in close contact with the children.

At the same time the girls began to have difficulty in school. The eldest was at school 3,000 miles away and began gradually to do less well academically. She became homesick, depressed, confused, and anxious about what might be going on at home. Her advisor suggested a year off. She had to return home until she felt able to study.

The younger daughter also began to have difficulty. She felt she really didn't like business, dropped out of school, and returned home at the same time as her sister. Then she, too, became depressed.

Relations between mother and daughters became tense. They argued about money, space, all household arrangements. Mrs. N became more and more depressed and anxious. She felt intruded on and frustrated that she and her husband were not alone. She constantly worried about the girls' dependency, but seemed to thwart every move they made toward help. She felt trapped; it seemed impossible to find a way out and the mutually hostile dependency seemed impossible to resolve. Her husband withdrew into the same relatively uncommunicative pattern of previous years. She then sought a consultation.

At that time she described her depression as very long standing, although previously less severe. Her father died several years after she had married and moved away. He had bought a farm, worked hard, and became ill just when the farm began to make money. In spite of the geographical distance she had been close to him and felt abandoned when he died. Her mother was living, but was more remote. A younger sister had been killed in an accident ten years ago. As she talked, she felt as if she was experiencing a recurrence of that earlier period of her life. Both deaths were reexperienced poignantly. She felt she had never mourned her father and sister before. Accompanying the anger at her daughters was a puzzling sense of loss, revived as she spoke of their leaving for school. She had never recognized that feeling as a loss before.

She had never completely dealt with the earlier separations, namely, the loss of the close family relationships when they moved, the death of her father, and the death of her sister. Her daughters' leaving home for college was the fulfillment of her own ambitions and hopes for them. However, she also experienced it as if they were abandoning her and she had subtly undermined their autonomous development. Their mutual attachment was strong; she encouraged their achievement, yet all had difficulty with the separation. The mother felt vulnerable and deserted. When the daughters returned, she resented their presence, yet could not let them go. Her husband's relative uninvolvement intensified the relationship among the women. Her own further growth was actually inhibited by the return of the children. However, the underlying problem was the unresolved original losses. None of the women were then able to develop without an undermining conflict emerging. Eventually, she was able to separate her feelings about her daughters from the losses of her family members and was better able to help them grow and separate. She herself changed her job, invested more in her own work, and with the diminished tension her husband's participation in the family increased.

Some women experience the period when the children leave as being "restored to themselves" and to their own development. Women depend much more than men on their relationships for their development, not only for their emotional comfort and security, but also for self-expression. The potential for autonomy, changes in relationships, the development of occupational skills, contacts, and self-image—all these may start after childbearing is over. An important aspect of the potential of middle age for women is the opening up of possibilities after family responsibilities are diminished. One has to recognize, however, that autonomy is often confused with aloneness, and separation with isolation. It is possible to achieve internal autonomy and independence without having to live alone.

Elderly Parents

Illness or death of a parent frequently ushers in the awareness of being middle aged. One becomes aware of being the person "in charge" as elderly parents become dependent and more helpless. The job of caring for elderly parents has by and large fallen to women because of their greater availability and their experience as caretakers and nurturers. This may create problems if the woman is also struggling for greater autonomy or is simply committed to work or school. Conflict between her own expectations and wishes and the demands of current commitments may lead her to give up the complicated process of entering the world of work or school or to delay doing so. If the work or school creates anxiety, this may be a relief. It gives the woman an "out" if she can return to a more familiar role of caretaker.

Years Alone

One predictable life situation for women is that they will most likely have to spend some years alone. Life expectancy for men is shorter, so many women will be widowed. A growing problem is the incidence of divorce among middle-aged and older couples, often leaving the woman alone. For the woman who has been abandoned at a time when she may be particularly concerned about her competence and attractiveness, the strain on her self-esteem can be intense. That widowhood is one of the greatest stresses in life has been documented repeatedly (see "Aging Healthfully," pp. 469–70). The initial reactions of numbness, disbelief, and grief give way to the difficult process of working through the loss and the equally difficult reorientation of one's life.

Women should prepare themselves for this possibility. They need to develop a sense of competence and autonomy. It is important to have some skills for employment or at least interests which are meaningful. It is important to develop social contacts which can provide later stimulation and support. It is also important to develop the ability to take care of oneself and some capacity for independence. The old model of the feminine role with its emphasis on compliance and passivity does not prepare women well for eventualities of middle age and later.

An additional stress for the middle-aged woman who finds herself alone is the return to a somewhat adolescent status in her relationships with men. "Dating" may be very uncomfortable and may revive social anxieties from her teens. Although there are singles clubs and many activities for unmarried people, they are often strained and the women outnumber the men. In spite of the increase in divorced and widowed women, many feel that social life is quite curtailed if they are not part of a couple. Support is often found from group discussion, from work (in spite of anxieties which may be involved in returning to the job market), and from further education, with its social contacts.

Returning to Work and School

Returning to work or school or starting to work for the first time after children are older has become the accepted pattern rather than the unusual event. Over 50 percent of women now work, including mothers of small children. Where formerly children were usually in college or at least high school, now inflationary pressures and the shift of expectations and opportunities for women have made it more usual for mothers of preschoolers to be working.

The woman who returns to work at midlife meets a combination of opportunity and stress. The older woman may be in a group where most are younger and she may have to learn skills and adapt to attitudes which are new. The competitiveness and aggression expected at work may run contrary to her training as a young girl to inhibit direct expression or even awareness of competition and aggressive feelings. Most women do not express wishes for fulfillment for themselves directly. It is hard to say, "I want this promotion" or "I want this reward for myself." It is easier and causes less conflict to seek rewards through doing things for others. Although this is changing to some extent, the woman in midlife who returns to work is likely to have been brought up with one set of values and find herself needing another set to function optimally, unless she is in a traditional work situation such as being a caretaker or facilitator. Old anxieties from school days may return. Successful resolution of these issues can lead to a sense of pleasure and accomplishment, even though some conflicts remain.

Families who have functioned with the mother fulfilling nurturant and organizing roles may find she is less available, and husbands and children may offer overt or covert resistance to her work demands or claims on her time. She may feel guilt and pressure to withdraw from work or to try to do everything and become exhausted. Sometimes inner conflict about the role change is projected onto the outer problems and demands or onto discrimination against women. The discrimination may be real, but blaming anxiety on external circumstances can also serve as a way to avoid dealing with the more complicated internal issues.

For the woman who is alone, work may offer a source of meaningful social encounters, a sense of being needed and important, and creative satisfactions, as well as necessary financial gains. During periods of unemployment women are likely to have more difficulty finding jobs, with consequent vulnerability to depression. In recent years a number of facilities have been organized to help women with these issues. Discussion groups, counseling offices and groups, and specific organizations which help women develop their assertiveness, strengths, job hunting skills, and even help find jobs, have emerged. Some of these are particularly responsive to the needs of middle-aged women reentering the job market. Others focus on understanding and expressing the feelings which have had little previous outlet.

CONCLUSION

The period of midlife has been compared to adolescence. The importance of separation, the change in relationship to the family, and the potential for further development of one's own interests are common to both. However, the differences are highly significant. At adolescence the separation is from parents. At midlife the separation is from children, if one has had them, and this experience often revives some sense of that earlier loss. For childless women midlife also contains the element of assessment, confrontation with finiteness, and sometimes a shift of goals, whether these involve personal and family possibilities or investment in work or other interests. The adolescent's perspective of infinite time and choices to be made differs from the sense of the finite and the midlife reassessment of choices which were actually made in the past. For example, women who are alone are less likely to find available appropriate men than are adolescents. The reality is that time is limited and that, although choices do exist or even increase, there is also a decreased range and variety. Physical health is very important. The emergence of an illness, impairment, or limitation, even a trivial one, can have a profound effect in confronting a woman with the finiteness of life.

Some women alter their physical appearance with a recognition of middle age. While those who have a strong investment in continuing to look young may have face lifts, dye their hair, and diet rigorously, others may relax some of these efforts, stop dyeing their hair, and choose a more "natural" look. This does not mean disregarding their appearance, gaining weight, or becoming inactive. In fact, increased understanding of the importance of physical fitness and exercise has made the old expectations of postmenopausal shapelessness and body "thickening" less the rule. There can be an acceptance of oneself without the pressure toward youthfulness, but with maintenance of vigor and sexual interest.

It is clear that for women in midlife, social changes have brought more options and sometimes more problems. Life patterns such as childlessness or working mothers, which were formerly rare or regarded as strange, are becoming more acceptable and will bring further changes in norms. It is also clear that growth and development goes on throughout life, and for women there is an interweaving of experiences related to their reproductive lives, establishment of personal identity, intellectual growth, relationship to work, and independence and autonomy.

REFERENCES

Barnett, R., and G. Baruch. "Women in the Middle Years: A Critique of Research and Theory." *Psychology of Women Quarterly* 3, no. 2 (Winter 1978).

Bart, P., and M. Grossman. "Menopause." *Women Health* 1, no. 3 (1976).

Butler, R. "The Facade of Chronological Age." *American Journal of Psychiatry* 119, no. 8 (February 1963): 722–728.

Friedman, E. "Pregnancy." In M. Notman and C. Nadelson, eds., *The Woman Patient: Medical and Psychological Interfaces*. New York: Plenum, 1978.

Levinson, D., C. Darrow, et al. *The Seasons of a Man's Life*. New York: Knopf, 1978.

McKinley, S., and M. Jeffreys. "The Menopausal Syndrome." *British Journal Preview Society of Medicine* 28, no. 2 (May 1974): 108–115.

Neugarten, B., and R. J. Kraines. "Menopausal Symptoms in Women of Various Ages." *Psychosomatic Medicine* 27 (1965): 266–273.

Neugarten, B. "The Awareness of Middle Age." In B. Neugarten, ed., *Middle Age and Aging*. Chicago: University of Chicago Press, 1968.

Perlmutter, J. "The Menopause: A Gynecologist's Views." In M. Notman and C. Nadelson, eds., *The Woman Patient: Medical and Psychological Interfaces*. New York: Plenum, 1978.

Weissman, M., and G. Klerman. "Sex Differences and the Epidemiology of Depression." *Archives of General Psychiatry* 34 (1977): 98–111.

FURTHER READING

Miller, J. B. *Towards a New Psychology of Women*. Boston: Beacon Press, 1976.

Neugarten, B. "Adult Personality: Towards a Psychology of the Life Cycle." In W. Sze, ed., *Human Life Cycle*. New York: Aronson, 1975.

Notman, M. "Pregnancy and Abortion: Implications for Career Development of Professional Women." In R. Kundsin, ed., *Women and Success*. New York: Morrow, 1974.

Notman, M., and C. Nadelson, eds. *The Woman Patient: Medical and Psychological Interfaces*. New York: Plenum, 1978.

Quigley, M., and C. Hammond. "Estrogen Replacement Therapy—Help or Hazard." *New England Journal of Medicine* 301, no. 12 (September 20, 1979): 646–648.

Rose, L., ed. *The Menopause Book*. New York: Hawthorn Books, 1977.

Rossi, A. "Transition to Parenthood." *Journal of Marriage and the Family* 38, no. 1 (1973): 92.

Sontag, S. "The Double Standard of Aging." *Saturday Review*, September 23, 1972, p. 29.

Aging is a topic of growing interest, as both the number and proportion of older people in our society are rapidly increasing. And it is of special importance to women, who constitute most of the older population and who frequently care for elderly family members. Geriatrics, the medical specialty concerned with aging and the conditions of the aged, and gerontology, the more general study of the process of aging, are both complex and rapidly developing fields.

The two following chapters discuss various aspects of aging. The first, Aging Healthfully—Your Body, concentrates on physical health; the second, Aging Healthfully—Your Mind and Spirit, focuses on mental health and related topics. Normal aging, prevention of disease, injury and disability, and management of conditions that have not been or cannot be prevented receive particular emphasis. Advice that is helpful to one woman may be inappropriate for another, for in the later years of life, the differences in physical condition among women of the same age are greater than at any other time. Nevertheless, most older women remain relatively healthy and active for many years. And application of our growing knowledge of aging may permit even more women to retain good physical and mental health.

EXTRA SURVIVORSHIP OF WOMEN

The Bureau of the Census predicts that the woman born today will live on average to approximately age 76, almost 8 years longer than her male counterpart. At present a woman who survives to age 65 can expect an average of 17.5 more years of life, but a man of the same age can anticipate only 13.4 more years. Thus, the older age groups are largely female. The U. S. population over age 65 currently contains only 69 men for every 100 women and that over age 85 includes more than twice as many women as men.

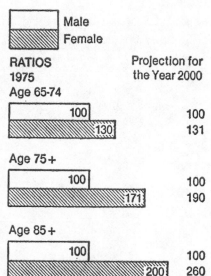

U.S. POPULATION AGE 65 AND OVER

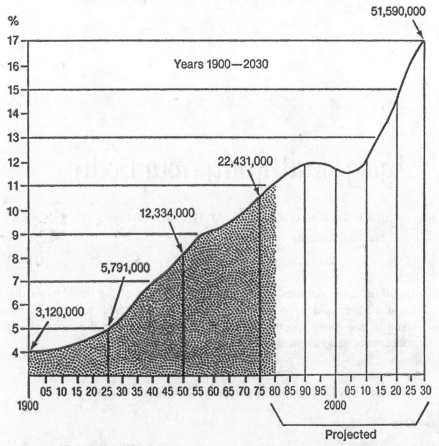

Years 1900—2030

51,590,000

22,431,000

12,334,000

5,791,000

3,120,000

%
17
16
15
14
13
12
11
10
9
8
7
6
5
4

05 10 15 20 25 30 35 40 45 50 55 60 65 70 75 80 85 90 95 | 05 10 15 20 25 30
1900   2000

Projected

Source: U.S. Census Bureau

The total number and the proportion of elderly are growing. In the United States in 1900 only 3.1 million persons, or 4% of the population, were over age 65. Today the aged number 24 million and represent 11 percent of the population. The drop in the projected estimate around the year 2005 reflects the lower birth rate during the depression of the 1930s. The Census Bureau predicts that by the year 2030, 52 million people or 13 to 21 percent of the population will be over age 65.

Aging Healthfully—Your Body

BARBARA GASTEL, M.D., M.P.H.
National Institute on Aging

Healthful aging requires attention to specific parts of the body, to particular disorders, and to general well-being. This chapter will first discuss some of the more specific topics, and then talk about the more general concerns of good medical care, medication, exercise, and safety.

AGE-RELATED CHANGES IN PARTS OF THE BODY

Skin

Neither beauty nor health is skin deep, but healthy skin can contribute greatly to both appearance and comfort in the later years of life. With age the skin becomes less elastic, its glands lubricate less effectively, and cells controlling its color often start to malfunction. Thus, wrinkles and "age spots" frequently occur. Although some age-related changes in the skin seem to be inevitable, others can be prevented or delayed.

Long hours of exposure to the sun, often called "the skin's worst enemy," accelerate aging of the skin and increase the risk of skin cancer. To prevent sun damage it is necessary either to avoid the sun or to guard the skin. Creams, oils, and lotions known as sun-screens help to protect the skin; many dermatologists and researchers believe that PABA (para-aminobenzoic acid) in an alcohol base and sulisobenzone are among the best sun-blocking agents now available.

Several other factors also can make the skin appear older. In winter cold weather and freezing winds, dry and overheated rooms, and even the use of electric blankets can make the skin scaly and inelastic. In summer air conditioning can have similar effects. Excessive alcohol intake, poor diet, and cigarette smoking also may damage the skin.

Although no method can completely arrest or reverse age-related changes in the skin, several approaches can contribute to attractive, healthy skin. One's own outlook is essential to others' perceptions. Aged skin does not mean lack of beauty. Many women feel that they are no longer attractive or even worthwhile once physical signs of aging begin to appear. However, attitudes are changing. As the population ages, so does our ideal of beauty; among women now considered most beautiful, many, for example Katharine Hepburn, Grace Kelly, and Elizabeth Taylor, are in or are approaching the later years of life. With women achieving more varied roles in society, other criteria are becoming more important than a youthful appearance.

Several mechanical procedures, including dermabrasion, chemical peel, and facelift, that can help to correct some types of age-associated skin damage are discussed in the chapter on "Cosmetic Surgery." Simpler approaches, including the use of "wrinkle creams," skin lighteners and bleaches, make-up, and moisturizers can also improve or conceal the appearance of aged skin. Wrinkle creams generally contain both oil to smooth the skin and an irritant to cause slight swelling and thus fill out small lines and creases. Skin lighteners and bleaches can help to fade darkened areas of skin; like medications, they must be used only as directed.

Moisturizers, among the most popular products for aging skin, temporarily improve the texture and appearance of skin and help to relieve dry, tight, itchy sensations. For moisturizers to be most effective, water should be patted onto the skin before their application. Generally, the effectiveness of a moisturizer is unrelated to its cost; many women find inexpensive products satisfactory, and moisturizers of different prices actually may contain similar ingredients.

Itching is a common problem in older persons. Several measures can help to relieve dry, itchy skin on the body. When bathing, use only mild soaps or cleansers, apply soap only to areas that need especially thorough cleansing (the underarms, pubic and anal areas, feet, hands), use warm rather than hot water, avoid long baths, and pat the skin dry gently instead of rubbing it briskly. After the bath, bath oil or another moisturizer should be applied to the moist skin. Addition of oil to the bath water is unwise, as the tub can become dangerously slippery. Humidification of the air, use of soft cotton flannel sheets, and addition of a small amount of bath oil to water used to rinse laundry also can be helpful.

Severe or persistent skin conditions such as rashes, sores, and unmanageable itching should be seen by a doctor. Some of the conditions may be relieved by locally applied measures, and others may be the first noticeable signs of a disease that affects the entire body and requires treatment. Growths on the skin should receive prompt attention to determine if they are malignant. The early removal of skin cancers almost always results in cure.

Eyes

Visual impairment becomes more common with age. Of the estimated more than 500,000 Americans who are legally blind, nearly half are above age 65. However, conditions affecting the eyes of older persons often can be treated successfully, and many special aids and services are available to individuals with irreversible visual impairment.

Even before middle age, the lens of the eye starts to become less elastic. By age 40 the reduced elasticity produces in most people a condition called presbyopia, or difficulty in focusing on objects at close range. Most persons over 40 require reading glasses or bifocals.

Another condition affecting the eye is cataract, in which the lens becomes opaque or cloudy and thus vision becomes unclear. Although 95 percent of persons over 65 may have some degree of cataracts, in only a small proportion is the condition severe enough to interfere significantly with vision and require treatment. At present, surgery to remove the cataract is the only treatment available, and it is successful in 90 to 95 percent of cases. After surgery replacement of the function of the individual's own lens is necessary, and special glasses or contact lenses are usually prescribed. A relatively new alternative to eyeglasses or contact lenses is the placement of a permanent plastic lens inside the eye during cataract surgery; the long-term safety and effectiveness of this procedure are still being evaluated.

Glaucoma, a condition characterized by increased pressure within the eye and loss of visual function, is a leading cause of blindness. In the most common type of glaucoma medication can usually control the pressure and prevent visual loss. However, surgery may be needed in some cases. All adults, especially those with a family history of glaucoma, should be checked periodically for this disease.

Diabetes, especially if present for many years, can damage the retina of the eye, and therefore diabetics require careful, frequent eye examinations. A treatment called photocoagulation, which uses a laser beam, can help to destroy abnormal tissue and blood vessels in the retina and thus preserve sight in some patients.

Senile macular degeneration, a poorly understood deterioration of the part of the retina responsible for sharp, clear color vision, affects about 10 percent of persons over 70 years of age and appears to be more common in women than in men. Individuals with this condition generally retain some vision and thus can continue to care for themselves. However, as senile macular degeneration produces a large blind spot in the middle of the visual field, it interferes with such activities as reading, sewing, watching television, and driving. The condition is associated with abnormal blood circulation to the retina, and photocoagulation may prove useful in some early cases, although this treatment has not yet been fully evaluated. Special low vision aids, including magnifiers, telescopic lenses, and closed circuit television that projects printed matter onto a screen, can allow some people with macular degeneration to continue many normal activities.

Numerous public and private organizations assist the visually handicapped of all ages. The Federal Government and each state and territory have offices to provide and coordinate such services, and the American Foundation for the Blind is a major nongovernmental source of information (see sources of information listed on page 484). Aids available to the visually impaired include large-type books, magazines, and newspapers; recorded literature; counseling; at-home instruction; special social security benefits and income tax concessions; and devices to facilitate daily living.

Ears

Ability to hear declines with age. Although often the loss is too slight to interfere with ordinary activities, an estimated one-third of all persons over 65 have significant difficulty hearing. Hearing loss is more common in men, perhaps in part because of greater occupational exposure to noise. Although little is known about prevention of age-related hearing loss, avoidance of excessive noise is advisable.

A wide variety of hearing deficits occur in the aged, but certain features are especially common. The elderly often have the most difficulty perceiving high tones. In addition, speech can sound loud enough but nevertheless seem unclear. Thus, older persons may say that others are mumbling and may remark "I can hear you all right, but I can't understand what you're saying."

The first step in managing a hearing impairment is identification of the specific problem. A general physician can examine the ears, perform basic tests of hearing, and manage some hearing disorders. For additional evaluation and treatment, he or she may refer the patient to an otorhinolaryngologist or otologist (a physician specializing in the ear) or an audiologist (a nonphysician specially trained to diagnose and manage hearing problems).

Often the diagnosis is presbycusis, which means hearing loss associated with aging. Although this condition cannot be cured, approaches such as hearing aids and special training can be very helpful. In other instances a reversible condition may be discovered. For example, treatment of an unsuspected ear infection or removal of wax clogging the ear canal can improve hearing.

Many older men and women find hearing aids helpful. Individuals are advised not to buy such devices without consulting a physician or audiologist, who can help select the most appropriate hearing aids and give advice as to their most effective use. Hearing aids make sounds louder, but they cannot correct hearing as precisely as glasses correct vision. A period of adjustment is often necessary, and sometimes a hearing specialist can help a patient to obtain hearing aids for trial periods of a few weeks each until a satisfactory device is found. Persons with conditions such as arthritis or stroke may find small parts of hearing aids difficult to handle; special hearing aids that compensate for some of these problems are available or are being developed.

Aids that may be especially helpful to hearing-impaired persons who live alone are attachments for telephones and televisions to amplify voices and devices that flash on a light when the doorbell or telephone rings. And now the American Humane Association is training "hearing dogs," which aid the deaf somewhat as seeing eye dogs help the blind.

Special training can help the hearing-impaired to make the most of their abilities. For example, "lip-reading," sensitivity to facial expressions and gestures, and use of appropriate questions can help the individual with a hearing loss to take an active part in conversation. Both individual instruction and classes in these skills are available in many communities. Family members, close friends, and employers may find attending such sessions along with the hearing-impaired individual useful in appreciating and dealing with the problem.

If you have difficulty hearing, the following suggestions may make communication easier.

· Ask people to face you.
· Keep background noise to a minimum.
· Ask people to speak clearly and loudly, but not to shout.
· Suggest that someone addressing you get your attention, for example by a gentle tap on the shoulder, before speaking.
· Ask to be told what is being discussed if you join a conversation already in progress.
· If you do not understand what someone is saying, ask the speaker to repeat the statement using different words.
· When you are given important instructions, be sure you understand the message.

Effective management of hearing problems in the elderly has social and psychological benefits. It helps the individual to retain or regain an active role in the family and the community. Likewise, it aids in combating the loneliness, boredom, and depression that can befall those who are unable to take part in conversation and to enjoy fully radio, television, movies, and other popular forms of entertainment.

Teeth and Gums

For years being old meant being toothless, a condition detrimental to nutrition, speech, and appearance. Today, however, increasing numbers of older persons are retaining their teeth or obtaining satisfactory dentures. Lifelong care of the teeth and mouth is essential to general health in old age.

With age the mouth undergoes several changes. Although the risk of tooth decay decreases with increasing age, tooth loss because of periodontal disease (disease of the gums and other tissues surrounding the teeth) becomes more common with age. Gum recession may loosen teeth and expose tooth roots which are then more susceptible to decay and do not hold fillings well because their softer dentine is not covered by enamel. In addition, age-related changes and certain medications can cause the mouth to become rather dry. Dryness causes discomfort, fosters decay, and makes dentures more difficult to retain. Because of factors such as tooth loss and a diminished sense of taste, many older persons choose soft, sweet diets, which promote root decay. Age-related bone loss can make old dentures uncomfortable and new dentures difficult to fit.

Throughout life and particularly in old age prevention of dental disease can be effective and more economical than treatment. Regular checkups, which should include detection of signs of local and systemic disease, prompt treatment of abnormal conditions of the teeth and mouth, and instruction in proper techniques of oral hygiene, are essential, although unfortunately not covered by many insurance programs. Daily mouth care, generally including both brushing and flossing, also is necessary. Devices such as electric toothbrushes and long-handled toothbrushes may help persons partially disabled by arthritis and other handicaps to maintain good oral hygiene. A well-balanced diet that provides plenty of chewing, is low in sugar, and includes sufficient fluid also promotes oral hygiene. As smoking predisposes to cancer of the mouth, avoidance of this habit is important.

Proper management and suitable diets can help to reverse or arrest incipient conditions that affect the teeth and mouth in later life. For example, prompt replacement of missing teeth helps to preserve oral structures and aids in maintaining good nutrition. Sipping plenty of water with meals and in some cases rinsing with specially prescribed mouthwashes can relieve dryness of the mouth. Because of age-related changes in the mouth and elsewhere in the body, both the older patient and the dentist sometimes need extra patience and effort to achieve the desired results.

Nervous System

Although mental impairment and other disorders of the nervous system are among the most feared conditions of old age, most people maintain a high level of mental competence and neurological function throughout life. Even after age 80 changes normally are slight and of little consequence. However, a significant minority suffer from disorders of the nervous system.

Any possible symptom of neurological disease, for example, partial paralysis, numbness, tremor, memory loss, or difficulty with speech, requires medical evaluation. In many cases examination will reveal a reversible condition such as depression, a vitamin deficiency, or a side reaction from a drug. In others, such as stroke, early diagnosis can help patient, family, and medical personnel to cope more effectively with the condition. Unfortunately, many neurological problems are poorly understood, difficult to manage, and frustrating to all involved.

An estimated 4 to 5 percent of Americans over age 65 have some degree of serious intellectual impairment. Such difficulties may be somewhat more common in women than in men, perhaps because women tend to live longer. Such impairment is commonly, but rather imprecisely termed "senility," a label that does not denote a specific disease, but rather stands for a wide variety of conditions, many of them curable.

Alzheimer's disease, a poorly understood condition believed to affect at least 500,000 Americans, is the most prevalent cause of mental decline in old age. A common early symptom is severe difficulty with short-term memory (not the slight forgetfulness that many people exhibit). Later the individual may have difficulty thinking, undergo personality changes, and become confused. Although much research is underway, effective treatments for Alzheimer's disease are not yet available. Physicians and other health personnel can help the individual to make the most of remaining abilities (for example, through the use of memory aids known as mnemonics) and can help the patient and family to cope with the condition. In both the United States and Canada families of patients with Alzheimer's disease are banding together to share support and information.

Over 100 other conditions, many of them curable, can produce signs and symptoms that mimic those of Alzheimer's disease. These underlying problems include depression, drug reactions, infections, heart disease, kidney failure, thyroid disease, head injury, and anemia. If such conditions are treated promptly, normal mental function may return. Therefore, a thorough medical evaluation, including history, physical examination, and laboratory tests, is essential for anyone who seems to have become "senile."

Stroke occurs when part of the brain suffers damage because of insufficient blood supply; blood clots and broken blood vessels supplying the brain can be responsible. Although various symptoms can occur, the most common is paralysis of part of the body, either alone or combined with impaired speech. In time and with promptly instituted, vigorous rehabilitative therapy, improvement often occurs. Special devices can help persons with lasting disability to perform everyday tasks independently.

At least 2 million people now alive in the United States have suffered strokes. They affect approximately twice as many women as men and are the third most common cause of death in this country. However, particularly in the elderly, strokes have become considerably less common in recent years. The cause for this reduction is unknown, but recent strides in controlling high blood pressure, which strongly predisposes to stroke, may be playing an important role.

Although information on how to prevent strokes is incomplete, control of high blood pressure and adherence to the measures recommended in this chapter's section on the heart and blood vessels appear to be wise. "Little strokes" (short periods of partial blindness, speech difficulty, paralysis, or other impairment) warn of the possibility of major stroke and thus demand medical attention. Of course, anyone with symptoms that may result from stroke should seek medical attention promptly.

Parkinson's disease is estimated to affect only 1 person in 1,000 in the general population, but 1 person in 40 over age 60. The three most common features of the disease are tremor, rigidity, and a bent posture. This condition's severity and rate of progression vary considerably from patient to patient.

Although the underlying cause of Parkinson's disease remains unknown, the condition is known to be associated with a shortage of dopamine in part of the brain. Since 1970 the drug levodopa, or L-dopa, which helps to replenish the supply of this substance, has been available by prescription. Although this medication has helped many patients, it is not totally and permanently effective, and often side effects eventually develop. Scientists are investigating several other agents in search of a medication that has fewer side effects and is more effective.

Most older persons escape the serious diseases just described, but the nervous system often becomes slightly less efficient with age. Generally, ingenuity and effort can overcome these limitations. For example, the use of lists and other reminders can compensate for minor difficulty with memory; attention to simple safety measures can prevent decreased balance and coordination from becoming hazardous; and a little extra time generally is sufficient for learning complex new tasks. With patience and a positive attitude, knowledge and skills can continue to grow impressively throughout life.

Indeed, perhaps the best advice for keeping the normally aging nervous system healthy is to keep it active. The individual who remains interested in the world, who continues to use and develop mental and physical skills acquired throughout life, and who continues amassing knowledge is most likely to remain young at heart—and young at nerve and brain.

Heart and Blood Vessels

Diseases of the heart and blood vessels account for most deaths, as well as much suffering in the older population. With age the heart muscle thickens and narrowing of the arteries is likely to occur. The healthy aged heart can still perform satisfactorily under normal conditions, but is less able to respond to extraordinary stresses. In addition, various cardiovascular disorders, including angina pectoris, myocardial infarction (heart attack), congestive heart failure, high blood pressure, and stroke, become more common with advancing age.

Research has suggested that the risk of cardiovascular disease is increased by smoking, high blood cholesterol levels, obesity, lack of regular exercise, high blood pressure, diabetes, and chronic excessive stress. Thus, not smoking, a well-balanced diet low in animal fat, maintenance of a normal weight, frequent and regular exercise, control of high blood pressure, and avoidance of unnecessary stress may help to prevent such conditions. Such measures also may help to avoid further, more serious damage in persons who already have cardiovascular disease.

Angina pectoris, a temporary but recurring chest pain caused by an inadequate supply of oxygen to the heart muscle, is usually a sign that the blood vessels supplying the heart have become narrowed. It tends to occur during exercise, stress, and other situations in which the heart must perform extra work. Anyone with chest pain should consult a physician who may determine if the condition is angina and, if necessary, prescribe medication such as nitroglycerin. Surgery to bypass the narrowed vessels is helpful in some cases.

Heart attack, technically known as myocardial infarction, occurs when part of the heart muscle dies because the artery supplying blood to it becomes blocked. The nation's number one killer, it is much more common in young men than young women, but rates in women increase considerably with age. Anyone experiencing symptoms of a possible heart attack —pain or pressure in the center of the chest that may spread to the shoulders, neck or arms, and sometimes dizziness, fainting, sweating, nausea, or breathlessness—should call for medical help immediately. With appropriate treatment most people can return to an active life after recovery from a heart attack.

Congestive heart failure, which occurs when the heart does not pump efficiently, can produce shortness of breath and swelling of the ankles. Medically prescribed measures including treatment of any associated heart conditions, drugs such as digitalis and diuretics, and a low salt diet may provide relief of symptoms. Adjustments in lifestyle to stay within the limits imposed by the condition can aid in coping with congestive heart failure. For example, a person who becomes breathless when climbing too many steps may wish to move to a one-story house, live in an apartment building with an elevator, or carry a magazine to read while pausing to rest at stair landings.

High blood pressure, or hypertension, especially essential (no known cause) hypertension, becomes more common with age. Among older persons it is found more frequently in women and tends to be especially common and severe among older black women. Although hypertension itself is painless and generally symptomless, it predisposes to heart attack, stroke, kidney damage, congestive heart failure, and other disorders. Every physical examination should include measurement of blood pressure. In treating hypertension a physician may suggest measures such as those described above in the discussion of prevention of cardiovascular disease, recommend a low-salt diet, and prescribe specific medications. Although vigorous treatment of hypertension is strongly recommended in youth and middle age, the benefits are uncertain of treating some types of mild or moderate hypertension in those over 65 without heart disease, and thus less aggressive management may be considered.

Stroke, a cardiovascular disease resulting from insufficient blood supply to part of the brain, already has been discussed in the section on the nervous system.

Perhaps because more people are observing the measures described at the beginning of this section, death rates from cardiovascular disease, including heart attack and stroke, have decreased considerably in recent years.

Varicose veins. Both being female and getting older increase the risk of developing varicose veins, enlarged or distorted veins often visible below the skin surface. Pregnancy leaves many women with this condition. With age the veins tend to become less elastic and the muscles supporting them generally weaken, thus predisposing to this disorder.

Although many cases of varicose veins merely are unsightly, others can result in serious complications such as leg ulcers if not properly treated. Therefore, anyone who has this condition and experiences leg pain or discomfort should seek medical care.

Doctors may recommend various measures, depending on the severity and type of varicose veins. The following suggestions for fostering good circulation are commonly made:

- Avoid round elastic garters, socks with tight elastic tops, and wearing elastic girdles for long periods of time.
- When possible, sit instead of stand. When sitting, do not cross your legs; instead elevate them on a chair or stool.

· Exercise your legs frequently. Walking and swimming are especially effective.
· When sitting for long periods of time, be sure to stretch your legs every hour or so.

To support the weakened veins, physicians sometimes prescribe elastic stockings or elastic bandages. In other cases, they suggest surgery, which may consist of such procedures as removing ("stripping") or tying off ("ligating") damaged veins.

Lungs

Although respiratory function declines with age, the normally aging lung has sufficient reserve to function effectively under ordinary conditions. However, cigarette smoking increases the age-related changes, sometimes to a dangerous extent. Chronic lung disease, especially that associated with smoking, makes activity and even breathing difficult for many older persons.

The chronic obstructive lung diseases, emphysema and chronic bronchitis, are considerably more common among smokers and tend to become evident between the ages of 45 and 65. In emphysema progressive damage to the smaller airways and to the air sacs may hinder the movement of air into and out of the lung and interfere with gas exchange. In chronic bronchitis the lung cannot obtain enough air because its passageways become blocked by swelling and by mucus and other fluids. These and other respiratory diseases, symptoms of which can include a persistent or recurring cough, "tightness" or pain in the chest, and a tendency to tire easily, require prompt medical attention. Measures such as stopping smoking, use of appropriate medications, good nutrition, sufficient rest, and pulmonary "toilet" (bending with head and chest down to promote lung drainage) can help to control chronic obstructive lung disease.

Lung cancer, mainly a disease of smokers and thus once largely a disease of men, is becoming more common among women. Today women are smoking more heavily, and women's death rates from lung cancer have increased 400 percent in the last 30 years. If present trends continue, this disease will become the leading cause of cancer deaths in women sometime during the 1980s.

The message of this section should be clear: avoidance of smoking is one of the most important factors in aging healthfully. Many harmful changes in the lungs, heart, blood vessels, and other parts of the body can be avoided or delayed by never smoking. Even in persons who have smoked heavily for many years, lung function often improves or its deterioration is halted or slowed after stopping smoking.

Digestive System

The digestive system usually ages successfully. Digestion of food generally remains adequate, but, as in other stages of life, upset and uncooperative stomachs are common.

In later life many factors can produce gastrointestinal distress. As at other ages, emotional stresses often produce abdominal discomfort and disturbances in bowel habits. Gallstones most frequently occur in women over 40, and cancers of the digestive tract generally become more common with age. Many other conditions, including ulcers, infections, and even back problems, can produce abdominal symptoms.

Because so many conditions can cause similar symptoms, self-diagnosis and self-treatment of digestive problems can be dangerous. Anyone with symptoms such as abdominal pain, vomiting, change in bowel habits, or blood in the bowel movements should seek medical attention. In many instances the condition can be treated successfully.

Constipation concerns many older people. Although it can result in part from age-related changes in the digestive system, lifestyle seems to be a more important factor. Inadequate fluid intake, faulty eating habits, frequent use of laxatives, lack of exercise, and depression all can contribute to constipation. A diet that is rich in fluids, whole grain cereals, fruits, and vegetables may help to control this condition. Laxatives should be taken only when prescribed by a physician.

Fiber, a largely undigestible food component that is abundant in bran and in many fruits and vegetables, recently has received considerable attention. Fiber helps to control constipation, and fiber-rich foods tend to be filling, but low in calories. However, it remains unclear whether, as some claim, a diet high in fiber also aids in preventing hemorrhoids, bowel cancer, heart disease, and other disorders.

For most individuals "an apple a day" and *not* keeping the doctor away when he or she is needed are basic to successful, comfortable aging of the digestive system.

Urinary and Reproductive Systems

The physical changes of the perimenopausal stage are described in "Midlife Transitions." In part because of postmenopausal changes in the reproductive system, some types of urinary problems become more common with age. Low estrogen levels may predispose to infections of the urinary tract. Furthermore, weakening of pelvic structures, particularly in women who have borne several children, can produce "stress incontinence," a leakage of urine during such activities as coughing, sneezing, and straining.

Special exercises often can help to control stress incontinence; in other cases medication or surgery may prove useful.

Menopause does not end the need for breast and pelvic examinations; their importance may even increase in the later years of life. Since older women no longer have the monthly menstrual reminder to do a breast self-examination, they should choose a specific date, for example, the first day or the day corresponding to one's birthday, on which to do it each month. The indications for special breast examinations, such as mammograms, are discussed in the chapter on "Breast Care." Breast tumors that appear later in life may tend to be less aggressive and more easily treatable than those occurring in younger women.

Regularly scheduled gynecologic checkups, as well as consultation with a physician whenever problems such as bleeding arise, continue to be important throughout life. Although in most cases of postmenopausal bleeding the underlying cause is benign, prompt medical attention is necessary to identify potentially serious conditions while they remain easily treatable.

Sexual Response

What actually happens to sexual functioning in old age? Basically, women and men experience a decrease in intensity and rapidity of sexual response. For a woman, this means that she may take as long as 5 minutes, compared to 15 or 30 seconds in younger years, to lubricate, but clitoral response remains the same. Between ages 50 and 70, the duration of her orgasm gradually declines from 8 to 12 contractions to 4 or 5. But there is no decrease in sexual arousability and there frequently is an increase. More important, women can still have multiple orgasms well into their eighties, an ability few men enjoy at any age.

As a man ages, the pattern is basically the same. Excitement builds more slowly; erection takes longer to attain. The plateau phase tends to last longer than during youth, making the older man better able to maintain erection without orgasm. When he does reach orgasm, it is usually briefer and less intense, and subsequent loss of erection may take just a few seconds compared to a younger man's minutes or hours. In other words, healthy men do not lose their ability to have erections and ejaculations as they age. But it takes longer to complete intercourse, which may be helpful, since older women also take longer to become sexually excited. Compared to women, men experience greater sexual changes with age, and tend to desire sexual intercourse less often.

Bones and Joints

Brittle bones and stiff joints are common as our bodies age. One condition, osteoporosis, in which the bones become thin and brittle, is mainly seen in women who have passed the menopause. In the United States an estimated 15 million persons, at least 75 percent of them older women, have osteoporosis. This condition usually remains silent until one of the weakened bones breaks. Fractures of the spine (vertebrae) and the hip (neck of the femur) most often result.

Prevention of osteoporosis and the resulting fractures is a field of active research but of little definite knowledge. Estrogens, diets high in protein and calcium (milk, milk products, and shellfish) and exercise appear to help maintain strong bones.

About 10.6 million older Americans, most of them women, have arthritis, which is not a single disease, but a class of several conditions affecting the joints. Pain, swelling, stiffness, and other joint symptoms demand medical attention, as the various diseases in the arthritis family require different treatments. Often the physician can reassure the patient that the symptoms are likely to remain mild and require little or no treatment. In other cases, rest, medication (commonly including aspirin), exercise, physical therapy, and sometimes surgery may be necessary to relieve pain and preserve function. Persons with arthritis should be wary of quack remedies and devices, which waste money and can cause permanent injury. Because arthritis generally comes and goes, these "cures" often are mistakenly considered effective. Devices such as long-handled combs and kitchen utensils, heightened chairs and toilet seats, and clothes without buttons or snaps can make daily activities easier and preserve independence for those partially disabled by arthritis.

When many people think of arthritis, they think of rheumatoid arthritis, a disease producing inflammation of the joints. This disease, most often seen in older people, affects about three times as many women as men.

Osteoarthritis, unlike rheumatoid arthritis, is not an inflammatory disease. It is much more common than rheumatoid arthritis, especially among the older population. Aging, irritation of the joints, and normal wear and tear all may contribute to this condition. Other risk factors include overweight, poor posture, injury, and physical strain at work or play. Generally, osteoarthritis is a slowly developing disease and is less severe than rheumatoid arthritis. In fact, most persons with X-ray evidence of the condition have no symptoms from it.

Gout is the best understood and most easily treated form of arthritis. Although most cases occur in men, some women develop gout after menopause. In this condition excess uric acid accumulates in joints, causing inflammation and pain. Specific drugs reduce the amount of uric acid in the body, thus preventing both the joint symptoms and the kidney damage that elevated levels of uric acid can produce.

Feet

Throughout life feet bear tremendous burdens. Year after year they support our weight; changing fashions, including towering heels, pointed toes, and tight shoes, create special stresses. Diseases such as diabetes and circulatory impairments increase the risk of serious foot problems.

Some foot conditions require the attention of a physician or a podiatrist (a specialist in foot care). For example, attempting to treat corns, calluses, and ingrown toenails oneself may be dangerous. Experts in foot care offer the following advice:

- Avoid decreasing the circulation to the feet. In particular, do not cross your legs, wear socks with tight elastic tops, use round elastic garters, or place your feet in cold water.
- Be careful to avoid injuring your feet. For example, test the temperature of the water with your hand before stepping into the bath; do not go barefoot, even at home; and do not apply hot water bottles or heating pads to your feet.
- Wash feet daily in warm, not hot, water and mild soap. Dry feet gently and thoroughly, especially between the toes.
- Inspect feet regularly for redness, rashes, injuries, and other abnormalities. Seek medical attention for such problems.
- Wear well-fitting stockings and shoes. Shoes should be comfortable and provide both support and protection. In order to avoid irritation of the feet, new shoes should be worn for brief periods at first, then for progressively longer intervals.
- Exercise your feet. Walking is the best exercise. In addition, doctors may prescribe specific exercises.

Diabetics are especially prone to serious foot disorders and must guard their feet carefully; they should obtain specific instructions from their physicians and podiatrists.

Diabetes

Diabetes, a condition in which excess sugar appears in the blood, is more common in later age and affects a greater proportion of older women than older men. Many new cases that occur in later life affect overweight persons, are relatively mild, and can be controlled by diet alone. Because diabetics are especially prone to foot disorders, eye problems, infections, diseases of the heart and blood vessels, and other conditions, both frequent medical care and attention to one's own health are important. Physicians and nurses, dieticians, associations dealing with diabetes, and the many books, including cookbooks, for diabetics can be valuable sources of information.

Infection

Infection is another threat to the older population. The usual signs and symptoms of infection may be absent in an older person. For example, an elderly individual with pneumonia may be tired and confused, but lack fever or chest pain. Medical attention should be sought for any symptoms, not just the classic indications of infection.

Good general health practices, including sufficient rest, a balanced diet, and avoidance of unnecessary exposure to contagious disease, may be helpful in preventing infections. As the elderly are especially prone to serious or fatal complications of influenza, annual vaccination against this disease is commonly recommended for persons aged 65 and above; the newly developed "flu shots" are more effective and less likely to cause side reactions than those available years ago. The recently developed pneumococcal vaccine, which helps to protect against some types of pneumonia, also may be advisable for some older persons.

GOOD MEDICAL CARE

Care by health professionals becomes increasingly important in the later years of life. Finding appropriate physicians, home and community services, and nursing homes is of great importance.

Until recently, few doctors in the United States had specific training in geriatrics. Today, however, more and more medical students, residents, and practicing physicians are studying the care of the aged. If a nearby medical school has a division of geriatrics, it may be able to recommend physicians who appreciate the needs of older patients; friends, family, and colleagues also can provide useful recommendations. In choosing a main physician, inquire about his or her interest and training in geriatrics and knowledge of the facilities available for the aged. Because many older persons are hospitalized at some time, information about the hospital to which the physician admits patients is also important.

Communication is basic to a good relationship with any health professional. A physician should show interest in understanding and helping the patient with his or her problems, explain illnesses and their treatment, discuss the patient's role in treating diseases and preventing accidents, and make clear that he or she will stick with the patient, no matter how difficult problems become. A helpful physician must be someone to whom a patient can and will talk openly about symptoms and problems, for providing such information is essential to receiving good health care.

In addition to a main physician, older persons often need the services of specialists such as cardiologists, neurologists, and rheumatologists. Also, routine care by ophthalmologists, gynecologists, dentists, and other specialists is often needed. When necessary, an individual's physician can refer him or her to skilled specialists in these and other fields.

Nonphysician services for the ill and disabled also are of great importance to the aged, as they can help to allow an older person to continue living at home. Such services include daily hot meal delivery, day care centers, visits by nurses, homemaker services, and daily phone calls to check whether help is needed. Some apartment buildings and communities especially for older persons provide this kind of help. Sources of information about such assistance include physicians and other health professionals, local health departments, government and private agencies concerned with aging, and religious and civic groups.

Sometimes health problems become so severe or home services are so limited that nursing home care is the only feasible approach. About 5 percent of the population over 65 resides in such institutions at any one time, and a much higher proportion of the population spends time in a nursing home at least temporarily during the later years of life. Almost three-quarters of elderly nursing home residents are women. For many older persons, the transition into a nursing home can be highly stressful. Likewise, many families and close friends experience feelings of guilt because they cannot care for an ill or disabled relative or lifelong friend. In many instances good nursing home care truly is in the best interests of the ill elderly individual, his or her family and friends, and their relationship. Finding a satisfactory nursing home can alleviate much of the stress and guilt.

Concern about good nursing homes should begin early. Attention to the type of care that older or sicker friends and relatives are receiving can be helpful. Interest in and, if possible, volunteer work at nursing homes in one's community both improves the facilities and provides an inside view. Participation in local organizations concerned with the quality of nursing home care achieves similar goals.

The Federal Office of Nursing Home Affairs has prepared an informative booklet, *How to Select a Nursing Home,* which concludes with a list of several dozen questions. Among items to consider in choosing a nursing home are:

· Does the nursing home seem to be a pleasant, friendly place to live? What do the current residents say about the home?
· Is the home clean, orderly, well-lighted, well-ventilated, and a comfortable temperature?
· Are residents' rooms attractive, conveniently furnished, safe, and sufficiently private?

- Does the nursing home have the required current license from the state or letter of approval from a licensing agency?
- Is the home certified to participate in the Medicare and Medicaid programs? Are you eligible for such coverage?
- Are necessary services, such as special diets and rehabilitative therapy, available?
- Is the nursing home safe for its residents, including the handicapped?
- What medical and dental services, including emergency care, are available?
- Does a qualified pharmacist supervise the pharmaceutical services?
- Is at least one registered nurse or licensed practical nurse on duty day and night?
- Are meals and snacks nutritious, appetizing, and sufficiently frequent?
- Is there a high-quality program of social and recreational activities?
- Does the nursing home have telephone service and indoor and outdoor recreational areas?
- Do the total estimated monthly costs and general financial policies compare favorably with those of other homes? Is the cost quoted inclusive, or are there extra charges for laundry, drugs, and special nursing procedures?
- Does the contract specify in detail such important aspects as costs, services, standards, and patients' rights?

MEDICATION

The 11 percent of the population over 65 uses approximately 25 percent of all prescription medication dispensed in this country, and the average older person receives 13 prescriptions, including renewals, each year. Drugs are the largest out-of-pocket medical expense for older persons living in the community.

Because the aging process and age-associated diseases can alter the body in various ways, reactions to certain medications can change with age. For example, age can affect the rates with which the body absorbs, processes, and eliminates certain drugs; thus, the doses required can change, often in a downward direction. Older persons also can experience different side-effects from drugs than younger persons do. Medications prescribed for one ailment can aggravate another. It is especially important for older persons to contact their physicians if a drug produces an unfavorable effect (such as sleepiness or nausea) or fails to work as it should.

Communication between patient and doctor is basic to good medical care. A physician cannot prescribe the proper amount of the right medication without correct, complete information. Questions especially important in determining what to prescribe include:

- Have you ever had an allergic reaction to any medication? For example, did any drug ever give you hives or make you dizzy?
- Are you taking any medications? Which ones? In particular, are you taking any drugs prescribed by other doctors? Are you taking any non-prescription drugs such as vitamins, laxatives, antacids or aspirin?
- Do you have any medical condition such as liver disease, kidney disease, or diabetes?
- Are you on a special diet, or do you have unusual eating habits?

Likewise, it is essential for the patient to obtain information about any drug that a doctor prescribes. Among the questions that the Federal Food and Drug Administration (FDA) suggests asking are:

- What is the name of the medication?
- What is the medicine supposed to do?
- What unwanted side effects might occur and should they be reported?
- Are there other medications that should be avoided while taking the medicine?
- How should the medication be taken? (How many times a day? Between, with, before, or after meals? At bedtime?)
- Is it necessary to take the medicine until it is all gone or just until the symptoms disappear?

Asking whether anything else is important to know about the drug also may be advisable.

Before visiting the doctor, you may wish to write out each of these questions and leave room to fill in the answers. Making several copies of the sheet (one for each drug) or a chart with room for information on several drugs can be helpful. Don't be disappointed if no drug is prescribed; in many conditions, medication is not helpful and even can be harmful.

In spite of efforts to record the important information about each drug, questions can remain. For example, you may return home and wonder: "I forgot to tell the doctor that I sometimes take sleeping pills; does that make a difference?" or "Is it safe to drive a car when I'm taking these capsules?" The best policy is to call the doctor's office for further information.

Your pharmacist can help answer questions about both prescription and nonprescription medications. He or she can discuss such subjects as how to save money on medications and whether to store various drugs at room temperature or in the refrigerator. Some pharmacists keep lists of all drugs that a customer receives; this practice can prevent the filling of two prescriptions for the same drug or of prescriptions for medications that should not be taken together. When requested, pharmacists also can place medications in containers that are easy to open.

Older persons often take several medications simultaneously, and keeping track of them can be difficult. The National Institute on Drug Abuse has prepared a booklet listing several approaches that may be helpful. It describes various types of charts on which to check off doses of medication. It also suggests placing the pills to be taken at each particular time of day in a separate container. For example, the compartments of an egg carton could be used to hold the pills to be taken together. However, before you store medications in other than their original containers, ask a physician or pharmacist whether it is safe to do so. Color-coding of medication bottles can help to prevent confusion.

Older patients, who often take several drugs simultaneously, should be especially aware of the way in which medications can affect each other's actions. Aspirin can dangerously increase the effects of drugs taken by mouth to thin the blood (oral anticoagulants); the effects of cold remedies can combine with those of sleeping pills or tranquilizers to make an individual perilously groggy; and alcohol can interact with many drugs in detrimental ways. Different medications can add to, distort, or cancel out each other's actions. Obviously, careful discussion of one's total drug profile—the use of nonprescription and prescription medications and alcohol—is necessary whenever a medication may be added.

Foods and drugs can interact negatively as well. Some foods can distort the effects of drugs; the antibiotic tetracycline, for example, may not be well absorbed if taken with milk products. Conversely, long-term use of some medications can affect nutrition; frequent use of mineral oil as a laxative can hinder absorption of vitamin D and other nutrients. Diuretics, which are commonly prescribed for older patients, can cause loss of potassium, an essential mineral; potassium-rich foods, such as tomatoes, oranges, raisins, prunes, and potatoes, help to replenish this vital supply. Therefore, discussion of diet also is important when drugs are being prescribed.

Drug costs also are of concern, especially to the many older persons with limited incomes. Comparison shopping, often most easily accomplished by calling various pharmacies and asking the prices of the drugs, can be helpful. In choosing a pharmacy, other factors, such as convenience of location, delivery service, and the keeping of complete medication records for each customer, also deserve consideration.

In many instances the prescription of generic rather than brand name drugs can save money. In general brand name and generic drugs are equivalent to each other. The best approach is to ask one's physician whether the drug being prescribed is available in generic form and whether a particular brand has any advantage for a specific condition. Some states now have laws that allow pharmacists to substitute generic drugs or less expensive brands for the specified product unless the prescriber forbids it. Other states now require prescribers to state on all prescriptions whether they approve of such substitution.

Here are several final suggestions for drug safety:

- Be especially careful if you must take medications during the night. Be sure to turn on the light. In order to avoid accidental overdoses, keep only one dose of medication at the bedside.
- Read labels on all medications carefully. Keeping a magnifying glass in or near the medicine chest can be helpful.
- Never exchange medication with anyone else.
- Store medications separately from other substances (such as cleaning solutions and seasonings) in order to prevent accidental poisoning. Also, separate medications to be taken internally from those that are only for external use. Persons with poor vision may wish to glue bits of sandpaper on bottles of substances that should not be consumed.
- Unlike humans, medications often may not age healthfully. Therefore, dispose of old or expired drugs.

EXERCISE

Several years ago a friend wrote to me about a woman whom she had seen on the tennis court one hot, muggy August day. Impressed that a person who appeared to be past 60 remained so vigorous and skillful, my friend approached the older woman and introduced herself. During the conversation the woman mentioned that she was 82 years old.

Few women past 80 can chase tennis balls in the 90 degree heat. But most older women can enjoy and benefit from frequent exercise. An exercise program specifically designed for women over 50 appears in the chapter on "Fitness." Many communities offer exercise classes for their older members. The decline in physical condition that occurs with age often results in part from lack of exercise. Appropriate exercise can help to prevent or reverse this process. It contributes to muscular function and to the health of the heart and blood vessels, as well as relieving tension and promoting a sense of well-being. Exercise also helps to maintain the figure and to decrease the risk of osteoporosis.

Certain types of exercise are specifically recommended for older women. Walking has been called the safest and best exercise for those both with and without heart disease. Because of the support that water provides, aquatic exercises often allow movement of joints and muscles in a manner impossible on land; in order to avoid potentially harmful changes in blood pressure, older women should enter and leave the water slowly. Physicians and physical therapists can prescribe special regimens for women with various disabilities.

Many older women can engage in more vigorous activities, such as jogging, bicycling, and swimming. However, before beginning such an exercise program, it is essential to consult a physician. In addition to evaluating general physical condition, the doctor may perform tests that measure the heart's response to exercise. Instructions regarding such matters as the maximum amount of exercise to be performed daily and the highest heart rate to be reached should be followed carefully in order to maximize benefit and minimize risks.

SAFETY

As people age, accidents remain common and become more dangerous. Problems such as impaired eyesight and hearing, poor coordination, weakness, and stiffness from arthritis can increase the risk of accidents. Sleepiness from medications and worries about personal problems can lead to carelessness. Accidental injuries often are more serious in the elderly; for example, a minor fall may only bruise a youngster, but may break an older woman's hip. In addition, older persons recover more poorly from injuries such as severe burns.

Many simple measures can help to prevent accidents. Slowing the pace of our daily activities is one way. As at all ages, people choosing and furnishing houses and apartments should pay attention to safety features.

Falls are the most common cause of accidental death in those over age 65. Suggestions for preventing such accidents include:

- Provide good, convenient lighting throughout and around the home.
- Place night lights in bedrooms and bathrooms or install remote-control switches that let persons in bed and elsewhere turn lights on and off.
- Light outdoor walkways and stairs.
- Wherever possible, place light fixtures and lamps so that bulbs can be changed without standing on a ladder.

- Pay special attention to stairways.
- Light steps well and provide light switches at both bottom and top of each flight.
- Have sturdy handrails—and use them.
- Use nonskid treads where possible.
- Firmly tack down carpeting on stairs.
- Place a gate at the top of stairway if you might walk near it at night.
- If moving, consider a house or apartment with few or no steps.

- Use nonslip floor waxes, avoid slippery throw rugs, and keep floors clear of objects over which a person could trip.

- Have grab bars over the bathtub and near the toilet, and place nonslip rubber mats or nonskid strips in the tub or shower.
- Keep outdoor walkways in good repair.
- Wear proper footwear. Well-fitting shoes with low, broad heels and nonslip soles and heels are best for everyday wear; keep them in good repair.
- Arise slowly from lying and sitting positions. Otherwise, faintness, dizziness, and falls can result. (Of course, anyone who becomes faint or dizzy often or for more than a moment should call a doctor.)

Safe use of medications already has been discussed.
Burns can be especially dangerous in later life. Safety measures include:

- Avoid smoking in bed. Do not smoke anywhere when drowsy.
- Wear tailored, closely-fitting clothes when cooking. (Loose garments, such as bathrobes and nightgowns, are likely to catch on fire.)
- Use ranges that have controls that are easy to see, reach, and use and elements or signal lights that glow when burners are in use.
- Set controls on water heaters or faucets to prevent water from becoming hot enough to scald the skin, and check water temperature with the hand before entering the bath.
- Have an emergency exit plan in case of fire.
- Use small, lightweight, easy-to-handle pots and pans for cooking.

Motor vehicle accidents are the most common cause of accidental death in the 65 to 74 age group and the second most common in older persons in general. Nearly one-fourth of all deaths to pedestrians occur in those aged 65 and over. Suggestions to reduce this risk include:

- At night wear white, beige, or fluorescent clothing or carry a flashlight.
- Give yourself extra time to cross slippery streets in bad weather.
- To allow plenty of time to cross the street, wait for a new green light before starting.

Several precautions should be taken to help prevent falls when using buses and other public transportation.

- Brace yourself when the vehicle is about to stop or turn.
- Because walking forward while the vehicle is slowing down is especially dangerous, move toward the door only when the vehicle is stopped or is moving at constant speed.
- Watch for slippery pavement and other hazards when entering and leaving the vehicle.
- Have fare ready in order to avoid losing your balance while fumbling for change.
- Use the vertical support bars when walking down the center aisle and if you must stand while the vehicle is moving.

• Do not overload yourself with packages; keep one hand free to hold on to railings.

Whether to continue driving a car and, if so, how to adjust driving habits, are important concerns. Age-related changes such as greater sensitivity to glare, poorer night vision, impaired hearing, diminished coordination, and slower reaction time can make driving more difficult. Older drivers tend to compensate somewhat for these problems by driving less often and more slowly and by driving less at night, during rush hours, and in the winter. Those considering stopping or limiting their driving may wish to discuss the matter with their doctors. Because older persons sometimes must stop driving, individuals looking for homes in which they may spend their old age should consider whether public transportation is available.

With age the body becomes less able to adjust to high and low temperatures. Therefore, care to avoid extremes of hot and cold is important. On hot days one should stay in a cool place and avoid strenuous exercise. In cold weather many older persons may be at risk of accidental hypothermia, a serious drop in body temperature. To avoid this condition:

• Keep the thermostat set at a temperature of at least 65° F. (Efforts to save energy by reducing room temperature can be a false economy for older persons.)
• Do not stay outdoors for long periods of time in cold weather.
• In cold weather wear plenty of clothing, including sweaters, robes, a cap or hat, and thick socks. Use enough blankets.

Momma   By Mell Lazarus

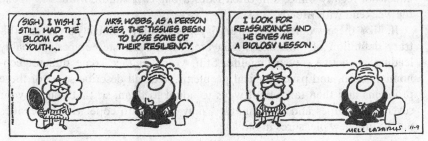

Courtesy of Mell Lazarus and Field Newspaper Syndicate.

The biology lesson is over; now for reassurance.

Aging Healthfully – Your Mind and Spirit

MAUREEN MYLANDER

National Institute on Aging

We see—perhaps only in our imaginations—the older woman walking slowly along a busy city street, sitting in a doctor's waiting room, or endlessly rocking on a front porch in a small town. But these images capture little more than a stereotype, noting only the slowing of life. They do not convey the warmth that encircles a 72-year-old widow who lives with her daughter's family in her own wing of a farmhouse; or the companionship and activity shared by a 68-year-old woman and her husband as they live in a rent-free guide's house and show visitors the beauties of a national park; or the independence of an 81-year-old nurse who has never married and who, legally blind, still often rides a bus two hundred miles to spend the weekend with friends.

If, like these women, you are 65 years or older (society's rather arbitrary definition of "old age") you are, despite the stereotypes, probably leading an active, rewarding life. Still, you will face some difficult economic, social, and psychological problems. We will describe some of these problems and then talk about ways to adapt to them, so that you, in your seventies, eighties and even nineties, may be able to cope with adversities and to find new pleasures in old age.

ECONOMIC, SOCIAL, AND PSYCHOLOGICAL PROBLEMS RELATED TO OLD AGE

Income

At one time or another, many of the country's current population of 13.9 million women over age 65 will probably have to manage on limited financial resources. Even those with substantial savings are apt to deplete their reserves if they live long enough. Inflation, fewer years in the labor market, reluctance of employers to hire old people, and inequities in social security and retirement benefits all lighten an older woman's purse and threaten to place her among the nation's poor. Indeed, the 5.7 million women aged 65 and older who lived alone or with nonrelatives in 1977 had median incomes of $3,762 a year, and 28 percent were below the official poverty level.

Women have, since World War II, increasingly entered the work force and have shifted from blue-collar to white-collar jobs. Yet their incomes are still half as much as men's, and women constitute only 2.3 percent of the workers who earn over $25,000 a year. Most women work for minimum wages in what one author calls "pink-collar ghettos"—beauty shops, department stores, restaurants, and offices. Only 5 percent of women aged 70 and older are employed even though age is a poor predictor of work performance. Numerous studies indicate that commitment, skill, and judgment are all very high for old people, men and women alike. Older women have been found more reliable than younger women at work, with lower rates of absenteeism and greater willingness to learn new tasks.

The social security system also treats today's women inequitably. Founded when most women worked in the home and were considered lifelong dependents upon their husbands, the system allowed no social security credit for their housework. Today 95 percent of the nation's aged receive social security benefits, but those paid to women are almost always lower than men's. Even when benefits are based on their own wages, women receive an average $230 a month, compared to $339 for men.

Many industries employing women offer no pension coverage. In those that do, benefits are generally lower for women, and survivors' benefits are virtually nonexistent in private pension plans. Even under the social security system, a widow cannot draw 100 percent of her deceased husband's social security benefits unless she is age 65. Pressure is growing for changes in these policies both in government and in private industry, and proposals are before Congress to give men and women equally fair and adequate social security benefits. Local social security offices have the latest information about these proposals, and about how much social security credit a worker has accumulated. For information about other federal programs to assist the elderly, contact a state or area agency on aging or the Administration on Aging (see p. 484 for address).

The older woman's economic plight is deepened by lack of formal education. In 1974 the average older woman had completed a median of 9.4 school years. This means half did not go beyond ninth grade. Moreover, these women attended school at a time when the school year was closer to six months than the present nine or ten. Some women in this age group have a poor knowledge of English, leaving them with few resources for coping with Medicare and social security forms, let alone jobs, mortgages, and higher finance. The trend, however, among younger women is toward rising education levels. Later this chapter will describe how older women and men are, in recent years, continuing their formal education through adult programs and other courses in community colleges and universities.

Housing and Transportation

Inadequate income colors every facet of an older woman's life, especially a woman who lives alone. Her housing, for example, tends to be older and of lower market value than houses of elderly couples. A greater proportion of her income is needed to cover basic housing costs than couples have to pay. She is more likely to live in a house lacking complete plumbing (hot and cold water, flush toilet, and tub or shower). Often she is forced to give up her house and move to a small apartment, hotel, trailer, or retirement home or community. If she can afford the latter, it may offer a sense of security, companionship, and shared activities, but it may also be an age-segregated, largely female environment sequestered from the rest of society in what some critics call "golden ghettos."

Wherever she lives, housing costs will consume an increasingly large share of her income. In states where older women tend to congregate—California, New York, Florida, Illinois, Ohio, Pennsylvania, and Texas—living costs are often high, making financial burdens even heavier. Yet some women have found ways to minimize such problems, and these will be discussed later.

Transportation problems can be as vexing as housing. Most elderly women living alone do not have regular use of a private automobile, because of expense or physical disability such as failing eyesight. Many never learned to drive and were unwilling or unable to assume this role when their husbands died. The consequences are especially severe in areas with inadequate public transportation systems. A trip to the food store, the doctor's office, or a friend's home can be not only difficult, but sometimes dangerous.

Crime

Old people are victims of crime more than any other age group, but the crimes tend to be of a certain type: theft, including purse-snatching and pocket-picking, consumer fraud, and con games. Property crimes, or theft, are the most frequent kind and usually occur when the property is unoccupied. Many old people, especially women, live on income delivered at predictable times, and their shopping, banking, and other errands fall into fixed patterns that a criminal can observe easily. Older women are especially vulnerable to violent crime, including rape, if they live in inner-city and low-income neighborhoods.

Fear of victimization is a major reason many elderly people restrict their activities and become withdrawn and isolated. Those who become victims are left with a lasting sense of invasion and fear that can make them withdraw into virtual self-imprisonment. To prevent this outcome, some communities and states have established victim assistance programs, and many communities are using older volunteers as assistants to the criminal justice system.

Widowhood

An overwhelming reality for women over 65, most of whom married when they were younger, is widowhood. More than one-half of all American women will lose their mates by age 65, three-fourths by age 85, and the gap in male-female life expectancy will continue to widen. By the year 2000, given present mortality rates, there will be ten women for every five men over age 75, and most women will live into their eighties and nineties.

The male-female imbalance and the tendency for men to marry younger women means older women are not likely to find another husband. Meanwhile, social taboos against older women marrying younger men remain largely (though not totally) unchallenged, and the average woman who marries a man two to three years older can expect about ten years of widowhood. Consider:

- If your husband is five years younger than you,
  your chances of widowhood are 6 in 12.
- If you and your husband are the same age,
  your chances of widowhood are 8 in 12.
- If your husband is five years older than you (most often the case),
  your chances of widowhood are 9 in 12.

Widowhood, from every standpoint, is one of the most stressful times in a woman's life. For many it follows a long period of caring for an ill and dying husband under incredible stress and threat to her own health. A woman whose husband has suffered a severe heart attack compared the stresses of taking care of him and of meeting family and work obligations ". . . to one of those ducks you see swimming in a pond: their feathers are all in place and they're gliding around smoothly, but underneath, their feet are paddling like mad." And a 61-year-old woman whose husband is dying of cancer writes, "I have grown to depend upon my husband socially and emotionally and cannot make plans or face the thought of what the future will be without him."

The Holmes-Rahe stress scale, which measures the emotional toll of various life events, ranks loss of spouse first, far above the stresses of birth, marriage, moving, or job change. The bereaved, regardless of sex, loses someone to whom she or he is emotionally attached, and grief is the inevitable reaction. Some widows mourn longer and harder than others; some fall seriously ill. Mortality rates, too, are higher among the widowed, especially during the first six months.

How does a widow reduce the threat to health and happiness? "Give sorrow words," as William Shakespeare said in *Macbeth*. "The grief that does not speak knits up the o'erwrought heart and bids it break." Delayed or suppressed grief severely hampers adjustment to widowhood, a process which usually takes up to two years. Widows find various ways to endure it. Some turn to their children and family for solace, others to a trusted friend or psychiatrist. The Widow-to-Widow program, a nationwide network of self-help groups that lend support to widows through group meetings, phone calls, and visits, is helpful to many women.

One of the most revolutionary approaches to easing the pain of death and dying is the hospice, an organization that cares for and counsels the terminally ill and their relatives. The first hospice was founded in New Haven, Connecticut, in the early 1970s and, as of this writing, about 75 operate throughout the United States. They are affiliated with hospitals or are independent and most provide home care and psychiatric help to the families of the dying, sometimes for as long as a year after the relative's death.

Widows often increase their stress and risk of illness by making rapid, major changes in their lives. They sell houses, change jobs, or move out of town soon after the funeral and only later realize the difficulty of making new friends and the pain of losing old ones. Some researchers believe that anticipation of a spouse's death makes it easier to adjust to the loss, because there is time to grieve beforehand.

One study of young widows and widowers under age 45 showed that good adjustment to widowhood was likely if the marriage was not critical to the widow's functioning and if she had adequate income, a satisfying career, and emotionally supportive friends. Self-sufficiency is an asset to the older widow as well. Indeed, many women report that they are happier, once they finish grieving, than when they were married. Their enjoyment stems from being, perhaps for the first time in their lives, free and independent persons.

Social Supports

What about an older woman's inner, emotional resources? People, regardless of sex or age, need a sense of security and belonging, nurturing, reassurance of worth, reliable assistance, emotional support, steady access to another person, and a network of social relationships. Indeed, people organize their lives around relationships that provide these emotional essentials. When death or other circumstance takes one of these relationships away, a person often turns to a social network or web of affiliations with kin, friends, friends of friends, co-workers, neighbors, and children. Neighbors and children, in particular, appear to play key roles in an older woman's network. They are important providers of social activities, personal assistance, and a sense that she is not alone in the world. But today's 70-year-olds belong to the famous "low fertility cohort" of women whose family size was limited by the Great Depression and who were too old for childbearing by the time their husbands returned from World War II. As a result, about a fourth of these women have no living children. Most of those who do have children see at least one on a regular basis, and these relationships remain an important source of continuity and support.

Older women who have no husband, kin, or friends to meet their day-to-day needs stand a higher risk of becoming institutionalized. Families provide 80 percent of all home health care to older members needing such attention. Thus, despite the myth that families abandon their old, families, and especially children, remain the ultimate caretakers of old people in this society.

This helps explain the statistic, surprising to many, that only about 5 percent of the nation's old people live in nursing homes at any given time. Of these, about 70 percent are older women, most of them widows. A large proportion of these women could survive successfully in the community with friends or family to take care of them.

Sex and Sensuality

A sense of emotional well-being also requires outlets for expressing sexuality. Mainly because of low numbers of males her age, any older woman without a mate is severely handicapped in finding such outlets. The persisting taboo against sex in old age does not help. Males who remain interested in sex are "dirty old men," while sexually interested older women are often considered pathetic, laughable, and perhaps crazy as well. This attitude is rooted in the not-so-ancient belief that women should not and do not seek sexual pleasure.

Some of these attitudes are relics of Victorian days, others stem from religious precepts that sexuality exists only for reproductive purposes. By this outmoded logic, sex after 60 is accepted for men, who can ostensibly still sire children, but not for postmenopausal women, who have no conceivable reason for indulging in sex. Some older women "lose" interest in sex to defend against the likelihood that they will probably not find sex partners anyway. Others, who might have sexual opportunities, fear risking outright rejection should their lover be repulsed by their aging bodies.

Meanwhile, scientific evidence proves that sexual interest and ability can persist into the ninth decade for men and women alike. Indeed, data from a longitudinal study at the Duke University Center for the Study of Aging and Human Development indicate that some women's interest in sex increases as they grow older. Studies by Kinsey, Masters and Johnson, researchers at Duke, the National Institute of Mental Health, and National Institute on Aging indicate that people who are sexually active in their early years tend to remain sexually active. Past enjoyment, interest, and frequency are key determinants of sexuality in old age. Although sexual decline is often caused by poor physical health, including alcoholism, anemia, diabetes, malnutrition, and fatigue, some studies show that even the terminally ill often retain sexual desire. At times it even increases, perhaps to counteract anxiety over dying.

For most people, sex is important to well-being, identity, and a sense of control over one's body. Even more important is sensuality, which is broader than sexuality and involves all the body's senses in the enjoyment of a partner. Best of all are loving relationships marked by intimacy and affection, of which sex and sensuality are but a part. Thus sexual "neutering" of old people denies the human need for pleasure, tenderness, warmth, and the satisfaction of body contact. Full sexual expression, on the other hand, can provide intimacy, love, commitment, self-assertion—all psychological reinforcements at a time when people most need them.

Self-Image

The myth of sexlessness parallels other misconceptions that aging is a disease, as *Newsweek* once suggested in an article asking, "Can Aging Be Cured?" Contrary to such headlines, most older people are in basically good physical health and able to cope with the demands of daily living. So-called senility is not an inevitable consequence of growing old, nor are old people, according to yet another myth, unproductive, apathetic, withdrawn, crotchety, childish, inflexible, bound to the past, uninterested in the present, and afraid of the future. Women bear an additional burden of myths, the worst being that wrinkles, gray hair, and the like are ugly. The beauty industry capitalizes on these stereotypes and broadcasts that older women must remain youthful, no matter what the cost in cosmetics, creams, fad diets, reducing salons, exercisers, hair dressers, and plastic surgery. So ingrained is the equation of youth and beauty that many women agonize about growing old at age 30, a startling thought considering that they have not lived half their current life expectancies of 76.7 years!

Depression

Susan Sontag has called growing old "a crisis that never exhausts itself." The crisis is mainly one of mind and emotions. While relatively little is known about emotional disorders in old age, it is known that the mental health of older people is affected by "cumulative deprivations," which involve an old person's ability to adapt to the stresses of aging. These, in turn, cause varying degrees of emotional distress.

Depression has not been studied adequately in older women, although it has been thought to be more prevalent among women than men, and this difference has been assumed to continue into old age. But recent studies suggest that rates of depression may equalize later in life.

Depressed people, regardless of age or sex, generally feel a strong sense of guilt, helplessness, sadness, low self-esteem, and hopelessness about the future. These feelings may be accompanied by frequent crying spells, loss of appetite and weight, constipation, sleep disturbances, fatigue, inability to concentrate, or other signs of physical distress. Depression in older people, especially those living alone, often is overlooked or mistaken for organic brain disease.

According to current theories, some depressions result mainly from external circumstances, others primarily from chemical changes in the brain. The major external causes of depression change with age. In young people they often relate to guilt and self-blame, while in old people depression commonly stems from loss—loss of youth, health, income, residence, status and, worst of all, of loved ones through death, relocation, or estrangement.

Women may be particularly predisposed to depression because of the psychological disadvantages of the traditional female role of "learned helplessness." Unlike men, women are taught that they cannot control what happens to them by any direct action, that they cannot do certain things, that they must be submissive to and dependent upon men, and that they must find satisfaction through nurturant relationships rather than through their own accomplishments. Younger women may be rejecting this kind of behavior, but many women in their seventies have been learning helplessness all their lives.

These are the women who have never written a check, have no idea how much money is in the estate, sell their property at a loss, and do not know what survivor benefits are due them. When they no longer have a husband, brother, or son to buffer them against the outside world, they fall apart. Many become depressed or succumb to a variety of other emotional impairments from sleep problems to suicide.

Sleep Problems

Many old people worry that lack of sleep will lead to serious illness, not realizing that what they see as a problem may be normal, age-related changes in sleep patterns. Sleep requirements change throughout life. A newborn infant needs 16 to 17 hours daily, while a healthy elderly woman may need 7 to 8 or even fewer hours.

Although sleep patterns and problems in old age are not well understood, it is known that sleep is lighter with more frequent awakenings. Some sleep problems in older people may result from physical illness such as degenerative diseases of the central nervous system. Other sleep disturbances stem from long-term dependence on hypnotics taken to relieve insomnia. Incompatible sleep schedules or physical illness of a bed partner may disrupt the sleep of both parties. And sleep disturbances may result from emotional conflicts and anxiety: a vague state of dread often accompanied by muscle tenseness, restlessness, rapid heart rate, and excessive sweating. In many cases sleep problems occur because older people expect that they will have trouble sleeping. Whatever the cause, sudden drastic changes in sleep patterns or prolonged trouble falling and staying asleep should be brought to a physician's attention.

Drugs and Alcohol

Sleeplessness by night and emotional distress by day cause many older people to turn to sleeping pills, mild tranquilizers, and other prescription and nonprescription drugs. These drugs can be of great benefit in relieving anxiety and other distressing symptoms, but when they are used continuously, as they are by many older people, they can cause undesirable side effects. Women are especially apt to use these drugs continuously because they generally use more over-the-counter and prescription drugs than men do.

Nobody knows how many older women have become unwitting drug abusers, although the National Institute on Drug Abuse estimates that 1 to 2 million women of all ages have problems because of prescription drugs. For example, 60 percent of all drug-related emergency room visits involve women and are the result mainly of suicide attempts or drug dependency.

Alcohol abuse in the elderly is somewhat better documented: of the nation's 10 million alcoholics, about 4 million are estimated to be women of all ages. Still, there is probably relatively little alcoholism among women over age 65 because many alcoholics die of their disease before reaching old age. Other people become alcoholics late in life to relieve the pain of the death of a loved one, loss of health and income, loneliness, boredom, and feelings of inferiority. Many women who drink, young and old, are hidden abusers: they take alcohol or drugs at home where nobody will see them. The families know, but ignore the problem because they feel ashamed or responsible. They also believe that men can drink and abuse drugs, but not women. There is tragedy in this attitude because drug and alcohol abuse, if recognized, can be treated like many other diseases.

Suicide

While some older people take drugs and alcohol to dull their despair, others resort to suicide. Many people think about committing suicide at some point during their lives, but each year from 5,000 to 8,000 Americans over age 65 turn such thoughts into deeds. These suicides represent 25 percent of the total number reported, even though the elderly constitute only about 10 percent of the population. The number of suicides among the elderly, moreover, is probably underreported, with perhaps twice this many occurring among people over age 65. Older men commit suicide five times as often as their female peers, who attempt it more often. Suicide rates are especially high among old people who lack spouses and jobs and who live alone in deteriorating neighborhoods.

Sometimes suicide takes subtle forms: accidental falls, overweight, heavy smoking, alcoholism, poor nutrition, neglect of routine medical examinations and treatment, failure to take life-saving medication, untreated vision and hearing problems, inadequate planning for possible medical emergencies, and uncontrolled psychological stresses. But the ultimate outcome—self destruction—is the same.

Psychotherapy and Personal Growth

An estimated 25 to 60 percent of the aged population may be affected by mild to severe psychiatric impairment. Yet, the aged receive very little psychiatric care on an outpatient, ambulatory basis. This occurs partly because members of this age group are not oriented toward psychotherapy. They grew up in an era when mental illness was shameful and when talking openly about personal problems, even to friends, simply was not done. Older people tend, like the rest of society, to accept emotional distress and mental deterioration as normal parts of aging. They accept the myth that they cannot develop further psychologically.

According to this myth, psychotherapy, a process in which a therapist helps a patient resolve mental distress, cannot benefit people over age 50 or 60. This attitude comes from numerous sources, among them Sigmund Freud, who maintained that old people are no longer educable, that treatment would continue indefinitely because of the mass of material to be covered in an old person's life, and that therapy for the young is more valuable because old people have fewer years to live.

Even today, many therapists cling to the misconception that the aged do not respond well to therapy. But not all. The American Association of Geriatric Psychiatry publishes a directory of more than 400 psychiatrists in 41 states who specialize in treating older people. A copy of the directory is available from Dr. Sanford Finkel, American Association of Geriatric Psychiatry (see p. 484 for address).

When old people do receive psychiatric help, they generally respond very well. Group therapy, in particular, succeeds with older patients because they become members of a social group which counteracts the effects of isolation. They learn to interact with others and to solve current problems, often with the help of another group member whose self-esteem is bolstered by being able to help. Rather than analyze childhood experiences or reconstruct personality, as therapy often does for younger people, the focus is on current concerns. Thus, the older patient might deal with grief, sexual and drug problems, fear of physical illness and disability, anxiety about death, and making new starts. One therapist has written that older people are better psychotherapy risks than the young, because the former can better postpone gratifications and acknowledge that you must perform to achieve.

ADAPTATION

The emotional problems of the elderly and their response to adversities of age are, in a sense, problems of adaptation. How, then, can they direct their efforts to adapt? How, more specifically, can older women begin to break the cycle of defeat and lead more rewarding lives? The final section of this chapter will offer suggestions, but ultimately each woman must act for herself. Society will offer little help because it conditions women to be wives and mothers and does not encourage changes of identity at any stage of life. Still there is much the older woman can do.

Earning Power

The older woman must first provide for her basic needs, the most basic being money. To ensure an adequate income for old age, a woman cannot rely solely upon social security income or retirement and pension plans. Paid work not only provides income, it provides a sense of accomplishment and worth when it relates to the needs of the rest of society. One 72-year-old woman has operated her husband's two-car taxi service since his death nine years ago. She is also treasurer for another cab company, is a notary public, and collects rent for several landlords. She teaches Sunday school, is a Cub Scout den mother, babysits, bakes cakes for friends, sews, and reads. Another woman, at age 68, drives a small tractor and works alongside her husband in their gardening and lawn-mowing business. A widow in Arlington, Virginia, started boarding dogs of neighbors in her home. Now she has a full-time pet hotel business and all the companionship, human and animal, that she needs. Another woman, lacking job market skills, decided at age 70 to put her culinary talents to commercial use. She cooks a week's worth of dinners at a time for customers' deep freezers.

Learning Power

To escape the trap of low-paying jobs, women need education and old age need be no barrier to receiving it. "Old men," T. S. Eliot once said, "should be explorers." This statement is even more true of old women, who are more numerous and who live more years in which to explore. A recently published book, *The Graying of the Campus,* suggests that college presidents and deans would do well to bolster enrollments, which are expected to decline by 4 million during the 1980s, with gray-haired students.

Freshmen already are getting older each year at colleges and universities throughout the United States. Fordham University in New York City has a College at 60 Program, Ohio State University has Program 60, and the University of San Francisco has the Fromm Institute of Lifelong Learning. Intellectual stimulation and adventure is also offered by Elderhostel, a nonprofit organization that offers low-cost, week-long residential academic programs for older people at about 230 colleges and universities in 38 states. Information about the program is available from Elderhostel, and area agencies on aging and the Administration on Aging (see p. 484 for addresses) have information about other educational opportunities for older persons.

From around the country come stories about women in their seventies taking degrees and starting new careers afterward. One woman returned to school at age 50 to earn a master's degree in social welfare. She now directs the Gerontology Program at the State University of New York at Stony Brook and is cofounder of the National Action Forum for Older Women. At one small college in North Carolina, an English major was, at age 80, elected homecoming queen.

The field of gerontology is open to older people even if they have no experience. Universities with gerontology programs include Duke University, University of Michigan, Columbia University, the New School for Social Research in New York City, and the University of Southern California.

Many women are learning self-sufficiency in adult education courses on car repairs, karate, or filing effective consumer complaints. In future years millions of women are likely to enroll for all kinds of learning experiences and may return periodically to school throughout the life cycle. For education is not just preparation for life; it is life itself.

Networks

Many paths besides jobs and education lead to new life for the elderly. Old people, like young, need to replace the loss of loved ones. The distinguished psychiatrist Dr. Ewald W. Busse writes that living alone and losing loved ones do not in themselves produce the social isolation that afflicts so many older women. Instead, it is failure to develop any significant *new* relationships that saps life satisfaction. Since individual effort can remedy this situation, no woman need remain socially isolated because of widowhood or any other loss.

One solution is to maintain close, emotionally supportive ties to others. The Widow-to-Widow program and the Unitarian Church's system of extended families, whose members act as one another's relatives, provide such ties. But older women also need to maintain networks of children, kin, friends, young people, co-workers, and members of the same organizations. Throughout life these networks can be an important source of support. They help members find jobs, housing, practical help, companionship, and emotional support. Because they offer so much, networks require much in return. They are a resource, like money in the bank, that women should maintain all their lives.

Loving

An important source of emotional support and pleasure in old age is sexuality. One couple, after 35 years of marriage, moved to an isolated house in the country where they spend most of their time working the garden, swimming, and making love. The 68-year-old woman, in an article in *Ms.* magazine, wrote that she hopes the honeymoon will last forever. "We are always touching. I'm glad I'm not like Mama was—she slept downstairs, Daddy slept up, and they never gave each other a good word."

Maggie Kuhn, who at age 65 launched an activist career that led to the founding of the Gray Panthers organization, includes maintaining an interest in sex and companionship with the opposite sex among her five new life styles for the elderly. She tells of a widow who for five years had been bedridden most of the time in her son's home. One day she received a letter from a man she had not seen in years. Next came a phone call. Shortly thereafter, she appeared downstairs fully dressed and carrying her suitcase. She told her astonished son and daughter-in-law that she was leaving to be married, gave them her love and a forwarding address, and left for a new life at age 82. She lived with her second husband until her death eight years later. In his book *Retirement Marriage,* Walter McKain wrote that marriage among older people is most likely to succeed when the bride and groom know each other well, when children and friends approve of the marriage, and when both bride and groom own a home, have sufficient income, and are reasonably well-adjusted individuals.

Unfortunately, few older women have opportunities to remarry. One solution to the shortage of older men is offered by author Anne Cumming in *The Love Habit: The Sexual Odyssey of An Older Woman*. Ms. Cumming advocates "intergenerational love" between older women and younger men—even men in their teens and twenties—and predicts that "my book will be required reading in the schools in 50 years' time."

More than 200 years ago Ben Franklin, a connoisseur of women to the end of his long life, offered similar advice. Franklin argued that older women (presumably, in those days, in their forties) and younger men (in their twenties) are ideally suited for one another, and that young men "in all (their) Amours . . . should *prefer old women to young ones.*"

Self-pleasuring is another sexual alternative, but many current older women find it difficult to enjoy masturbation. Their generation tends to feel guilty about it and to believe that sexuality should be shared only with a husband or partner of long-standing commitment. Many of these women also share a culturally induced difficulty loving their own aging bodies. An even more controversial sexual outlet for older women is relationships with other women. This may be unthinkable to some people, but the possibilities are likely to be explored, more and more, by women of all ages who are in the midst of changing expectations about their sexuality.

One physician specializing in geriatric medicine advocates a change in the structure of marriage itself, that is, group marriage of two, three, or even five older women to a man over age 60. This arrangement would give women unable to find matés more family life, better diet because of added incentive to cook, pooled funds, better living conditions, mutual help during illness, shared housework and activities, and—admittedly controversial —access to sex. Proponents of this idea argue that males are polygamous by nature, and a variety of partners could bring many men back to life sexually. Jealousy, to be sure, might become a problem among the women, but what marriage, proponents argue, is without troubles? Opponents say men would be using women in such an arrangement. Still, group marriage, even without sex, might solve many problems stemming from an older woman's aloneness in the world. Alvin Toffler predicts in *Future Shock* that "geriatric communes" or group marriages of elderly persons will become increasingly common vehicles for companionship and mutual assistance.

Other programs offer old people physical affection devoid of all sexual connotations. One is the Foster Grandparents program, sponsored by the Administration on Aging in Washington, D.C. Elderly men and women spend time each week with brain-damaged children, many of whom have been abandoned by their parents and have little physical contact beyond essential care. The hours a child spends being held and cuddled on the lap of a foster grandparent provide comfort, security, and warmth to both. In another program, Mother-in-Deed, older women live with families whose mother has died or is absent. These substitute mothers often live with the families several years until the father remarries or the children leave home. In Ann Arbor, Michigan, and other cities older women are acting as volunteer aides in elementary school classrooms.

Group Living

Age-integrated living arrangements are also becoming more popular. Challenging the notion expressed by the sixteenth-century poet that "Crabbed Age and Youth Cannot live together," one elderly woman shared her home with several young medical students who helped her maintain it. This kind of living arrangement redefines the family as a group of people united not by blood or marriage, but by mutual needs and interests. Another woman, after her husband's death, subdivided their large old house into six apartments, lived in one, rented out the others to friends, and paid her mortgage and repair bills from the proceeds. Communal living arrangements of several women living together can provide companionship, mutual help and protection from crime. More important, such arrangements help keep older people out of nursing homes.

Exercise

Some people become convinced as they grow older that traveling and other exertions are bad for their health. But the human body is a marvelous machine that thrives on use. More than 2,000 years ago the physician Hippocrates suggested that functions which are not used become atrophied. Several hundred years later Cicero listed four factors which adversely affect aging—being barred from useful activity, being weakened physically, being deprived of pleasure and aware of the nearness of death. More recent theories of successful aging add lack of proper sleep and diet, smoking, and heavy drinking to the list of harmful factors. Other studies validate the importance of exercise, not only in maintaining physical health, but in preventing or counteracting depression, possibly because exercise increases your sense of well-being.

It is never too late to start exercising, although the amount and type of exercise should depend on your state of health—and nerve. One woman, described by author Jane Howard in her book *Families,* learned to swim at the age of 75 and before long was diving off the high board.

Life Work

Mental activity may be even more important than physical. Margaret

Mead, who remained a working anthropologist until she died of cancer at age 76, used to say, "I know I can't live forever. I'm just not ready to go yet." She kept a journal of observations on the progress of her cancer and remained until her death passionately involved in life even as she was losing it.

Many older women find rewarding activities, although filling the hours is a major problem for some. Mere "busy work" seldom satisfies anybody. Simone de Beauvoir once said, "The only solution to the problems of old age is for each old person to go on pursuing ends that give existence meaning." One woman decided at age 70 to fulfill a lifelong dream of living in San Francisco. She invested her savings in a bus ticket and despite limited social security income of $160 a month and a lame leg, successfully settled in a strange city where she had no friends or family. Today she plays in a band at a senior center and has walked across the Golden Gate Bridge six times. Another woman, at age 72, founded an organization called Neighbors Helping Neighbors, in which volunteers provide rides to doctors' offices, hospitals, and clinics for disabled people with no other means of transportation. For eight years she ran this enterprise from her small cottage in Sharon, New Hampshire, before turning it over to a new manager. Looking back, she says, "Who would have thought my seventies would be the happiest years of my life?" In her nineties another woman began to write essays about aging. Asked why she took up writing, she replied, "I'd be bored to death if I didn't have something to do." Octogenarian author Faith Baldwin maintains a full writing schedule and believes that the best approach to life is to continue doing the things she's always done.

Charles Schulz, creator of *Peanuts*, once suggested in cartoon form another way old people could remain assets to society. Lucy, while reading a composition to her class, concluded:

> "And so World War II came to an end. My grandmother left her job in the defense plant and went to work for the telephone company. We need to study the lives of great women like my grandmother. Talk to your own grandmother today. Ask her questions. You'll find she knows more than peanut butter cookies! Thank you!"*

Lucy, in effect, recommends "life review," an autobiographical process which allows an old person to take pride in the past by talking or writing about it, reading diaries or letters from an old lover, attending a reunion, or visiting one's birthplace. When an older person is encouraged to reminisce, perhaps by a grandchild with a notebook or tape recorder, the listener gains wisdom and experience, and the reminiscer discovers that somebody cares enough to listen.

* Text from PEANUTS by Charles M. Schulz; © 1976 United Features Syndicate, Inc.

Leverage

Old people can be heard in other ways too. Wrinkled faces are appearing in Pepsi Cola ads, including one for a new diet soda being marketed for victims of "middle-aged spread." The older population, as *Business Week* acknowledged back in 1971, "travels, buys cars, dines out at fancy restaurants, buys presents for the kids and grandchildren, and spends a growing share of its retirement dollar on goods and services." More recently, data from the Census Bureau shows that people aged 60 years and older, who represent about 10 percent of the population, earned about $207 billion in 1977 or nearly 20 percent of the income. These figures show that the older population of men and women has considerable purchasing power. While poverty is still prevalent among the old, it is not universal nor, with women increasingly entering the job market, is it likely to remain so.

Another way old people can wield power is at the voting booth. In 1978 some 56 percent of the population over 65 voted, the highest proportion of all age groups except the 55 to 64 group. Yet only rarely do older voters cast their ballots in a bloc. It is encouraging, however, that increasing numbers of old people are making themselves heard as members of such activist groups as the Gray Panthers, a coalition of young and old who oppose age discrimination and age stereotyping and other dehumanizing forces in our society.

A final way of exercising power, in this case over one's self, is through living wills, which give you legal control over your own and your relatives' bodies. These documents enable you to decide, while you are still healthy and legally competent, whether you wish others to prolong your life by artificial means and heroic measures despite the indignity of deterioration, dependence, and hopeless pain. The growing movement toward hospice care provides the terminally ill with a pain-free, humanistic environment in which to spend their last days.

Society continues to view old people, even while they are still healthy, more as a problem than as a valued social, economic, and political resource. At a Conference on the Older Woman in September 1978, Dr. Robert N. Butler, Director of the National Institute on Aging, commented on the survivorship of the old: "I for one am somewhat tired of hearing about the 'aging problem.' We are talking about a major human triumph in this century." Despite the litany of problems an older woman faces, she has great strengths and potentials. For example, she has the opportunity to:

- Become, perhaps for the first time in her life, an independent being, undominated by others and in full control of her life.

- Fulfill her own expectations, not society's.
- Enjoy good friends and leisure pastimes.
- Keep physically active and fit.
- Continue to discover and use her talents.
- Remain curious and interested in life.
- Remember that what is frowned upon in a girl of 20 is applauded as "character" in a woman of 80.
- Remain passionately involved with life, enjoying each day as it comes.

The older woman who does even a few of these things will begin to see a different person when she looks in the mirror, not a wrinkled facade, but a successful individual who knows there still is work to be done, dreams to be dreamed, pleasure to be enjoyed. Older women who can view the aging process in this manner could serve as role models for women now in their fifties, forties, thirties, and even twenties. The women most likely to adapt successfully to the stresses of old age will be those who have adapted well to stresses of equal or greater severity throughout their lives. What is past is prologue.

LOOKING AHEAD

The 50-year-old woman of today has not been hardened to adversity like the 70-year-old who learned in the Great Depression to deal with problems similar to those encountered in old age. Yet these younger women have more education than ever before, and when they reach age 70, they will have more earned pensions and financial resources of their own. They will have more children and grandchildren to support them economically and emotionally in old age. Family ties will be extended, with parent-child bonds lasting 50 years or more, and grandparent-grandchild bonds 30 years or more. In sum, women now in their fifties and younger are likely to experience old age differently than the women who preceded them, and the experience will, on balance, be better.

If, to restate the proverb, "A woman resembles her times more than her mother," the prospects are even brighter for women now in their twenties, thirties, and forties. They will be even better educated, better paid, and healthier physically and mentally. They will have more models of accomplished women to emulate, as younger women look to their 50-year-old mothers *and* their peers for inspiration.

A study of three generations of women, aged 10 to 92, makes this final point. Grandmothers in the study had practically no formal education in their youth and had conventionally moral upbringings, although they had strong desires to achieve creativity. Their granddaughters were less bound by conventional morals and more oriented toward achievement, control of their own destinies, and influencing others. This group, in every sense, represents changes in American womanhood over the last century. To return to an opening theme of this chapter, if women are to outlive men and, in that sense, inherit the earth, they might as well make the most of it. And, judging from those who are coming along, they will.

SOURCES OF INFORMATION AND HELP

Many organizations and publications provide information on healthful aging. A brief list of agencies addressing topics of importance to older persons follows. Many of these organizations answer inquiries, provide and recommend publications and services, and refer individuals to other groups catering to more specialized needs. Several publications that may be especially useful also are listed.

Administration on Aging, U. S. Department of Health and Human Services
    330 Independence Avenue, SW, Washington, D.C. 20201
Alcohol, Drug Abuse, and Mental Health Administration
    5600 Fishers Lane, Rockville, Md. 20857
    Components include: National Institute of Mental Health; National Institute
    on Drug Abuse; National Institute on Alcohol Abuse and Alcoholism
Alliance for Displaced Homemakers
    3800 Harrison Street, Oakland, Calif. 94611
Alzheimer's Disease and Related Disorders Association
    32 Broadway, New York, N.Y. 10004
American Association of Geriatric Psychiatry
    230 North Michigan Avenue, Suite 2400, Chicago, Ill. 60601
American Association of Retired Persons
    1909 K Street, NW, Washington, D.C. 20049
The American Diabetes Association, Inc.
    1 West 48 Street, New York, N.Y. 10020
American Foundation for the Blind
    15 West 16 Street, New York, N.Y. 10011
American Heart Association
    7320 Greenville Avenue, Dallas, Tex. 75231
Displaced Homemakers Network
    2012 Massachusetts Avenue, NW, Washington, D.C. 20036
Elderhostel
    55 Chapel Street, Newton, Mass. 02160
Gray Panthers
    3635 Chestnut Street, Philadelphia, Pa. 19104
National Action Forum for Older Women: Center on Aging
    University of Maryland, College Park, Md. 20742
                        or
Health Sciences Center
    State University of New York, Stony Brook, N.Y. 11794

National Association of Area Agencies on Aging
   1828 L Street, NW, Washington, D.C. 20036
National Caucus on the Black Aged
   1730 M Street, NW, Washington, D.C. 20036
National Clearinghouse on Aging
   330 Independence Avenue, SW, Washington, D.C. 20201
National Council of Senior Citizens
   1511 K Street, NW, Washington, D.C. 20005
National Hospice Organization
   765 Prospect Street, New Haven, Conn. 06511
National Institutes of Health
   9000 Rockville Pike, Bethesda, Md. 20205
   Components of particular interest to older persons include: National Insti-
   tute on Aging; National Cancer Institute; National Heart, Lung, and
   Blood Institute; National Eye Institute; National Institute of Allergy and
   Infectious Diseases; National Institute of Arthritis, Metabolism, and Diges-
   tive Diseases; National Institute of Dental Research; National Institute of
   Neurological and Communicative Disorders and Stroke
National Safety Council
   444 North Michigan Avenue, Chicago, Ill. 60611
Office of Nursing Home Affairs
   5600 Fishers Lane, Rockville, Md. 20857
President's Council on Physical Fitness
   400 6th Street, SW, Washington, D.C. 20201
Sex Information and Education Council
   137 Franklin Avenue, Hempstead, N.Y. 11550

FURTHER READING: "AGING HEALTHFULLY—YOUR BODY"

Chronic Obstructive Lung Disease: Emphysema and Chronic Bronchitis. DHEW
   Publication No. NIH 77-614. Washington, D.C.: U. S. Department of
   Health and Human Services, 1979.
Guide to Fitness After Fifty, edited by Raymond Harris and Lawrence J.
   Frankel. New York: Plenum Press, 1977.
How to Cope with Arthritis. DHEW Publication No. NIH 76-1092. Washing-
   ton, D.C.: U. S. Department of Health and Human Services, 1976.
How to Select a Nursing Home. DHEW Publication No. OS 76-50045. Wash-
   ington, D.C.: U. S. Department of Health and Human Services, 1976.
An Older Person's Guide to Cardiovascular Health. Dallas, Tex.: American
   Heart Association, 1977.
Using Your Medicines Wisely: A Guide for the Elderly. Rockville, Md.: Na-
   tional Institute on Drug Abuse, 1979.
Varicose Veins. Dallas, Tex.: American Heart Association, 1969.
A Winter Hazard for the Old: Accidental Hypothermia. DHEW Publication
   No. NIH 78-1464. Washington, D.C.: U. S. Department of Health and
   Human Services, 1978.

REFERENCES AND FURTHER READING:
"AGING HEALTHFULLY—YOUR MIND AND SPIRIT"

Blank, Marie L. "Raising the Age Barrier to Psychotherapy." In U. S. Department of Health and Human Services, National Institute of Mental Health, *Readings in Psychotherapy with Older People* (DHEW Publication No. ADM 77-409, 1977).

Block, Marilyn R., et al. *Uncharted Territory: Issues and Concerns of Women Over 40.* Silver Spring, Md.: University of Maryland Center on Aging, 1978.

Busse, E. W., and Eric Pfeiffer. "Functional Psychiatric Disorders in Old Age." In E. W. Busse, *Behavior and Adaptation in Late Life.* Boston: Little Brown, 1977.

Butler, Robert N., and Myrna I. Lewis. *Sex After Sixty: A Guide for Men and Women for Their Later Years.* New York: Harper & Row, 1976.

Cumming, Anne. *Love Habit: The Sexual Odyssey of an Older Woman.* Indianapolis, Ind.: Bobbs-Merrill, 1978.

Franklin, Benjamin. *The Papers of Benjamin Franklin.* Vol. 3, January 1, 1745 through June 30, 1750. New Haven, Conn.: Yale University Press, 1961: 30–31.

Howard, Jane. *Families.* New York: Simon & Schuster, 1978.

Kassel, Victor. "Polygamy After 60." *Geriatrics,* 21 (April 1966): 214–218.

Kuhn, Margaret E. "New Life for the Elderly." *Enquiry,* rev. ed. Crawfordsville, Ind.: Geneva Press, 1974.

Lazar, Joyce B., and Betty H. Pickett. *Final Report of the Workshop on the Older Woman: Continuities and Discontinuities.* National Institute on Aging and National Institute of Mental Health, Bethesda, Md., September 14–16, 1978.

Lebowitz, Barry D. "Statement on crimes against the elderly before House Subcommittee on Domestic and International Scientific Planning, Analysis, and Cooperation." U. S. Congress, House Committee on Science and Technology, *Hearings,* January 31, 1978.

Lehr, U. "Preparation for Old Age—More Than Just a Medical Problem." *Triangle,* 16 (1977): 93–103.

Lewis, Myrna I., and Robert N. Butler. "Why Is Women's Lib Ignoring Old Women?" *International Journal of Aging and Human Development,* 3 (1972): 223–231.

Martin, Cora A. "Lavender Rose or Gray Panther?" *Aging,* nos. 285–286 (July–August 1978): 28–30.

McKain, Walter. *Retirement Marriage.* Monograph No. 3. Storrs, Conn.: University of Connecticut, 1969.

National Institute on Aging and National Institute of Mental Health. *The Older Woman: Continuities and Discontinuities.* Summary of conference on the older woman held September 14–16, 1978, Bethesda, Md.

Nowak, Carol A. "Socialization to Become an Old Hag." Paper presented at

85th annual convention of American Psychological Association, San Francisco, Calif., August 26–30, 1977.

Patterson, Robert D., et al. "Preventing Self-Destructive Behavior." *Geriatrics* 29 (November 1974): 115–121.

Stueve, Ann, and Claude S. Fischer. "Social Networks and Older Women." Paper presented at conference on the older woman held at National Institutes of Health, Bethesda, Md., September 14–16, 1978.

Tavris, Carol. "The Sexual Lives of Women Over 60." *Ms.* 6, no. 1 (1977): 62–65.

Troll, Lillian E. "Different Types of Older Women." Paper presented at conference on the older woman held at National Institutes of Health, Bethesda, Md., September 14–16, 1978.

Weg, Ruth B. *The Aged: Who, Where, How Well.* University Park, Calif.: University of Southern California, Ethel Percy Andrus Gerontology Center, 1978.

Weg, Ruth B. "More Than Wrinkles." In Lillian E. Troll, et al., *Looking Ahead: A Woman's Guide to the Problems and Joys of Growing Older.* Englewood Cliffs, N.J.: Prentice-Hall, 1977.

Weg, Ruth B. "Normal Aging Changes in the Reproductive System." In Irene M. Burnside, *Nursing and the Aged.* New York: McGraw-Hill, 1976.

Weg, Ruth B. "The Physiology of Sexuality in Aging." In Robert L. Solnick, ed., *Sexuality and Aging,* rev. ed. University Park, Calif.: University of Southern California, Ethel Percy Andrus Gerontology Center, 1978.

Weinstock, Ruth. *The Graying of the Campus.* New York: Educational Facilities Laboratories, 1978.

Weiss, Robert S. *Marital Separation: Managing After a Marriage Ends.* New York: Basic Books, 1977.

Weissman, Myrna M. "Sex Differences and the Epidemiology of Depression." *Archives of General Psychiatry* 34 (January 1977): 98–111.

Weissman, Myrna M., and Jerome K. Myers. "Depression in the Elderly: Research Directions in Psychopathology, Epidemiology and Treatment." Paper presented at conference on the older woman held at National Institutes of Health, Bethesda, Md., September 14–16, 1978.

You, Your Doctors, and the Health Care System

FRANCES DREW, M.D., M.P.H.

Professor of Community Medicine and Associate Dean
for Student Affairs, University of Pittsburgh School of Medicine

The health care system today neither begins nor ends with physicians. The vastly improved health education offered daily in all media has drawn us, the patients, the public, the "consumer," into an awareness of and responsibility for our own health. Dr. Benjamin Spock's book on babies began an ever-expanding "do-it-yourself" movement. All of the women's magazines have columns about health maintenance and health problems, and their informational quality is generally high. Most newspapers have both a "Dear Abby" and a "Dear Doctor" letter-answering column, though here the information tends to be a bit more shopworn. Television has had some excellent documentaries, but its regular medical programs exploit the drama and the horrors. Many books have been written for the lay public, running the gamut from excellent and informative to tedious and overtechnical to downright quackery. Clearly, this torrent of information is responding to a perceived public interest, perhaps spurred on by the complexities of the health care system.

Not only have words tumbled forth. Numbers of self-help groups have arisen, whose goals are to alert people to their own ability to cope with illness. Women's cooperative clinics are one fine example, a group like Reach for Recovery for mastectomy patients is another. The patient is acquiring a growing sophistication about health which is all to the good.

The result of all these trends is a new participation by the patient in a system which used to operate on a strictly authoritarian basis. In the next decade both physicians and patients will expect to deal with each other in a more equal way, both knowing that the better informed patient will be healthier, will recover faster, and will be more gratifying to treat.

Women have a special responsibility. In our culture, as in most others, it is the women who are the custodians of the skills needed to nurse the sick and care for the children and the elderly. Yet at present we have no teachers. While our mothers learned this art from their mothers who lived nearby, we are nomads and our neighbors are rarely ever related to us. We must master the knowledge by ourselves—and many of us need help. How does the woman today find a physician for herself, her family, her child? How can she get the best available care? This chapter will attempt to serve as a guide to our present health care system.

CHOOSING YOUR DOCTORS

Choosing a Primary Physician

Many people decide fairly suddenly that they "want a doctor," perhaps because an illness is upon them or because they have just read an article suggesting the dangers of eating Brand M or because they must immediately produce a bona fide health report. Little thought is given ahead of time to choosing wisely and well. Inquiries are made of a friend who recommends Dr. Blow because the friend "likes" Dr. Blow or found Dr. Blow accessible to the nearest supermarket or got an instant appointment when Dr. Zilch couldn't see her for two months. Dr. Blow has been stumbled upon, not chosen. You have no knowledge of this doctor's abilities, qualifications, areas of special competence, hospital affiliations, referral patterns, and all of these will become important to you at a later time. Getting away from Dr. Blow is a great deal harder than making the original connection, so an effort to avoid a mismatch in the first place is rewarded over and over again in the succeeding years. Rule 1, therefore, is: Choose, don't stumble, and choose when you are well, when you have time to wait for a convenient appointment, when your first visit will be for a check-up rather than for treatment.

Geography. Convenience to both you and your physician is important. Neither of you wishes to travel long distances if you need care. On the other hand, the nearest doctor isn't necessarily the best.

If you live in a suburb or a semirural area you may not have much choice. You know where your nearest hospital is located and you will want a physician affiliated with the staff of that hospital.

If you live in a metropolitan area, your choice widens considerably. You may wish to have a physician on the staff of a Catholic or Jewish hospital because of your religious beliefs; you may wish to get your care from a university complex; you may have strong preference for one or another hospital because of friends who have been there. The next step is to call either the hospital or a county medical society and ask them to give you the names of physicians in a given discipline on the staff of that hospital. You can then look them up in the telephone book and make inquiries about the lag time until they will see new patients.

Qualifications. When you call a new doctor for the first time, you have every right to ask about his credentials. Nearly every physician under 50 today is board certified in some discipline. Certification in either family practice or internal medicine indicates that the physician provides primary care rather than concentrating on the treatment of specific conditions.

Style of Practice. If you are satisfied with qualifications, the next question might be whether the office is a group or solo practice. Most younger physicians are reluctant to enter solo practice for a number of reasons, of which the most important is night and weekend calls. The solo work year of seven days a week, twenty-four hours a day, palls and drains. Another important reason is the sharing of equipment and support staff, costly outlays for a single physician who does not use them to capacity. The pattern of group practice has grown enormously over the past decade and few physicians entering practice even consider going it alone.

Apart from the advantages to the physician, there are many to the patient. In an office with several physicians someone is always on call and always available. It may not be the person you see regularly, but your record is there. If the group is a fairly large one, it comprises more than one area of practice. There may be an obstetrician/gynecologist, there probably is a pediatrician, there may be a surgeon, there certainly will be a contract with a radiologist, and there will be clear referral patterns to other specialties. Your record will be immediately available to all of them and you will be spared the time-consuming job of being a completely "new" patient over and over again.

AGE, PERSONALITY, AND SUBCULTURE

Patients are as varied as physicians, and no one is equally comfortable with everyone. Much has been written about why patients choose a particular physician and one of the most readable, accurate, and interesting studies is Earl Lomon Koos's *The Health of Regionville.* The author looked at a town in upper New York State in which five physicians practiced, asking patients of different backgrounds why they preferred their physician. The reasons given were that their physician (1) had served the family in the previous generation, and they saw no reason to change; (2) was known to them socially; (3) was recommended by a relative or friend; (4) was generally known in the community as a "good doctor"; (5) made home calls; (6) was "willing to spend time with you"; (7) didn't press for payment; (8) charges moderate fees; (9) was "just liked as a person"; (10) was "the most available"; and (11) had "good equipment."

You will recognize many of these reasons as topics already discussed, but there is no gainsaying that past commonality of experience may make both the physician and the patient more comfortable and their interaction more effective, particularly if social or family pressures are contributing significantly to the ill health. You may need only technical expertise in a one-time visit to a specialist, but you should give extra weight to compatibility if your psychological as well as physical needs are to be met. For example, a 60-year-old woman may be initially uncomfortable discussing her psyche or her sexuality with a 30-year-old man, and a teenager may be seriously mismatched on these same topics with a physician of grandfather's age. The physician's expertise and attitudes can sometimes overcome these initial obstacles, but time is lost in the process. As another example, the intelligent, informed patient is impatient with the physician who simply expects orders to be carried out and refuses to give answers of substance to questions, and the patient who expects authoritative treatment is equally put off by a physician who says, "I don't quite know what is wrong with you, but let's start here."

The only way to establish whether or not you trust and are comfortable with a physician is to try the relationship out. If you find yourself ill at ease or lacking in confidence, pay your bill and find someone else.

SEX OF PHYSICIAN

Some women prefer male physicians, some are indifferent, and some vastly prefer a woman. Preferences are apt to be particularly strong in seeking an obstetrician-gynecologist. While recent years have brought a sharp increase in the number of young women in all specialties and especially in family practice, the medical world is still predominantly male. If you feel strongly enough about finding a woman, the county medical society will give you names, but you may have to pay an extra price in convenience of location. With approximately 25 percent of each current class of graduates being women, this gap will close and the difficulties will lessen.

CHANGING DOCTORS

Everyone knows that marriage is easier than divorce, that many marriages are sustained on inertia rather than on compatibility or love. The same is true of doctor-patient relationships, and the techniques of "divorcing" your doctor are nearly as awkward as divorcing your husband. It can be done and in the long run should be, and, if we continue the analogy to marriage, annulment is easier than divorce. The sooner you get out, the better off you are.

If you are moving to another city, the situation is easy. The most comfortable solution is to find a physician in your new locality (Dr. Y) and then write your former physician (Dr. X) asking to have your record or a summary of it sent to Dr. Y. If Dr. Y requests the record from Dr. X, you will be asked to sign a waiver. This process is often facilitated by a conference with Dr. X before you move, in which you ask about physicians near your new residence. Each specialist is apt to have a list of all members of that specialty board in the United States, giving age, university, perhaps even residency training sites, and from this you can together cull some likely names.

If you want to change physicians within a group or to a new office, embarrassment may glue you to the chair. Most people see the change as quite different from returning a dress to a department store, but while techniques differ, the motivation is the same—you are dissatisfied with your choice. If you are enrolled in a group practice, you are apt to have seen more than one primary physician over time because of vacations, on-call schedules, and the like. If Dr. A was your original physician, but the last time you had the flu you saw Dr. B with whom you felt more comfortable, you need only make your next appointment with Dr. B through the secretary. If you happen to be seeing Dr. B, you can easily say that you would really prefer to continue this relationship, and Dr. B can then manage the problem in the office with no fuss at all.

You encounter only slightly more difficulty in changing completely to another office. Here the routine is exactly the same as when moving to another town. You choose your new physician, say that you have been seeing Dr. A who has your record, sign a waiver, and let Dr. B write requesting it from Dr. A. If your only contacts with Dr. A were for routine check-up or upper respiratory conditions, the record will contain very little important information and you can forget about asking for its transfer. On the other hand, if you have had any chronic or complicated condition or much laboratory data has accrued (the usual levels of some chemical values or what your chest X-ray looked like a year ago, etc.) your new physician needs and deserves to know all of these facts. *No amount of embarrassment should prevent you from getting this information into the hands of your new physician.*

Payment Plans

You may be a member of an employee group which offers prepaid medical care as a fringe benefit or you may be fortunate enough to live in a community which has a prepaid plan open to the public. You may even have a choice among groups offering such plans. Many people prefer prepayment, assuming that the physicians offering it are of high quality, since it is easier to budget for a fixed sum each month than to worry about the cost of seeing a physician if a medical problem arises. A number of studies have shown that illnesses are seen earlier and treated more effectively when money is not an obstacle. Once you have joined such a plan, the group has the responsibility to care for you and the lag time to an appointment is shorter.

If your employee benefits include Blue Cross/Blue Shield as either the only coverage or as an alternative to a prepaid plan, read the contract carefully, compare the benefits, estimate what your out-of-pocket costs would be for ordinary illness. With these plans you are free to continue with your own physician, but many office charges are not covered even if your physician is a Blue Shield participant. For covered procedures Blue Shield may be billed and their fee accepted as full payment, or because of your higher income, you may be charged an extra amount. If your physician does not participate, there is probably a mechanism in the contract which will reimburse you for charges.

If you are eligible for Medicare, you must again find out what benefits are allowed, and you may well discover that private care is still out of your financial reach. The overwhelming majority of physicians will accept Medicare as payment in full for a patient they have cared for over the years, but they may not do the same for a new patient. This will necessitate your seeking alternative care as an outpatient (see below). Obviously this limits in some measure your "free choice" of physician but the financial benefits are great and all such plans deal with group practices so that you have choice among the physicians in the group.

Blue Cross offers a "65+" contract for which you pay a fee, but which augments your coverage considerably and assures you more hospital days covered. Medicare has an annual deductible so that you will pay some money before coverage begins, but this is a comparatively modest amount. There are, however, a number of items not covered, among them glasses, dentures, prescriptions. Medicare alone, without the added Blue Cross, will probably leave you with almost 50 percent of your total medical costs. If you are eligible for Medicaid, because of a low income, you are in theory totally covered, though this varies greatly from state to state. Many physicians will not accept the lower fees derived from these plans and your best, and perhaps only, recourse is to seek care in a hospital out-patient department.

If your health insurance contract includes "major medical," you have a bolster against catastrophe. If you or a family member is disabled, there are other sources of payment. The important point to remember is to read your contract carefully so you are not taken by surprise by deductible amounts or items not covered. Hospitals, clinics, and group practices all have someone available to explain the variations of coverage and will help you in wending your way through the complications.

Having established exactly what your coverage includes, you should discuss with your physician or someone in the office what additional charges may occur and under what circumstances. You must not be embarrassed to ask exactly what your care will cost you for a routine visit, for laboratory tests, for a house call. If you know these facts, you will avoid the irritation and dissatisfaction of receiving a "surprise" bill far higher than you expected, even though your expectation may have been unreasonable.

Hospital Outpatient Departments

The word "clinic" (unless labeled Mayo, Menninger, Lahey, or Joslin) conjures up an image of crowded benches, offhand care, students as the only doctors—a medical Ellis Island. Today the facts are quite different.

Many university clinics are run in tandem with private doctors' offices and there is no way of telling who is the public patient and who the private. If you go to a clinic for your general medical care, it is certainly likely that you will have more than one physician over a five-year period, since much of the care is provided by residents, and it is also true that you are apt to encounter a medical student first. However, you must understand one point about illness. Approximately 80 percent of visits to physicians are precipitated by either self-limiting illness (flu) or problems easily diagnosed and easily treated (rashes, sprains, headaches, ulcers, hypertension). Even when surgery is required (gallstones, appendixes, hernias, hemorrhoids), the procedure is usually a straightforward one. Appreciating this, recognize that the chairman of medicine is as powerless to treat flu as is the medical student—aspirin and plenty of fluids to tide you through is still the best treatment. However, if you should acquire a complex disease like leukemia, you can be certain that you will be seen by the chief of hematology in that institution and you can't improve on *that* quality of care. If you need surgery, you can sleep quietly through the anesthetic knowing that while the scalpel may be held by the chief resident in surgery, that resident has had five years of postgraduate training and a faculty member is scrubbed and standing by to supervise. In short, while it is difficult to consider a clinic as "your doctor," the care provided is of the highest quality, you have the advantage of continuity of records, and referrals are available to all specialties.

While a number of nonuniversity clinics are excellent, particularly in hospitals which have family practice programs or are situated in areas distant from an urban center, there is nonetheless a wide variation in quality. If you have a choice in a large, metropolitan area, choose a clinic associated with a medical school. You can then be confident that there is an approved residency training program, which means that there are an adequate number of appropriately trained faculty members to supervise. If you must choose between two community hospitals, phone and ask whether their residency training program is approved in medicine, surgery, or whatever. If it is not, go elsewhere, because the clinic will be manned by staff of the hospital who consider it a chore to be disposed of as rapidly as possible and it may well *be* Ellis Island.

Choosing a Specialist

Almost every primary physician establishes personal patterns of referral to known and trusted specialists. If you happen to have heard that Dr. Zilch is a fine dermatologist and you ask to be referred, your physician has two choices: immediate agreement, even though this is not the usual pattern, or demurral with another suggestion. Many interpretations can be put on this latter action: your physician may know that although Dr. Zilch is "nice," his competency level is not very high; Dr. Zilch may simply be unknown, whereas other physicians in the usual office referral pattern are both known and competent; of course, your physician may be splitting fees, but that is both illegal and unlikely. What is fairly certain is that if your physician is competent and you have chosen well in the first place, your specialists will in turn be chosen well for you.

Your relationship to a specialist need not be as close as to your primary physician, unless you anticipate that your condition will require a great deal of interaction over a long period. We all would prefer dealing with charming, congenial people at every turn of the medical road, but if you need a fracture set or a mole removed, you need technical skill more than congeniality. Your physician can, and should, be asked, "What kind of a person is Dr. Blow?" The honest reply may be something like, "Well, not very attractive, a little gruff, but superb in the operating room." If you know that much, you will accept a less than prepossessing manner because you are assured that this is the best person to deal with your problem. In short, if you are confident in your choice of primary physician, you can let the choice of specialists be part of your doctor's responsibility to you.

One specialty area deserves particular comment—pediatrics. If your primary physician is in family practice, this may well include pediatrics. If you are receiving care from a group practice, there is probably a pediatrician in it. If you need to find a new doctor to care for children, recommended names will come from many sources, from your obstetrician, from your internist, from friends. Again, you need to know relationships to hospital staffs. All of the questions you asked before choosing your physician apply as well to the physician for your child, but there are differences. You must feel confident that this person *likes* children, that your child will be comfortable, and that you can establish a cooperative relationship. More than any other specialist, the pediatrician relies on you to handle minor problems yourself while being instantly alert to danger. Young children can get very sick very quickly. You must feel comfortable about calling to raise any questions and to report symptoms you observe, but at the same time you must let yourself be educated in handling your own child, in learning to distinguish between the minor problems and signs of danger, and in understanding your child's pattern of response to illness.

BEING A WOMAN AND A PATIENT

The medical as well as lay literature has been exploding recently with objections about the ways male physicians treat (or mistreat) women. There is certainly much to what is said and a knowledgeable woman patient should be aware of the areas of danger.

A single case history will illustrate the problem better than any analysis. A friend, the mother of three daughters, two of whom were twins born fourteen years before when she was 35, mentioned casually to me in a social setting that she had not menstruated since the twins were born, at which time she had bled profusely and been in serious condition for two days. A few more questions made it very clear to me that she had, at that time, suffered pituitary hemorrhage which had left her debilitated and chronically ill. Throughout the period she had seen both her internist and her obstetrician on many occasions and each had checked her blood count, listened to her symptoms of lassitude, weakness, lack of menses, and then said something like, "There, there, dear, you'll have that boy yet" or "It's just change of life" or "It's all your nerves." She was spending nearly a third of each day in bed, while still managing to get her children off to school and the dinner ready. She had been a vigorous and active woman before her illness, but had been forced to be nearly a recluse after it. The most distressing part of the story came after my diagnosis.

For another three years she did nothing because she didn't want to offend her family physician by seeking other care and because by this time both doctors had indeed convinced her that it was in her head. When she finally went to a prestigious medical center in another city, she became a classic case presentation of serious pituitary deficiency. Her physician there told me later that she would forever be the paragon of a nonneurotic patient because, at the conclusion of the tests, he came into her hospital room, stupefied at the extent of her illness and the lag time to treatment, and said, "Mrs. S, I can't really understand how you have managed all these years." She replied, "Doctor, I couldn't have done it without coffee!"

While this may be an extreme instance, it has the virtue of being true and it illustrates all of the societal biases against women as well as the acceptance by a woman of a diagnosis of neurosis or menopause in the face of serious illness. Women are expected to be weak, are expected to complain of vague symptoms like fatigue. Beyond that, there is always the menopause to blame. The best thing that could happen to women would be the abolition of the menopause, not because it is intolerable, but because it's a wastebasket into which all manner of unexplained symptoms are pitched. In contrast, were a man to complain of equal fatigue, he would probably be hospitalized instantly for a complete work-up and a diagnosis would be made within a week.

An excellent paper, "Alleged Psychogenic Disorders in Women" by K. J. Lennane, lists the complaints of women which physicians routinely impute to neurosis even in the face of ample evidence of organic cause. Nausea of pregnancy, premenstrual tension, and the menopause come readily to mind, but the list also includes infantile colic attributed to the mother's neurosis. That these are reflections of a male-oriented society and a male-dominated profession is certainly clear to any woman. The pertinence of discussing them in this chapter rests with their warning value. If your physician murmurs about a symptom being psychosomatic, you should neither accept nor deny this suggestion until you have given it some thought. Look closely at your complaint, and ask yourself whether it is stress dependent. Question your life style and your sleeping and drinking habits; look yourself in the eye. Look particularly carefully at whether your complaint serves as an excuse for you at home or at work, allows you to be treated differently, protected more or excused from unpleasant tasks. Such secondary gains frequently maintain symptoms in even well-adjusted, dynamic women. The body readily expresses the psyche's unconscious needs, and those "sick headaches" or recurrent fatigue or "bad colds" give many a woman a little more attention at home or a little more respite at work. After you have done all this and have come to the conclusion that you had the same stress last year and you didn't feel this way, go back to your physician and say so. Say you have looked at it, describe the factors you have considered, and then insist that you wish to explore further.

EMERGENCY CARE

Suppose that you are in a strange city and you suddenly become ill. Carry it further, and you are ill in a foreign country. What do you do? You know no one; you are unfamiliar with the hospitals and perhaps even the language. Most likely you will turn to the hotel manager and he will supply the name of a physician with whom he deals regularly. If your problem is a simple one, this may suffice, but if it is serious and requires hospitalization, you must be prepared to make your own choices. My general rule is to ask to be taken to the university hospital if there is one. This at least assures the highest quality of care in that community. Once in the emergency room, you will be seen first by a resident who will assess the situation and perhaps say that you need to be seen by a surgeon. Your next question should be, "If you needed a surgeon for your daughter in this hospital, whom would you call?" This question is entirely different from "Whom would you suggest?" because if the resident happens at that moment to be rotating through the service with Drs. A, B, and C, he will feel compelled to name one of them. However, all residents know well who are the competent (and incompetent) physicians in that hospital in their discipline; each hospital has at least one "doctor's doctor" who somehow has all the medical and nursing staff families as patients because they know who is the best. If you ask the right question, you'll find that person and that's who you want.

But suppose you are in an automobile accident and find yourself in a hospital in a community alien to you. You are there not by your own choice, but because that is where the ambulance driver took you. Immediate care will lessen the urgency—bleeding will be stopped, intravenous fluids begun, some assessment of the gravity of the situation will be made. If the hospital is small and rural, it will be ill-prepared to deal with serious injury of the head, chest, or abdomen, and once your medical condition is stabilized, they will suggest and arrange for transfer to a more appropriate hospital. Here again, you will be offered some choices, and if you are too far away from your own physician and hospital, the wisest decision is to request transfer to the nearest university health center complex. Some hospitals other than university centers provide excellent care for the most complicated problems, but you have no way of knowing which they are, and you certainly wish to avoid a second transfer later.

If you have any condition which requires constant therapy, such as diabetes, allergies, or epilepsy, make sure that you *always* wear an identification tag, such as the Medic-Alert emblem, which gives the diagnosis and a collect call telephone number for additional information. (Write Medic-Alert, Turlock, California 95380 for further information.) An unconscious person cannot give a history, and your prior illness may be either the cause of your admission or may be seriously complicating it.

One last word about emergencies—they occur at home as well. If an accident happens or a family member suddenly becomes acutely ill, do not bother to telephone your physician. This will take costly minutes and the physician will almost certainly say, "Go immediately to the emergency room at the hospital." You should save the time of the call and go directly there. Your physician knows, and you should know, that the little black bag and a medical presence are almost impotent in any true emergency and that a house call would do little except waste time. What is needed is immediate access to an X-ray machine, intravenous fluids, medications which a physician is unlikely to carry, and often sophisticated equipment housed only in a hospital.

Orders should be left in your house which specify exactly which hospital is to be used for which family member, the hospital(s) on which your pediatrician, internist or general practitioner has staff privileges. The resident in the emergency room will phone the physician, but in the meanwhile the patient is being cared for in the best place with the best facilities and staff.

HOSPITALS

To the public the most frightening area of medicine is the hospital. It has unfamiliar machines and smells, it contains seriously ill and dying people, it is impersonal, it is above all mysterious. Processions of people in different uniforms troop through your room, each punching or poking or stabbing you for a different reason, until finally you lose track and simply submit. Once you submit, you have become "institutionalized"; you have accepted your own depersonalization. If you are seriously ill, this matters very little, but if you are comparatively well, it disturbs you. What are your defenses?

The American Hospital Association has published a patient's bill of rights to which all accredited hospitals must accede. The list is as follows:

1. The patient has the right to considerate and respectful care.
2. The patient has the right to obtain from her physician complete current information concerning her diagnosis, treatment, and prognosis in terms the patient can reasonably be expected to understand.
3. The patient has the right to receive from her physician information necessary to give informed consent prior to the start of any procedure and/or treatment.
4. The patient has the right to refuse treatment to the extent permitted by law and to be informed of the medical consequences of his action.
5. The patient has the right to every consideration of her privacy concerning her own medical care program.
6. The patient has the right to expect that all communications and records pertaining to her care should be treated as confidential.
7. The patient has the right to expect that within its capacity a hospital must make reasonable response to the request of a patient for services.
8. The patient has the right to obtain information as to any relationship of her hospital to other health care and educational institutions insofar as her care is concerned.
9. The patient has the right to be advised if the hospital proposes to engage in or perform human experimentation affecting her care or treatment.
10. The patient has the right to expect reasonable continuity of care.
11. The patient has the right to examine and receive an explanation of her bill regardless of source of payment.
12. The patient has the right to know what hospital rules and regulations apply to her conduct as a patient.

Armed with this information, the patient should feel considerably less helpless. She *can* ask what is being done to her, she *can* refuse treatment, she *can* ask to have her room changed.

If you are traveling, and in a new hotel, *you* ask who provides which service, *you* discover what a concierge does even if you never heard of one before. In a hospital tasks are clearly assigned and you should ask what any given person is responsible for. A laboratory technician may know only that blood is to be drawn, an X-ray technician only that a chest film has been ordered, but the floor nurse or the resident or your physician can and should tell you the entire game plan. If you are to have an X-ray of your stomach the next day, you have a right to know that you will be given a laxative and will be allowed no food or fluids the night before. If you have been depersonalized, you don't bother to ask and your fear heightens.

The costs of a private room in most hospitals are very high and are not covered by Blue Cross, so your purse will favor your having a roommate. By and large this contributes to your comfort and decreases your anxiety. You have someone to talk to, you have a mutual aid source, you have company. The drawbacks come when your roommate is a chronic complainer or a groaner or when she is very ill and the traffic in the room exceeds your tolerance. Under any of these circumstances you should speak with the head nurse and ask to be changed to another room. Discharges occur every day and within a reasonable time you should be relocated. Such requests are not unusual nor, if done with courtesy, are they interpreted as griping.

Both your phone and your visitors maintain your connections with the outside world; you will gradually sort out the staff and greet some of them with pleasure and enthusiasm; you will begin to understand the routines. All these lessen your anxiety and improve your state of well-being. Since most admissions are less than a week in duration, you will not have suffered inordinately and your next admission will be fraught with considerably less apprehension. If your condition or treatment requires a longer hospitalization, you will find that you adapt quite well to the restrictions imposed on you by the hospital, just as you adapted when you first went to camp or to college. The difference is that your psychic strength has been sapped by your illness and your elasticity does not compare with that of a healthy person.

At the time of admission for more serious conditions, many patients and families worry about whether they should engage a "special duty" nurse. Will the floor nurses come when one rings the bell or will they be too busy? Can the nursing station down the hall respond adequately to the patient's personal needs? The way to find this out at admission is to ask the nurses how they feel about the matter. The extent of nursing required will be a large factor, the number of patients on the floor another. In most situations there are enough nurses to meet all the needs of the patients, and they are highly skilled in dealing with the equipment and procedures required for the specialty clustered on that floor. If, for any reason, you feel that extra care is needed, the hospital has a roster of both registered nurses and licensed practical nurses who are available for special duty. The cost of a registered nurse is considerably greater than a practical nurse and in most situations there is no need for the former since the goal is largely to meet needs of creature comfort. Occasionally a physician feels that extra assistance is needed and has a particular nurse whose skills are appropriate to the case. You should accept this advice.

If you have worries about your convalescent period, if you will need further help at home or further treatment or whatever, ask to be seen by a member of the social service department. All of the community facilities are at their finger tips and they can be very helpful in arranging for the best post-hospital care.

The intensive care unit is far and away the most distressing hospital area. Patients are submerged under equipment, sleep is disturbed by constant monitoring, privacy is nonexistent, relatives usually may visit only five minutes every hour. Families wait for each hourly visit wondering what they will find and what to say and often the patient is too ill to know or care whether someone visited an hour ago. The visiting rules were made to insure optimal care, to limit the number of people hovering around a bed when patient monitoring must be done repeatedly. If a member of your family is in such a unit and your life is being torn to tatters by these waits and unsatisfactory visits, do not be afraid to tell the nurse exactly what you intend to do—you will be back at six o'clock, you can be reached at such-and-such a number. Ask her to reassure the patient that you were there and will return. If the unit is comparatively quiet, she may allow you to stay longer than the five minutes if it will comfort the patient.

WHAT YOU HAVE A RIGHT TO EXPECT FROM YOUR PHYSICIAN

Clearly, you expect your physician to provide good medical care, of which many facets have been covered above. But you have other expectations as well, some you may not consciously recognize. Above all, you want *help*. If you are threatened with a serious illness, you not only want to be confident that you have been referred to the most competent specialists, but you want some time to discuss the threat as well.

Let us assume that you have just discovered a lump in your neck and your doctor has confirmed that indeed it is a cause for further investigation, probably surgery. These are the facts, but many other things are whirling through your mind. Benign or malignant? How much surgery? How many hospital days? How much time off work? Who will look after the children? Will I have a disfiguring scar? Why do I have a lump at all? How much will it cost and how will we find the money? If I am hospitalized for a long time, what will it do to my marriage, my relationship? Who will look after me as I convalesce? If it is a malignancy, how will I face it? You may be tempted to play the courageous role and say nothing out loud, and unless your physician brings up the subject of your anxiety, you simply leave the office and continue to whirl at home, in bed, at work. You may not even wish to share this with your husband or best friend because you don't wish to "worry them." The result is a load of unnecessary anxiety piled on top of the realistic amount which the unsettling news brings you, and you may enter the hospital having lost both sleep and weight, with your blood pressure twenty points above its normal level.

Such courage is not only unnecessary, but unwise. Your physician owes you help just as much as you are owed laboratory results, and you have every right to discuss all of these questions. It may well be that the schedule is too tight at that moment to cover the ground, but you should ask whether you can make another appointment in the very near future only to talk. Often you can be immediately reassured that the overwhelming odds are against malignancy and that, if it is benign, surgery is simple and hospitalization short. But, the "ifs" still lurk in the back of your mind and should be handled on top of the table.

Of course, many of your questions are not for the physician to answer. No matter how frankly you have discussed your marital situation, no other person can predict how your spouse will react nor can you be told how to find money or a babysitter. But you can, and should, have every question answered about the medical situation and can then be referred to a social worker or a community agency to help in arrangements for children and for convalescence.

Once you enter the hospital for surgery, the surgeon rather than your physician will probably be your "physician of record." However, your physician will undoubtedly come to see you frequently when making rounds and, because of personal knowledge, will be able to allay any new anxieties as well as interpret any findings which other physicians have left unexplained. It is possible that your doctor will also be in the operating room (whether you know it or not), anxious to find out what the status is, and will see you again the next day. There will have been discussions with the surgeon and a plan of action for the future will have begun to unroll.

Now let us suppose that you have a malignancy, that the surgery was far more radical than anticipated, the hospitalization longer, the cost greater, the scar wider, the convalescence more stormy and fraught with new symptoms from X-ray or chemotherapy. The worst has happened and more decisions must be made. There will be conferences between your physician, the surgeon, and the radiologists and a plan of medical action will be formulated; the social service department will assist in sorting out the family and financial problems. Even so, your anxiety about *you* is high. What can you expect then?

You can expect, and should receive, comfort and honesty. Any question which you ask about your future should be answered. That last sentence is very carefully worded, and the appropriate analogy is to the sex education of a child. There is substantial agreement that in childhood sexual questions should not be answered before they are asked, that the child's unconscious or preconscious adapts the question to the amount of information which can be assimilated. Similarly, in questions of malignancy and death the patient virtually always asks the questions she wants answered, and no others. If your physician tells you that today most malignancies are treatable and many curable, you are not being conned; this is the truth. You should not dwell on all the frightening things that may or may not happen; you must participate actively in your own recovery. On the other hand, active participation depends on full information, so you will be told, for instance, that you should not return to work while getting radiation because you will probably be nauseated for a few weeks. The path of your immediate future can be accurately charted, but you cannot expect to be told what will happen in two years because no one knows. You and your doctor will be a team for that period, making decisions as you go in the light of what is known about medicine and about you.

While one example does not cover all exigencies, it should indicate the dimensions of your physician's responsibility to you under the worst of circumstances and you can extrapolate from it what you should expect in other, less anxious situations. Without question your physician should accept with grace any request for a second opinion; in difficult cases such a consultation usually is welcomed as either a new slant on the problem or confirmation. Any situation which offers a choice of therapies with different risks and side effects must be completely discussed; this is the essence of "informed consent." If a new approach to your problem is available only in another city, your physician should discuss appraisal of the treatment and, if you wish it, refer you to that site. Such a referral assumes that a complete record of your illness and laboratory findings will be sent prior to your appointment.

You also have every right to expect complete confidentiality from your physician, and this includes responsibility not to discuss anything in your record without your permission, even with your family. There will, however, be times when you will not only allow such a family discussion, but will ask to have one. If, for instance, you will have to restrict your activities, it is important that your family understand why this is so and exactly what you can and cannot do. Their cooperation will be more complete if their information is first hand rather than through your interpretation. Furthermore, you may not be trustworthy to relay exactly the message you have been given, since you may feel obligated to spare your family extra tasks. While the analogy to a "team" is shopworn, nonetheless, persons other than the patient have a responsibility to carry out a regimen of cure and everyone does this best when fully informed of the rationale of the tasks.

You have one further right—dignity. To be called "honey" or "dearie" is to be robbed of your identity by patronization. To be called by your first name without your permission is to establish a relationship in which you have been immediately cast as the meek, the docile. Some patients prefer being called Mary to Mrs. Brown, but the initiative should rest with the patient. State your preference but beware of an office in which first names are bandied around by physician and staff alike. You will never be treated as a colleague by such a group; you will always be the helpless little girl regardless of your age.

WHAT YOU SHOULD NOT EXPECT FROM YOUR PHYSICIAN

Your physician is neither your parent nor your best friend, even though often you have confided more intimate facts than you have to anyone else. To survive as a good physician objectivity must be maintained. You have no right to expect "love," in the sense of protection from all evil, nor should you ask advice on personal matters which have nothing to do with your physical health. Whether you should break off a relationship with your alcoholic lover or husband, whether you should buy a house instead of renting, whether you should change your job—these are your decisions. Granted that each of these may cause you anxiety and be reflected in your physical condition, the physician has only two responsibilities. If there are community resources which can help you untangle the dilemma, such as Al-Anon or a marriage counselor, you should expect encouragement to seek them out. The only other responsibility is to point out to you that you are getting too little sleep, that you are run down, and that solving your problem will improve your health. In acute situations, such as death in the family, a tranquilizer or a sleeping pill may be prescribed to tide you over, but you should not press to continue such drugs indefinitely. Anxieties are uncomfortable, but they are part of living and growing. Solutions enlarge one's capacities to face the next crisis (and there certainly will be one), and the only way to solve a problem is to address it head on. Supportive drugs postpone solutions.

Some patients feel that they have a right to manage their own illnesses and demand treatments which they have read about—multivitamins, laetrile, acupuncture, the newest diet. These therapies may be pharmacologically innocuous even though ineffective and costly, but they may, as well, be particularly contraindicated in your case. Your physician can and should explain to you why such treatment will not be prescribed for you, whether because you wish to substitute it for more effective (but more discomfiting) medication or because you are using the medicine as a crutch to prevent yourself from facing reality. Even sophisticated patients may try to pressure a physician into prescribing antibiotics so that they can feel that something is being done, even when antibiotics are ineffective, as in viral infections. They also involve needless costs, and they may have side effects, such as allergic reactions. Once you have trusted yourself to a physician's knowledge and judgment, you should accept advice without pressing for something else.

You also have no right to invade your physician's personal time. Phone calls at off hours which could be easily postponed until morning, demands for unnecessary house calls, phoning for an "emergency" appointment when, in fact, there is no emergency—these are sure ways to antagonize your physician, even to the point where capabilities to treat you are diminished.

A particularly sensitive and difficult area is encountered when your physician feels that your anxiety level is serious enough to require either more help or more expert help than is feasible in that office. The suggestion will be made that you see a counselor or a psychiatrist. This may startle you, you may respond with anger because "I'm not crazy," you may feel rejected. However, you must accept this judgment in such situations. You are *not* being told you are "crazy"; you are being told that your psyche is interfering with your body at a level of intensity which your physician feels unprepared to handle. Suggesting such a referral is (and should be) no different from asking that you see a surgeon. What is wanted is another opinion or a kind of treatment which requires a different kind of skill.

Each physician has a few patients for whom "demands" are a way of life. Often they are well-to-do and take the position that if they "pay" they can "demand." Implicit in this behavior is the assumption that the physician is their servant. These patients (more often women than men) have no insight that they are behaving much as infants do when they are hungry, or that they are making a profession out of being "ill" in order to manipulate their environment, whether this be the physician or the spouse or the children. They disrupt an office routine, they cause the physician to groan when their name is on the day's appointment list, they are the ones who take particular umbrage at being referred to a psychiatrist. Parenthetically, they are usually extremely difficult to treat, even at the top level of psychiatric expertise, because they have built an almost impregnable cocoon of behavior in order to guard their neuroses and they discard them with enormous reluctance and only after long periods of therapy. They have filled their lives with ill health as a substitute for something more productive which would demand effort and discipline on their part, and they are quite satisfied with the arrangement.

When they have used up the tolerance of one physician, they move to the next; their charts are thick, their bathroom cabinets full of pills, they frequently see more than one physician at a time without revealing this.

Unwittingly, they are receiving the worst possible medical care because they will not accept good care. Physicians are also aware that one can die from "hysteria with metastases," because the hypochondriacal complaints finally confuse and mask a serious new illness. Because of this awareness the physician will send the patient to specialists just to "rule out" a new organic disease, and this, of course, feeds the fires of the process. It also results in a good deal of unnecessary surgery because one cannot ever be "sure" and the complaints of the patient finally acquire an insistency which leads to agreement among physicians that the only way to become "sure" is to operate. Surgery is never completely innocuous and over the long run there are after-effects such as adhesions or malfunctions which, again, feed the fire of the complaints and justify still more referrals or visits or surgery. The viciousness of this particular circle taxes the family and the physicians and results in both poor care and poorer health. The only hope of reprieve is acceptance of in-depth psychiatric care.

WHAT YOUR PHYSICIAN HAS A RIGHT TO EXPECT FROM YOU

A doctor-patient relationship is a two-way street, and you also have responsibilities. At its best, the relationship is between allies; you are partners in dealing with situations about which you have unequal information, but in which you both have rights.

Patient responsibilities include a number of niceties which you would never ignore with a friend, but are often ignored in physicians' offices. If you cannot keep an appointment, phone as far ahead as you can so that another patient can be scheduled in that time. If you must be late because the babysitter didn't come, phone the office before leaving home so that the choice is given the physician between seeing you later that day or rescheduling. You would not want a guest to come an hour late for dinner and your physician doesn't need a patient crowding the end of a day.

Bills are for paying, not for filing away in the desk because the telephone company is threatening to disconnect your phone and that seems more urgent. Granted that few if any physicians refuse to see a patient because of outstanding fees, but, nonetheless, a service has been provided which has a worth to you and the bill should be paid promptly. If you cannot muster the total amount at that moment, every office will listen sympathetically and allow you to pay the bill in monthly installments. The important thing is to tell them your intentions so they can plan rather than send bill after bill until they finally turn it over to a collection agency.

While some offices seem to run chronically behind schedule and patients pile up in the waiting room, most schedule realistically. No matter how smoothly an office runs, there will be emergencies which prevent your physician from seeing you promptly. You must be tolerant of this; you must not make angry, threatening noises to the staff. If you cannot wait, say so politely and make another appointment.

The key word in all of these situations is consideration. The physician is neither a servant nor a master, but rather a colleague. Any courtesy which you grant without thinking to a friend is due here as well.

THE COMMUNITY OF HEALTH CARE

The physician is not the only source of health care; the network of health services stretches far beyond the physician's office and may provide as much as 90 percent of the total care. One good example is the area of vision. You see an ophthalmologist who tells you that your child has amblyopia, a condition of muscle imbalance of the eyes which interferes with efficient focusing. If this condition is of moderate extent, surgery will not be suggested, but you will be referred to a clinic where special muscle exercises are taught and progress checked. The ophthalmologist will check the status of the condition in six months, but in the interim you will be receiving excellent and important health care continuously.

Take a more serious situation. You are a diabetic and your ophthalmologist has told you for a number of years that your retinae are deteriorating; you obviously know this because your vision is decreasing. There comes a point when you can no longer manage your job or your housekeeping or your transportation. The physician has done everything known and is powerless, but the resources of the community haven't yet been touched. Referral to a center whose entire purpose is the retraining of the blind can be made, and you will embark on an educational experience of which your physician does not know the details or the techniques, but only knows the results and the availability.

The number of paramedical universes is vast and no physician is aware of them all. The accident or stroke victim who requires months of rehabilitation deals almost entirely with physiotherapists and not with doctors; the mastectomized patient gains more ongoing help from Reach for Recovery than from her surgeon; the multiple sclerosis victim is bolstered by the MS Society and its members though her physician is supervising her medications. The examples are innumerable, but almost all of these groups help to establish a way of dealing with a new problem or to minimize difficulties with a long-standing one. In any of these areas your physician's responsibility rests with knowing which facilities relate to your problem and then referring you to the proper ones.

One other rather different community resource available in nearly every community is the Visiting Nurse Association. These groups offer a variety of nursing services, from skilled nurse to homemaker, that may provide a much needed respite for the family member responsible for a chronically ill patient. All too often physicians take for granted that if you are looking after your bedridden parent, no one but you is needed. They have never had such a responsibility and cannot conceive of the daily drain, of your need to get out of the house two or three times a week to walk in the park or go to a movie or visit a friend. If the physician does not suggest a visiting nurse, explore the idea yourself, and then ask for authorization which probably will be willingly given.

The only group whose responsibility it is to know *all* of these resources is the social service department of a hospital or community. If you are the victim of a chronic illness or the caretaker of a patient with one, it is well worth exploring with such a department some means of making the burden more tolerable.

Over the past decade a number of new categories of health practitioners have appeared, and one, the midwife, has reappeared. She is the prototype for the others, a professional taught to deal competently with normal pregnancies and to recognize those abnormalities which should be referred to a physician. Physicians' assistants, pediatric and adult nurse practitioners, while doing different tasks, have the same orientation. Well-child care, monitoring of chronic disease, treatment of minor complaints, carrying out assigned tasks which they have been specially taught to perform—these are some of the ways in which they function as physician extenders. The school nurse, the industrial nurse, the "medic" are examples which come readily to mind. Many clinics and group practices include one or more of such professionals and you should not feel that you have been cheated if you see them and not the physician. If they were not competent to deal with your problem, your physician wouldn't have given it to them. Any untoward or unusual turn of events will be immediately reported to the physician.

Other professionally trained people lay claim to curing disease and these groups should not be clumped as a lunatic fringe of medicine. Osteopaths currently have very similar training to physicians and some excellent hospitals are staffed entirely by them. They can prescribe drugs, they can operate, they are fully licensed. In communities with both osteopaths and physicians there is apt to be some snobbery on the part of the medical profession about their "inferior" colleagues, but so far as patients are concerned, osteopaths are legitimate givers of care.

Dentists and podiatrists are examples of sister professions to medicine, sharing the same principles of belief and the same methods of treatment. They limit their practice to one area of the body and in these areas have a competence far exceeding physicians. They have comfortable relationships with the medical profession and referrals flow easily both ways.

Chiropractors have a limited area of skill—the manipulation of the musculoskeletal system, where, they believe, most disease originates. Many a physician sends his patients with backaches to them after being assured that there is no underlying disease which should be treated surgically or by some other means, and many patients get a great deal of relief from pain. Nonetheless, the danger lies in the philosophic underpinnings of the profession. Medicine believes and teaches that there are multiple causes of disease and each should be treated in a particular fashion; chiropractic does not share this belief. A patient who deals first or exclusively with a chiropractor may get relief from pain for the moment, but may harbor a disease which should be treated in quite another fashion.

Beyond these groups lie a wide range of "healers," and it is not uncommon to find patients dealing both with a physician and a nonmedical healer, particularly when the culture of the patient is alien to that of the physician. In many underdeveloped countries two-system healing exists. The patient goes to the clinic in the morning and to the herbalist, witch doctor, or medicine man, in the evening; this is simply hedging the bets! In our own society the same behavior often applies. The patient, particularly if her disease is life-threatening, will follow the physician's orders scrupulously while at the same time going to revival meetings or seeking an herbalist. The wise patient discusses this with her doctor who, it is hoped, can accommodate comfortably to such a dual track once assured there is no harm involved.

Many people are intimidated by physicians and the world of illness and hospitals, and thus they forget that this territory is no different from any other. In a department store you have no hesitation in asking for directions, in pointing out inadequacies of merchandise or service. When you travel, you expect the maps to be accurate and the hotels as advertised; you assume (perhaps groundlessly) that trains and planes will be on schedule. The land of medicine should be no different. The maps should be as accurate and the directions as clear, and if you want to get from Here to There, you should follow them. No worlds are without detours or accidents or frustrations, but one need not add to the vicissitudes by ignorance or false expectations. If you ask questions and directions courteously, intelligently, and with concern, you have every right to get the best of medical care.

FURTHER READING

Belsky, Marvin S., and Leonard Gross. *How to Choose and Use Your Doctor.* New York: Fawcett World, 1976.

Freese, Arthur S. *Managing Your Doctor.* New York: Stein and Day, 1975.

Levin, Arthur. *Talk Back to Your Doctor.* New York: Doubleday & Co., Inc., 1975.

Neirenberg, Judith, and Florence Janovic. *The Hospital Experience: A Guide to Understanding and Participating in Your Own Care.* New York: Bobbs-Merrill, 1978.

REFERENCES

Koos, Earl Lomon. *The Health of Regionville.* New York: Columbia University Press, 1954.

Lennane, K. J., et al. "Alleged Psychogenic Disorders in Women—a Possible Manifestation of Sexual Prejudice." *New England Journal of Medicine* 288: (1973): 288–292.

Part Two

ENCYCLOPEDIA OF HEALTH AND MEDICAL TERMS

AA *See* ALCOHOLICS ANONYMOUS.

abdominal pain Acute pain or persistent ache in the region between the chest and the pelvis is a symptom that may be difficult to diagnose. Since the abdominal cavity contains the stomach, liver, spleen, gallbladder, kidneys, appendix, intestines, ovaries, and during pregnancy the expanding uterus, a disorder, dysfunction, or infection of any of these organs may be the source of the discomfort.

Pain that disappears within a few hours and doesn't recur may be due to indigestion. If accompanied by nausea and diarrhea and it subsides within a day or two, it may be due to a comparatively harmless virus infection of the intestinal tract.

Two possible causes of severe upper abdominal pain are the onset of a heart attack and food poisoning; both require emergency medical treatment. The formation of gallstones leading to gallbladder inflammation will produce pain ranging from mild and recurrent to acute enough to require hospitalization. A serious gallbladder which has affected the liver may produce symptoms of jaundice and hepatitis and pain that occurs only when pressure is applied to the upper right side of the abdomen.

An acute pain accompanied by a cough may be a symptom of pleurisy or pneumonia. Although these diseases cause inflammation in the chest, the pain may travel along the nerve pathway to the upper abdomen. Colitis is likely to produce abdominal cramps and attacks of diarrhea; a peptic ulcer manifests itself in a burning pain a few hours after meals. Gastritis, an inflammation of the stomach wall, may be a temporary condition caused by tension, overeating, or too much alcohol, and its characteristically severe pain may subside with a return to a normal routine. However, the chronic pains of gastritis associated with alcoholism or emotional disturbance require accurate diagnosis and systematic treatment.

Cramps in the lower abdomen sometimes occur immediately before or during the first day of menstruation, and for some women menstrual pain may spread to the back and down the leg. Among other causes of lower abdominal pain are endometriosis or endometritis (disorders of the uterus), infection of the fallopian tubes, ectopic pregnancy, and intestinal obstruction.

Persistent pain localized in the lower right part of the abdomen is a characteristic signal of the onset of appendicitis. Self-treatment of appendicitis may worsen the condition. Enemas, laxatives, heating pads, and unprescribed medicines should be avoided in favor of a call to the doctor.

abortion, induced The expulsion of a fetus through medical intervention before the twentieth week of pregnancy, well before it can live outside the uterus.

Induced (often called therapeutic) abortion is still one of the most common methods of birth control worldwide, with an estimated one pregnancy in three deliberately terminated. Since January 1973, when the U. S. Supreme Court declared the abortion laws of two states to be unconstitutional, the decision to terminate a pregnancy during its first trimester (up to 12 weeks) has been a private matter between a woman and her doctor. Abortion is now the most frequently performed operation in the United States and one of the safest. Since legalization, there has been a dramatic decline in maternal deaths associated with abortion. The mortality rate for legal abortions is 3 per 100,000; the mortality rate for illegal abortions is 50 to 150 per 100,000.

Which of the various methods currently in use is suitable in a particular case is usually determined by how far the pregnancy has proceeded, the preferences of the doctor in charge, and other individual circumstances.

A woman seeking an abortion should carefully consider the facilities available to her. If she can't afford the private services of a gynecologist, she should get professional advice about the best alternative within her means. Referral services that charge fees should be avoided. Information on abortion can be obtained from local offices of Planned Parenthood or by writing Planned Parenthood Federation of America, Inc., 810 Seventh Avenue, New York, New York 10019. The local state health department or the county medical association can often provide reliable information about free-standing clinics, clinics associated with hospitals, as well as private physicians.

Anyone about to undergo an abortion has a right to inspect the credentials and licenses of the doctors and the facilities. In addition to the required preliminary tests, the patient should have a blood test for the Rh factor. There should also be a straightforward discussion about the fee and whether it covers anesthesia, emergency treatment, and a postoperative checkup. Counseling, contraceptive information, cleanliness, and, above all, human decency should be provided by any reputable and well-run abortion center.

Many questions have arisen about the legal rights of parents and male partners as well as those of patients and doctors. The answers to these and similar questions should be available in official documents on public library shelves. *See also* "Contraception and Abortion."

abortion, spontaneous The expulsion of a dead embryo or fetus from the body of a pregnant woman; also known as miscarriage. Since many miscarriages are not recognized, it is difficult to estimate the number of pregnancies that terminate in this way. Doctors, however, estimate the figures at one in ten. Of these, most occur between the sixth and tenth week of pregnancy. At least half of the total of spontaneously aborted fetuses are abnormal in some way. The abnormalities may be caused by genetic defect, poor health of the mother, maternal infections of syphilis, medications, a serious accident, and an emotional trauma affecting hormone production. Evidence is accumulating that excessive caffeine intake in coffee and cola beverages, excessive alcohol, and heavy smoking during the early months of pregnancy may cause the type of fetal damage that leads to miscarriage. The typical symptom is vaginal bleeding with or without cramps. If the blood flow is only a matter of staining, the embryo or fetus may still be alive and miscarriage not inevitable; if it is heavy, miscarriage is probably inevitable. In either case, the doctor should be called at once. If there is a possibility of averting the miscarriage, absolute bed rest may be ordered and sedatives administered until the crisis is past. If a miscarriage does occur, the uterus should be scraped clean of all retained products of conception by dilatation and curettage (D&C). This is essential if infection is to be prevented. In most cases, any subsequent pregnancy is a normal one. Women who have experienced more than one spontaneous abortion should consult a gynecologist to attempt to determine and correct the underlying causes. *See also* "Pregnancy and Childbirth."

abscess An accumulation of pus in an area where healthy tissue has been invaded and broken down by bacteria. An abscess may form anywhere in the body that might be vulnerable to bacterial infection—around a hangnail or splinter, around an infected tooth, in the breast, in the middle ear, in the lung. Many abscesses can be cured with antibiotics, but some require surgical incision and draining.

When harmful bacteria begin to destroy tissue, blood rushes to the spot to provide the white blood cells and antibodies necessary for fighting off the infection. The resulting mixture of blood cells, bacteria, and dead tissue is called pus. Pain is caused by the inflammation of adjacent tissues and the accumulation of pus pressing against the adjoining nerves. The blood concentration causes redness.

A simple abscess beneath the skin may break through the surface, drain, and heal itself. A skin abscess should never be squeezed or cut open by an untrained person. A doctor or the emergency services of the nearest hospital must be consulted at once if the redness that surrounds an abscess begins to travel in a visible line towards a gland.

abuse *See* "Rape and Spouse Abuse"

Achromycin Brand name of one of the tetracycline group of antibiotics.

acidity and alkalinity Acids and alkalies (alkalies are also called bases) are produced by the body for various metabolic purposes. For example, the stomach produces hydrochloric acid which is essential in protein digestion; the kidneys produce the alkali ammonia to neutralize body chemistry. An upset in the acid-base balance of the body may produce symptoms that require medical attention. Seemingly harmless medication is sometimes responsible for a serious imbalance. Small amounts of the alkali sodium bicarbonate (bicarbonate of soda, baking soda) can remedy mild hyperacidity of the stomach, but an overdose can cause metabolic alkalosis. The overuse of diuretics as a way of losing weight may result in excessive loss of acids through the urine. An overdose of aspirin may cause salicylate (acid) poisoning. The balance may also be disturbed by conditions of the body such as kidney malfunction or loss of essential chemicals due to diarrhea.

Like most body tissues, the lining of the vagina is normally acid. It becomes alkaline at the time of ovulation in order to keep the alkaline sperm alive. In cases of infertility caused by an invariable acid environment of the vagina, chemicals are prescribed to produce vaginal alkalinity.

acne A skin disorder occurring mainly in association with the hormonal changes of adolescence. The increased amounts of androgen produced by both the male and female sex glands stimulate the sebaceous (oil) glands of the hair follicles to produce an increased amount of the fatty substance called *sebum* which is normally discharged through the pores to lubricate the skin. The overproduction of sebum results in oily skin. The characteristic pimples, pustules, and blackheads of acne are formed when the pores become plugged by the sebum that has backed up, mixed with the skin pigments, and leaked into surrounding areas.

Acne is not caused by junk food or faulty hygiene; the chief cause is the onset of puberty combined with the hereditary factors that govern the oiliness of the skin. The condition may be controlled—not cured—by keeping the skin clean and avoiding any particular food that makes it flare up. Mild cases of acne usually clear up by themselves. Emotional upsets, the onset of the menstrual period, and humid weather often cause the problem to worsen. Vitamin A acid cream (resorcinol), sun lamp treatments, and tetracycline pills may be beneficial. Current experiments indicate that a synthetic derivative of vitamin A (13 *cis* retinoic acid) administered in pill form over several months drastically reduces the amount of sebum produced in acne patients, thus controlling the chief cause of acne lesions. This treatment is still being studied for long-term effectiveness and the possibility of adverse side effects.

If acne has left scars and blemishes, a dermatologist can be consulted about the advisability of removing them by the skin-planing technique known as dermabrasion. *See* "Cosmetic Surgery."

ACTH Adrenocorticotrophic hormone, a hormone secreted by the anterior lobe of the pituitary gland; also known as adrenocorticotrophin and trophin. ACTH is carried by the blood to the adrenal glands. When it reaches the outer layer or cortex of these glands, the adrenals secrete a number of vital hormones grouped together as corticoids. Since the development of adrenal steroids which can be taken orally and have fewer side effects, ACTH is rarely used for treatment, but it is sometimes used in a diagnostic test of adrenal function.

acupuncture A therapeutic technique based on the theory that key points in the body are related to specific disorders or pain elsewhere in the body and that these conditions can be healed by stimulation at the key points by the insertion and rotation of needles. Acupuncture has been practiced for at least 5,000 years in the

Orient and is now gaining increased acceptance for certain purposes among Western doctors.

Although cures of various ailments have been reported, the most verified benefits of acupuncture have been in the field of anesthesia and analgesia. American medical teams who have witnessed major operations performed by Chinese hospitals have been impressed by the effectiveness of acupuncture as a means of controlling pain reception without inducing unconsciousness. These analgesic properties are currently being explored, with varying degrees of success, in many hospitals in the United States and Europe, especially in pain-control experiments.

Before embarking on acupuncture treatment for any disorder, it is advisable to examine the practitioner's medical credentials and legal status. State-chartered acupuncture centers in various parts of the United States will provide detailed information about their activities on request.

acute symptom A symptom of a disorder which has a sudden onset and runs a comparatively brief course such as an "acute" asthma attack as opposed to a persistent, or chronic, manifestation of a disorder. "Acute" should not be confused with "fatal."

addiction Physical dependence on a drug; adaptation of the body to the presence of a drug so that its continued use is required by the user just to feel well and to continue to function physiologically. *See* "Drugs, Alcohol, and Tobacco."

Addison's disease A rare disorder whose immediate cause is failure of the adrenal glands. It was first identified by the English physician Dr. Thomas Addison (who also identified pernicious anemia) in the mid-nineteenth century. The disease usually occurs in people in their twenties or thirties. The glandular underfunction is sometimes the result of tuberculosis. Other causes may be a tumor, hemorrhage, or any injury that interferes with hormone production. Addison's disease, once fatal, is now treated with cortisone and other forms of hormone replacement therapy in the same way that diabetes is treated with insulin.

adenoma A usually benign tumor composed of glandular tissue.

adhesion The union of two internal body surfaces that are normally separate. The term also refers to the formation of the fibrous, or scar, tissue that connects them. The scar tissue that forms around a surgical wound during the healing process may cling to adjoining areas causing them to fuse. Lung adhesions may occur after inflammation and scarring of the pleural membrane; abdominal adhesions may occur following peritonitis. Although most adhesions are painless and without consequence, they may occasionally cause an obstruction or malfunction that requires surgical correction. The incidence of postoperative adhesions has dramatically diminished as a result of early ambulation after surgery.

adoption Adoption laws differ from state to state, and only an accredited agency can advise you about the circumstances and qualifications that govern a legal adoption in your state. Persons eager to offer a child warmth and acceptance into their family are always preferred to those who talk only about privileges and luxuries. Agencies do not approve of too great an age disparity—no more than forty years —between parents and child.

As soon as a congenial pairing has been worked out, the adoption must be legalized by the courts. This can take six months to a year, and during this "trial period" the agency provides help and advice to the family. During all court proceedings, adoptive parents should have the counsel of a reputable lawyer so that future legal complications will be avoided.

adrenal glands   A pair of glands situated at the upper part of the kidneys. The adrenals, like other components of the endocrine system, secrete hormones into the bloodstream for transportation to other parts of the body. Each adrenal consists of two separate glands that manufacture different classes of hormones: the cortex, or outer shell, secretes adrenocorticosteroids or corticoids for continuous regulation of bodily processes such as fluid and salt balance, protein metabolism, antibody formation, and the repair of damaged tissue; the medulla, or inner core, secretes epinephrine (adrenalin) and norepinephrine which are released in stress situations, mobilizing the body to deal with combat or flight at maximum efficiency.

adrenalin   One of the hormones produced by the medulla or inner core of the adrenal glands; also known as epinephrine. This hormone maximizes the body's physiologic response to stress. The large quantities of stress-secreted adrenalin result in increased heart rate and blood pressure. By transforming the glycogen in the liver into glucose, the adrenalin also provides the muscles with a quick source of energy so that they can perform effectively without suffering fatigue. Adrenalin dilates the pupils of the eyes for more effective vision and expands the bronchial tubes for more effective respiration. When the body sustains a wound, adrenalin increases the clotting capacity of the blood.

Adrenalin was originally extracted from animal glands, but it is now produced synthetically and is widely prescribed as an emergency medication in heart arrest, acute asthma and other allergy attacks, shock, and severe bleeding.

afterbirth   *See* PLACENTA.

air pollution   *See* POLLUTION.

air sickness   *See* MOTION SICKNESS.

Al-Anon   An organization which, though separate from Alcoholics Anonymous, provides the same kind of help, support, and therapy for the family of the alcoholic that AA provides for the alcoholic. Alcoholism is considered a family disease because the alcoholic affects the mental and physical health of other members and their response in turn affects the alcoholic.

A person who suspects that any member of the household, including teenage children, is an alcoholic may find that going to Al-Anon meetings is an effective first step toward recognizing the illness for what it is and beginning to deal with it in a realistic way.

Alateen, a subsidiary of Al-Anon, is a fellowship for the adolescent children of alcoholics. Further information about both organizations is available by writing to Al-Anon Family

Group Headquarters, P.O. Box 182, Madison Square Station, New York, NY 10010.

alcohol Any of a group of related chemical compounds derived from hydrocarbons. Ethyl alcohol, also called ethanol or grain alcohol, is the intoxicating ingredient of fermented and distilled beverages. Methyl alcohol, also known as wood alcohol or methanol, is widely used in industry as a solvent and a fuel. Taken internally, it is a poison that can lead to blindness and death. Rubbing alcohol, used on the skin as a cooling agent or disinfectant, may be ethyl alcohol made unfit for consumption by the addition of chemicals known as denaturants (denatured alcohol) or it may be another compound called isopropyl alcohol.

alcoholic beverages Drinks that contain ethyl alcohol, the substance that results naturally from the fermentation of carbohydrates (sugars, such as those in grape mash, molasses, and apples, or starches, such as those in wheat, rice, barley, and other grains). Hard cider, beer, and ale contain about 3 to 5 percent alcohol; table wines about 10 percent; fortified wines like sherry about 20 percent. Beverages of higher alcoholic content, such as vodka, bourbon, and brandy, are called liquors or "hard" liquors and are produced by distilling the alcohol from the fermented mash. Liqueurs like Benedictine or Cointreau may contain as much as 35 percent alcohol, and whiskey and rum as much as 50 percent. The concentration of alcohol in a beverage is usually given in terms of "proof." Half of the proof number is the percentage of alcohol by volume; thus a 90-proof

vodka is 45 percent alcohol, with the remainder made up of water, flavoring, and other ingredients. In assessing alcohol intake, it should be kept in mind that a 12-ounce can of beer contains four-fifths as much alcohol as a 1½-ounce jigger of 80-proof whiskey, 6 ounces of wine equals 1½ ounces of vodka, and 6 ounces of sherry contains almost twice as much alcohol as a 1½-ounce jigger of whiskey.

Alcohol is metabolized to produce a substance that provides high energy, but no other nutritional value. It enters the bloodstream very quickly, and unless it is consumed very slowly and in combination with food, the alcoholic content of the blood rises rapidly. It is a depressant and sedative that has a marked effect on the central nervous system. Intoxication occurs when the alcohol concentration in the blood is about $\frac{1}{10}$ of 1 percent; a concentration of twice that amount results in marked intoxication; and at $\frac{4}{10}$ of 1 percent the drinker usually passes out.

It is estimated that about 80 million Americans drink alcoholic beverages and about 10 percent of these suffer from alcoholism. However, in terms of health and safety, all people who drink at all should observe certain rules and precautions. Anyone with chronic gastrointestinal disorders shouldn't drink unless allowed to do so on special occasions by their doctors. Anyone taking tranquilizers, antidepressants, or barbiturates should observe *to the letter* the doctor's and pharmacist's instructions about alcoholic intake. A hostess should never offer a last drink "for the road" to the guest who is about to drive a car. Anyone on a weight reduction diet should cut down on or eliminate alcohol; a glass of whiskey contains 120 calories with no nutritional value, and alcoholic beverages simultaneously increase the appetite and weaken the will to diet. Alcohol in any form generally should not be given as a first aid measure or as emergency treatment unless a doctor has issued the instruction. See "Drugs, Alcohol, and Tobacco."

Alcoholics Anonymous A worldwide community resource for dealing with the problem of alcoholism. AA is a fellowship of men and women who help each other stay sober and who share their recovery experience freely with all those who have the desire to stop drinking. It is an integral part of the tradition that no member may violate another member's anonymity. Although its members may cooperate with other organizations that help alcoholics, AA is not affiliated with any sect, denomination, political group, or institution.

Membership is estimated at about 1 million people. Since 1971 one out of every three new members is a woman. Approximately 28,000 local groups meet in 92 different countries. Meetings are held once or twice a week, and each group is self-supporting through voluntary contributions.

The telephone directory of most towns and cities contains an AA listing. Where such information is not available, write to General Service Office, P.O. Box 459, Grand Central Station, New York, NY 10017. This name, rather than any AA designation, will appear on the wrapper containing the requested material.

alcoholism Compulsive drinking, now recognized as a disease—not a moral disorder—by the American Medical Association, the U.S. Public Health Service, and the World Health Organization. The National Council on Alcoholism estimates that there are at least 5 million women alcoholics in the United States. Experts agree that the qualitative difference between the "heavy" or "hard" drinkers and alcoholics is that the former, unlike alcoholics, can control their drinking if and when they choose to. Another way of expressing the difference is: social and heavy drinkers like alcohol but can do without it; alcoholics need alcohol, and their addiction becomes progressively worse.

The National Council has reported a number of significant facts in regard to women alcoholics. Regardless of their life style, women drink primarily in relation to life crises and to relieve loneliness, inferiority feelings, and conflicts about their sex role. Women alcoholics tend to become involved with other drugs such as tranquilizers. Just as many teenage females drink as teenage males. Maternal alcoholism can harm fetal development and cause addiction to alcohol in the newborn. The husband and children of a woman alcoholic are more likely to "protect" her (and themselves) from public exposure than to encourage her to seek help. The woman alcoholic is abandoned by her husband in nine out of ten cases, whereas the male alcoholic is abandoned by his wife in only one out of ten.

Although many theories have been advanced for the cause of alcoholism, it is now generally agreed that there is no single explanation and that the disorder is usually the result of a combination of physical, psychological, and circumstantial factors. Current research also indicates that once a person develops an addiction to alcohol, the body chemistry becomes different from that of a nonalcoholic, and that even though the disease can be treated, the alcoholic can never return to "normal" drinking.

Even though alcoholism, like peptic ulcers, may be evidence of psychological stress, it must be understood that, also like peptic ulcers, alcoholism itself can be fatal. Fortunately, many of the physical effects of alcoholism—on the liver, heart, and kidneys and on resistance to infection —are reversible through sobriety and rehabilitation therapy.

Medical care may involve the doctor's supervision of diet, vitamins, and, in some cases, drugs to ease the transition to total abstention. Psychotherapy, especially in groups whose members are mutually supportive, helps the alcoholic face problems and deal with them realistically. Membership in AA is recommended by most specialists, and since the role of the family is extremely important in the treatment of the alcoholic, participation in groups such as Al-Anon can be very helpful.

Because alcoholism is now recognized as one of this country's major public health problems, the U.S. Department of Health and Human Services has established the National Institute on Alcohol Abuse and Alcoholism. Information on all aspects of the disease, as well as state-by-state listings of most public and private counseling and treatment facilities may be obtained by writing to the Institute's National Clearing House for Alcohol Information, P.O. Box 2345, Rockville, Maryland 20852. *See also* "Drugs, Alcohol, and Tobacco."

allergy Hypersensitivity to a substance such as food, pollen, animal dander, or medicine or to a climatic condition such as sunshine or low temperature which in similar amounts is harmless to most people. Literally the word means an altered capacity to react. It is known that allergy can occur anywhere in the body: on the skin, in the eyes, in the lungs, and so on. The offending substance contains an allergen that signals the body of the allergic person to manufacture antibodies as a defense. In this process chemicals known as histamines are released into the bloodstream, and these chemicals are the immediate cause of the allergic symptoms. Histamine can produce two main effects. First, by increasing the permeability of the small blood vessels, it causes the fluid portion of the blood or serum to leak into the tissues. Second, it causes spasm of particular muscles, especially in the bronchial tubes. The first condition produces swelling, blisters, and irritation of some tissues such as the eyes, nose, and skin; the second produces labored breathing and asthmatic episodes. In extreme cases hypersensitivity to penicillin or nonhuman antitoxin serum or to the venom in an insect sting produces sudden shock (anaphylactic reaction) which can be fatal.

Most allergies are treated by identifying the offending substance and avoiding it. This is relatively simple in the case of a cosmetic that causes a rash or a cantaloupe that brings on diarrhea or a long-haired pet that produces an asthma attack. In many instances, however, identification can be extremely difficult. Specialists have evolved various scratch tests and patch tests that are painless, time-consuming, and not always helpful.

For cases in which avoidance is not possible and relief from symptoms is necessary there are desensitizing treatments that can build up a resistance to the allergen once it is identified. Medicines such as antihistamines, cortisone, ephedrine, and aminophylline, alone or in combination, may be effective in controlling the symptoms and reducing discomfort. Self-medication with any of these drugs, prior to identifying the problem, is always inadvisable. Because emotions play a prominent part in many allergies, some reactions, especially asthmatic attacks, may be eliminated by psychotherapy.

alveoli The smallest air sacs of the lungs. Each alveolus is a microscopic structure covered by a capillary wall through which oxygen in the air and carbon dioxide in the blood are exchanged in the respiratory process. The hundreds of millions of alveoli form grapelike clusters. When their function is disordered by bronchitis, pneumonia, or a cardiocirculatory attack associated with heart failure, treatment is essential.

AMA *See* AMERICAN MEDICAL ASSOCIATION.

amenorrhea The absence of the menstrual flow. Primary amenorrhea is the failure of menstrual periods to begin by the age of 18. The cause is usually endocrine (glandular) in nature. Secondary amenorrhea is the cessation of menstrual periods after they have begun. It occurs normally during pregnancy, nursing, and following the menopause. When none of these circumstances accounts for the interruption of menstruation, it may be a symptom of malnutrition, alcoholism, glandular disturbance, or tumors. It may also be psychogenic in

origin and related to a severe emotional disturbance, to a prolonged psychotic episode, or to an emotional condition such as anorexia nervosa (obsessional refusal to eat resulting in extreme weight loss, usually occurring in young women). When there is no obvious explanation for either primary or secondary amenorrhea, a doctor should be consulted.

American Medical Association (AMA) A professional organization made up of county and state units, with approximately 210,000 members—about 75 percent of all practicing physicians. It was founded in 1847 with the purpose of improving medical education and eliminating quackery. Together with the American College of Surgeons and the American Hospital Association, it accredits hospitals, inspects medical schools, and approves residency and intern-training programs.

The AMA publishes the American Medical Directory which lists the professional credentials of all licensed physicians, including nonmembers. The directory, organized by states, is usually available in the reference collection of local libraries.

In recent decades, the AMA has been increasingly criticized for its outspoken opposition to practically all government-initiated public health programs as well as to the extension of social security benefits, health insurance plans, and group medical practice.

amnesia Loss of memory. Amnesia may be partial or extensive, temporary or permanent. With total amnesia (very rare), practically all mental functions would necessarily cease. Memory loss may result from brain damage caused by injury, tumor, arteriosclerosis, stroke, or alcoholism. It may also be caused by the psychological mechanism of repression. Amnesia following an accident or acute emotional shock may cause the victim to black out and forget the event itself, but remember all details leading up to it. When serious memory lapses due to an overriding anxiety neurosis interfere with normal functioning, some form of psychotherapy may be helpful. Except for the amnesia associated with senility, memory loss that wipes out past identity occurs more frequently in fiction than in fact.

amniocentesis A diagnostic procedure in which a small amount of the amniotic fluid that surrounds the fetus during pregnancy is withdrawn and examined to assess genetic and other disorders. The technique, developed in the 1960s, is accurate and relatively safe and requires only a local anesthetic. A needle similar to a hypodermic needle is inserted through the abdomen into the womb. The extracted fluid contains cells shed by the fetus, and when these cells are grown in laboratory cultures, it is possible to detect fetal chromosomal abnormalities.

Amniocentesis may be performed for a variety of reasons. If either parent is known to have a transmissible defect for certain diseases, amniocentesis can determine if that defect has been transmitted to the fetus. When a mother is 35 years of age or over and therefore is at increased risk of having a child with Down's syndrome (trisomy 21 or mongolism), amniocentesis can determine if the fetus is normal. It is also done to assess Rh complications and fetal maturity. To protect both fetus and mother, amniocentesis should be done by medically accredited specialists. *See* "Pregnancy and Childbirth."

amnion The tough-walled membrane that forms the protective sac in which the embryo is contained within the uterus during pregnancy. The amnion and its contents (amniotic fluid) are commonly known as the bag of waters. During labor contractions the bag generally breaks and the fluid leaks out. When the amnion remains intact and envelops the head of the newborn baby, it is known as a caul. It then has to be broken by the person delivering the baby. A caul was once regarded as an indication of great good fortune for the offspring.

amphetamine A category of drugs, including Benzedrine, Dexedrine, and Methedrine, which act as stimulants to the central nervous system. Formerly prescribed somewhat indiscriminately as antidepressants and aids in overcoming obesity, the widespread abuse of amphetamines in the form of "pep" pills and diet pills, the increased tolerance developed by some users, and the freak aftereffects experienced by athletes, dancers, students, and others who seek to perform at the peak of their powers through amphetamine intake have led to a greater control over the use and availability of these drugs. Their therapeutic use should be limited to cases of narcolepsy and to counteracting the effects of an overdose of sedatives. *See also* "Drugs, Alcohol, and Tobacco."

ampicillin Generic name of one of the forms of penicillin.

analgesic Substance that temporarily reduces or eliminates the sensation of pain without producing unconsciousness. The most common over-the-counter analgesics are aspirin and acetaminophen (such as Tylenol). Narcotic analgesics derived from opium, such as codeine and morphine, as well as similar synthetic substances should be prescribed with caution since they are habit-forming. Analgesia may be produced by means other than drugs such as hypnosis and acupuncture. *See* ANESTHESIA.

analysis *See* PSYCHOANALYSIS.

androgens The male sex hormones that determine the secondary sex characteristics of men. Although the two chief androgens, testosterone and androsterone, are manufactured mainly by the male testes, they are also produced to a lesser extent by the adrenal glands of both sexes and by the female ovaries. In males they are responsible for the deepening of the voice and the development of the beard at puberty, and they account in part for the greater size and muscular development of men since they also stimulate the growth of muscles and bones. An overproduction of androgen in women accounts for the presence of these essentially male characteristics. The administration of androgens in postmenopausal anticancer therapy is an extremely complex matter and should be approached warily by both doctor and patient. The hormones are used in replacement therapy for men suffering from testicular malfunction.

androgynous Having both male and female sex characteristics. True androgyny is extremely rare and can be corrected in part by a combination of hormone therapy and surgery.

anemia A condition in which there is a deficiency in the number of red blood cells, hemoglobin, or the total amount of blood. Anemia, whether acute or chronic, is not a disease in itself, but rather the result of an underlying disorder: chronic malnutrition, industrial poisoning, bone marrow disease, heavy bleeding, intestinal parasites, kidney disease, or a defect in the body's ability to absorb iron. Since treatment varies according to the cause, accurate diagnosis is extremely important. The symptoms of a mild deficiency may be vague: listlessness, general lack of vitality, and fatigue following little effort. When the condition is more severe, the inability of the anemic blood to supply oxygen to body tissues can result in shortness of breath, rapid pulse, and the sensation that the heart is work-

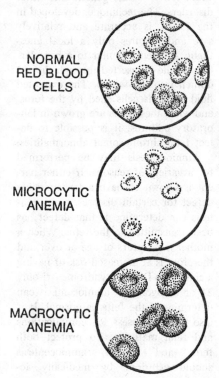

NORMAL
RED BLOOD
CELLS

MICROCYTIC
ANEMIA

MACROCYTIC
ANEMIA

ing harder or faster. Visible indications are the paleness of the lining of the eyelids and of the area under the fingernails. When the blood has sufficient hemoglobin, these parts of the body are a healthy pink.

Anemia should never be self-diagnosed for the purpose of self-treatment with tonics, vitamins, pills, or herbal remedies. It is a specific condition which can be diagnosed accurately only by laboratory analysis of blood samples. In these tests the number, size, color, and shape of the red blood cells are determined, and the amount of hemoglobin in the sample is measured. When anemia is clearly present, other tests may follow. A sample of bone marrow may be taken in order to find out whether defective cells are produced at the source. Other laboratory procedures may be used to establish the fragility of the cells. If there is suspicion of bleeding within the body, usually within the gastrointestinal tract, additional tests may be essential.

There are several types of anemia. The most common form, deficiency anemia, is a deficiency of iron essential for the body's manufacture of hemoglobin. It may result from insufficient iron in the diet or from chronic blood loss from excessive menstrual flow or internal bleeding due to an ulcer or some other gastrointestinal disorder. When diet deficiency is the cause, foods high in iron content as well as supplementary medicine containing iron will correct the anemia. When chronic bleeding is involved, the basic cause must be dealt with if the anemia is to be corrected.

Pernicious anemia, also known as Addison's anemia, is a serious disease characterized by a breakdown in the mechanism of red blood cell formation, usually traceable to a deficiency

of vitamin B_{12}. In addition to the symptoms of deficiency anemia, this disorder produces the following symptoms: the skin becomes pale yellow, the tongue is bright red and sore, and a resulting malfunction in the nervous system may produce a chronic tingling sensation in the fingers and toes. The disease is most often a result of the absence in the body of the substance necessary for the absorption of vitamin B_{12}. Therapeutic amounts of the vitamin with or without folic acid (another B complex vitamin) are administered for a lifetime. The disease may also result from a dietary deficiency of vitamin B_{12}, although this is rare because the amount required by the body is easily obtained from small amounts of animal products. It may sometimes occur among the strictest vegetarians unless their diet is supplemented by the vitamin in capsule form.

Hemolytic anemia results from the destruction of red blood cells, which may occur because of Rh incompatibility, mismatched blood transfusions, industrial poisons, or hypersensitivity to certain chemicals and medicines. This type of anemia may also accompany other diseases, especially certain types of cancer. Severe cases require immediate hospitalization for determination of the underlying cause and suitable treatment, including blood transfusions.

Aplastic anemia is caused by a disease of the bone marrow, the part of the body where red blood cells are manufactured. While some cases result from bone marrow cancer, others follow excessive radiation exposure or contact with a long list of substances that have the same destructive effect (the chemicals in certain insecticides, antibiotics, medicines containing bismuth and other heavy metals). In addition to the usual symptoms of anemia, this type results in dark discolorations of the skin and, in extreme cases, bleeding from the nose and mouth. Hospitalization is mandatory, with prompt treatment of blood transfusions and in some cases cortisone injections.

Hemoglobinopathies are forms of anemia of genetic origin. Included in this category are sickle cell anemia, thalassemia (Cooley's anemia), and hemoglobin C disease. When such a congenital trait is known to exist, genetic counseling is advised before pregnancy.

anesthesia Partial or total loss of sensation or feelings. Analgesia, one category of anesthesia, refers specifically to loss of sensation of pain. The great advances in surgery have gone hand in hand with modern methods of anesthesia and the discovery of a variety of anesthetics (substances capable of producing anesthesia). Until the nineteenth century opium and alcohol were the only available painkillers. Ether, nitrous oxide (called "laughing gas" because it produces a kind of euphoria), and chloroform were all discovered in the 1840s, and since that time many more effective and less dangerous methods have been perfected. The study of these substances and their application is known as anesthesiology. An anesthesiologist is a doctor who specializes in this branch of medical science. An anesthetist is not a doctor, but usually a nurse with advanced training.

The following are among the procedures that produce anesthesia and analgesia. They may be used separately or in combination. *Intravenous injection* of sleep-producing drugs such as sodium pentothal produces light an-

esthesia. The injection of light anesthetics often precedes the use of longer lasting methods when major surgery is involved. *Inhalation* of gases such as nitrous oxide, cyclopropane, or Halothane is used to anesthetize the whole body. *Spinal injection* of one of the cocaine derivatives does not produce sleep, but deadens the nerves in a specific part of the body. *Rectal administration* by a light enema of paraldehyde, a sleep-inducing drug that is quickly absorbed by the body, is used for patients who are especially difficult to deal with, such as alcoholics, psychotics, or those who are extremely apprehensive. More limited procedures are *local freezing, nerve block,* such as the injection of procaine for dental surgery, and *surface or topical analgesia,* such as the use of cocaine-related drugs for eye surgery. *Hypnosis* is being used successfully in situations such as childbirth and pediatric dentistry. *Acupuncture* is being evaluated scientifically for its analgesic applications.

aneurysm An abnormal widening or distension of an artery or vein, forming a sac which is filled with blood. Aneurysms may be congenitally caused by a deficiency in the vessel walls, or they may be acquired through injury or disease, especially atherosclerosis and the late stages of syphilis. When the sac wall is composed of one or more intact layers of the blood vessel tissue, it is known as a true aneurysm; when the whole vessel has given way and the blood is contained by the surrounding fibrous tissues, the condition is known as false aneurysm.

Both kinds may exist for many years without any symptoms and may be detected only as a result of an

X-ray taken for some other reason. Aneurysms in the arteries of the brain or in the aorta may make themselves known by pressure in the surrounding area, for example on the optic nerve or on an organ in the chest.

When the swelling is detected in a small artery or vein, the vessel can be tied off so that the flow of blood is redirected to healthier channels. The repair of larger vessels has recently been made possible by organ banks that provide vascular replacements, both plastic and those available from smaller mammals. Rupture of an aneurysm requires emergency hospitalization and treatment.

angina pectoris Literally, pain in the chest, and the signal of an interference (generally reversible) with the supply of oxygen to the heart muscle. The pain is rarely confused with any other; it characteristically produces a feeling of tightness and suffocation beginning under the left side of the breastbone and sometimes spreading to the neck, throat, and down the left arm. Angina pectoris is more common among men than women, but women, especially in their late fifties and sixties, may suffer from the condition, especially if they smoke or are overweight, hypertensive, or diabetic.

The onset of an angina attack is likely to follow strenuous exercise, exposure to cold and wind, eating and digesting a heavy meal, or a strong emotional experience such as a quarrel or a frightening dream. In such circumstances the heart works harder and pumps faster and therefore needs an extra supply of blood and oxygen. When circulation is impaired in any way, especially by atherosclerosis, the blood supply does not reach the heart muscle cells quickly enough. The resulting lack of oxygen is the immediate cause of the pain.

An angina attack is usually brief and subsides upon resting. Nitroglycerine in the form of quickly dissolving tablets is an effective medication available by prescription. The nitroglycerine promptly dilates the smaller coronary vessels, thus increasing the supply of blood and oxygen to the heart. Since angina pectoris is a signal that the heart is under stress, the underlying causes should be explored and corrected or minimized wherever possible.

angiography A diagnostic procedure in which radiopaque substances are injected into the blood vessels so that any abnormalities or displacements are visible on an X-ray film. This type of radiological picture is called an angiogram.

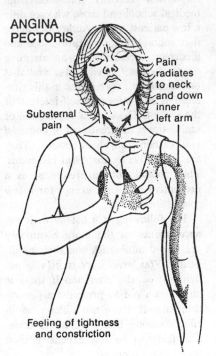

ANGINA PECTORIS

Pain radiates to neck and down inner left arm

Substernal pain

Feeling of tightness and constriction

animal bites Any animal bite, even by a family pet, that breaks the surface of the skin requires attention. It should be washed at once with soap under running water. Medical attention should be sought for deep or severe bites and for any bite by a wild animal. Although rabies and tetanus are comparatively rare, they should never be excluded. Not only dogs and cats, but squirrels, horses, mice, bats, foxes, and other warm-blooded animals are capable of spreading diseases through bites. If the offending animal can be caught, it should not be killed, but rather turned over to a veterinarian or a health authority. *See* RABIES.

ankles, swollen The tissues around the ankle may swell for various reasons: heart disease, kidney or liver malfunction, and pregnancy. Women who spend lots of time on their feet, such as salespeople, artists, waitresses, housewives, are especially susceptible to this complaint in hot weather, not because of disease but because of insufficient venous return. When the puffy condition persists in spite of sitting with the feet extended and raised or a warm bath before bedtime, a doctor should be consulted.

Antabuse Brand name of the drug disulfiram developed in Denmark for the treatment of alcoholism. Antabuse affects the metabolism of alcohol so that the patient becomes so sick after drinking that he or she may stop taking alcohol. A responsible doctor does not use Antabuse alone in treating alcoholism. At best it is an emergency measure that should be combined with more basic and supportive therapy.

antacid A substance that relieves acidity. *See* ACIDITY and ALKALINITY.

antibiotic A chemical substance produced during the growth of various fungi and bacteria that has the capacity to kill or inhibit the growth of other bacteria or fungi. Since the discovery of penicillin in 1929 and its mass application during World War II, literally thousands of antibiotic substances have been isolated and studied. As disease-causing bacteria develop strains that are resistant to a particular antibiotic, new drugs are developed to counteract the adaptation.

While antibiotics have saved many lives, there is increasing concern about their indiscriminate prescription by doctors who rely on drug advertising rather than the more objective information in scientific journals. Surveys indicate that doctors most up-to-date about how to prescribe antibiotics are those most recently graduated from medical school and those who see only a few patients a day. Authorities agree that antibiotics are overprescribed and incorrectly prescribed to an alarming degree in the United States and that one of the best correctives to this situation is the informed self-interest of the patient. The correct application of antibiotics is the treatment of *bacterial* and certain fungal infections. They are ineffective against viral infections. They should not be prescribed as a preventive medicine, except for a few special conditions.

The following is a list by their generic names of the more commonly prescribed antibiotics and their application. You have every right as a patient to ask the physician if there is any reason not to prescribe a generic drug and if there are differences in effects among brands. Generic drugs are likely to be less expensive than brand-name products.

The penicillin group of antibiotics includes penicillin G potassium, penicillin V, and ampicillin. The first two drugs are both most frequently prescribed for streptococcus infections of the ear and throat, sinus infections, gonorrhea, syphilis, pneumococcal pneumonia. Ampicillin is prescribed for middle ear and urinary infections. Allergic reactions to penicillin may range from a mild rash, diarrhea, or nausea to severe shock. Any history of adverse reactions to penicillin in any form should be pointed out to a doctor, especially in an emergency situation involving a possible injection.

The tetracycline group includes tetracycline HCL (hydrochloride), chlortetracycline, oxytetracycline, and some new drugs in the same family. These are commonly prescribed under various brand names for bronchitis, acne, pneumonia, and, in cases of penicillin allergy, for syphilis and gonorrhea.

Erythromycin is an antibiotic developed for those patients who are allergic to penicillin or who should not be given tetracycline because of pregnancy or possible side effects on bone development.

Chloramphenicol is sold under the brand name of Chloromycetin. It should be prescribed only for typhoid fever and a few other special situations since it has been found in some cases to interfere with the production of blood cells in the bone marrow.

antibody A component of the immune system produced by cells called plasmocytes in the presence of an antigen (any substance foreign to the body) to destroy or neutralize that antigen; a specific antibody is produced for each antigen. This specificity is the basis of immunization by vaccination; the introduction of a controlled

ANTIBODIES

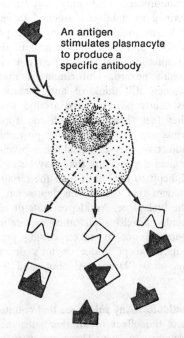

An antigen stimulates plasmacyte to produce a specific antibody

amount or variety of a disease-producing organism stimulates the plasmacytes to develop the antibodies necessary to fight the organism in advance of an uncontrolled invasion of the body. In addition to warding off disease and controlling infection, antibody activity also results in the rejection of grafts, transplants, and prostheses and in Rh disease in which Rh negative maternal antibodies destroy Rh positive fetal blood cells.

antidepressant A class of mood-changing drugs which counteract some of the immobilizing effects of depressive illness. While antidepressants do not cure mental illness, they have largely replaced electroshock therapy as a means of helping certain withdrawn or hysterical patients benefit from psychotherapy. In cases of agitated depression or hysteria antidepressants may be combined with tranquilizers. They may also be prescribed to stabilize a suicidal patient.

These medications were once prescribed and used with a lack of discrimination that constituted a major health hazard. Unfortunately, many women still think of antidepressants as handy pills to have around when they feel "low." Although antidepressants are not known to be physically addictive, they can establish a psychological dependency that may be more difficult to deal with than the circumstances that caused the depression in the first place. Antidepressants of any kind—as well as all other medication —should not be taken during pregnancy except under doctor's orders. *See also* "Drugs, Alcohol, and Tobacco."

antidote Any substance that counteracts the effect of another substance, usually a poison. There are very few specific antidotes, and since ridding the body of a poison is a complicated matter, a local poison control center should be consulted immediately for emergency care.

antigen Any substance that stimulates the production of antibodies. Antigens are present in bacterial toxins, pollens, immunizing agents, blood, and other substances.

antihistamine Any of various drugs that minimize the discomfort of hay fever, hives, and other allergic reactions caused by the body's release of chemicals known as histamines. Depending on the nature of the allergy, antihistamines may be prescribed in the form of drops for the nose or eyes, a salve or topical ointment to be used on the skin, or pills to be taken orally. They may also be an effective remedy for motion sickness. Whether antihistamines are helpful in relieving the symptoms of a cold is debatable. Many researchers feel that such relief is the result of a placebo effect or is an indication that an allergic situation coexists with the cold.

Continuous and indiscriminate use of these drugs may have unpleasant effects and should be avoided. Since antihistamines produce drowsiness, caution is advisable while driving a car and when alertness at a job or at household tasks is essential for proper functioning and well-being. They should not be used by pregnant women for morning sickness. Nonprescription "daytime sedatives," widely advertised for their effectiveness in diminishing tension and anxiety, actually contain little more than an antihistamine that causes drowsiness and perhaps serious adverse consequences.

antiperspirant A mixture of chemicals that diminish the amount of perspiration that reaches the skin and reduce the rate of growth of the odor-creating bacteria. (Deodorants only reduce the speed with which bacteria multiply). Antiperspirants are considered drugs and their ingredients must be listed on their containers. They may contain irritants to the skin so it may be necessary to experiment with different brands to find one that does not produce a rash. Those packaged in spray cans contain propellants harmful to the lungs and should be rejected in favor of a cream or roll-on product.

antiseptic A substance that inhibits or slows down the growth of microorganisms; in more recent usage the term conveys the meaning of bactericide, that is, a substance that kills bacteria. Disinfectants are included under the general heading of antiseptics, although they are too strong to be applied to body tissues and are meant to make surfaces germ-free in kitchens, bathrooms, and sickrooms. The English surgeon Joseph Lister's application of the principle of antisepsis to surgery was one of the major medical accomplishments of the nineteenth century, eliminating a significant number of fatalities caused by infection.

antitoxin A type of antibody that neutralizes the specific toxin released by a disease-causing agent. Antitoxins may be manufactured by the body's immune system or they may be injected as a defense against diseases such as tetanus, diphtheria, or botulism.

anus The opening at the end of the alimentary canal (at the end of the rectum, which is the last segment of the large intestine). The action of the anus in bowel evacuation is controlled by valves of two ringlike voluntary muscles known as anal sphincters.

anxiety A feeling of threat or danger in which the threat cannot be clearly identified; a response to stress in which the condition creating stress is not fully known. *See* "Your Mind and Feelings."

aorta The largest and most important artery, carrying blood from the heart to be distributed throughout the body. The aorta begins at the left ventricle of the heart, curves over and downward into the chest, and then penetrates the diaphragm for entry into the abdomen where it ends opposite the fourth lumbar vertebra. The branches of the aorta supply arterial blood to all parts of the body.

aphasia Loss of speech (motor aphasia) or the ability to comprehend speech (sensory aphasia). Aphasia is usually the result of damage by disease or injury to those parts of the brain concerned with language formulation rather than comprehension. Since brain function rather than mind function (the formulation of thoughts and ideas) is involved, rehabilitation of speech can be accomplished in many instances, especially if the patient, the therapist, and the family are optimistic and persistent. When aphasia occurs as a form of hysteria, psychotherapeutic techniques, including hypnotism, can be effective in restoring the ability to speak.

aphrodisiac A substance that purportedly increases sexual desire and potency. Aphrodisiacs may be celebrated in song, story, overheated imaginations, and "health food" literature, but scientific investigation has yet to validate the claims of any of them. Where sexual incapacity exists, a good physician should be consulted for treatment.

apoplexy *See* STROKE.

appendicitis Inflammation of the appendix, the 3- to 6-inch appendage or sac that lies in the lower right portion of the abdominal cavity at the junction of the small and large intestine. Appendicitis accounts for at least half the abdominal emergencies that occur between the ages of 10 and 30. The critical aspect of an attack of acute appendicitis is that the inflammation may result in a rupture leading to peritonitis (infection of the abdominal lining).

Appendicitis is not caused by swallowing fruit pits or nut shells. However, hard bits of matter in food being digested, intestinal worms, or some undetermined element may plug up the tubelike appendix, hindering normal drainage and increasing the likelihood of bacterial infection. If the body's defenses do not stop the multiplication of colon bacilli and streptococci, inflammation results, causing three main symptoms: pain in the lower right side, nausea or vomiting, and fever. If one or all of these symptoms persist, see a doctor promptly.

If they become acute and no doctor is available, call an ambulance to take you to the nearest hospital's emergency room. Under no circumstances should anything be taken by mouth without professional instructions: no food, no fluid, no medicines, and especially *no laxative or cathartic.* Self-treatment with an enema or a hot-water bottle is equally ill-advised.

APPENDICITIS

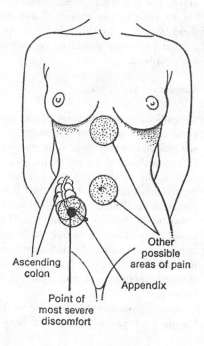

Ascending colon

Point of most severe discomfort

Appendix

Other possible areas of pain

An appendectomy performed under the best medical conditions has a very low mortality rate. Even when postoperative complications occur, they can be overcome with antibiotics.

So-called chronic appendicitis is considered to be a designation with little medical validity. Constant complaints of discomfort in the lower right part of the abdomen should be investigated for the correct cause.

appetite The natural desire for food, usually conditioned by psychological factors such as eating habits, pleasant memories, and the stimuli of the sight and smell of particular foods. Hunger, on the other hand, is a physiological phenomenon resulting from the contractions of an empty stomach. An infant's cries for food are an expression of hunger, not appetite.

When appetite is active and intense beyond the apparent physical needs of the body, diabetes or a thyroid disorder may be responsible. More frequently, an insatiable appetite that leads to compulsive overeating may originate in an emotional problem that requires attention.

People occasionally experience a loss of appetite in the presence of unattractive surroundings or uncongenial company. Emotions such as fear, anger, or anxiety affect the flow of stomach juices and diminish the appetite. A continuing loss of appetite, technically known as chronic *anorexia* (not to be confused with anorexia nervosa), may indicate kidney malfunction or cancer. When a lack of interest in food occurs in old age, it may be related to depression and withdrawal from life.

A doctor's guidance is advised when someone's appetite needs to be stimulated or reduced.

areola Any round, colored area surrounding a raised center, such as the inflamed area surrounding a pustule or the pigmented area of the breast in which the nipple is centered.

arteriosclerosis A disease of aging, also called hardening of the arteries, in which the walls of the arteries thicken and lose their elasticity. It is more prevalent among men than women. *See* ATHEROSCLEROSIS.

arthritis Inflammation of a joint. The term is broadly used to cover almost 100 different conditions many of which do not necessarily involve inflammation, but do result in aches and pains in the joints and connective tissues all over the body. The designation rheumatism is often incorrectly used for such aches and pains. The

Arthritis Foundation estimates that about 20 million Americans suffer from some form of arthritis severe enough to require medical attention and that among the sufferers women far outnumber men.

Arthritis is a chronic condition, but it may be less of a problem if its symptoms are recognized early enough for prompt and proper treatment. The typical warning signs of the onset of one of the arthritic diseases are: stiffness and pain in the joints on getting up in the morning; tenderness, soreness, and swelling in one or several joints; tingling sensations in the fingers and toes; fatigue and weakness unconnected with any other disorder. Authorities emphasize that the mountain of misinformation about arthritis has been the cause of a great deal of unnecessary suffering and misman-

ARTHRITIS OF THE ELBOW JOINT

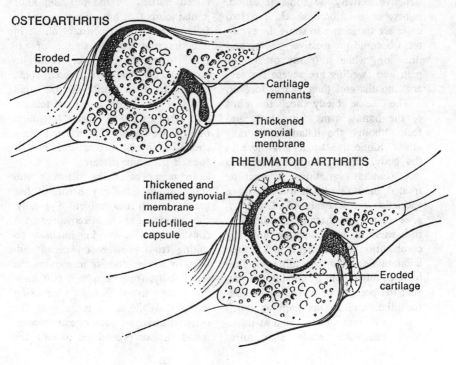

OSTEOARTHRITIS

Eroded bone

Cartilage remnants

Thickened synovial membrane

RHEUMATOID ARTHRITIS

Thickened and inflamed synovial membrane

Fluid-filled capsule

Eroded cartilage

agement of the various arthritic diseases. It is *not* true that most women have arthritis as they get older and there's nothing to be done about it. It is *not* true (loud and persistent claims to the contrary) that diet is an important factor in arthritis. It is *not* true that home treatments are just as effective as professional medical care. This last misconception is the most dangerous of all since it can lead to a delay in getting an accurate diagnosis and effective treatment early enough to avoid irreversible joint damage.

Rheumatoid arthritis is the most serious—and the most mysterious—of the arthritic diseases. Although no one is immune to it, 80 percent of all cases occur between the ages of 25 and 50, with three times as many women affected as men. The current theory about the cause is that viruslike organisms remain dormant in the body until they are triggered into destructive activity by some infection, injury, or emotional shock. No two cases are the same: in some the symptoms become progressively worse and disabling, while in many others the pain and swelling are severe for several months and then vanish forever.

The disease chiefly affects the joints of the hands, arms, hips, legs, and feet, although the inflammation may attack connective tissue anywhere in the body. Since rheumatoid arthritis has so many variations, it must be treated on an individual basis by a specialist who is aware of all the possible forms of therapy: medication, rest, exercise, heat, surgery, and any combination of treatments to keep the inflammation from spreading, to eliminate as much pain as possible, to prevent the occurrence of irreversible deformities, and to maintain as much joint movement and function as possible. Analgesics such as aspirin (which also is anti-inflammatory) are helpful in mild cases. Corticosteroids are used for their anti-inflammatory effect in more severe cases. The use of combinations of these drugs plus newer, more powerful ones in very severe cases may require hospitalization. Recent developments in surgical techniques—plastic surgery, fusions, and artificial implants—are achieving good results in overcoming deformities and disabilities.

Osteoarthritis, also known as degenerative joint disease, is the most common form of arthritis, usually an accompaniment to aging and rarely disabling. Mild aches and stiffness are likely to settle in those joints that have received the most use and weight stress; women are especially vulnerable to osteoarthritis of the hip, knee, big toe, and the end (or distal) joints of the fingers. Overweight is clearly a contributing cause since it places an added burden on the hip and knee joints; joints that have been injured in falls or have taken constant abuse in athletics may be the source of arthritic discomfort; heredity seems to be a factor that predisposes some women to osteoarthritis in the small joints of the fingers and toes; tension that takes its toll in muscle fatigue is one of the factors that has led some specialists to call osteoarthritis one of the self-punishing diseases.

In many cases the disorder will show up in an X-ray before it has caused much discomfort. Typically, the symptoms are localized soreness, a constant pain of varying intensity resulting from pressure on nerve endings, or some difficulty in moving the joint easily, for example, a stiff knee or pains in the hip ("creaking joints"). While there is no cure for osteoarthritis, a doctor can recommend various procedures to ease the discomfort and to prevent further deterioration of tissue.

The national office of The Arthritis Foundation, 3400 Peachtree Road NE, Suite 1101, Atlanta, Georgia 30326, supplies information on request about local specialists and treatment centers. It also offers free literature covering many aspects of the disease and current research activities.

artificial insemination The transfer of semen into the vagina by artificial means for the purpose of conception. The procedure known as AIH (artificial insemination by the husband) is used in cases where normal sexual intercourse and ejaculation cannot be achieved. The husband's semen is injected into the vagina by syringe on three or four successive days around the time of ovulation. If the husband is sterile, the same procedure may be followed with semen from a donor.

artificial respiration Any of several techniques whereby air is forced into and out of the lungs when natural breathing has ceased. None of the techniques requires special equipment, so they are first aid measures that almost anyone can master. Since brain death occurs four to six minutes after breathing has stopped, artificial respiration must be administered at once in such circumstances as a near-drowning, an almost lethal electric shock, suffocation from smoke inhalation. It is therefore crucial to learn the techniques *before* the need arises in order to function swiftly and competently. Local Red Cross chapters or other community organizations should be contacted for information about courses that cover instruction in first aid for common emergencies.

ascorbic acid Chemical designation of vitamin C.

aspirin Common name for the pure chemical acetylsalicylic acid; originally the brand name invented by the Bayer Drug Company, but now a generic term. Aspirin is always aspirin no matter what company packages it; therefore, there's no reason not to buy the least expensive brand. Aspirin is one of the greatest discoveries of all times because of its many benefits. It is a painkiller (analgesic); it lowers fever (antipyretic); it reduces some of the destructive consequences of arthritis (anti-inflammatory); and recently it has been reported to play a role in controlling the mechanism that causes blood to form clots (anti-coagulant).

The addition of certain chemicals to aspirin may be profitable to the manufacturer, but of questionable value to the consumer. Aspirin combined with caffeine? It probably costs less to have plain aspirin with a cup of coffee. With phenacetin? In large doses this is an ingredient likely to produce stomach upsets and kidney problems.

Aspirin itself can be a stomach irritant and should be avoided by anyone with ulcers or gastritis. It can be "buffered" by combining it with an alkalizer such as a bicarbonate of soda pill or a half glass of milk. When aspirin causes an allergic response, acetaminophen (Tylenol or other aspirinlike analgesics) should be substituted.

Children should be given a recommended dose of plain aspirin, not "candied" aspirin. Medicine is medicine and candy is candy. Confusing the two has caused many tragedies.

Headaches, ringing in the ears, and drowsiness are signs of aspirin overdose. Severe cases of aspirin poisoning, with symptoms of vomiting and delirium, require emergency treatment.

asthma A respiratory disorder in which the air tubes of the lungs are constricted by tightened muscles, mucous plugs, and inflamed tissue, causing breathing to be mildly or severely labored; technically known as bronchial asthma. While most asthma victims are children, it is also common among adults, with men and women affected in equal numbers. Asthma is a disease that occurs in "attacks" or "episodes." Asthmatics are said to have lungs that are abnormally sensitive to certain stimuli, ranging from cat hairs to chemicals to sudden changes in temperature to virus infections. The offending stimulus (in most cases an allergen that causes the body to produce histamines) triggers muscle tightening, mucous secretion, and tissue swelling in the bronchial passages that transport oxygen into the lungs. The victim of the attack begins to wheeze, cough, and gasp for air. An attack may subside in a few minutes or it may continue intermittently for hours.

Asthmatics who know exactly what substances or circumstances precipitate an attack but cannot easily avoid the stimulus should be desensitized. If the episodes are of mysterious origin, the American Lung Association recommends that a doctor be consulted before taking any medicines. Since no environment is pollen-free, pollutant-free, dust-free, or mold-free year round, moving is rarely a final solution. For some the answer is as simple as avoiding other people's cigarette smoke; for others it is as difficult as giving up smoking themselves.

Attacks that are triggered by ten-sion or anxiety may be eliminated after a period of productive psychotherapy.

astigmatism A defect in the curved surface of the lens or the cornea that results in blurred vision. When the refracting surface is not truly spherical, rays of light coming from a single spot are not brought into sharp focus. Astigmatism is a common disorder of vision that is easily corrected with properly fitted eyeglasses.

atherosclerosis A thickening and decreased elasticity of the arteries combined with the formation of fatty deposits (plaquer) on or beneath their inner walls. When these plaques become large enough to block the flow of blood, the tissue beyond the block dies (infarcts). This blockage of blood flow is what causes the brain damage in most strokes and the heart muscle damage (myocardial infarction) in most heart attacks. Similar blockage may occur in other blood vessels, resulting in such conditions as kidney failure and gangrene in the legs. Atherosclerosis is the major cause of cardiovascular disease which is the immediate cause of about half of the deaths in the United States each year.

The causes of atherosclerosis are not sharply defined. Because the disease is rare in undernourished populations, some specialists blame overeating, especially of animal fats. Because the disorder is not a major problem in agricultural countries, other specialists blame the stresses of industrial society, especially since its incidence is greatest among male business executives. Because between the ages of 35 and 40 the death rate from atherosclerosis is almost 500 percent higher for men than for women, researchers

ATHEROSCLEROSIS

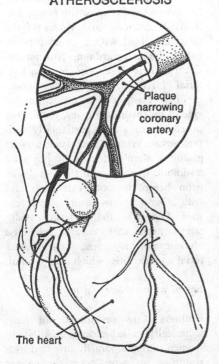

Plaque narrowing coronary artery

The heart

into a small computer for analysis. The loudness and pitch indicate the degree of narrowing caused by the fatty deposits. Phonoangiography can be conducted on an out-patient basis as a screening test when dangerous degrees of atherosclerosis are suspected.

athlete's foot *See* FUNGUS INFECTIONS.

atrophy The wasting away, degeneration, or shriveling up of any part of the body through disuse or lack of nourishment. A healthy muscle will atrophy if the nerve that controls its function is irreversibly damaged.

Aureomycin Brand name of one of the tetracycline group of antibiotics.

auscultation A means of examining the body by listening. A doctor may do this by placing his or her ear against various parts of the body or, more commonly, by using a stethoscope which makes binaural listening possible without the distraction of outside sounds. Auscultation is used to determine the condition of the heart and lungs, to discover possible disorders within the abdominal cavity, to determine the health of the fetal heart, and to make a prenatal determination of twins.

have begun to explore the role of sex hormones in its development.

Although simple hardening of the arteries (arteriosclerosis) is a concomitant of aging, the fatty deposits (atheromas) are not. Medical science has recently discovered special constituents, known as HDL (high density lipoproteins), in the blood of certain people that seem to break down cholesterol instead of allowing it to remain and clog the arteries.

Yearly checkups should include diagnostic blood tests as insurance against the sudden onset of a preventable disease. One of the recently developed diagnostic procedures for assessing arterial disease is phonoangiography. This procedure records the noise produced by the blood flow in a constricted artery and feeds the sound

autoimmune responses The body's production of antibodies against its own tissues. The autoimmune mechanism is one of the most important areas of present-day medical research because it is thought to be responsible for various diseases such as rheumatoid arthritis and for many allergic responses. If the autoimmune mechanism is triggered by an infection such as mumps, it may explain the onset of encephalitis. Since this response is also the cause of rejected grafts of tissue that are essential in successful transplants, a better understanding of autoimmunity will represent an important medical advance.

backache The discomfort of backache, sometimes called lumbago, can in most cases be reduced by appropriate exercises and by rectifying such causes of the problem as poor posture, ill-fitting shoes, an improper mattress. Upper back pain can often be traced to stress and anxiety, and lower muscles may be strained for many reasons such as lifting heavy objects. Backache may be connected with osteoporosis of the spine in older women, with premenstrual internal pressures in younger ones, and with a kidney disorder or an ovarian cyst in some cases.

When acute back pain interferes with normal activity and all efforts have been made to eliminate apparent external causes, a doctor should be consulted.

bacteria Single-cell microscopic organisms, essentially a form of plant life without chlorophyl, that occur everywhere in nature. Some bacteria are harmless, many are useful, and some cause disease. Bacteria are classified by their shape: bacilli are rod-shaped, spirochetes spiral, vibrios hooklike, and cocci round. Cocci are also classified by the way they are grouped: diplococci occur in pairs, streptococci run together in a chain, and staphylococci are clustered.

The development of antibiotics was based on the observation that there are substances in nature, produced by microorganisms and fungi, that can destroy disease-producing bacteria.

bacterial endocarditis A serious infection of the lining of the heart. The internal chambers and valves of the heart are lined with a delicate tissue called the endocardium. Normal endocardium is usually immune to bacterial infection, but where abnormalities exist, either congenital or caused by rheumatic fever, the danger of endocarditis is a particularly serious threat. Women with such a heart disability should discuss prophylactic antibiotic therapy with their oral surgeon before a tooth extraction and with other surgeons before any procedure. Otherwise the bacteria, usually streptococci, that escape into the bloodstream may cause subacute bacterial endocarditis, which can be fatal.

bag of waters *See* AMNION.

baldness Loss or absence of hair; technically called alopecia. Although women may temporarily lose hair as a result of an acute fever, anticancer chemotherapy, tuberculosis, thyroid disorder, or pregnancy, they are spared the characteristically male baldness that is permanent. When women's hair begins to thin out with age, hormone replacement is not effective. Although chemicals in hair dyes or constant "permanents" may cause hair to break off, unless the root is destroyed, hair will grow back.

barbiturate A class of sedative and hypnotic medicines derived from barbituric acid that have a depressant effect on the central nervous system. Depending on the type and amount prescribed, barbiturates produce sedation, sleep, or anesthesia. An overdose may result in coma, respiratory failure, and death.

Short-action barbiturates such as sodium pentothal are injected intravenously as anesthetics. Sodium pentobarbital (Nembutal) and sodium secobarbital (Seconal) are slower acting; an oral dose of 100 mg produces about six hours of sleep. Phenobarbital, one of the slowest acting barbiturates, may be prescribed with other drugs for the control of epileptic seizures.

The indiscriminate prescribing of barbiturates and their consequent overuse have come under severe criticism. Sedatives and sleeping pills that contain no barbiturates have become available in recent years. Barbiturates should be used only when and as prescribed and should be prescribed only when there is an authentic need for them. These drugs not only can be physically and psychologically addictive, but can produce the kind of confusion responsible for accidental overdose. The combination of alcohol and barbiturates can be lethal. Sudden and total withdrawal can also be lethal and should *never* be attempted without medical supervision.

The victim of acute barbiturate poisoning should be given strong, black coffee at once and hospitalized for emergency treatment. Low-level chronic poisoning may be evident in poorly coordinated movements, sluggishness, memory lapses, and slurred speech. If these symptoms appear, professional help is essential. *See also* "Drugs, Alcohol, and Tobacco."

barium test A diagnostic test for the exploration of gastrointestinal disorders by X-ray. Barium sulfate, a harmless chalky substance, is administered to the patient. The opacity of the barium causes the gastrointestinal (GI) tract to stand out in a white silhouette on the fluoroscope or X-ray plate, making visible to the diagnostician ulcers, tumors, and various other disorders of the stomach, duodenum, or intestines. The barium, mixed with water and a drop of flavoring, is taken orally for an examination of the upper tract. A barium enema is administered for an X-ray examination of the lower bowel and colon.

Bartholin's glands A pair of glands situated on each side of the vaginal opening. They are named after the Danish anatomist who first described them. Their function is not known, but they are presumed to provide some of the lubricating liquid that facilitates intercourse. These glands cannot be seen or felt unless they become inflamed or abscessed.

basal metabolism test A procedure for measuring the body's energy output by recording its rate of oxygen intake and consumption. The test for BMR (basal metabolism rate) measures the rate at which the body uses energy in order to carry on its basic life processes such as respiration, circulation, and temperature maintenance. The test calculates this rate by measuring the oxygen intake and comparing its consumption with a norm based not on weight, but on age, sex, and body surface area. The results of the test express the BMR as a percentage indicating its variation from the normal rate for a woman of the same age and size. Thus a result of minus 20 means that the patient's BMR is 20 percent slower than average, plus 5 that it is 5 percent faster. The BMR is no longer the most accurate indicator of the proper functioning of the thyroid gland and is seldom used for that purpose.

bed sore Patch of degenerating skin tissue, technically called decubitus ulcer, caused by prolonged and uninterrupted pressure of the bedding on the skin of a patient immobilized during an illness or postoperative convalescence. Elderly women and women with diabetes or heart disease are especially susceptible. The parts of the body most vulnerable are the area over the heels, the shoulders, the elbows, the buttocks, and the ankles. The first symptom of the sore is redness of the skin; continued interference with circulation produces a blue appearance of the affected area and then the formation of ulcers. Preventive measures are advisable as bed sores heal with great difficulty and are susceptible to infection. Bed linens should be soft, smooth, and dry. The patient's skin should be washed and powdered each day and the vulnerable areas cushioned with cotton pads. If possible, the bedridden patient should change body position every few hours.

bee stings *See* INSECT STINGS AND BITES.

Bell's palsy Paralysis of the muscles of one side of the face caused by inflammation of the facial nerve to a point where it becomes incapable of transmitting impulses. It generally is caused by an inflammation of the ear canal with resultant pressure on the facial nerve. The condition causes loss of the blink reflex, inability to close the eyelids, a flow of tears from the affected eye, and the dribbling of saliva from the immobilized side of the mouth. Food may also collect inside the cheek.

Recovery is based in part on treating the cause, if known, or stimulating the nerve electrically. Until the blink reflex is restored, the eye must be protected from excessive dryness and foreign particles. In most cases the condition subsides in a few weeks. At its very worst the deformity caused by Bell's palsy can be partially corrected by cosmetic surgery.

Benadryl Brand name of an antihistamine.

Benzedrine Brand name of an amphetamine.

bifocals *See* EYEGLASSES.

bile A yellow-brown fluid with a greenish tinge secreted by the liver and concentrated and stored in the gallbladder until needed for the digestive process, especially for the digestion of fats. The channel known as the biliary duct carries bile into the small intestine for this purpose. When the gallbladder has been removed, bile passes directly from the liver into the duodenum through the biliary duct. Among the constituents of bile are cholesterol, bile salts, some proteins, and the emulsifier lecithin. When the balance of these contents is upset, a common type of gallstones, which are actually a precipitate of cholesterol, may form. In some instances such gallstones can be treated medically by dissolution rather than surgically. Blockage of bile ducts by inflammation or other abnormal circumstances is one of the causes of discoloration of the skin and whites of the eyes that characterize jaundice.

biofeedback A still largely experimental technique, also called biomedical feedback, whereby a person learns how to achieve a state of relaxation that minimizes arteriolar constriction in her body in order to ward off headaches, particularly vascular headaches, and other symptoms of stress. A sensitive device that measures skin temperature, which in turn reflects blood flow, is used in biofeedback training.

biopsy The microscopic examination of small fragments of tissue cut from an organ of the body. The term is usually applied to the removal and evaluation of cells to determine whether they are cancerous.

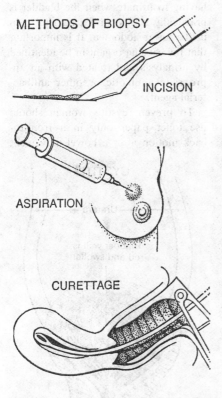

METHODS OF BIOPSY

INCISION

ASPIRATION

CURETTAGE

birth control *See* "Contraception and Abortion."

birth defect Any disorder or disease which is either genetically determined (inborn or inherited) or congenitally caused by chemicals, drugs, virus infection, injury, or malnutrition that affect the normal physical and mental development of the fetus before birth.

birth injuries Damages sustained by a baby during the birth process, beginning at the onset of labor and ending when the newborn has been delivered. Thanks to new obstetrical procedures, new medicines, and new monitoring techniques of blood and oxygen supply to the baby, the number of birth injuries has been dramatically reduced. Ultrasonic apparatus can determine the exact placement of the fetus and position of the head, so that complications of delivery can be anticipated. Electronic monitors can record the fetal heartbeat during labor and any cutoff in oxygen supply is immediately corrected before brain damage can occur. Injuries and fatalities to the newborn that result from heavy sedation of the mother during labor have also been reduced. Advances in anesthesiology and the increasing number of women taking courses in childbirth have combined to hold sedation in the delivery room to a minimum.

birthmarks Congenital skin blemishes visible from birth. The most frequent type of birthmark, commonly called a strawberry mark and technically known as a hemangioma, is a collection of small red or purplish blood vessels appearing on the skin surface. Most of these marks disappear by the time a child is 3 or 4. If they do not or if they grow and ulcerate, they can be removed by radiotherapy or surgery. The mark known as a port wine stain is formed by a combination of blood vessel clusters and erratic pigmentation. This blemish does not disappear spontaneously, but it may be treated with diatherapy or effectively hidden under cosmetics prepared for this purpose.

bisexuality Sexual attraction to both men and women. An increase in the number of people who consider themselves bisexual may be due to the fact that more men and women feel free to acknowledge their bisexual feelings. *See* "Sexual Health."

black eye Discoloration, swelling, and pain of the tissues around the eye, usually caused by a bruise that has ruptured tiny blood vessels under the skin. An icepack or cold compress applied immediately after the blow will slow subcutaneous bleeding, thus reducing the symptoms. A warm, wet compress applied on the following day will help absorb the discoloring fluids. If a blow to the eye is followed by persistent blurring of vision or severe pain, an ophthalmologist should be consulted promptly.

blackhead A skin pore in which fatty material secreted by the sebaceous glands has accumulated and darkened, not because of dirt, but because of the effect of oxygen on the secretion itself. Blackheads usually accompany the acne of adolescence and may occasionally trouble older women whose skin is oily. Their occurrence may be reduced by keeping the skin clean and dry. When blackheads do appear, the temptation to squeeze them should be resisted in order to avoid infection. Blackheads can be removed with a device designed for this purpose and available at most drugstores.

bladder disorders The urinary bladder is joined to the kidneys by tubes called ureters and to the outside of the body by the urethra. Cystitis, the technical term for infection of the bladder, is caused by multiplication of bacteria in the urine. Women are more prone to bladder infections than men because the female urethra is shorter, facilitating the entry of bacteria, particularly from the rectal area. Although the condition is rarely serious, it can be very annoying. It has a tendency to recur intermittently and the symptoms are a burning sensation during urination, a frequent feeling of having to urinate when the bladder is practically empty, and a nagging pain in the lower abdomen. It is important that the causing organism be identified by urinalysis and treated with an appropriate antibiotic or other antibacterial agent.

To prevent cystitis women should use toilet paper only in a front-to-back motion after a bowel movement

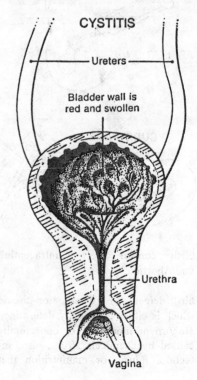

CYSTITIS

Ureters

Bladder wall is red and swollen

Urethra

Vagina

and wash their genital area daily. Since bacteria can enter the urethra during sexual contact, it is a good idea to urinate afterward to "flush" them out.

Blood-streaked urine unaccompanied by pain may be an indication of a tumor in the bladder or kidney or of kidney stones. Although the tumor may be nonmalignant, surgical removal may be recommended to eliminate discomfort. Surgery is also the only way of removing stones that are not passed with urination since there is, as yet, no medical way of dissolving them.

Surgical correction is the usual procedure for dealing with the type of hernia resulting from a difficult delivery during which the weakening pelvic tissues have allowed the bladder to protrude into the vagina.

bleeding *See* HEMORRHAGE.

blister A collection of fluid (lymph), usually colorless, that forms a raised sac under the skin surface. A common cause of blisters is friction on the skin. Improperly fitted shoes should be stretched or discarded and gloves should be worn to protect the skin when using tools which may blister the hands. Mild burns, such as overexposure to the sun and scalding with steam or hot water, will cause the skin to blister. Minor injuries that do not break the skin may rupture a tiny blood vessel beneath the skin and cause a blood blister. Blisters are also associated with various allergic reactions such as poison ivy sensitivity and eczema, with infections caused by the herpes simplex virus (fever blisters or cold sores), and with fungus invasions such as ringworm.

Blisters caused by an illness usually vanish as the illness improves. Small surface blisters should be left to heal by themselves since the unbroken skin protects against infection. A large and painful blister may be drained in the following way: sterilize a needle by placing it in a flame, swab the area with soap and water, prick the outer margin of the blister, press the inflated skin surface gently with a sterile gauze to remove the fluid, and apply a sterile bandage. Any inflammation or accumulation of pus around a blister that has ruptured is a sign of bacterial infection and should be examined by a doctor.

blood The principal fluid of life; the medium in which oxygen and nutrients are transported to all tissues and carbon dioxide and other wastes are removed from tissues. Blood maintains the body's fluid balance by car-

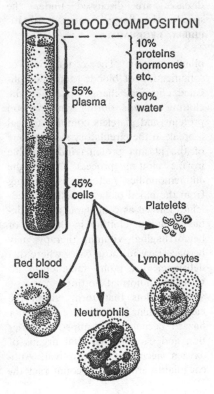

BLOOD COMPOSITION

10% proteins hormones etc.

55% plasma

90% water

45% cells

Platelets

Red blood cells

Lymphocytes

Neutrophils

rying water and salts to and from the tissues. It contains antibodies that fight infection, delivers hormones from the endocrine glands to the organs they influence, and regulates body temperature by dispersing heat in the form of perspiration. Every adult body contains about 1 quart (1,000 cc) of blood for every 25 pounds of weight. About 45 percent of blood composition consists of red cells that contain hemoglobin, white cells that fight infection, and platelets essential for the clotting process. The remaining 55 percent of blood composition is plasma. Blood plasma consists of water (over 90 percent) and proteins, hormones, enzymes, and other organic substances. Dissolved in the plasma are such proteins as globulins, fibrinogen, and albumen. *See also* BLOOD SERUM, HEMOGLOBIN. Blood diseases are discussed under the specific headings: ANEMIA, HEMOPHILIA, LEUKEMIA.

blood clotting The coagulation or solidification of blood. Many complicated chemical changes occur in the clotting process during which blood proteins and platelets combine to seal a break in the circulatory system. One of the plasma proteins indispensable in the clotting process, AHF (the *anti*hemophilic *f*actor), is missing from the blood of hemophiliacs. Medicines known as coagulants are available to hasten clotting in the case of hemorrhaging; vitamin therapy may be necessary in those cases where diet deficiencies or faulty metabolism interfere with normal clotting.

Blood clots that form within the cardiovascular system are a major hazard because they impede circulation and can deprive vital organs of oxygen necessary for survival. Anticoagulants are used to counteract the formation of dangerous blood clots that may accompany diseases of the veins (phlebitis) or arteries (arteriosclerosis). Heparin, a drug until recently used only in high doses to reduce the possibility of clotting in high-risk patients after surgery, injury, or childbirth, is now being used preoperatively in low doses by some surgeons. It has also been discovered that aspirin, in addition to its many other properties, is an anticoagulant since it depresses platelet activity.

blood pressure The amount of pressure exerted against the arterial walls when the heart contracts (systolic pressure) and when it relaxes between beats (diastolic pressure). These measurements vary according to changes in the rate at which the heart beats and changes in the dilation or constriction of the blood vessels. The pumping action of the heart and the efficiency of the arteries in circulating the body's five quarts of blood are affected by many factors: general health of the heart muscle, elasticity and smoothness of the arterial walls, emotional stress, overweight, ingestion of drugs, alcoholic intake, time of day, and so on.

Blood pressure is measured by a device called a sphygmomanometer. It consists of a rubber cuff which can be blown up by squeezing an attached rubber bulb. The cuff is connected to a mercury-filled glass tube or to a gauge calibrated in millimeters. The cuff is wrapped around the brachial artery of the upper arm and inflated. As the cuff begins to put pressure on the artery, the mercury indicator rises. The doctor or nurse places a stethoscope on the crook of the elbow where the sound of the arterial pulse can be heard, while continuing to inflate the cuff until the arterial blood flow is momentarily halted. The air pressure in the cuff is then released so that the blood flow resumes, producing a rhythmic tap. As soon as this tap is heard, the pressure registered on the gauge is recorded. This number is the systolic pressure. The cuff is then deflated slowly until the sound becomes so faint that it can scarcely be heard. The number registered by the gauge at this moment is the diastolic pressure.

The figures 120/80 are sometimes called an average reading, but they should not be considered a rigid norm. Normal readings for age ranges are: 17 to 40 years, up to 140/90; 41 to 60 years, up to 150/90; 61 years and older, 160/90. Lower limits of both systolic and diastolic pressures vary and their significance, if any, must be individually determined. When the readings go up and stay up for several months, medicines may be prescribed to reduce them.

blood pressure, high *See* HYPER-TENSION.

blood serum The clear, yellowish liquid which separates from whole blood when it clots. It contains proteins, enzymes, hormones, and chemicals such as glucose and sodium—in fact all the constituents of whole blood except hemoglobin and fibrinogen. Albumin protein can be fractionated out from the serum (or plasma) of human blood and used to treat people who need more albumin in their blood. Also, protein antibodies (gamma globulins) present in the blood naturally or subsequent to active immunization can be fractionated out from serum, concentrated, and injected intramuscularly into another person to provide passive (short-lived, not more than 6 months) immunization against such diseases as hepatitis and measles. The general term for serum from humans used for this purpose is Immune Serum Globulin (Human). Serum from people who are convalescing, or have been immunized recently against a specific disease is given a more specific name, for example, Tetanus Immune Globulin (Human), Measles Immune Globulin (Human). The more specific the preparation, the more effective it is. Animal serum also is used, but many people are allergic to it.

blood test Laboratory analysis of the blood which provides information for the diagnosis of a disorder or disease. If only a small amount of blood is required, it is taken from the fleshy cushion of a finger. When a large amount is needed for several different laboratory tests, blood is usually taken from a vein in the crook of the arm.

A patient entering the hospital for surgery is often given several blood tests. These are necessary for diagnostic purposes as well as to establish the patient's blood type in the event a transfusion is required during or after the operation. Blood tests for hemoglobin, cholesterol, and glucose are among the routine procedures of a comprehensive annual checkup. Blood tests can indicate the presence of diabetes, anemia, kidney disorder, or glandular disorder.

blood transfusion The infusion of blood into the veins of a patient from an outside source. Transfusions had unpredictable results until the beginning of the twentieth century when blood groups were discovered. The accurate matching of blood is necessary for a successful transfusion.

The replenishment of blood is a

lifesaving measure in such circumstances as hemorrhage resulting from accident, tissue injuries caused by severe burns, or blood loss attendant on surgery. While whole blood may be desirable in most cases, it may not be essential in instances of shock, when the crucial requirement is blood plasma or serum. These components can be accumulated without regard to type since they are universally compatible. They can be stored frozen in large amounts and drawn on in emergencies involving large numbers of victims, such as a plane crash.

Among the most recent developments in blood transfusion are two techniques with broad application. Plateletpheresis involves taking blood from a healthy donor, removing the platelets which are the component essential for clotting, and immediately returning the remainder—the red cells, white cells, and plasma—to the donor. The transfusion of platelets can extend the lives of patients with certain types of anemia, leukemia, and other malignant diseases for whom bleeding episodes might otherwise be fatal. This procedure in no way endangers the donor's blood supply since platelets in the body of a healthy person are automatically replaced within two days. The second innovation in transfusion is a technique whereby white blood cells can be supplied to cancer patients who are receiving drugs that temporarily suppress the ability of the bone marrow to manufacture them. In this way patients undergoing anticancer chemotherapy are provided with the white cells necessary for fighting infection.

blood types For many years it had been observed that some blood transfusions were successful and some were not, but it was not until the twentieth century that the riddle of incompatibility was solved. It is now known that the blood of all humans, regardless of skin color, race, country of origin, or sex, can be classified under four main groupings: A, B, AB, and O. Blood type O (the "O" stands for zero) is composed of red cells that can blend with any type of plasma. Because of this compatibility, a person with O type blood is a universal donor. Conversely, anyone with AB type blood is a universal recipient. Of each 100 individuals, approximately 45 will be type O, 40 will be type A, 10 will be type B, and 5 will be type AB. There are many minor subtypes which are inconsequential for most people. *See also* RH FACTOR.

body odors Natural odors associated with the human body. Fresh perspiration from a healthy body is practically odorless. Most unpleasant body odors are caused by the presence of bacteria or fungi that multiply in areas where perspiration can accumulate, such as the genital area, the armpits, and between the toes, and by stale perspiration absorbed by clothing. Regular scrubbing with soap and water and regular changes of clothes should keep the body clean and odorless. It should be noted that vaginal sprays can be quite harmful to the delicate membranes they are supposed to deodorize.

boil A painful bacterial infection, usually staphylococcal, of a hair follicle or sweat gland, often occurring on the face, neck, shoulders, breast, or buttocks. The infected lump, technically called a *furuncle,* may be as small as a cherry pit or quite large. Since the infection can easily spread, a boil should be treated promptly. Moist, hot compresses should be applied several times a day. The boil should then be covered with an antibiotic salve such as bacitracin ointment and protected by a sterile gauze bandage. A boil should never be squeezed, especially one on the nose, ear, or upper lip, since some of the bacteria may invade the bloodstream, instead of going to the lymph glands or being exuded to the skin surface, leading to possible blood poisoning. Boils that do not drain naturally following the application of heat and moisture may have to be incised surgically. Those that occur in groups (carbuncles) or that recur may be the result of faulty habits of personal hygiene, low resistance, diabetes, or a strain of bacteria requiring a newer antibiotic. Such cases should be treated by a doctor.

bone The hard tissue that forms the major part of the skeleton. The 206 bones in the human body are connected by ligaments at the joints and are activated into movement by muscles secured to the bones by tendons. Bones are covered by a thin fibrous membrane called periosteum which sheathes and protects them and supports the adjacent tendons. The periosteum stops at the joints which are covered by a layer of cartilage. The fibrous layer of tissue directly under the periosteum gives bones their elasticity. Next are the dense hard layers called compact tissue within which are encased the porous materials known as spongy tissue. The innermost cavity of bone contains the marrow, which is the source of red blood cell production. Every layer of bone is crisscrossed by blood vessels. Bone tissue also contains a large number of nerves.

The hardness and strength of the skeleton result from the mineral content—calcium phosphate. This mineral, plentiful in milk, is essential for the transformation of cartilage into the calcified part of bone during childhood and adolescence. Bone tissue, even when fully formed in adulthood, constantly renews itself, but since the rate of renewal slows with age, the bones of the elderly become more brittle as they become more porous and less elastic.

The health of bones may be impaired by dietary deficiency of the mother during pregnancy or of the child during the years of growth, by infectious diseases (osteomyelitis), degenerative diseases (osteoporosis, osteoarthritis), tumors, and a rare form of primary cancer (sarcoma). The most common bone injury is a fracture, and bones may also bleed internally after sustaining a severe bruise.

boric acid An antiseptic in the form of a powder dissolved in water and once commonly used as an eyewash or for application to minor skin irritations. Since it is highly poisonous when swallowed, it should be discarded in favor of equally effective and less dangerous substances.

botulism A form of food poisoning caused by bacteria that produce a toxin that attacks the nervous system. The causative bacterium, *Clostridium botulinum,* thrives in low-acid, low-sugar substances where there is no oxygen. It is typically found in improperly preserved foods, such as canned vegetables, meat, or smoked fish, and the contaminated food rarely smells, tastes, or looks spoiled. Faulty procedures in home canning are responsible for a significant number of cases, as many as half of which are fatal. Diagnosis is simplified by the fact that several people, including household pets, are likely to be affected at the same time.

Nausea and vomiting occur generally in less than 24 hours and may or may not precede the central nervous system symptoms which are caused by the toxin and whose onset usually is from 12 to 36 hours after eating. These symptoms are double vision, puffy or drooping eyelids, and paralysis that impedes swallowing and breathing. The victim must be hospitalized at once for treatment to nullify the toxin and to prevent respiratory failure. Anyone who has eaten the spoiled food must be treated without delay with botulinus antitoxin.

With more and more families growing and preserving their own vegetables, the U.S. Department of Agriculture has issued warnings about the dangers of careless food processing. The department issues bulletins on home canning that are often available in libraries and can be ordered by mail.

brain The central organ of the nervous system, interpreting all sense impressions, controlling the activities of over 600 of the body's voluntary muscles, regulating the autonomic nervous system, and through its capacity for storing and recalling the messages received by its billions of cells, functioning as the memory bank that we call the mind.

The human brain is made of soft, convoluted, pinkish-gray tissue that weighs about 3 pounds and fits within the confines of the skull. Enveloping the brain and separating it from its bony encasement are three tough membranes, collectively called the meninges, which also sheathe the spinal cord. Between two of these membranous layers is the cerebrospinal fluid which may be tapped for accurate diagnosis of such diseases as cerebrospinal meningitis. The portion of the brain that has come to be synonymous with the mind is the cerebrum whose outer layer, the cerebral cortex, is fissured, furrowed, and wrinkled into "gray matter." The deepest fissure divides this part of the brain into two distinct halves: the nerves in the right hemisphere control the left side of the body and vice versa. Emerging from the cerebrum at the middle of the skull and extending down the back of the neck into the spinal cord is the brain stem; on either side of the brain stem are the two halves of the cerebellum. The cerebellum is the portion of the brain whose essential function is the coordination of muscular activities.

Because the activities of the brain are manifested by the transmission of electrical impulses, normal and abnormal brain wave patterns can be charted by an instrument called an encephalograph. This enables neurologists to diagnose such disorders as epilepsy and tumors and to explore the various stages of sleep by the different brain wave patterns they produce. The brain responds to electrical stimulation from the outside, thus revealing the particular function of different areas.

The brain also functions as a gland, manufacturing substances similar in chemical composition to morphine which have the same effect on the body as synthetic painkillers. These hormonelike substances are called endorphins and enkephalins. The amounts in which they are produced and released are presumed to define the body's sensations of pain and pleasure as well as to account for the symptoms of some forms of mental illness.

Epilepsy is the most common disease that originates in disordered electrical impulses of the brain without affecting the function of the mind. Parkinsonism is a disease originating in an abnormality of brain function in which, for the most part, the mind remains unaffected also. However, in the degenerative hardening of the arteries of the brain or in cerebrovascular stroke, both brain physiology and mind physiology are intimately involved. Brain/mind function may also be irreversibly damaged by the late stages of alcoholism, by tertiary syphilis, or by a hemorrhage within the skull. Many brain tumors which were previously untreatable or inoperable can now be reduced by radiation or completely removed due to advances in the techniques of hypothermia and microsurgery. Legal death is now often defined not by the cessation of the heartbeat, but by the death of the brain resulting from oxygen deprivation.

breast In the human female, the milk-producing glands and surrounding duct, fat, and connective tissue. *See* "Breast Care."

breast examination *See* "Breast Care."

breech delivery Childbirth in which the baby emerges buttocks or feet first instead of head first. *See* "Pregnancy and Childbirth."

Bright's disease An obsolescent term for nephrosis, or the nephrotic syndrome. *See* KIDNEYS AND KIDNEY DISORDERS, GLOMERULONEPHRITIS.

bromides Compounds of bromine which until recently were used as anticonvulsants in the treatment of epilepsy, as sedatives to reduce tension, and as headache remedy. Bromides have largely been replaced by medicines that are equally effective and less likely to cause unpleasant side effects in the form of rashes and boils. Another reason for eliminating bromides is that use over a long period has a cumulative toxic effect. Bromine poisoning is a condition characterized by mental confusion, listlessness, and, in serious cases, hallucinations.

bronchitis Inflammation of the lining of the bronchial tubes, the air passages that connect the windpipe and the lungs. In its acute form the inflammation may be an extension of an upper respiratory viral infection or may be caused by a bacterial infection following an upper respiratory illness. Such an attack is accompanied by fever and coughing up of the excess mucus secreted by the inflamed membranes. Bed rest and an expectorant medicine that loosens the sputum rather than one that suppresses the cough are the standard treatment. Antibiotics are used if the infection is diagnosed as bacterial. Chronic bronchitis is a much more serious matter, since the recurrent or persistent coughing and spitting up can lead to irreversible lung injury and an increased vulnerability to emphysema and heart disease. The American Lung Association estimates that of the approximately 6½ million Americans who suffer from this debilitating disease, the great majority are smokers. The typical sufferer is a middle-aged male (men are three times as likely as women to have the disease), who lives in a city where respiratory problems are exacerbated by pollutants in the air. The victim coughs and spits up yellow mucus, especially in the morning and evening, and eventually the condition becomes irreversible.

Too many patients take early symptoms for granted and wait until the disease approaches a disabling stage before seeing a doctor. The first and indispensable aspect of treatment is to stop smoking. In some cases rehabilitation may involve a change of job. In others the symptoms may gradually disappear after strict adherence to a wholesome regimen: proper diet, mild exercise, rest and relaxation, and avoidance of lung irritants.

bruise An injury in which small subcutaneous blood vessels are damaged, but the skin surface remains intact; also called a *contusion*. When the skin is broken, the injury is called an abrasion or a *laceration*. In a bruise the escape of blood into the surrounding tissues causes pain and swelling as well as the characteristic discoloration of the skin. The effects of a bruise may not be visible when a blow is sustained by a muscle, a bone or an ear. Healing is usually hastened and pain reduced by the use of cold compresses just after the injury to slow down the bleeding. An injured arm or leg will cause less discomfort and mend more quickly if it is elevated. The application of heat to the bruised area the following day is likely to hasten the reabsorption of the blood. If symptoms increase rather than abate, a doctor should be consulted, especially where deeper internal bruises are suspected.

Some women bruise more easily than others; some parts of the body look worse than they feel when bruised, for example, a black eye or a puffy lip. Since constant bruising and slow healing may be an indication of an arterial disorder, a disturbance in the blood-clotting mechanism, or a vitamin deficiency, the condition should be discussed with a doctor.

bunion A deformity of the foot that occurs when the big toe deviates from its natural position because of inflammation at the joint connecting the toe to the foot. Continuing pressure results in the hard swelling at the base of the toe and the development of the bunion. Discomfort is best relieved by correcting the footwear that causes the problem. In mild cases, with shoes that fit properly, the condition may be eliminated without further treatment. When the pain is severe enough to interfere with normal functioning even when wearing shoes with an orthopedic correction, surgery may be the only practical solution.

burns Injuries resulting from contact with dry heat (fire), moist heat (scalding by steam or liquid), electricity, chemicals, or the ultraviolet rays of the sun or a sunlamp. Whatever the cause, the injury is classified according to the extent of tissue damage. A first-degree burn is one in which the skin turns visibly red; a second-degree burn causes the skin to blister; a third-degree burn damages the deeper skin layers and may destroy the growth cells in the subcutaneous tissues. Even a first-degree burn is potentially dangerous if a large area of the body has been affected, especially if the victim is very young or very old. Until professional help is available a person who has sustained a serious burn should lie down and liquids should be administered, but only if they can be consciously swallowed. Ice cold water can be gently applied to the burned area. *Do not* give any alcoholic beverage. *Do not* disturb blisters. *Do not* attempt to remove clothing adhering to burnt skin. *Do not* apply oily salves or ointments or antiseptic sprays except in cases of superficial burns involving a small area.

bursitis Inflammation of a bursa, one of the small fluid-filled sacs located at various joints throughout the body for the purpose of minimizing friction. Bursitis most commonly occurs at the joints receiving the most wear and tear: at the hip, shoulder, knee, and elbow. "Housemaid's knee" and "tennis elbow" are the result of bursa inflammation. A bunion is the result of inflammation of the bursa that lubricates the joint between the big toe and the foot. An acute, and acutely painful, attack of bursitis may occur after an accident, following unusual exertion connected with moving heavy objects, or as a concomitant of a systemic infection. Although such an attack may be self-healing within a week or ten days, the process can be

BURSITIS OF THE SHOULDER

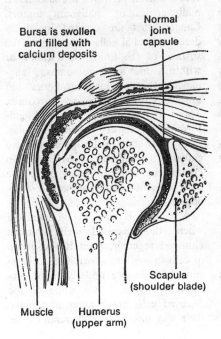

Bursa is swollen and filled with calcium deposits

Normal joint capsule

Scapula (shoulder blade)

Muscle   Humerus (upper arm)

eased and hastened by taking aspirin or some other analgesic and immobilizing the affected joint in a sling or a flexible bandage. When the sudden onset of bursitis is connected with bacterial infection, antibiotic treatment usually eliminates the discomfort. Chronic bursitis is best treated by reviewing the circumstances that bring it about and modifying them.

caffeine A drug that stimulates the central nervous system, the heart, and the kidneys. *See* "Drugs, Alcohol, and Tobacco."

calcium A metallic element essential to life. *See* "Nutrition and Weight."

Improper metabolism of calcium during the growing years may result in osteoporosis, a disorder in which the bones are excessively brittle and weaker than normal. This condition commonly occurs during aging, especially in women, and is caused by the loss of calcium associated with the cessation of estrogen production. A diet deficient in calcium and vitamin D, during pregnancy or at other times, may cause muscle cramps, especially in the legs. If the symptom persists in spite of proper nutrition, it may indicate faulty calcium metabolism, necessitating the injection of the calcium or the vitamin directly into the bloodstream. This particular malfunction may be due to underactivity of the parathyroid glands. Overactivity of the glands may cause excessive amounts of calcium in the bloodstream, which in turn may encourage the formation of kidney stones and increase the likelihood of bone fractures. In either case diagnostic blood tests are a guide to proper treatment.

calculus Technical term for stone formation in the body. Calculi may develop in the gallbladder or in the kidneys. Gallstones are usually composed of cholesterol, minerals, and bile pigments. Stones in the kidneys, which may migrate to the urinary tract, are composed of mineral salts. Cholesterol stones can now be disposed of with medicines; kidney stones still have to be removed surgically.

calendar rhythm method A means of contraception based on the avoidance of sexual intercourse during those days of the month when a woman is most likely to conceive. See "Contraception and Abortion."

callus An area of the skin that has thickened as a protection against repeated friction; also an irregular bump on a bone that has formed when the recalcification process closes a fracture. The calluses that form on the hands as a result of constant friction or repeated pressures can best be prevented by wearing protective gloves. Most of those that form on the soles of the feet or around the outer rim of the heels can be eliminated by wearing proper footwear. Calluses of this type become painful when they are thick enough to transfer pressure exerted on them to a bone. Calluses can be reduced by rubbing them with pumice or an emery board, or they can be carefully shaved after softening them by soaking in warm, soapy water. The shaving should not be attempted by anyone with diabetes or a circulatory disturbance.

A callus on the bone originates when the bone-forming cells multiply in order to repair a break in the tissue. This "knitting" of the bone takes about a month, after which the callus decreases and the bone resumes its normal shape. The bump formed by the bone callus may become permanent if a fracture is improperly set or if the break or splinter of the bone was so minor as to escape attention.

calorie A unit of energy measurement used in both physics and in the study of nutrition. Food is the fuel that provides the body with the energy essential for carrying on the life processes. The potential energy provided by various foods as they are metabolized by the body is measured in calories. In dietetics 1 calorie is equal to the amount of heat (energy) required to raise the temperature of 1 kilogram of water by 1 degree centigrade.

cancer The general term for a disease process in which the cells in a particular part of the body grow and reproduce with abnormal rapidity. This defect in the controls that govern normal cell growth characterizes about 200 different diseases known as cancers, most of which are also called malignancies or malignant tumors. Cancers that are created by disordered epithelial cells and arise on the surface of the lining of a tissue or within a duct are carcinomas. Malignancies that originate in bones and muscles are known as sarcomas. Those that originate in the blood-forming organs are called leukemias. Those that start in the lymphatics are called lymphomas. Malignancies created by the cells that carry the dark pigment melanin are called melanomas.

A cancer is said to be localized when the diseased cells remain clumped together, even if the group of cells grows into a visible mass large enough to invade underlying or surrounding tissue. When some of the diseased cells break away and make their way into the bloodstream or the lymphatics, eventually reaching other parts of the body, the cancer is said to have metastasized. *See also* CARCINOMA, SARCOMA, LEUKEMIA, METASTASIS.

candidiasis A yeastlike fungus, also called moniliasis or thrush. *See* Yeast Infections, "Sexually Transmissible Diseases."

canker sore An ulceration of the mucous membrane at the corner of the mouth or inside the lips or cheeks. The cause of canker sores is uncertain, but it may be virus infection, stress, sensitivity to particular foods, or mechanical irritation by a rough-edged tooth or filling or ill-fitting dentures. Most canker sores are occasional and self-healing. Recurrent canker sores of unknown origin should be discussed with a physician.

car sickness *See* MOTION SICKNESS

carbohydrates Any of a number of chemical substances, including starches, sugars, cellulose, and gums, containing only carbon, hydrogen, and oxygen in varying amounts with the ratio of hydrogen to oxygen usually being two to one as in water. Carbohydrates are present in many foods, primarily in grains and potatoes as starch and in fruits and vegetables as sugar. They are an indispensable source of animal (human) energy. Dietary starch and polysaccharide (complex) sugars—maltose, sucrose, and lactose—are converted into glucose in the digestive tract and are absorbed in that form into the bloodstream. Monosaccharide (simple) sugars—glucose, fructose, and galactose—are absorbed into the blood unchanged. Some of these absorbed monosaccharides are used immediately to provide energy. The rest are converted into glycogen by the liver and stored primarily in the liver and muscles for later energy or are converted into fat. Many factors, including diseases, influence the rate and amount that is absorbed. The most common disease which interferes with normal carbohydrate metabolism is diabetes mellitus. *See* DIABETES, GLUCOSE, SUGAR. *See also* "Nutrition and Weight."

carcinogen Any agent (tobacco smoke, X-rays, asbestos fibers, DES) capable of causing changes in cell structure (mutagenesis) and therefore a potential cause of cancer.

carcinoma One of the two main groups of cancers; the other is sarcoma. A carcinoma originates in epithelial cells located in glandular structures, mucous membranes, and skin. Practically all malignancies of the skin, tongue, stomach, uterus, and breast come under this heading.

cardiologist *See* DOCTORS

cardiopulmonary resuscitation (CPR) An emergency lifesaving technique in which oxygenated blood is sent to the brain and other tissues of the victim of cardiac arrest by the simultaneous administration of artificial respiration and external manipulation of the heart. CPR must be initiated at once following a heart attack, electric shock, or any other circumstance in which the lack of circulation has begun to deprive the brain of oxygen. Because of its proven effectiveness when administered by a properly trained individual, the Red Cross and the American Heart Association are encouraging ordinary citizens, including teenagers, to take the six- to twelve-hour CPR courses being offered under their auspices. Authorities in first aid techniques stress the fact that anyone who weighs 90 pounds or more can accomplish a rescue once the skills have been mastered.

carotene A plant pigment especially plentiful in carrots and also found in yellow, orange, and red fruits and vegetables in smaller amounts. Carotene is essential in the diet since it is converted into vitamin A in the body. It is also one of the weaker pigments in human skin. Its yellowish tone is generally masked by the melanin pigment in dark-complexioned women, but a fair complexion will take on an orange hue if the diet contains an excessive amount of carrots.

cartilage The tough, whitish elastic tissue which, together with bone, forms the skeleton. There are three different types of cartilage. Hyaline cartilage forms the extremely strong slippery surface of the ends of the bones at the joints, acting as a shock absorber. It is also the material of which the nose and the rings of the trachea are made. Fibrocartilage is densely packed with fibers and forms the disks between the spinal vertebrae. Elastic cartilage is the most flexible, forming the external ear and the larynx. The stiffness in the joints that characterizes osteoarthritis is associated with a deterioration of cartilage. A knee injury resulting in severe damage to the two sections of cartilage at the edges of the joint may cause the knee to lock in one position. This condition, sometimes referred to as a trick knee, may require surgical repair or removal of the torn cartilage.

CAT Computerized axial tomography. *See* SCANNING MACHINES.

cataract Opacity or cloudiness that develops in the crystalline lens of the eye. When the lens becomes so opaque that light can no longer reach the retina, loss of vision results. Fortunately, restoration of eyesight is accomplished safely and successfully in 95 percent of the hundreds of thousands of cataract operations performed every year in the United States. Although a few types of cataracts are congenital or are caused by injury or infection, the largest number by far are senile or degenerative cataracts, those that develop after the age of 60. They are one of the leading causes of blindness among the aged.

In many instances the cloudiness develops so slowly that no significant change in vision is detectable. Annual visits to an ophthalmologist for a glaucoma check after the age of 40 are the best way to find out about incipient cataracts and to plan ahead for their removal. However, for most people the first awareness of a cataract comes with blurred or dimmed vision, double images, and a scattering of light beams when looking directly at a street lamp or at the headlights of an approaching car. As soon as any of these symptoms occur, an ophthalmologist should be consulted. The only effective treatment for the condition is surgery. Since there is as yet no magical method for "dissolving" cataracts with "special medicines," all such claims should be regarded as quackery and, if possible, reported to the proper authorities for investigation.

A cataract operation consists of the removal of the degenerated lens and its replacement with an artificial lens in the form of eyeglasses, contact lens, or more recently, for certain patients, an intraocular lens. Whether the surgery is the conventional method that removes the cataract by lifting it out in one piece or the newer method that pulverizes the lens with an ultrasonic probe, recovery is considerably faster today than in the past. Even in cases where there is some difficulty in adjusting to the artificial lens, it rarely takes more than a few months for the transition to occur.

Since people who develop a cataract in one eye are likely to have the same problem with the other eye, it is considered advisable to schedule early treatment of the damaged eye without waiting for the cataract to develop fully, so that the unaffected eye can provide unimpaired vision following the operation.

cathartic Any medicine in liquid, tablet, or suppository form that stimulates intestinal activity for the purpose of bowel evacuation. Cathartics, also known as physics and purgatives, are stronger than laxatives and should never be used to treat constipation without a doctor's recommendation. They should be avoided when there is the slightest suspicion of appendicitis. A cathartic should not be used as a countermeasure against poisoning without consulting a doctor.

catheterization The procedure in which a tube is inserted through a passage in the body for the purpose of withdrawing or introducing fluids or other materials. Catheters have been used for centuries, but since the introduction of plastics they are less costly to manufacture and give minimal discomfort to the patient. In the more common applications, a catheter is introduced into the urethra for draining urine from the bladder; an intravenous catheter is used for "tube-feeding" following surgery; a nasogastric tube is used for withdrawing samples

of material from the stomach as a diagnostic clue. Catheterization is essential in the administration of oxygen through the nose, and it can effectively remove stones lodged in the ureter, the passageway connecting the kidney and the bladder. Cardiac catheterization is routinely used to detect and measure critical abnormalities caused by circulatory disorders.

cauterization The burning away of infected, unwanted, or dead tissue by the application of caustic chemicals or electrically heated instruments. Cryosurgery used in the treatment of certain types of tumors is a form of cauterization; the removal of surface moles with an electrical needle is another. Cauterization of cervical tissue to prevent the spread of erosion is a common gynecological practice.

cavities *See* DENTAL CARIES.

cell The structural unit of which all body tissues are formed. The human body is composed of billions of cells differing in size and structure depending on their function. In spite of these differences every cell includes the same basic components, chiefly, an outer limiting membrane which regulates the transport of chemical substances into and out of the cell; a mass of cytoplasm containing substances involved in metabolism and genetic transmission; a nucleus whose membrane contains the concentration of RNA and which encloses the DNA that determines the hereditary transmission of genetic characteristics. The study of normal cell structure and behavior is basic to cancer research, since all cancers are characterized by aberrational cell growth and reproduction.

cerebrovascular accident *See* STROKE.

cervix The neck or narrow portion of any organ, but generally used to refer to the hollow end of the uterus that forms the passageway into the vaginal canal. The cervix is approximately 2 inches in length. Under normal circumstances it has the diameter of a quarter with an opening (*os*) which has the diameter of a drinking straw. At the time of delivery the cervix dilates to a diameter usually given as 10 centimeters or five fingers. Dilatation to this size marks the end of the first stage of labor; the baby is ready to come down the birth canal, and the cervical opening has become large enough to permit passage of the infant's head.

Women who use a diaphragm should be aware of the position of the opening of the cervix, since the diaphragm is inserted across this opening as a barrier against the passage of sperm toward the ovum.

During pregnancy natural processes deposit a thick layer of mucus across the cervical entrance, sealing off the womb against invasion by infectious organisms.

Infections of the cervix—cervicitis—are quite common at other times. Among the chief causes are viruses, fungi, and bacteria, especially gonococci. In some women cervical tissue may be chronically inflamed by the use of birth control pills. The first symptom of cervicitis is likely to be a vaginal discharge that becomes more abundant immediately following menstruation. Other signs may be bleeding, pain during intercourse, a burning sensation during urination, or lower back pain. Such symptoms should be brought to the attention of a gynecologist. Examination of the cervix by insertion of a speculum usu-

ally indicates the source of the trouble. A culture of the discharge may be necessary to identify the infectious agent, especially if the infection does not respond to antibiotic medicines or fungicides. Where tissue erosion has occurred, cauterization by electricity, chemical application, or freezing may be necessary.

Another cause of bleeding, especially in middle-aged women with a history of cervical infections, is the presence of fleshy growths called polyps. Although these growths are easily removed and generally benign, a tissue biopsy is performed to rule out the possibility of cancer. The best safeguard against cervical cancer, one of the leading causes of cancer deaths in women over 40, is an annual pap test. This simple and painless procedure is based on the microscopic examination of a cervical smear to identify abnormalities before they produce any symptoms.

cesarean section A surgical procedure in which an incision is made into the uterus through the front of the abdominal wall to facilitate the delivery of the baby. At a time when many women feel that conscious participation in the birth experience is an inalienable right and when many fathers want to share as much of the experience as the hospital will allow, cesarean deliveries sometimes cause feelings of deprivation, depression, and guilt. A Massachusetts-based organization has been formed with chapters across the country to provide literature, films, and, above all, supportive reassurance to those women who are concerned about having a cesarean section or who want more information about it. The organization is called C/SEC (Cesarean/Support, Education, Concern) and is located at

66 Christopher Road, Waltham, MA 02154. It offers information on local chapters and will mail literature on receipt of a request which includes a stamped self-addressed envelope. *See* "Pregnancy and Childbirth."

chafing Inflammation of the skin caused by the friction of one body surface against the other or of clothing against a body surface. Chafing is especially common in hot weather when sweating increases irritation, particularly in the fleshier parts of the body.

The chafed area is likely to itch and burn, and without treatment the inflamed skin may crack or blister, increasing the possibility of bacterial or fungoid infection. Diabetics and obese women are particularly vulnerable to chafing. The irritation can be relieved by medicated powders to promote dryness, topical ointments to reduce itching, or cold compresses to alleviate the inflammation. In acute cases the doctor may prescribe a cortisone salve and a sterile dressing. The most effective way to prevent chafing is to keep the skin clean and dry, especially in hot weather, and to wear clothing that is loose and comfortable.

chancre An ulcerated sore in the area of bacterial invasion that is the first sign of the primary stage of syphilis. *See* "Sexually Transmissible Diseases."

chapping Irritation and cracking of the skin, usually due to dryness resulting from overexposure to cold or wind. In cold weather the lubricating glands of the skin are less active, and as the outer layer of the skin loses its oily secretion, it becomes dry and vulnerable to cold and to the irritating effects of strong soaps and detergents.

Chapping can be prevented or reduced by the use of protective creams, lotions, and bath oils. Once the irritation has occurred, the chapped areas of the skin should be cleansed with a mild soap substitute and tepid water and blotted dry with a soft towel. A layer of lotion or cream containing lanolin should be applied before bedtime, and exposure to irritating housecleaning chemicals should be kept to a minimum until the chapped skin has healed.

chemotherapy The treatment of illness by the use of specific chemicals. The term was used originally to describe the use of medications effective against particular organisms with minimal damage to the patient. One of the earliest such treatments was the use of quinine against the malarial parasite. This was followed by Dr. Paul Ehrlich's discovery in 1910 that salvarsan effectively destroyed the spirochete that causes syphilis and by later development of sulfa drugs and antibiotics. More recently, the meaning of the term chemotherapy has been expanded to include the use of the medication to relieve the effects of disease, for example, the application of such drugs as chlorpromazine in controlling some of the symptoms of mental illness.

At present treatment of various cancers by chemotherapy has increased survival rate in a significant number of cases. Especially dramatic results have been achieved by postsurgical multiple-combination chemotherapy in cases of advanced breast and ovarian cancers and by chemotherapy combined with radiation in the treatment of certain types of cancer. Pharmacologists and medical chemists are concerned in their research not only with finding new chemical agents to combat disease, but with minimizing adverse side effects, mainly, destruction of healthy tissue. In order to do so it is necessary to find the right agent and the critical dose that will cure without causing secondary complications.

chest pains Discomfort in any part of the thorax, usually caused by a disorder of one of the organs within the thoracic cavity enclosed by the rib cage, by an injury to a rib, or by a strained muscle. The site of a disorder may be the heart, lungs, large blood vessels, esophagus, or part of the trachea. Any viral or bacterial infection of the respiratory system may be accompanied by pain which may become acute when constant coughing is involved. Various allergies to mold, dust, animal dander, chemical pollutants may be another cause. Pain might be referred to the chest by the nervous system from areas outside

ORIGINS OF CHEST PAINS

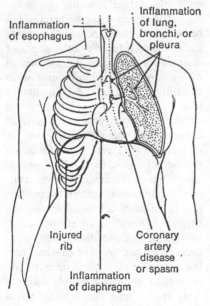

Inflammation of esophagus

Inflammation of lung, bronchi, or pleura

Injured rib

Coronary artery disease or spasm

Inflammation of diaphragm

the thoracic cavity. For example, certain types of indigestion produce a pain that may be mistaken for a heart attack. In most cases, however, the pain resulting from cardiovascular problems is the feeling of tightness and suffocation characteristic of angina pectoris. Almost all chest pains that originate in respiratory or circulatory disorders are intensified by smoking. Persistent chest pains should always be diagnosed and treated by a doctor.

childbirth *See* "Pregnancy and Childbirth."

chilblains Inflammation of the skin, accompanied by burning and itching, usually caused by exposure to cold. Special vulnerability to chilblains may result from poor circulation, inadequate diet, or an allergic response to low temperatures. The affected areas are commonly the face, hands, and feet and less frequently the ears. The areas swell and turn reddish-purple.

The condition is easier to prevent than to treat. Anyone sensitive to the cold should always wear warm clothes, especially woolen or partly woolen socks (never 100 percent synthetic), fleece-lined boots, and woolen gloves. Wet garments should be removed at once on coming indoors and the skin dried gently (never rubbed or massaged) with a soft towel. When chilblains have occurred, no attempts should be made to "stimulate" circulation by applying extreme heat or cold to the affected areas. In most cases a warm dry environment will bring about a return to normal. If the symptoms persist or if blisters form on the skin surface, a doctor should be consulted for further instructions.

chills A sudden onset of shivering or shaking, accompanied by the sensation of cold and by uncontrollable chattering of the teeth; the technical term for the condition is rigor. It should not be confused with feeling "chilly" because of a sudden draft or drop in the temperature. Chills are usually followed by fever as a symptom of infection, most commonly by the bacteria that cause pneumonia, "strep" throat, food poisoning, or kidney infection. They are also associated with various tropical diseases, especially malaria. Since chills and fever are a warning of a disorder that may need prompt treatment, the doctor should be called. Until a regimen is prescribed, the patient should get into bed, remain under the covers, and keep a record of temperature readings.

chiropodist *See* PODIATRIST.

chiropractor A practitioner of a therapeutic system based on the theory that disease is caused by subluxations, that is, partial dislocations, of the vertical bones that cause pinching of the nerves emanating from them. The pinching of the nerves impairs the function of vital organs and is corrected by spinal adjustment. Chiropractors are licensed to practice in all 50 states, but since they are not medical doctors, they are forbidden by law to write prescriptions. Chiropractic fees can be reimbursed through Medicare and in most states through Medicaid and Workmen's Compensation. Although many people claim to have found relief from various symptoms, particularly back pain, through chiropractic treatment, this specialized approach to disease has yet to be scientifically proven right or wrong.

chlorine A chemical element widely used to purify public water supplies and disinfect swimming pools because it is cheap, easily manufactured, and effective against bacteria, viruses, and fungi. An excessively chlorinated swimming pool will cause temporary eye discomfort. Household bleaches containing chlorine should be kept out of the reach of children since they can cause serious damage to the membranes of the mouth and stomach if swallowed.

chloroform An easily inhaled, volatile, colorless liquid introduced as a general anesthetic around 1850 and in widespread use until replaced by equally effective and less damaging substances.

Chloromycetin Brand name of the antibiotic chloramphenicol. *See also* ANTIBIOTICS.

chlorpromazine The first of a new class of drugs now categorized as major tranquilizers. Chlorpromazine (brand name, Thorazine) was discovered in 1949 in connection with antihistamine research and successfully used in 1952 by two French doctors as a means of forestalling the onset of acute psychotic episodes in schizophrenic and manic-depressive patients. It has since been widely used in the treatment of mentally ill patients, not as a cure, but to control their disturbance. This application of chemotherapy has largely replaced electroshock treatments, previously used for the same purpose. Although chlorpromazine was also used at one time as an antidepressant, it has been replaced for this purpose by other more effective drugs.

A patient taking Thorazine on a regular basis must be given periodic tests to ascertain whether the liver is being affected adversely, whether there is any white cell aberration, and whether other negative side effects are evident. None of these effects seems to be irreversible; however, close medical supervision is necessary with the use of this medication.

choking Obstruction of the air passage in the throat by a swallowed object that has gone into the windpipe instead of into the esophagus. When food is being swallowed, an automatic mechanism closes the flap at the top of the trachea (windpipe). It is not unusual, however, for a morsel of food or, in the case of a small child, a foreign object such as a button to "go down the wrong way." This is apt to happen when a sudden intake of breath caused by laughing, talking, or coughing occurs while a person has food in her mouth. The immediate signs of choking are an inability to speak or breathe. In minutes the skin turns bluish, and unless emergency assistance is prompt, the results can be fatal.

If an infant is choking, hold the body upside down by the torso and strike its back lightly several times between the shoulder blades. For an older child or an adult use the Heimlich maneuver, a lifesaving technique illustrated in entry under HEIMLICH MANEUVER.

cholesterol A crystalline fatty alcohol found in animal fats, blood, bile, and nerve tissue. Cholesterol is synthesized in the liver and is the material from which the body's steroids, including the sex hormones, are manufactured. It is also one of the chief constituents of biliary gallstones which can now be dissolved by a drug that reduces the liver's synthesis and secretion of cholesterol.

It has been demonstrated that very high levels of cholesterol in the blood serum increase the likelihood of atherosclerotic disease and the possibility of heart attack. However, these levels can be determined only on the basis of an individual blood test, and until a doctor recommends that animal fats or eggs be eliminated from the diet, no one need eliminate these foods. *See* "Nutrition and Weight."

chorea A disorder of the nervous system characterized by involuntary jerking movements (the term comes from the Greek word meaning "dance" as in choreography); also known as St. Vitus's dance. There are two types of the disease, each named for the doctor who described it. Sydenham's chorea is an acute disease of childhood often associated with rheumatic fever, but usually there is no known explanation. Huntington's chorea is an incurable hereditary disease in which the motor disturbances usually become manifest in middle age and are associated with mental deterioration. When there is a family history of Huntington's chorea, genetic counseling is advisable before considering having children.

chromosomes Stringlike structures within the cell nucleus that contain the genetic information governing each person's inherited characteristics. Normal human body cells contain 46 paired chromosomes composed of DNA (deoxyribonucleic acid). An ovum contains 22 autosome and 1 sex (X) chromosomes. A sperm contains 22 autosome and 1 sex (X or Y) chromosomes so that when they combine during reproduction the off-

HEREDITY

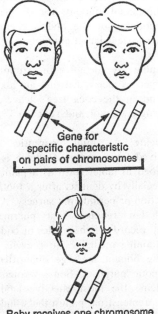

Gene for
specific characteristic
on pairs of chromosomes

Baby receives one chromosome
from each parent for each pair

spring cell receives its full complement of 46 "message carriers."

The sex of an offspring is determined by the combination of the sex chromosomes designated as X and Y. If an egg is fertilized by a sperm carrying the X chromosome, the offspring will have two X chromosomes and will therefore be female (XX). If an egg is fertilized by a Y-bearing sperm, the offspring will have one of each and will be male (XY).

Chromosomal abnormalities vary in significance, the more serious ones being responsible for birth defects, mental retardation, and spontaneous abortion.

The possibility of abnormalities severe enough to warrant abortion can be determined through prenatal genetic counseling. Research in recent years indicates that environmental and occupational exposure to various chemicals can cause irreversible damage to chromosomes, leading to genetic mutations in the offspring. Possible effects of various drugs are discussed in the chapter "Drugs, Alcohol, and Tobacco." *See also* SEX-LINKED ABNORMALITIES.

chronic symptom Symptom of a disorder that lasts over a long period of time, sometimes for the remainder of the patient's life, such as the fatigue associated with most cancers or the joint pains characteristic of rheumatoid arthritis.

circulatory system The heart and network of blood vessels throughout the body. *See* "The Healthy Woman."

cirrhosis Degenerative disease of an organ, in rare cases the heart or kidney, but generally the liver, in which the development of fibrous tissue with consequent hardening and scarring causes the loss of normal function. Cirrhosis of the liver is most frequently associated with chronic alcoholism. However, the condition may also occur after infectious hepatitis or, more rarely, as a consequence of toxic hepatitis in which liver cells are damaged because of sensitivity to such drugs as chlorpromazine (Thorazine) or chloramphenicol (Chloromycetin).

Cirrhosis is insidious because it may be asymptomatic until it has resulted in irreversible damage. When symptoms are manifest, they include abdominal swelling with fluid, soreness under the rib cage, swollen ankles, weight loss, and general fatigue. In advanced cases the signs are jaundice evident in the yellowing of the skin and the eyes and possible vomiting of blood leading to collapse.

When alcoholic cirrhosis is treated promptly at an early stage, the liver may repair and rehabilitate itself. Total abstention from alcohol and a diet rich in proteins and supplementary vitamins are essential to recovery.

claustrophobia An irrational, persistent, and often insurmountable fear of enclosed places such as elevators, windowless rooms, and the like.

climacteric The time in a woman's life when her childbearing capabilities come to an end; the menopause. The so-called male climacteric is characterized by the psychological stresses that accompany aging rather than the loss of reproductive potential.

clinics Medical establishments that offer treatment on an outpatient basis. A clinic may be publicly supported or privately owned; it may be free-standing or part of a hospital's many services. Special clinics exist for special functions, for example, prenatal and baby care, eye and ear, abortion, psychiatric. Medicaid clinics exist to provide treatment for the indigent.

clitoris The female genital organ located at the upper end of the vulva. The clitoris is the counterpart of the male penis and although it may vary in size and placement, it is a direct source of orgasm for most women. During sexual intercourse it becomes firm and engorged with blood. Penile, oral, manual, or other manipulation of the clitoris may be essential to the achievement of orgasm.

coagulation See BLOOD CLOTTING.

cobalt A metallic element that produces the radioactive isotope cobalt 60 used with beneficial effect in some types of cancer radiation therapy. It is also one of the elements essential in infinitesimal amounts for the healthy functioning of the body's chemistry, but is toxic in larger amounts.

cocaine A drug with stimulating properties derived from an alkaloid found in the coca tree's leaves. See "Drugs, Alcohol, and Tobacco."

codeine A mild narcotic drug derived from opium. Codeine is prescribed in tablet form as a painkiller, especially by dentists after a tooth extraction or periodontal surgery. A federal law requires that pharmacists keep records of their sales of codeine-containing medicines to prevent their being bought in large quantities for narcotic purposes. Some women find codeine the most effective analgesic for premenstrual pain; others find that it produces side effects of nausea and constipation. See "Drugs, Alcohol, and Tobacco."

coffee A beverage containing varying amounts of caffeine and producing such side effects as insomnia and heartburn, and in some people, withdrawal symptoms of headaches, irritability, and fatigue. Coffee itself, and not other caffeine-containing substances such as tea and cola beverages, is now circumstantially connected with cancer of the pancreas. This type of cancer causes about 20,000 deaths a year in the United States. Previous studies have indicated some link between coffee-drinking and diabetes, the disease caused by faulty insulin production by the pancreas. See also "Drugs, Alcohol, and Tobacco."

coitus interruptus The withdrawal of the penis before ejaculation as a means of preventing pregnancy. As a contraceptive method its failure rate is high.

cold sores *See* HERPES SIMPLEX.

colitis Inflammation of the colon (large intestine). The type most frequently encountered is mucous colitis, also known as spastic colon. Mucous colitis produces lower bowel spasms with or without cramps, accompanied by an alteration of diarrhea and constipation. Since in such cases the bowel itself has no organic impairments, the disorder is called functional colitis. A far more serious condition is ulcerative colitis, in which there is tissue impairment. A mucus and blood mixture is often found in the feces of persons with ulcerative colitis. The onset of this form of the disease typically occurs among young

adults of both sexes, eventually producing disabling attacks of diarrhea. Cancer of the colon or rectum develops in up to 10 percent of those who have had colitis for ten years or more.

The cause of colitis in any of its manifestations is presumed to be emotional stress produced by anxiety. Unfortunately, it is an illness in which cause and effect produce a vicious circle, making it difficult to treat medically. In practically all cases of ulcerative colitis psychotherapy in one form or another is indispensable to the abatement of the more disturbing symptoms. Since patterns of remission and relapse are usual, the disease must be treated with patience and care, including supervision of diet, bed rest, and elimination of as many tension-producing factors as possible. Where complications of weight loss, anemia, or infections develop, medicines with the least number of adverse side effects must be administered. In extreme cases removal of the diseased portion of the bowel is essential as a lifesaving measure.

colon *See* INTESTINES.

colostomy A surgical procedure by which an artificial anal opening is created in the abdominal wall. A colostomy may be performed as a temporary measure after bowel surgery or it may have to be a permanent procedure. Patients who have undergone a colostomy usually must regulate their diets to control the character of their stool.

colostrum The thin, pale yellow substance exuded by the breasts late in pregnancy and immediately following delivery. Colostrum contains proteins, minerals, and antibodies and provides

ULCERATIVE COLITIS

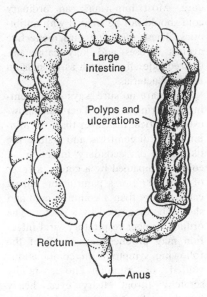

Large intestine

Polyps and ulcerations

Rectum

Anus

Mucus and blood excreted in feces

COLOSTOMY

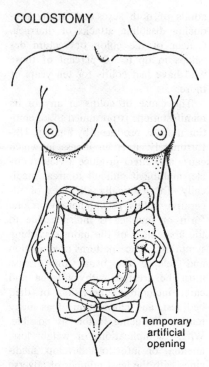

Temporary
artificial
opening

adequate nourishment for the new-born baby before breast milk becomes available, usually about the third day after birth. Mothers who do not wish to breast-feed their babies should discuss with their doctor the importance of providing them with colostrum for the two days following delivery.

colposcopy A diagnostic procedure in which a magnifying device (colposcope) is used to examine the cervix and vagina. Colposcopy requires no anesthesia and can be done in a doctor's office.

coma Deep unconsciousness resulting from, among other circumstances, injury to the brain, stroke, poisoning by barbiturates or alcohol, overdose or underdose of insulin, coronary thrombosis, or shock. Expert care should be obtained without delay, and if the victim is suffering cardiac arrest, cardiopulmonary resuscitation should be initiated.

common cold The designation for any of a large number of brief and relatively mild virus infections of the upper respiratory tract which may produce uncomfortable symptoms in the nose (rhinitis), throat (pharyngitis), or voice box (laryngitis). Since allergies to grasses and pollens produce certain overlapping symptoms, they are often mistakenly labeled "summer colds." The development of a cold vaccine has so far proved impractical because the symptoms are caused by more than 150 different viruses.

Scientific investigations have exploded many myths about colds: the infection is less contagious than once thought, taking a laxative does not dispose of cold germs, sweating does not drive the germs out of the pores of the skin, staying in bed is not a cure. Most important: an ordinary cold should *not* be treated with antibiotics. These medicines are ineffective against viruses and may cause undesired side effects such as changes in normal bacteria.

There are no sure ways of preventing or curing a cold. There are, however, practical measures that can minimize the discomforts and reduce the likelihood of secondary infection. A cold accompanied by a cough, a fever of over 100°, or a painful sore throat can be more than a common cold and should be diagnosed by a doctor. The ordinary upper respiratory viral infection may produce any or all of the following symptoms in combination: stuffed or running nose, mildly scratchy throat, teary eyes, heavy breathing, fits of sneezing, some impairment of the sense of taste and smell, mild headache, and a general feeling of lassitude. Many healthy adults do not bother to treat these symptoms and go about their business until the cold goes away, usually within three or four days. Others buy over-the-counter medicines containing antihistamines, often exchanging drowsiness for unclogged nostrils and dry eyes. The occasional use of nasal decongestants may be harmless and somewhat helpful, but overuse can have a destructive effect on delicate mucous membranes.

Whether vitamin C taken daily is effective to prevent colds is an unsettled issue. The dose usually taken for this purpose is 1 to 4 grams per day for several days. It appears that the action of vitamin C is similar to that of interferon, a substance produced in the body which suppresses virus growth. It is this protein substance that scientists hope to synthesize eventually as the most generalized and effective method of fighting the many viruses that produce common cold symptoms.

compulsion The expression of inner emotional stress through the involuntary and repetitive performance of a particular action. Compulsive behavior generally provides a certain relief from the anxiety generated by unconscious, and therefore unexpressed, feelings of rage against an individual or repressed sexuality.

conception The fertilization of the ovum by the sperm. *See* "Pregnancy and Childbirth."

concussion, cerebral Impairment of brain function resulting from a blow to the cranium or jaw. In a mild concussion there is temporary loss of consciousness with possible amnesia and emotional instability. In severe concussion there is prolonged unconciousness with possible loss of both the respiratory reflex and vasomotor activity and dilation of the pupils.

condom A protective sheath, generally made of thin rubber, that is used to cover the penis during sexual intercourse as a way of preventing sperm from entering the vagina and also as protection against venereal disease. *See* "Contraception and Abortion."

conjunctivitis Inflammation of the conjunctiva, the thin membrane that lines the eyelid and covers the front of the eye. The disorder is commonly called pink eye. Conjunctivitis may be caused by bacteria or a virus or it may be an allergic response to a new brand of eye makeup, a reaction to a chemical pollutant in the air or water, or the result of irritation from an ingrown eyelash in the lower lid. An inflammation caused by bacteria or a virus is highly contagious, and precautions should be taken to prevent its spread to others and to minimize self-reinfection. For example, the patient should use disposable paper towels to dry the face after washing. When an infectious organism is the cause, an ophthalmic antibiotic ointment is usually the effective treatment. In some cases the application of hot wet compresses several times a day will eliminate the inflammation. If it persists or shows no sign of improvement within a few days, the condition should be treated by a doctor.

consciousness-raising groups Informally organized sessions at which discussion is directed toward disclosing and confronting feelings and problems previously buried or suppressed. In the exchange of ideas and airing of emotions the participants often achieve a sense of shared purpose as well as a clearer sense of who they are, what they want, and how best to achieve it. *See* "Your Mind and Feelings."

consent laws State legislation that covers the following circumstances. (1) *The age of consent:* the age of a woman before which sexual intercourse with her is considered statutory rape whether or not she has given her consent to the act. (2) *Consent to an abortion:* some states require the written consent of a parent before a legal abortion can be performed on an unwed minor. Other laws require the consent of the husband. These are being struck down by various courts. (3) *Hospital consent forms:* a patient undergoing surgery or some other potentially hazardous procedure must sign a statement consenting to the operation. In the case of a child (defined differently in different states) or an incapacitated adult the form must be signed by a responsible member of the family. In an emergency responsibility is assumed by the hospital staff after consultation.

constipation A condition in which the fecal matter contained in the bowels is too hard to eliminate easily or in which bowel movements are so infrequent as to cause physical discomfort. The body may take from 24 to 48 hours to transform food into waste matter, and the frequency with which this waste is normally eliminated may vary from once a day to once a week, depending among other things on age, diet, amount of exercise, emotional health, and general personality traits.

The most common causes of chronic constipation unaccompanied by any organic disorder are faulty diet, insufficient exercise, emotional tension caused by the repression of anger and resentment, and chronic dependence on laxatives. Attention to these factors will generally prevent its occurrence. When constipation does occur, a cleansing enema is usually more effective than a dose of a laxative. However, the regular use of enemas or laxatives is likely to be self-defeating since it causes the bowel to depend on artificial stimulation rather than on natural signals.

The feelings of bloat, nausea, and general malaise that usually accompany constipation have nothing to do with the body's absorption of "poisons"; they are caused by messages from the nervous system reacting to a distended rectum. When these symptoms persist after elimination or when constipation itself persists in spite of all common sense treatments, the possibility of an organic disease or obstruction should be investigated by a doctor.

contact dermatitis Any skin disorder produced by substances that come in contact with the skin and cause redness, swelling, itching, hives, or other symptoms of allergic response. When the offending substance touches the skin, the blood vessels dilate, becoming more and more porous and permitting cellular fluid to seep under the skin surface. This accumulation of fluid forms blisters which eventually break. As the area dries out, crusts are formed which thicken and then flake off. Less extreme cases involve no more than a rash that itches and burns.

The first step in treatment is to eliminate the substance causing the response. Once the irritant has been removed, the skin heals eventually. In severe cases, especially where the skin is broken and vulnerable to infection, the affected surface should be covered with an antibiotic salve or ointment containing corticosteroids. If the symptoms persist even with this treatment, the doctor may prescribe cortisone to be taken orally.

contact lenses Corrective lenses placed directly on the eyeball. There are two types of contact lenses—hard and soft. Both are designed in such a way that the natural flow of tears to the surface of the cornea is unimpeded. Of the two types, hard lenses correct a larger number of sight disorders, are simpler to care for, and cost less; soft lenses are more comfortable and the wearer usually adapts to them more quickly. Because soft lenses follow the natural curve of the eye, there is less chance that foreign bodies will reach the cornea than when the cornea is covered by a hard lens. The disadvantages of soft lenses, in addition to the greater expense, are their fragility and the complicated disinfecting routine they require. An ophthalmologist or an optometrist fits contact lenses, explains exactly how they should be used, and informs the wearer as to what services and follow-up procedures are covered by the professional fee. The occasional need for small adjustments requires frequent checkups in order to safeguard the health of the eye.

contraception The prevention of conception following coitus; birth control. *See* "Contraception and Abortion."

contraceptives Chemical or mechanical means to prevent conception following coitus. Chemical methods are hormonal (oral contraceptive) or spermicidal (foam, cream, jelly, vaginal suppository, and the medicated intrauterine device). Mechanical methods are the condom, diaphragm, and nonmedicated intrauterine device. *See* "Contraception and Abortion."

contraction The action of the muscular walls of the uterus by which the infant is propelled from the uterus through the birth canal. *See* "Pregnancy and Childbirth."

convalescence The transitional period between an operation, injury, or illness and the reestablishment of normal health, strength, and emotional equilibrium. Many convalescents try to push themselves beyond their actual stage of endurance. They may do so to prove to others that they are well or because they feel guilty about not being able to accomplish daily activities for which they are normally responsible. It is most important not to try to do too much as it only postpones or jeopardizes full recovery. The doctor is the one who should decide when a normal routine can be resumed.

A prolonged convalescence following a critical illness, major surgery, or an accident often requires special attention and long periods of bed rest. A visiting nurse or a nurse's aide may be needed to provide sufficient home care, but should the convalescent require constant supervision, an extended care facility connected with the hospital may be a more practical solution. A woman in charge of the convalescence of another family member should work out ways of sharing responsibilities, explaining to each person exactly what is expected.

convulsions Violent and abnormal muscular contractions or spasms that seize the body suddenly and spontaneously, usually ending with unconsciousness. Convulsions are almost always a symptom of a serious disorder and they are the classic manifestation of the grand mal seizures of epilepsy. They are not uncommon among children during infections of the nervous system or during generalized infections that cause a very high fever. Convulsions in late pregnancy are a sign of the toxemia known as eclampsia and usually are preceded by other warning signs. Convulsions are one of the critical consequences of unsupervised and sudden withdrawal from barbiturates following heavy and habitual use. They may also occur in adulthood from a tumor or from diseases that attack the brain and central nervous system, especially encephalitis and meningitis.

At first sign of seizure the mouth should be opened (forced open if necessary) and something (a knotted handkerchief, a wadded piece of sheet, or a smooth stick) put between the upper and lower teeth to keep the mouth open so that an airway can be maintained and to keep the patient from biting his tongue. If the tongue is swallowed, keep the mouth wide open and free the tongue with a finger. Then seek medical attention.

cornea The transparent tissue that forms the outer layer of the eyeball, covering the iris and the lens through which vision is achieved. It is a continuation of the tough sclera (the "white" of the eye). The most serious disease that affects the cornea is herpes simplex keratitis; it causes more loss of vision in the Western world than any other corneal infection. When this virus attacks the tissues, painful ulcers form and to date there is no successful cure for the condition. The infection may recur frequently causing progressive impairment each time.

Corneal dystrophy is an inherited disease in which there is a progressive loss of vision resulting from an increasing cloudiness of the tissue. Corneal dystrophy as well as vision impairment caused by damage to the cornea can be corrected by a corneal transplant.

corneal transplant The removal of an impaired cornea and its replacement with a clear, healthy one. This operation, which originated in the 1920s, is the most successful of all tissue transplants. Ideally, a cornea should be removed within 6 hours of death and transplanted within 24 hours. The Eye Bank for Sight Restoration, of which there are chapters throughout the world, receives donor eyes through bequests and can preserve them for 2 to 3 days. Most large cities have ophthalmological specialists who can perform corneal transplants. Some operations are scheduled well in advance; others are performed under emergency conditions. The patient is given either local or general anesthesia before the transplant and full vision is usually restored no more than three days after surgery.

corns An area of thickened skin (callus) that occurs on or between the toes. There are two types of corns: hard corns which are usually located on the small toe or on the upper ridge of one of the other toes; soft and white corns which are likely to develop between the fourth and fifth toe. The hard core of both types of callus points inward and when pressed against the surrounding tissue causes pain. Corns are the result of wearing shoes that are too tight, and unless proper footwear is worn they will recur.

Treating corns at home with razor blades or with strongly medicated "removers" can injure surrounding tissues, resulting in additional discomfort and sometimes in serious infection. The sensible course is a visit to a podiatrist.

coronary artery disease *See* HEART ATTACK.

corpus luteum The ovarian follicle after it releases its ovum. The corpus luteum produces the hormone progesterone which prepares the lining of the uterus for possible implantation of a fertilized ovum and is essential to the maintenance of pregnancy. If conception occurs, the corpus luteum continues to produce progesterone for a short time until the placenta takes over this function. If conception does not occur, the progesterone level drops, the corpus luteum degenerates, and menstruation starts.

corticosteroids A group of hormones produced from cholesterol by the adrenal cortex; now also synthesized in the laboratory. The original biochemical designation for these hormones was adrenocorticosteroids. At least 30 of these substances have been identified, of which the best known is cortisone. Among their many functions are regulation of the water and salt balance of body fluids and assistance in protein metabolism, antibody formation, and repair of damaged tissue.

The fact that these steroids suppress inflammation of the joints and reduce the destructive effects of rheumatic fever and kidney inflammations has provided successful treatment for a large number of disorders formerly unresponsive to drug therapy. For people suffering from Addison's disease (nonfunction of the adrenal cortex) they play the same vital role in lifetime replacement therapy as insulin does for some diabetics. Overproduction of cortical hormones causes Cushing's syndrome.

cortisone *See* CORTICOSTEROIDS.

cosmetic surgery *See* PLASTIC SURGERY; "Cosmetic Surgery."

cosmetics Preparations designed to enhance the appearance. Cosmetic preparations must meet the standards of the Food and Drug Administration for health protection. On occasion there is a justifiable concern over an ingredient in a particular product: a potential cancer-causing red dye found in a lipstick, dangerous amounts of asbestos dust in an expensive dusting powder, a lung-damaging chemical in a spray-on hair lacquer. The purchaser should make a habit of reading the fine print and warnings that appear on all packages and in the enclosed printed material. This is usually the only way to find out whether the manufacturer has been required by the FDA to indicate that some ingredient "may be harmful to health."

Cold creams, cleansing creams, lubricating lotions, and moisturizers should be judged on their merits and individual suitability, not on their cost or expensive packaging. Cosmetics advertised as containing "secret formulas" or special medications should be checked out with a knowledgeable person or doctor to make certain the product is not harmful. Any product which produces an allergic reaction, such as a rash or puffy eyelids, should, of course, not be used. Special hypoallergenic cosmetics and soaps are available for those who require them. Since infections can be spread by powder puffs, lipsticks, or makeup brushes, articles of this type should not be borrowed or lent.

coughing A reflex action for the purpose of clearing the lining of the air passages of an excessive accumulation of mucus or disturbing foreign matter. A cough is achieved by the following mechanism: a deep breath is drawn; the glottis which controls the passage of air through the windpipe is closed; pressure is built up in the chest by the contraction of muscles; the glottis suddenly opens causing an explosive release of air to sweep through the air passages. The air expulsed carries with it foreign irritants such as dust, particles of food, or abnormal secretions that are irritating the larynx, trachea, or bronchial tubes. Coughing may also be a psychological manifestation of boredom or a means of attracting attention.

Medicines that loosen the secretions resulting from an inflammatory condition of the mucous membranes and make it easier to cough them up are called expectorants. The congestion may also be loosened and coughed up after treatment with hot tea, hot lemonade and honey, or steam inhalation. It is advisable to rid the air passages of the accumulated mucus by coughing it up, but if coughing interferes with sleep, the doctor may decide that a cough suppressant is necessary. Suppressant medicines often contain codeine or some other opiate which requires a prescription.

Coughs associated with common colds may last two to three weeks after all other symptoms have disappeared. A cough that lasts longer or causes pain in the chest is the sign of a chronic condition that should be discussed with a doctor. Early diagnosis of the underlying cause of a chronic cough followed by proper treatment and no smoking can help prevent the onset of emphysema, lung cancer, or other respiratory disease.

crabs Parasites, also known as pubic lice, that infest the genital and anal hairs, causing extreme itching and irritation. *See* "Sexually Transmissible Diseases."

cramps *See* ABDOMINAL PAIN.

cryosurgery Operations in which tissues are destroyed by freezing them, usually with supercold liquid nitrogen or carbon dioxide. Cryosurgery is frequently used for the removal of hemorrhoids, warts, and moles and for treatment of cervical erosion. Cryosurgical instruments are also used successfully in certain types of delicate brain surgery.

curettage A procedure in which the walls of a body cavity are scraped with an instrument called a curette in order to remove a tissue sample for examination or to remove unwanted tissue.

Cushing's syndrome A group of symptoms caused by the presence in the body of an excess of corticosteroid hormones. Formerly, Cushing's syndrome was a rare disorder resulting in most cases from overactivity of the adrenal cortex because of a glandular tumor or from hyperfunction of the pituitary gland. It has become more common, now resulting from the side effects of medication containing steroids prescribed as long-term therapy for chronic diseases of the kidneys, the joints, etc.

Early symptoms include weakness, facial puffiness ("moon" face), and fluid retention, followed by general obesity and an interruption of menstruation.

When Cushing's syndrome is attributable to glandular malfunction caused by a tumor, surgery is essential. If total removal of the gland is indicated, replacement therapy of the corticosteroid hormones is necessary for the remainder of one's life.

cuts *See* FIRST AID.

cyanosis A blue appearance of the blood and mucous membranes caused by an inadequate amount of oxygen in the arterial blood. A cyanotic appearance is one of the first signs of a number of respiratory diseases in which lung function is so impaired that the blood cannot take up a sufficient amount of oxygen. Cyanosis is also a characteristic of certain heart diseases characterized by abnormal shunting of blood. The cyanotic characteristic of the so-called blue baby is due to a congenital heart defect that leads to an excess of unoxygenated arterial blood. Surgery often is helpful in correcting such defects.

cyst An abnormal cavity filled with a fluid or semifluid substance. While some cysts do become malignant, most are harmless and are often reabsorbed by the surrounding tissues, leaving no trace of their existence. A benign cyst that interferes with the proper functioning of an adjacent organ, such as a gland, is removed in an operation called a cystectomy.

There are several categories of cysts. Retention cysts occur when the opening of a secreting gland is blocked, causing the secretion to back up and form a swelling. In this category are several different types. Sebaceous cysts cause a lump to appear under the skin. Mucous cysts are commonly found in the mucous membranes of the mouth, nose, genitals, or inside the lips or cheeks. Breast cysts may result from a chronic mastitis that causes the ducts leading to the nipples to be blocked by the development of fibrous tissue. Kidney cysts are a congenital defect eventually proliferating to the point where they interfere with kidney function.

Pilonidal cysts form in the cleft between the buttocks. They are called "pilonidal," which means literally resembling a "nest of hair," because the folding over of the skin in the cleft between the buttocks results in ingrown hairs that block the pores of the ducts leading outward from the sebaceous glands. When the retained secretions accumulate and back up, the affected area becomes swollen and painfully inflamed. When the cyst is small, treatment need be no more complicated than warm sitz baths to open and drain the abscess. The open cyst is covered with an antibiotic ointment to prevent the complication of bacterial invasion. A pilonidal cyst that becomes chronic and recurs with uncomfortable frequency may require surgical removal.

When a retention cyst develops in the Bartholin's glands in the vagina, infection and inflammation may occur blocking the gland and its secretions and surgical removal of the gland may be recommended to prevent the development of an abscess. Other cysts are formed by the slow seepage of blood into a tissue, forming a pocket similar to a tumor. These are called hematomas and can be under the skin, under a fingernail, in a muscle, or elsewhere.

Parasitic cysts are caused by certain types of tapeworms which enter the body in the form of eggs. Once the eggs hatch in the intestines, the microscopic embryos settle in the kidneys or liver, forming cysts large enough to be dangerous and to require prompt surgical removal. Parasites, such as those responsible for amebic dysentery and trichinosis do not cause a cyst to develop in the tissues of the human host, but form and encase themselves in their own cysts as part of their life cycle.

The category referred to as ovarian cysts includes a variety of different types. *See* "Gynecologic Diseases and Treatment."

cystic fibrosis An inherited, disabling respiratory disease of early childhood. The disease is genetically transmitted to offspring when both parents are carriers; when only one parent is a carrier, some of the offspring may also be carriers. Although there is no known cure for cystic fibrosis, new treatments have increased the life expectancy of patients with the disease. Prenatal genetic counseling can detect the presence of the disease in the fetus, thus giving the parents the option of an induced abortion at an early stage of the pregnancy.

cystitis *See* BLADDER DISORDERS.

cystocele A hernia in which part of the bladder protrudes into the vagina. A cystocele causes a feeling of discomfort in the lower abdomen and may produce bladder incontinence. The abnormal position of the bladder results in an accumulation of residual urine that increases the possibility of bacterial infection. Surgical correction is therefore advisable.

cystoscopy A diagnostic procedure in which the inner surface of the bladder is examined by an optical instrument called a cystoscope. The procedure, usually performed by a specialist known as a urologist, consists of passing the cystoscope through the opening of the urethra into the bladder. The doctor can detect inflammation, tumors, or stones by means of an illuminated system of mirrors and lenses and can obtain tissue samples. If diagnostic X-rays are to be taken during a cystoscopy, a catheter may be passed through the hollow tube of the instrument in order to inject radiopaque substances into the bladder.

D&C *See* DILATATION AND CURETAGE.

D&E *See* DILATATION AND EVACUATION.

DTs *See* DELIRIUM TREMENS.

dandruff A scalp disorder characterized by the abnormal flaking of dead skin. The underlying cause of the condition is not known, but it is directly related to the way in which the sebaceous glands function. There is no evidence that dandruff is triggered by an infectious organism.

Normal skin constantly renews itself as dead skin cells are shed. Oily dandruff is the result of overactivity of the tiny oil glands at the base of the hair roots, accelerating the shedding process. The hair becomes greasy and the skin flakings are yellowish and crusty, similar to the flakings that characterize "cradle cap" in infants. A dry type of dandruff occurs when the sebaceous glands are plugged, causing the hair to lose its natural gloss and the flaking to be dry and grayish. In either type of dandruff it is important not to scratch the scalp, as broken skin may lead to infection.

There are several medicines that can control dandruff and sometimes eliminate it. If over-the-counter shampoos containing tar, salicylic acid, or sulfur prove ineffective, treatment by a prescribed medication may be necessary.

deafness *See* HEARING LOSS.

death Traditionally, the end of life was presumed to have occurred when breathing ceased and the heart was still. The increasing technological means for prolonging life and the concern of the medical profession as to precisely when a donor's organs should be removed for transplantation have created a compelling need for a "redefinition" of death in terms acceptable to both the legal and medical professions. Various state legislatures have statutes in which death is equated with the irreversible cessation of brain function. The criteria for brain-death are generally accepted by the medical profession throughout the world. The creation of similar state laws is essential for the prevention of civil or criminal liability suits against a hospital or a doctor that signs a patient's death certificate. Passage of brain-death legislation has the active support of the three major religious denominations as well as the most prestigious organizations of the legal and medical professions.

Following the lead of California, several states are enacting a "right-to-die" law which gives people the opportunity to make out living wills prohibiting the use of unusual or artificial devices to prolong their lives if they become terminally ill. More and more frequently, doctors are discussing the subject of dying among themselves, with their patients, and with the families of terminally ill patients. Many communities have organized patients' rights movements and death-with-dignity organizations to facilitate the passage of laws like the California law. Group activity of this type can be gratifying and a means for the living to confront their own mortality.

deficiency disease A disorder caused by the absence of an essential nutrient in the diet. Not until the twentieth-century discovery of the vital role of vitamins was this category of disease understood, although before that time people had discovered through trial and error what foods or extracts appeared to prevent particular disabilities, such as the control of rickets with cod liver oil (rich in vitamin D) and the control of scurvy with citrus juice (rich in vitamin C). Pellagra was once prevalent in areas where meat, eggs, or other foods containing niacin were precluded, due to poverty, from the diet. This deficiency disease has practically disappeared through the use of synthesized niacin as an additive in commercially processed foods. Certain types of blindness and skin ulcers, once thought to be infectious ailments, were discovered to be the result of diets deficient in liver, eggs, and other foods rich in vitamin A. Margarine and many other widely used items are now fortified with vitamin A. Beriberi, a deficiency disease that produces gastrointestinal and neurological disturbances, is caused by a lack of fresh vegetables, whole grains, and certain meats, all of which contain vitamin B_1 (thiamine). Mild beriberi symptoms are likely to appear among people on restricted diets, among alcoholics, and among crash dieters who fail to take supplementary doses of this essential nutriment. All of these deficiency diseases, however, are rare in the United States, in large part due to the multivitamin fortification of bread.

degenerative disease A category of disorders having in common the progressive deterioration of a part or parts of the body, leading to increasing interference with normal function. Among the more common of the degenerative diseases are the various forms of arthritis, cerebrovascular disabilities caused by the dystrophy diseases that impair neuromuscular function, arteriosclerosis, and the many disorders connected with progressive malfunction of the heart and lungs.

dehydration An abnormal loss of body fluids. Deprivation of water and essential electrolytes (sodium and potassium) for a prolonged period can lead to shock, acidosis, acute uremia, and, especially in the case of infants and the aged, to death. Under normal circumstances water accounts for well over half the total body weight. The adult woman loses about 3 pints of fluid a day in urine; the amount of water in feces is variable, but may account for another 3 or 4 ounces; vaporization through the skin (perspiration) and the lungs (breath expiration) account for another 2 pints. Normal consumption of food and water generally replaces this loss. A temporary increase in the loss of body fluid due to heat, exertion, or mild diarrhea is usually accompanied by extreme thirst or a dry tongue and can be rectified simply by drinking an additional amount of liquid. Salt pills are not always necessary as an aid to fluid retention.

The body becomes dehydrated if the daily fluid intake cannot compensate for fluid loss. Dehydration results from an extraordinary loss of fluids for reasons such as accident or illness; excessive perspiration through fever, extreme heat, or overactivity; or excessive production of urine due to the use of diuretics. Severe dehydration may require intravenous fluid replenishment. The fever, diarrhea, and vomiting that are characteristic in cases of gastroenteritis and cholera (and, to a lesser degree, dysentery) can cause dehydration that is severe enough to be fatal if it is not treated by intravenous fluid and electrolyte replacement. Dehydration that accompanies the acidosis signaling the onset of diabetic coma or of certain kidney diseases requires prompt hospitalization and treatment. Severe dehydration should be reported to a doctor for proper medical attention.

delirium tremens (DTs) Literally, a trembling delirium; a psychotic state observed in chronic alcoholics as a result of withdrawal of alcohol. The condition is characterized by confusion, nausea, vivid hallucinations, and uncontrollable tremors. The victim of delirium tremens may become obstreperous and therefore should be hospitalized for self-protection as well as for the treatment of chronic alcoholism. Until a doctor or ambulance arrives, the victim should be confined to a well-lighted room that is free of sharp or breakable objects and calmly reassured that help is imminent.

delivery See "Pregnancy and Childbirth."

delusions False and persistent beliefs contrary to or unsubstantiated by facts or objective circumstance; one of the symptoms of mental illness. Delusions are false beliefs, as differentiated from hallucinations which are false sense impressions. As an example, an individual suffering from paranoid schizophrenia may have delusions of being destroyed by people who are thought to be enemies. In true paranoia the delusion becomes the focus of all activity. Some delusions are difficult to recognize and the person is merely thought of as an eccentric. When a delusion takes the form of ordering the individual to commit an inappropriate act, hospitalization is mandatory.

Demerol Brand name of the sedative and analgesic drug meperidine, a synthesized crystalline narcotic.

dental care The strength or weakness of one's teeth begins with one's genetic inheritance combined with the prenatal health and diet of one's mother. (Pregnant women please note.) However, good health, good habits of oral hygiene, and periodic dental checkups are the most important factors in preventing the decay of teeth. Tooth decay is incurable and irreversible, and prompt treatment of cavities is essential. A cavity should be filled before decay advances beyond the enamel. Otherwise bacteria may penetrate the dentin and attack the pulp chamber of the tooth. This may produce an infection that not only kills the tooth, but, in extreme cases, may spread throughout the body causing bacteremia and possibly bacterial endocarditis, a serious inflammation of the lining of the heart.

A vaccine immunizing against tooth decay is one of the long-range goals of the National Institute of Dental Research. Until such a vaccine is available, the most effective means of preventing dental caries is through regular visits to the dentist for checkups and cleanings and proper home hygiene. X-rays should be taken only when absolutely necessary. The American Dental Association makes the following recommendations. Rinse your mouth thoroughly after eating anything containing starch or sugar. Plain water will do, or you may use a mouthwash of ¼ teaspoon of baking soda or ½ teaspoon of salt dissolved in ½ glass of water. Deposits of food should be removed after each meal or, at the very least, before bedtime by using a brush with properly resilient bristles to clean every surface of every tooth and by using unwaxed floss to remove accumulations between the teeth.

Since dental fees vary considerably, not only in different parts of the country, but in the same city or town, it is wise to discuss fees with the dentist prior to treatment. The latest American Dental Association national survey of dentists indicates that the following charges are typical:

Examination	$10.00
Cleaning	$15.00
Complete mouth X-ray	$25.00
Single extraction	$15.00
One surface amalgam (permanent filling)	$15.00
Gold-inlay restoration (one surface)	$100.00
Root-canal therapy (molar, one canal, excluding filling)	$200.00
Porcelain crown	$200.00
Complete upper or lower denture with six months' post-delivery care	$300.00

dental caries Tooth decay, in particular cavities caused by bacteria. *Streptococcus mutans,* a microorganism that induces cavities, is related to the bacterial agent that causes strep throat. Some people appear to inherit an immunity to caries. The decay results from bacteria feeding on sugar and producing a corrosive acid. There are billions of bacteria in the saliva, but only *S. mutans* appears capable of creating an adhesive out of sucrose that adheres to the enamel tooth surface gradually destroying it. *See* DENTAL CARE.

dentin The hard calcified tissue that forms the body of a tooth under the enamel surface. When bacterial decay spreads from the enamel into the dentin, a toothache is likely to occur. If this symptom is ignored, the bacteria will eventually invade the pulp and increase the probability of the death of the tooth.

dentures Artificial teeth used to replace some or all natural teeth. Dentures may be removable or permanently attached to adjacent teeth. While preventive dentistry has reduced the number of women who need dentures at an early age, the loss of some teeth is almost inevitable with advancing age. Teeth should be replaced promptly to avoid the possibility of a chewing impairment, a speech impediment, or the collapse of facial structure caused by the empty spaces. In addition, missing teeth imperil the health of the adjacent natural ones. Dental materials and techniques used today make it virtually impossible to distinguish between a person's artificial and natural teeth.

deodorants Over-the-counter products containing chemicals that slow down the bacterial growth in perspiration, thus diminishing the likelihood of unpleasant body odor. Unlike antiperspirants, deodorants do not inhibit the amount of perspiration itself. Vaginal deodorants advertised for "feminine daintiness" should be avoided because of their irritating effect on tissue. Daily use of a pleasantly scented mild soap is a safer, cheaper, and sufficiently effective way of keeping the genital area clean.

deoxyribonucleic acid *See* DNA.

depilatory *See* HAIR REMOVAL.

depressant A category of drugs that produce a calming, sedative effect by reducing the functional activity of the central nervous system. *See* "Drugs, Alcohol, and Tobacco."

depression A feeling that life has no meaning and that no activity is worth the effort; profound feelings of sadness, discouragement, or self-deprecation. *See* "Your Mind and Feelings."

dermabrasion A procedure in which the outermost layers of the skin are removed by planing the skin with an abrasive device. *See* "Cosmetic Surgery."

dermatitis Inflammation of the skin, often accompanied by redness, itching, swelling, and a rash. Inflammation caused by direct contact with an irritant is called contact dermatitis; inflammation caused by psychological stress is called neurodermatitis. Types caused by viruses, bacteria, fungi, or parasites are called infectious dermatitis; they are discussed under entries entitled BOIL, FUNGUS INFECTIONS, HIVES, and IMPETIGO. Other forms appear under the headings CHILBLAINS, FROSTBITE, and HIVES. *See also* CONTACT DERMATITIS, RASHES.

DES (diethylstilbestrol) A synthetic nonsteroidal estrogen hormone. DES was first prescribed in the 1950s to prevent miscarriage. In 1971 it was discovered to be the specific cause of a rare type of vaginal cancer found at a young age in a few female offspring of women who took the hormone. This cancer, previously rare in women under 50, is called adenocarcinoma; it is an *iatrogenic* cancer, that is, a cancer inadvertently caused by prescribed medication.

Approximately 4 to 6 million people (mothers, daughters, sons) were exposed to DES, mainly in the 1950s. Of the daughters born to these women ("DES daughters"), about 1.4 per 1,000 to 10,000 developed clear cell adenocarcinoma of the vagina or cervix. Less than 200 such cases (often effectively treatable) have been identified in the United States. Other DES daughters, perhaps about the same number, may develop squamous cell cancer of the vagina or cervix. A larger number of DES daughters have developed minor vaginal abnormalities, called adenosis, which apparently have no functional or other effect on the women. Some of these daughters have uterine conditions that cause miscarriages and problems during labor. DES daughters should be examined periodically by a gynecologist starting in their early teens. The possible effects of DES on the male offspring of DES mothers are not completely understood, but seem to be related to an abnormal urethra. Some of these sons have reduced fertility. For DES mothers, there is a suspected risk of breast and gynecologic cancers. For further information on DES contact DES Registry, Inc., 5426 27th Street, NW, Washington, D.C. 20015.

desensitization A process whereby an individual allergic to a particular substance is periodically injected with a diluted extract of the allergen in order to build up a tolerance to it.

detoxification A form of therapy, usually conducted in a hospital, whereby the patient is deprived of an addictive drug and given a substitute one in diminishing doses. Alcohol detoxification produces severe withdrawal symptoms which can be eased by the use of sedatives on a transitional basis. When detoxification has

been accomplished, a program of physical and psychological rehabilitation is usually essential.

Dexedrine Brand name for dextroamphetamine, a drug that has a greater stimulating effect on the central nervous system than amphetamine by itself.

dextrose A variant of glucose. *See* GLUCOSE.

diabetes A chronic hereditary disease characterized by the presence of an excess of glucose in the blood and urine due to an inability to metabolize glucose normally, usually as a result of an insufficient production of insulin by the pancreas. Although the basic cause of diabetes is still unknown, the condition can be controlled if treated

DIABETES

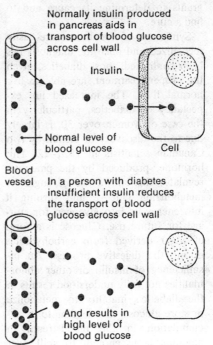

Normally insulin produced in pancreas aids in transport of blood glucose across cell wall

Insulin

Normal level of blood glucose

Cell

Blood vessel

In a person with diabetes insufficient insulin reduces the transport of blood glucose across cell wall

And results in high level of blood glucose

correctly. The full name of the disease is diabetes mellitus, roughly translatable from the Greek and Latin as "a passing through of honey."

According to the American Diabetes Association, the number of diabetics is increasing, with approximately 10 million Americans being affected at this time. Of this number, 6 million are aware of having the disease and are under treatment; the other 4 million are unaware of their diabetic condition or are not being treated for it. Adult onset diabetes is the direct cause of at least 38,000 deaths a year and is considered to be the indirect cause of an additional 300,000 deaths. Thus it can be considered the third highest cause of death in the United States. Concern about this major health problem has resulted in the allocation by the federal government in recent years of about $75 million in annual research grants to determine its cause and to find a cure.

Symptoms of the disease are easily recognized and once the diagnosis has been confirmed, most diabetics, given the proper treatment, are able to live normal lives. The increased life expectancy of diabetics, particularly in the case of women over 30, is largely due to the discovery of insulin by two Canadian scientists in 1921–22. This hormone, produced by the pancreas, regulates the body's use of sugar by metabolizing glucose and turning it into energy or into glycogen for storage for future use. Glucose is a form of sugar derived from carbohydrates during the digestive process. An insufficiency of insulin or other abnormalities not fully understood results in the diabetic's inability to metabolize or store glucose, thus leading to its accumulation in the bloodstream in amounts large enough to spill over

into the urine. This metabolic aberration causes the characteristic symptoms of diabetes: frequent urination due to the abnormal amount of urine produced to accommodate the excess glucose that the kidneys filters out of the blood, chronic thirst, an excessive hunger. Dramatic weight loss occurs because, being unable to use glucose, the diabetic must use body fat and protein as a source of energy. In order to reach the proper balance of insulin production and glucose conversion, which is constantly being regulated by the normal body, each diabetic must be individually stabilized through a controlled regimen of medication, diet, and energy output.

In addition to the previously mentioned symptoms, other symptoms that indicate the possibility of diabetes are drowsiness and fatigue; changes in vision; repeated infections of the kidneys, gums, or skin; intense itching without a known cause; and cramps in the extremities. Any woman with symptoms suggesting diabetes should have a urine and blood sugar test. There is also a simple laboratory procedure, the glucose tolerance test, that can identify prediabetics, thus alerting the doctor and patient to the possible onset of the disease.

When medication is essential to maintain normal blood sugar levels, the amount of insulin needed is determined initially by the level of glucose in the blood. Thereafter it usually can be determined by the level of glucose in the urine which is tested regularly by the patient. Variations in the results of the urine tests are the guide to necessary adjustments in diet, medication, and exercise. The use of oral drugs that stimulate the pancreas to produce its own insulin is now being reevaluated, especially since many of these drugs have been removed from the market by the FDA after a significant number of fatalities resulted from their side effects.

With the combined efforts of patient and doctor, satisfactory control can be attained and is reflected in the patient's general feeling of well-being, the maintenance of normal blood sugar and negative urine tests, and a minimal fluctuation of weight. Many authorities now believe that less severe cases of diabetes can be controlled successfully by diet and exercise alone.

Control is essential in order to avoid two specific reactions: hypoglycemia, a condition in which the blood sugar level is too low, and hyperglycemia, in which it is too high.

Hypoglycemia is likely to occur if the diabetic does not eat additional food to compensate for physical exertion, skips a meal, or takes too much insulin. Onset is sudden, the symptoms being nervous irritability, moist skin, and a tingling tongue. The situation can be corrected quickly by promptly eating or drinking anything containing sugar—a spoonful of honey, a glass of orange juice, a piece of candy, or a lump of sugar.

Hyperglycemia accompanied by acidosis and diabetic coma was the chief cause of early death in diabetics before the discovery of insulin. While rare today, hyperglycemic reaction does occur when the diabetic fails to take the necessary amount of insulin. Blood sugar builds up to a point at which the body begins to burn proteins and fats, a process that ends in the formation of chemicals known as ketones. When the accumulation of ketones leads to a critical imbalance in the body's acid concentration, the result can be diabetic coma. This condition is characterized by a hot dry skin, labored breathing, abdominal pain, and drowsiness. The patient should be hospitalized immediately so that the correct doses of insulin can be administered. A diabetic should carry cubes of sugar and wear a diabetic identification tag or bracelet at all times. *See* MEDIC ALERT.

A woman with diabetes may be concerned about whether she can or should become pregnant. While fertility is generally unaffected, once conception occurs, the blood sugar level of a diabetic woman may rise precipitously and behave erratically throughout the pregnancy. It is therefore essential that urine tests be made three or four times a day and that the blood sugar level be checked during prenatal visits as a guide to adjusting the dose of insulin. If the mother-to-be takes proper care of herself, there is every reason to expect a normal, healthy baby. Although diabetes is a genetic disease, the pattern of inheritance appears more complicated than originally assumed, making it impossible to predict the likelihood of transmission. Genetic counseling can be most helpful in this regard.

Diabetes that develops after having a baby or at middle age may not present the usual symptoms of urine frequency, thirst, and excessive appetite, but may be discovered because of a persistent skin infection or in some other way. In women over 60 a comparatively asymptomatic diabetes may lead to arteriosclerosis and in turn to a stroke or heart attack. Related disorders of vision, kidney function, and the nervous system may also develop in cases of delayed or improper control of diabetes.

Most diabetics lead a productive and fulfilling life, both on a personal and professional level. Women applying for jobs are protected by a federal law which prevents employers from discriminating against applicants solely on the basis of this disorder. Diabetics should be in touch with their local chapter of the American Diabetes Association. This organization provides information on current research, job options, travel possibilities, summer camps, and international affiliations. It publishes a bimonthly magazine called *Diabetes Forecast* containing practical material on menu planning and medical equipment and providing a forum for an exchange of ideas on living as a diabetic or with one. If there is no listing in the telephone directory, write directly to American Diabetes Association, 600 Fifth Avenue, New York, N.Y. 10020.

diabetic retinopathy An abnormal condition in the retina occurring among diabetics who have had the disease for a prolonged period of time. Diabetic retinopathy was practically unknown until the lives of diabetics were extended by the use of insulin. Leakage of blood and fluid from the retina's tiny blood vessels is the cause of the condition and the degree of vision impairment depends on the extent of the leakage. If the retinal hemorrhage is extensive and leads to a proliferation of "new" vessels and obstructive fibrous tissue, surgery is essential to prevent sight deterioration. Photocoagulation is the treatment in which a laser beam is directed at the diseased retinal tissue in an attempt to destroy it and prevent it from activating new obstructive tissue growth.

dialysis The separation of waste matter and water from the bloodstream by mechanical means, usually in cases of kidney failure. This form of "blood washing" prolongs the life of many thousands of patients who might otherwise die of renal failure. The dialysis machine, which may be installed in the home of the patient or used at a hospital or special clinic, is connected to the body by a complex arrangement of tubes. Blood containing impurities and wastes, that would normally be filtered out by healthy kidneys, runs through one set of tubes past a thin membrane. On the other side of the membrane is a solution which extracts salt wastes, excess water, and other substances from the blood by osmotic pressure. The cleansed blood is then returned to the body through another set of tubes. This procedure is routinely followed at least three times a week and takes about four hours per treatment.

The machine that serves as an artificial kidney to accomplish this procedure is costly, and patients using it require medical supervision for the rest of their lives. There are over 22,000 people in the United States on dialysis programs. The number increased considerably after Congress passed a law in 1973 amending the Social Security Act to extend Medicare funds to anyone under 65 suffering from kidney failure.

diaphragm A rubber, dome-shaped cap inserted over the cervix to prevent conception. *See* "Contraception and Abortion."

diaphragm The large muscle that lies across the middle of the body, separating the thoracic and abdominal cavities. The diaphragm is convex in shape when relaxed. Approximately 20 times a minute, upon receiving signals from the area of the brain that controls the respiratory process, it tenses and flattens so that the thoracic cavity enlarges, thus enabling the lungs to expand each time a breath is taken.

Many nerves pass through this muscle and it also contains large openings to accommodate the aorta, the thoracic duct, and the esophagus. When there is a weakening of the muscle structure that surrounds the esophagus, the stomach may push upward into the hole, causing the disorder known as a diaphragmatic or hiatus hernia. Involuntary spasms of the diaphragm are the cause of hiccups.

diarrhea Abnormally frequent and watery bowel movements usually related to an inflammation of the intestinal wall. The inflammation may follow infection caused by microorganisms that produce food poisoning or dysentery. Causes of diarrhea may be food, alcohol, a new medication, too strong a cathartic, an allergy, excitement or emotional stress. Some women have mild diarrhea with the onset of menopause, and practically all women have diarrhea before the onset of labor. At times it is accompanied by stomach cramps, nausea, vomiting, and a feeling of debility due to loss of body fluids and salt.

Chronic diarrhea may be a symptom of any of the following: thyroid disturbance, especially hyperthyroidism, nonspecific ulcerative colitis, a cyst or tumor of the bowel, low level chemical poisoning, and alcoholism.

The weakening effects of a brief siege of diarrhea can be remedied by the replacement of lost fluids and a bland diet. If the condition persists, the doctor may request a stool sample for laboratory analysis. If no infectious agent is discovered, diagnosis may involve internal examination with a proctoscope (a lighted tube which is passed into the rectum) or sigmoidoscope (a similar device for examining the sigmoid colon), blood tests, or a barium test.

diathermy Treatment by heat generated within the body by tissue resistance to the passage of high frequency electric current. The machines that produce the current are designed with various attachments shaped to fit the parts of the body that need treatment. Medical diathermy makes use of slight heat for purposes of muscle rehabilitation and tissue healing as one of the aspects of physical therapy. Surgical diathermy generates enough heat to coagulate and destroy body cells. As a procedure for removing warts and moles or for cauterizing cervical erosion, it has largely been replaced by cryosurgery.

diet pills See AMPHETAMINE, DIURETIC.

diethylstilbestrol See DES.

dieting The systematic attempt to lose weight by cutting down on caloric intake. It is generally agreed by health authorities that any woman who weighs 20 percent more than the norm for her age and body build ought to go on a diet. Reducing need not be supervised by a doctor unless the individual is extremely overweight or special medical circumstances are involved, such as diabetes. The most effective weight reduction program is a self-motivated change in eating habits sustained over a protracted period of time. See "Nutrition and Weight."

digestion The transformation of food into nutrients that can be absorbed into the blood and assimilated by the cells; the digestive, or gastrointestinal system involves the alimentary canal and related organs (liver, gallbladder, and pancreas). *See* "The Healthy Woman."

Digestion may be temporarily impaired or chronically affected by obstructions, bacterial or chemical poisoning, alcoholism, and infections such as dysentery, typhoid fever, cholera, and influenza. Emotional states of fear, excitement, anxiety, and anger are all known to be causes of acute or chronic digestive disorders, ranging from an attack of nausea to the development of a peptic ulcer. Any abdominal pain of an unknown nature should be brought to the attention of a doctor for proper diagnosis and treatment.

digitalis A substance derived from the dried leaves of the foxglove flower (*Digitalis purpurea*) and used in the treatment of heart disease. For several hundred years digitalis has been used effectively as a means of stimulating the action of the failing heart muscle, while at the same time slowing down the heartbeat. Digitalis is chemically purified so that doses can be measured with meticulous accuracy. Patients in need of immediate results may be given a dose that is close to being toxic; others may be placed on a daily maintenance program. Since the medication may have to be increased or decreased over a patient's lifetime, continuing medical supervision is mandatory. Symptoms suggestive of toxicity such as nausea, loss of appetite, headache, diarrhea, and irregular pulse should be reported to a doctor promptly.

dilatation and curettage (D&C) The expansion of the cervix by the use of surgical dilators and the removal of tissue from the lining of the uterus with a curette. The D & C procedure is used in early pregnancy as an abortion method; following a miscarriage to remove unexpelled tissue; in diagnosing uterine cancer, abnormal bleeding, or other discharge; and in certain cases of infertility to improve the general condition of the uterus. *See* "Contraception and Abortion," "Gynecologic Diseases and Treatment."

dilatation and evacuation (D&E) The expansion of the cervix with surgical dilators and the removal of the contents of the uterus by suction. *See* "Contraception and Abortion."

disc, slipped The dislocation or herniation of one of the gellike, cartilaginous rings that separate the spinal vertebrae from each other. The column of 33 bones that make up the spine bears much of the body's weight above the hips. The vertebrae themselves are constantly being subjected to stress and sudden shock due to lifting, bending, and performing other activities that are part of one's daily routine. The discs between the vertebrae are the built-in shock absorbers. These resilient and somewhat spongy structures are held in place by rings of tough, fibrous tissue. When one of the discs slips out of position, it may press on a spinal nerve, causing acute pain to spread through the pathway of the nerve. In some cases the pain may radiate from the lower back into the buttocks, through the thighs and calves, and into the feet. When the pressure on the nerve is not as intense, the symptom may be restricted to lower back discomfort.

The point at which the pain origi-

SLIPPED DISC

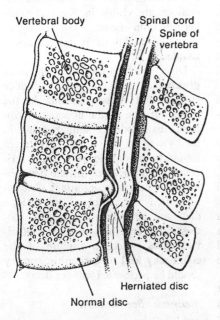

Vertebral body

Spinal cord
Spine of vertebra

Herniated disc

Normal disc

nates is located by X-rays of the spine. The first aspects of treatment usually consist of bed rest on a hard mattress, analgesics to mute the pain, and traction. The condition may also be substantially improved by wearing an individually adjusted surgical corset with a back brace or a neck collar. In about 20 percent of slipped disc cases relief sufficient to make mobility possible can be achieved only by an operation known as a laminectomy; a piece of the vertebra is removed and the protruding piece of the disc that is causing the pressure is eliminated. Recovery is usually complete in a couple of weeks. A more radical operation is a spinal fusion involving bone graft. This procedure requires a long stay in the hospital and the use of a body cast and brace until fusion has been accomplished. It is an operation that is performed only as an alternative to painful disability.

discharge An abnormal emission signifying an infection or disorder, such as pus from a boil or an ear infection or the leukorrhea that characterizes cervical erosion. Normal emissions, such as the waste matter of the menstrual flow or the lubricating secretions of the vaginal membranes during sexual excitation, are not usually called discharges. Discharges of various composition are usually the first sign of vaginal infection. The color, odor, and consistency of the discharge depends on the nature of the infection. When the organism is a yeastlike fungus as in candidiasis, the emission is thick and white and has a yeasty smell. When the inflammation is caused by the parasite responsible for trichomoniasis, a greenish-gray discharge with a strong unpleasant odor is characteristic. Bacterial infections of the cervix, vagina, or other genital areas produce a foul-smelling yellowish discharge compounded of mucus, pus, and sometimes streaks of blood. Any unusual discharge should be called to a doctor's attention for evaluation, analysis, and treatment.

dislocation Specifically, the displacement of a bone from its normal position in the joint; also called subluxation. Dislocations most commonly occur in the fingers and shoulder and less frequently in the elbow, knee, hip, and jaw. A dislocation does not necessarily involve a break in the bone, but it almost always involves some damage, either slight or serious, to the surrounding ligaments and muscles. Anyone may experience a dislocation as a result of a fall or a blow, but it is a routine hazard among dancers and athletes. Dislocations are also more apt to occur to women whose joints are flexible rather than stiff, who consider themselves to be "double-jointed." Once the displacement occurs, particularly if the site is the shoulder or elbow, it is likely to recur because of the stretching of the sac and the ligaments that hold the joint in place. After several recurrences surgery is usually recommended to tighten the tissues.

A sudden dislocation can be extremely painful, and since the possibility of fracture as well as injury to surrounding nerves and blood vessels must be taken into consideration, prompt medical attention is essential to ensure restoring normal function. To minimize pain and swelling, cold compresses should be applied to the injured area. The injured joint should be immobilized while transporting the victim to the doctor or hospital.

The layman should never attempt to reset a dislocated joint; such an effort can result in serious irreversible injury.

diuretic Any drug that increases urinary output. The increase is called diuresis. Diuretics are indispensable in the treatment of heart failure to prevent fluid accumulation. They are often used in treating high blood pressure and certain kidney and liver disorders. Since diuresis involves the loss of vital salts such as potassium as well as water, patients receiving a daily dose of this type of medication are advised to consume extra potassium. Common substances such as coffee and alcohol have a diuretic effect.

diverticulosis The presence of diverticula, an abnormal mucous membrane pouch, in any part of the gastrointestinal tract, but especially in the colon. Diverticulosis may be entirely without symptoms and is most commonly found in middle-aged and elderly women with a history of chronic

constipation. Since the diverticula formations are visible in X-rays following a barium enema, accurate diagnosis of diverticulosis is comparatively simple.

Diverticulitis is the inflammation of diverticula and it may produce cramps and muscle spasms in the lower left side of the abdomen. (Appendicitis produces similar pains in the lower right side.) Treatment should be prompt to prevent the serious consequences of fistula development or complete intestinal obstruction. Bed rest, a bland low-residue diet, and antibiotics are usually successful therapy. In severe cases of diverticulitis, where a rupture of the colon may lead to peritonitis, surgery should be performed without delay.

dizziness *See* VERTIGO.

DNA One of the basic components of all living matter; the molecular material in the nuclear chromosome of the cell responsible for the transmission of the hereditary genetic code. The designation DNA stands for the chemical compound deoxyribonucleic acid, the molecules of which are connected in an arrangement known as the double helix. The discovery in 1962 of the molecular composition of DNA is the foundation on which the comparatively new field of genetic medicine is based.

doctor The term doctor or physician designates persons who have either the degree of Doctor of Medicine (M.D.) or Doctor of Osteopathy (D.O.). The term doctor, but not physician, is also used to designate persons who have completed training and earned a degree in specific areas of treatment such as chiropractic, podiatry, and optometry. In order to practice medicine, a doctor must be licensed by the state in which the office is to be located.

Physicians usually work as hospital interns for one or two years before they become general practitioners (GPs). Most doctors who intend to specialize remain in an accredited hospital as resident physicians for several additional years in order to gain the necessary experience for certification in the specialty. This certification involves passing an examination given by a board of specialists in the selected branch. It is unfortunate—and a warning to the unwary—that any doctor may set himself or herself up as a specialist without having received certification through examination.

Information about a doctor's special qualifications is conveyed in the initials that follow the M.D. designation on a bill or prescription form. The designations indicate further credentials and peer recognition. The more common initials are:

F.A.C.C.   Fellow of the American College of Cardiology
F.A.C.P.   Fellow of the American College of Physicians
F.A.C.G.   Fellow of the American College of Gastroenterology
F.A.C.O.G. Fellow of the American College of Obstetrics and Gynecology
F.A.C.R.   Fellow of the American College of Radiology
F.A.C.S.   Fellow of the American College of Surgeons

The most recent designation is P.C. which stands for Professional Corporation and must appear after the other credentials attached to the name of any doctor whose medical practice has been incorporated. *See also* "You, Your Doctors, and the Health Care System."

Although there are now as many as 50 different specialties, all with subdivisions, the medical profession officially certifies specialists in these fields.

Anesthesiology. The anesthesiologist is a physician who is responsible for choosing the proper means for the safe and effective anesthetizing of a patient before and during surgery. This choice is based on an assessment of detailed information of the patient's medical history and present condition. An anesthetist is not an M.D., but a specialized nurse who may administer the anesthesia under an anesthesiologist's direction.

Emergency medicine. A discipline recognized and approved in 1979 and defined by the American Board of Medical Specialties as "the split-second recognition, evaluation, stabilization, and care of trauma, illness, and emotional crisis." The American College of Emergency Physicians has a membership of over 10,000 doctors, most of whom practice in the emergency departments of hospitals and other institutions.

Family practice. The specialist in family practice is trained to give basic and comprehensive medical care to any individual of any age. This is one of the most recent areas of specialization for which there is approved hospital-residency training and certification. The development of training programs for this specialty is an updating of the concept of the general practitioner.

Internal medicine. An internist (not to be confused with an intern, a medical school graduate practicing under supervision to acquire practical experience) is trained in all areas of medical diagnosis and treatment. This practitioner may, however, refer a patient to another doctor who is a specialist in the treatment of a specific ailment. Most internists develop their own subspecialization, and they may limit their practice to a particular field. Among the best known of the subspecialists are: allergist, endocrinologist (glandular and hormonal problems), hematologist (disorders of the blood), cardiologist (heart disease), and gastroenterologist (digestive disorders).

Neurology. A neurologist diagnoses and treats organic disorders and diseases of the nervous system, spinal cord, and brain.

Obstetrics and gynecology. The obstetrician is concerned with pregnancy and delivery; the gynecologist with disorders of the female reproductive system and with matters relating to birth control. A doctor who has had specialized training in both areas may decide to practice in both fields or in only one.

Ophthalmology. The ophthalmologist specializes in diagnosis and treatment involving the structure, function, and diseases of the eye. This specialist not only prescribes corrective lenses and eye medicines, but also performs all types of eye surgery.

Orthopedics. The orthopedist is trained to handle all diseases and injuries affecting the skeletal system, including joints, muscles, ligaments, tendons, and bones.

Otolaryngology. Commonly known as an ENT specialist (for ear, nose, and throat), the otolaryngologist is trained in the medical and surgical treatment of these particular organs as well as the cavities of the head, excluding those containing the brain (the skull) and the eyes (the eye sockets). An otolaryngologist is the specialist who usually performs tonsillectomies.

Pathology. The pathologist is essentially involved with the causes and behavior of particular diseases as revealed in laboratory research. They investigate bodily reactions to disease in tests on tissue, blood, urine, and other specimens. They do the tissue analysis in biopsies and also perform autopsies.

Pediatrics. The pediatrician is a specialist in child care, including immunization. Some pediatricians treat patients until their late teens; others consider the onset of puberty as the time young people should transfer to a family practitioner. A recent subspecialty in the pediatric field is neonatology. A neonatologist, usually a member of a hospital's staff, specializes in the care of the newborn, especially premature infants and those born with birth defects.

Physical medicine and rehabilitation. This specialist works to rectify disabilities of patients who have had a stroke, an injury, or a disease that affects the normal function of a certain part of the body.

Plastic surgery. The plastic surgeon deals with the repair, restoration, or replacement of malformed, damaged, or missing parts of the body resulting from injury or from congenital defect, for example, repair of cleft palate, skin grafting after major burns, reconstruction of facial bones damaged in an accident, and replacement of a joint or limb with a prosthesis. Cosmetic surgery is that branch of plastic surgery concerned with changing appearance solely for esthetic reasons.

Preventive medicine. This specialist is usually associated with community health programs and public health measures involving the anticipation and prevention of disease and injuries.

Proctology. The proctologist specializes in medical and surgical treatment of disorders of the anus and rectum.

Psychiatry. The psychiatrist is a medical doctor who deals with the mind and feelings. There are many categories of psychotherapists, but among them only those who are licensed

M.D.s are legally permitted to write prescriptions for medication. A psychoanalyst is a psychotherapist who bases therapy on Freudian principles and who may or may not be a medical doctor. A psychologist is a person who has an academic degree in psychology. Psychologists with a Ph.D. may be called doctor, but they are not medical doctors nor are they legally permitted to dispense prescription medication. The term psychotherapist or therapist is a catchall for anyone from a psychiatrist to someone with no professional training or recognized credentials.

Radiology. A qualified radiologist uses X-rays, sonography, radioactive substances, and other forms of radiant energy in the diagnosis and treatment of disease.

Surgery. A general surgeon is qualified to perform any type of operation. Most surgeons specialize in a particular type of operation. For example, the thoracic surgeon performs operations involving the lungs and heart. Neurosurgeons are called upon for the removal of brain tumors, repair of nerves following injury, and similar operations.

Urology. A urologist specializes in medical and surgical treatment of disorders of the urinary tract.

dog bites *See* ANIMAL BITES.

dopamine A substance in the brain that is essential to the normal functioning of the nervous system. A decreased concentration of dopamine is assumed to be the underlying cause of Parkinsonism. Symptoms of this disorder are dramatically alleviated by chemotherapy with dopamine in the synthesized form known as L-dopa.

douche *See* VAGINAL CARE.

Down's syndrome A form of inherited mental retardation caused by defective chromosomal development in the embryo. It is also referred to as mongolism due to the downward curve of the affected offspring's inner eyelids and as Trisomy 21 because there are 3 instead of 2 number 21 chromosomes. In addition to retardation, these children often suffer eye disorders and have a tendency to develop leukemia.

The incidence of Down's syndrome increases with the age of the mother from 1 birth in 1,000 among women between 20 and 25 years of age, to 1 birth in 100 among 40-year-olds, to 3 births in 100 among women 45 years old or older. The role of the father is uncertain. Amniocentesis is advised for women at risk to determine if the defect is present.

Dramamine Brand name of the chemical dimenhydrinate, an antihistamine effective against motion sickness and vertigo. Since it induces drowsiness, it should never be taken before driving or engaging in any activity requiring mental alertness.

drugs *See* "Drugs, Alcohol, and Tobacco"; Brand Name Drugs and Generic Equivalents, p. 742.

duodenal ulcer An open sore in the mucous membrane lining of the duodenum, the portion of the small intestine nearest to the stomach. *See also* ULCER.

dysentery An infectious inflammation of the lining of the large intestine characterized by diarrhea, the passage of mucus and blood, and severe abdominal cramps and fever. There are two types: bacillary dysentery is caused by several different types of bacterial strains; amebic dysentery is caused by amebae. Both types are endemic in parts of the world where public sanitation is primitive. Dysentery is spread from person to person by food or water that is contaminated by infected human feces and by houseflies that feed on human excrement containing the infectious agent. It may also be spread by food handlers who transmit the disease by way of unwashed hands.

When bacillary dysentery is diagnosed in the very young or very old or in anyone with diabetes or some other chronic condition, hospitalization is usually recommended so that dehydration can be prevented or treated. In milder forms of dysentery, rest combined with a prescribed dose of an antibiotic or other medication is a common course of treatment. Close supervision is important in the case of amebic dysentery since the infection can become chronic if amebic abscesses are formed in the liver.

Travelers to parts of the world where infection is an everpresent hazard should take the necessary precautions against dysentery by drinking only bottled water or other bottled beverages, avoiding raw fruit and vegetables, and, if possible, inspecting the facilities where food is prepared to make sure that the premises are screened against flies. If symptoms of the disease occur, a local doctor should be consulted promptly.

dysmenorrhea Painful menstruation. The discomfort is usually felt in the lower abdomen, extending into the lower back, and in some cases into the lower part of the legs. Dysmenorrhea may occur with or without headaches and may be the result of tension.

If there is no recognized organic disease, such as endometriosis, that is thought to be responsible for the dysmenorrhea, it is referred to as primary dysmenorrhea. The causes of this are not fully understood, but one explanation is that the painful uterine contractions are caused by excess prostaglandin effect. See PROSTAGLANDIN. Recently several anti-prostaglandin drugs have become available (proprietary names are Indocin, Motrin, and Ponstel) which generally are effective though they may cause some nausea. Various analgesics and small amounts of distilled alcohol often are helpful. Since after a pregnancy the problem often subsides, another form of treatment has been oral contraceptives which suppress ovulation and thus create a "pseudo" pregnancy.

Secondary dysmenorrhea is treated, if possible, by treating the organic disease thought to be causing it. See "Gynecologic Diseases and Treatment."

dyspareunia Painful sexual intercourse caused by physical or psychogenic factors or a combination of both. Women for whom intercourse is so painful that it interferes with their sexual life should consult a gynecologist. Among the many organic reasons for the pain are endometriosis, cervicitis, cystitis, and cysts in the Bartholin's glands.

One of the most common circumstances resulting in coital pain is the first occasion of penetration when the penis may cause lacerations of vaginal tissue due to insufficient natural lubrication. In such cases the difficulties are compounded by the involuntary spasm of the vagina that follows the original trauma. Older women may experience the gradual onset of discomfort during or following intercourse as a consequence of the degeneration of vaginal tissues and a drying out of the lubricating mucus. An organic anomaly, such as a tipped uterus, may turn out to be the underlying factor. When there appears to be no organic explanation for the pain and no sign of infection, a woman should seek psychological counseling either with or without her sexual partner.

dyspepsia *See* INDIGESTION.

dysplasia An aberration of cellular development that may occur in the cervix, lung, and other places. In the cervix it is diagnosed by a pap smear. Although cervical dysplasia usually does not progress to cancer, women in whom it has been diagnosed need to be examined regularly. Some cases of dysplasia clear up without treatment; others require cauterization or other treatment.

dyspnea Labored breathing; the feeling of being "out of breath." Dyspnea is a symptom or sign of insufficiently oxygenated blood resulting from an obstruction in the air passages such as occurs in chronic respiratory diseases; a reduction in the capacity of the lungs to carry on the normal oxygen-carbon dioxide exchange because of areas of scar tissue; certain forms of heart failure in which the lungs fill with fluid; chronic anemia. An acute breathlessness may accompany asthma, bronchial pneumonia, the sudden onset of an allergic response that causes the swelling of the windpipe, and myocardial infarction. It is also one of the most distressing manifestations of an anxiety attack. Shortness of breath that often accompanies obesity can be rectified by loss of weight. When dyspnea is accompanied by chest pain or when it is chronic, medical evaluation is indicated.

ear The organ of hearing and equilibrium. The ear is divided into three parts: the outer ear consists of the visible fleshy auricle that collects the sound waves which are then transmitted through the ear canal; the middle ear contains the three bones of hearing; the inner ear is the site of the organ of hearing and the organ of balance. The thin layer of tissue known as the eardrum, also called the tympanus or tympanic membrane, forms the barrier between the outer ear and the middle ear. The bones of hearing in the middle ear, called the ossicles, are named for their respective shapes —the hammer, anvil, and stirrup. They are connected to the bone surrounding the middle ear by ligaments. When loud noises strike the eardrum, tiny muscles attached to the ossicles limit the vibrations of the eardrum by

MIDDLE AND INNER EAR

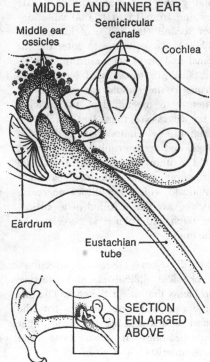

Middle ear ossicles

Semicircular canals

Cochlea

Eardrum

Eustachian tube

SECTION ENLARGED ABOVE

contracting, thus protecting it and the inner ear from damage. Equal pressure is maintained on both sides of the eardrum because the eustachian tube connects the middle ear to the upper rear part of the throat. The organ of hearing within the inner ear is called the cochlea, a spiral-shaped organ whose name means "snail" in Latin. The cochlea covers the nerves that sort out various sound messages and sends them on to the auditory center of the brain. The organ of balance, made up of the three semicircular canals situated in three different planes of space within the inner ear, maintains the body's equilibrium in relation to gravitational forces. Any disturbance or infection of the semicircular canals results in vertigo and imbalance.

The hearing process works in the following way. Any vibrating object that pushes air molecules at a rate ranging from 15 to 15,000 vibrations per second (the range of human audibility) causes waves to enter the ear canal and strike the eardrum. The vibrations are transmitted by the eardrum to the middle ear where their intensity is magnified by the ossicles. The waves are then sent through a membranous window behind the third bone, and are transmitted through the fluid within the cochlea. Hairlike structures within the cochlea communicate with the auditory nerves in such a way that a sound of a particular pitch and volume is perceived by the brain.

ear disorders Diseases, infections, mechanical difficulties, and pressure problems that affect the ears. The disorders directly responsible for the onset of deafness are discussed under the headings HEARING LOSS and OTOSCLEROSIS.

Discomfort within the ear may range from irritation due to dermatitis of the outer ear to a feeling of pressure caused by congestion in the eustachian tube to acute pain resulting from bacterial infection of the middle ear. Until the discomfort is diagnosed, it may be temporarily relieved with aspirin and the application of heat. Any sharp pain in the ear, an earache that lasts more than a day, an earache accompanied by a discharge, or chronic pain resulting from exposure to dangerous sound levels should be investigated by a doctor immediately.

Because the ears are directly connected to the nose and throat by the eustachian tube, a head cold is likely to cause the ears to feel "stuffed." The symptom may be remedied by the supervised use of nosedrops. Precautions should be taken to prevent the entrance of infectious material into the ear through the eustachian tube. Nostrils should not be held closed when blowing the nose, because closing both at once may force such material into the ear. Similar precautions should be taken while swimming. Air should be breathed in through the mouth and exhaled through the nose; if the mouth or nose fills with water, it should not be swallowed, but rather sniffed into the back of the throat and spat out. Earplugs may be worn. If water enters the ear, it can usually be drained by the force of gravity when lying down with the ear to the ground.

Otomycosis, a fungus infection of the outer ear, results from swimming in polluted waters and causes itching, swelling, and pain. It is often accompanied by crusted sores that must be kept dry in order to cure the condition. Fungicidal ointments and antibiotic salves are usually effective treatment.

Infections of the middle ear, more common in childhood than in later years, can be brought under control by antibiotics.

An earache caused by sinusitis or a diseased tooth will usually diminish as the underlying condition is treated. An infection that spreads from the middle ear to the inner ear will affect the sense of balance and cause vertigo. Several ear disorders are accompanied by a temporary "ringing in the ears" known as tinnitus.

The eardrum is susceptible to damage. A sudden and dramatic change in air pressure as occurs in an airplane or while swimming at great depths may lead to a ruptured or perforated eardrum. Probing the ear to remove wax or to relieve itching with any object, other than a twisted wad of cotton, may also cause perforation of the eardrum. This condition is usually accompanied by pain and bleeding and should be attended to without delay. The chief danger of a perforated eardrum is that it increases the possibility of middle ear infections. Anyone with this condition should be especially careful about protecting the ears while swimming.

echogram A recording produced on an oscilloscopic screen that shows the difference between the wave patterns of healthy and diseased tissue which cannot be distinguished by X-rays. Echocardiograms provide tracings of the ultrasonic waves reflected back from the internal heart tissues. The echoencephalogram provides similar material for the diagnosis of brain disorders.

eclampsia An acute condition occurring during pregnancy characterized by elevated blood pressure, convulsions, and coma; also known as toxe-mia of pregnancy. *See* "Pregnancy and Childbirth."

ectopic pregnancy The implantation of the fertilized ovum in a fallopian tube, the cervix, or the abdomen instead of within the uterus. *See* "Pregnancy and Childbirth."

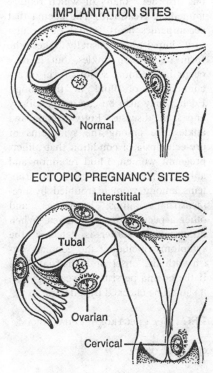

IMPLANTATION SITES

Normal

ECTOPIC PREGNANCY SITES

Interstitial

Tubal

Ovarian

Cervical

eczema A skin disorder characterized by itching, a rash, and scaling. The eczematous symptoms may result from an allergy to a particular food, medicine, or pollen or from contact dermatitis. Eczema is also associated with varicose veins, since this circulatory disturbance can be responsible for local hypersensitivity of the skin, particularly of the ankles. Eczema is treated by eliminating the underlying cause and by topical creams that reduce discomfort and hasten healing.

When flareups are traced to emotional stress, psychotherapy may be helpful.

edema Swelling caused by the abnormal accumulation of fluid in the tissues. The archaic term for edema is dropsy, derived from the Greek word *hydrops* from *hydros,* meaning "water." Edema is a symptom of various disorders, many of which require immediate treatment. The edema that accompanies heart failure or circulatory impairments usually takes the form of swollen ankles, but it may occur in the more serious form of accumulation of fluid in the lungs. Edema may also be caused by kidney and liver diseases. Puffy eyelids and ankles are among the symptoms of pre-eclampsia, a condition that afflicts pregnant women. Fluid retention and a bloated feeling are common problems among women troubled by premenstrual cramps, headaches, and other aspects of dysmenorrhea. When no organic disorder is detected, the symptoms, including the edema, vanish with the onset of menstrual flow. If the edema persists between periods, it should be checked by a doctor.

EEG *See* ELECTROENCEPHALOGRAM.

egg *See* OVUM.

ejaculation The reflex action by which semen is expelled during the male orgasm. Premature ejaculation, usually psychogenic in origin, is a circumstance in which the male reaches orgasm relatively rapidly and sooner than he or his partner desires. Rapid ejaculation may occur occasionally because of stress, a long period of abstinence, or several other factors. When it is chronic, a reputable therapist specializing in such problems should be consulted by both partners.

EKG *See* ELECTROCARDIOGRAM.

elastic stockings Hosiery reinforced with elastic thread in order to provide support for or to help prevent the formation of varicose veins. Elastic stockings are often recommended where circulation in the legs is affected by pregnancy or by work that necessitates standing in one place for long periods of time.

elective surgery *See* SURGERY.

electrical injury Any accident involving the transmission of electrical current through the body, either by a conductive apparatus or by being struck by lightning. If the voltage is sufficiently high, a fatal cardiac arrest can occur. To prevent electrical injuries in the home, electrical equipment should be inspected on a regular basis.

electrocardiogram (EKG) A tracing that represents the electrical impulses, that is, changes in electrical potential, generated by the heart as measured by an instrument called an electrocardiograph. The instrument magnifies the current about 3000 times. This magnified current provides the power to propel a lever in contact with a moving paper on which the wave pattern is recorded. The pattern indicates the rate of the heart rhythm, tissue damage that may have occurred following a heart attack, the effect of various medications on the heart muscle, and other valuable information for the diagnosis of cardiac disorders.

electroencephalogram (EEG) A tracing by an electroencephalograph of the electrical potential produced by the brain. Electrical impulses picked up by electrodes attached to the scalp surface are amplified so that they are strong enough to move an electromagnetic pen to make a record of brain wave patterns. This procedure is quick and painless. It is used routinely to diagnose tumors, brain damage, and neurological disorders such as epilepsy.

electrolysis   *See* HAIR REMOVAL.

electroshock therapy   A procedure in which a controlled amount of electric current is passed through the frontal area of the brain of a mentally ill patient. The physical response is convulsions and unconsciousness. Electroshock is not a cure for any form of mental illness, but when treatments are given in series, they may temporarily relieve some of the more anguishing emotional symptoms and thereby make the patient accessible to other forms of psychotherapy. It has largely been replaced by antidepressant drugs and tranquilizers.

elephantiasis   Abnormal swelling of the legs and abdomen that occurs as a late stage of the tropical and subtropical disease filariasis, caused by a parasitic worm that invades the lymphatic system.

embolism   Obstruction of a blood vessel by material carried in the bloodstream from another part of the body. The material, or embolus, is most often a blood clot, but it may also be a fat globule, air bubble, segment of a tumor, or clump of bacteria.

embryo   The term by which the developing human organism is known from conception to the end of the eighth week of pregnancy. After that time and until delivery, it is known as the fetus.

emetic   Any substance that causes vomiting. A safe and fast emetic is a mixture of 2 tablespoons of salt in a glass of warm water.

emotional problems   *See* "Your Mind and Feelings."

emphysema   A severe respiratory disease, incurable but treatable, characterized by the air-filled expansion of the lungs. Emphysema is more prevalent among men than women and is most commonly observed in heavy cigarette smokers living in an area with a high level of air pollution. The disease develops gradually and is usually preceded by a chronic cough and intermittent bouts of bronchitis. Symptoms often become apparent between the ages of 50 and 70, as the lung's functioning surface area is progressively diminished by the destruction of the walls that separate the air spaces. This creates a disruption in the exchange of oxygen and carbon dioxide so that the lungs become inflated by an accumulation of stale air. Cigarette smoking aggravates emphysema since it places a burden on the lungs to oxygenate the blood. A first sign of the disease is difficulty in breathing after a minimum amount of exertion. As breathing becomes more labored, the heart is forced to work harder to increase the blood supply to the lungs.

To counteract the debilitating effect of emphysema, proper breathing techniques must be established in order to enhance lung capacity. Other aspects of treatment include a proper diet to counteract weight loss, supplementary oxygen, elimination of environmental irritants, immunization against respiratory infections, and medications that dilate the bronchial passages. Above all, people suffering from emphysema should never smoke cigarettes.

empyema A collection of pus within any body cavity; generally used to describe pus in the pleural spaces around the lungs as a consequence of infection. Pus within the chest cavity may follow pleurisy, pneumonia, pulmonary tuberculosis, or a chest wound or tumor. When possible, the fluid is drained off by a technique called thorocentesis: a hollow needle attached to a syringe is inserted into the pleural cavity and the pus withdrawn by suction. When the pus is too thick, surgical drainage may be required. In either case antibiotics are prescribed to halt the further development of abscesses.

encephalitis Inflammation of the tissues covering the brain. One form of the disease, encephalitis lethargica, was epidemic from 1915 to 1926 and was generally called sleeping sickness. The brain inflammation may be associated with such virus infections as measles, mumps, and herpes. It may be produced by lead poisoning, or it may follow the infectious bite of certain ticks and mosquitos. The disease may occur at any age. Typical symptoms are fever, vomiting, headache, and in some cases convulsions. Correct diagnosis is made by laboratory tests of the blood, spinal fluid, and stools and by an electroencephalogram. There is no specific cure. Treatment consists of bed rest, medication to keep the fever down, and antibiotics in cases where the infectious agent is bacterial.

endocrine system A physiological system that includes the ductless glands whose secretions, the hormones, are delivered directly into the bloodstream. *See* "The Healthy Woman."

endometrial aspiration A technique in which suction is applied to remove the lining of the uterus (the endometrium). *See* "Contraception and Abortion."

endometriosis A condition in which tissue normally found in the lining of the uterus (the endometrium) begins to grow in the ovaries, fallopian tubes, bladder, or between the rectum and vagina. *See* "Gynecologic Diseases and Treatment."

COMMON SITES OF ENDOMETRIOSIS

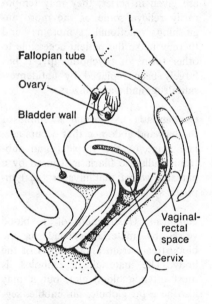

Fallopian tube
Ovary
Bladder wall
Vaginal-rectal space
Cervix

endometritis Inflammation of the endometrium (the lining of the uterus), caused by bacterial infection which may follow a normal delivery, a cesarean section, an induced or spontaneous abortion, or irritation resulting from an IUD. Symptoms include pain in the lower abdomen, discharge, and fever. Acute endometritis is usually treated with antibiotics. Where the condition is caused by an IUD, a reevaluation of birth control methods should be considered. Chronic cases that do not respond to medication may require curettage.

endorphins A group of morphine-like chemicals produced by the brain and thought to control the activity of the pain-receptor nerve cells. *See* PAIN.

endoscopy Examination of a hollow cavity or an internal organ with an illuminated optical instrument (endoscope). Among the more commonly used instruments are the cystoscope for examining the bladder, the proctoscope for examining the lower portion of the intestine and rectum, and the bronchoscope for locating the origin and extent of respiratory disorders.

enema The injection of a fluid into the lower bowel by means of a tube inserted into the rectum; also, the fluid injected. A barium enema is administered prior to X-rays of the lower gastrointestinal tract, a sedative enema may be used for a calming effect, and a warm water or special solution enema is often recommended in special cases of constipation. The habitual use of enemas as a means of bowel evacuation is not recommended because they are apt to impair the natural responses involved in the normal process of elimination. Disposable enema units are a convenient substitute for the more traditional equipment which must be washed and stored.

energy The capacity for activity. Energy may take mechanical, electrical, chemical, or thermal form. All fuel is stored energy, and the body's fuel is food. The chemical energy stored in food is transformed by the metabolic process. The three essential sources of human energy are proteins, fats, and carbohydrates. "Lack of energy" may be traced to faulty diet, chronic illness, or emotional conflict.

ENT The initials that designate *e*ar, *n*ose, and *t*hroat as an area of medical specialization. The doctor who is an ENT specialist is known as an otolaryngologist.

enterocele A hernia in which a loop of the small intestine protrudes into the vaginal wall. The condition may reveal itself when X-rays are taken to diagnose pain. Surgical correction is the usual treatment.

enuresis Involuntary bedwetting while sleeping; more specifically, by a child past the age at which bladder sphincter control is expected.

enzyme An organic substance, usually protein, manufactured by the cells of all living things and acting as a catalyst in the transformation of a complex chemical compound into a simple or different one. The human body produces hundreds of different enzymes, each with a specific function: some are related to the chemistry of muscle function; three main groups of digestive enzymes are essential for the normal metabolic processing of proteins, fats, and carbohydrates; particular enzymes are involved in maintaining normal respiratory function.

ephedrine A chemical derived from an Asian shrub, ephedra, or produced synthetically. For centuries the Chiese have recognized its medicinal properties which include dilating air passages, shrinking mucous membranes of the nose and throat, increasing blood pressure, and speeding up the heartbeat. In its synthesized form ephedrine is a component of various medicines that relieve nasal congestion and counteract the effects of an asthmatic attack. It must be used with discretion by anyone with a heart condition or with high blood pressure.

epiglottis The leaf-shaped flap of cartilage covered with mucous membrane that lies between the back of the tongue and the entrance to the larynx and the trachea (windpipe). In the act of swallowing, the epiglottis folds back over the opening of the larynx which contains the vocal apparatus (in the glottis) and channels the food from the back of the tongue to the esophagus. The disruption of this mechanism, such as by a person's laughing while eating, may allow food to enter the windpipe, leading to a coughing spell and in more serious cases to choking.

epilepsy A disorder of the nervous system in which an imbalance in the electrical activity of brain circuitry leads to convulsive spasms, loss of consciousness, and in some cases abnormal behavior. The seizures vary in magnitude and duration. There are approximately 4 million epileptics in the United States. The disorder is not contagious nor is intelligence affected. Some epilepsy is attributed to brain injury, but usually the basic cause of the disorder is unknown. It cannot be cured, but the seizures can be controlled in approximately 80 percent of all cases with anticonvulsant medicines.

Temporal-lobe epilepsy is a form of the disorder that may cause abnormal behavior without the characteristic seizures. When this form of the disease exists, it is important that the cause of the aberrant behavior be properly diagnosed as physical rather than psychological so that it can be treated medically or surgically rather than with psychotherapy.

Through its local affiliates, the Epilepsy Foundation of America, whose national office is located at 1828 L Street, Washington, D.C., 20036, will supply information through literature, films, and speakers on all aspects of the disorder including how to recognize a seizure and deal with it in an emergency.

episiotomy An incision made in the perineum from the vagina downward toward the anus during the final stage of labor. *See* "Pregnancy and Childbirth."

EPISIOTOMY

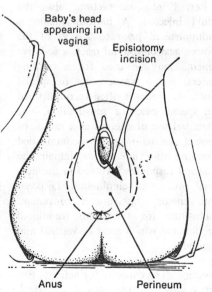

Baby's head appearing in vagina

Episiotomy incision

Anus

Perineum

epithelioma A tumor composed of epithelial cells, usually benign; the former term for skin cancer. One of the more common causes of this type of growth is overexposure to sunlight, especially among women with fair complexions. Another cause is overexposure to X-rays. Where the epitheliomas are confined to the outermost layers of the skin, they may seem to be no more than scaling patches. When they are more deeply buried, they appear to be pimples. Any such growth, especially if it suddenly begins to enlarge and is also bounded by a shiny border, should be removed. Even though this type of tumor is not generally cancerous, its continuing growth may interfere with the normal function of other vital organs.

Equanil Brand name of a chemical compound meprobamate, prescribed as a tranquilizer for the control of mild anxiety. It may produce side effects of drowsiness and a skin rash. There are indications that Equanil (or Miltown, another brand name of the same chemical) taken during the first twelve weeks of pregnancy increases the possibility of birth defects.

erection The swelling and stiffening of the penis or increase in length, diameter, and firmness of the clitoris resulting from sexual arousal. The stimulus may be psychological (sexual fantasies), visual (the sight of a sexually appealing person), or physical (touch).

There is no correlation between the size of the flaccid penis and the same penis in erection, which may range on the average from 5 to 7 inches. There is no correlation between body size and the size of the erect penis nor between the size of the erect penis and

sexual prowess. Inability to have an erection is called impotence.

erogenous zone Any area of the body, especially the oral, genital, and anal, that is the source of sexual arousal when stimulated by touch.

erysipelas An acute streptococcal skin infection, formerly called St. Anthony's fire because of the bright red patches that appear on the affected areas. While erysipelas may affect any part of the body, it usually originates through a lesion on the face or hands; once contracted, it is virulent and dangerous, especially to the very young or old. In addition to the changed appearance of the skin, other symptoms include headache, fever, and vomiting. Untreated, the red patches swell, spread, and cause the adjacent skin to blister. Erysipelas is a disease that requires prompt administration of antibiotics and a supervised regimen including lots of liquids, simple foods, and bed rest until recovery is complete.

erythema The reddening of the skin resulting from a dilation of the capillaries. An erythematous condition may be caused by allergy, bacterial or viral infection, superficial burns, chafing or chapping, or response to certain medication. Blushing is an erythematous response to an emotional situation.

erythrocytes The red blood cells. Each cubic millimeter of blood normally contains about 5 million erythrocytes. They are the smallest cells in the body and are constantly being manufactured in the bone marrow. Erythrocytes live for about 100 days. Any change in their number, size, shape, color, or density, which can be determined by microscopic examination, indicates a deviation from the normal health pattern.

erythromycin Generic name for an antibiotic commonly prescribed to patients with a penicillin allergy and to pregnant women and young children when the tetracycline antibiotics are considered inadvisable.

esophagus The muscular tube that transmits food from the mouth to the stomach; the gullet. This portion of the alimentary canal is approximately 10 inches long; it extends from the pharynx through the chest and connects with the stomach just below the diaphragm. Between the esophagus and the stomach is a muscular ring, the cardiac sphincter, that opens to permit food to leave the esophagus and descend into the stomach.

estrogen A sex hormone, primarily a female hormone, which is produced in the ovary, adrenal gland, and placenta. Males also produce estrogen in much smaller amounts in their adrenals. Estrogen regulates the development of the secondary sex characteristics in women and is involved in the menstrual cycle and the implantation and nourishment of a fertilized ovum. Synthetic estrogen is widely used in birth control pills and in estrogen replacement therapy to treat symptoms of menopause. For a full discussion of the use of synthetic estrogens, *see* "Contraception and Abortion" and "Midlife Transitions."

eustachian tube The canal that connects the middle ear with the back of the throat and equalizes the pressure on either side of the eardrum. Swallowing is the mechanism by which air is forced into the tube, correcting the stuffy sensation in the ears produced by a change in air pressure as occurs in an elevator or airplane. The eustachian tube is also the pathway through which infection may travel from the nasal passages into the middle ear.

eye The organ of vision. The eyes are contained in bony sockets of the skull. The extent of their movements depends on six delicate muscles attached to the top, sides, and bottom of each eyeball. The movements of the lids, which serve to protect the eyes, are controlled by other muscles that are both voluntary and involuntary.

The front of the eyeball is covered by the translucent tissue called the cornea. It is a continuation of the tough fibrous sclera, the white of the eye that protects the delicate structures within. Under the cornea is a middle, pigmented layer that forms the iris which is responsible for the color of the eyes and which is densely supplied with blood vessels. The iris functions in much the same way as the diaphragm of a camera, narrowing or widening in response to varying light conditions to expand or contract the pupil, the opening through which light enters the eye. The dilation of the pupil is influenced by various chemicals as well as by light intensity.

The light that passes through the pupil is focused on the retina, the expanded end of the optic nerve extending into the middle of the brain. Within the retina are the nerve cells, the light- and color-sensitive rods and cones, and the many connections that supply information to the occipital lobes of the brain where stimuli are transformed into the images called "seeing." The information the eyes continuously send to the brain may

THE EYE IN X-SECTION

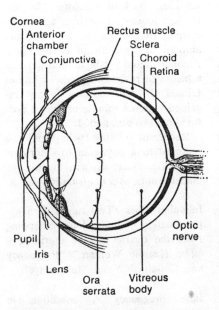

Cornea
Anterior chamber
Conjunctiva
Rectus muscle
Sclera
Choroid
Retina
Optic nerve
Pupil
Iris
Lens
Ora serrata
Vitreous body

be acted upon immediately or may be stored away as memory for future recall.

The main part of the eyeball is filled with a transparent jelly called the vitreous humor, and the area in front of the lens is filled with a watery substance called the aqueous humor. The eyes are constantly lubricated, cleansed, and protected from infection by the tears secreted through the lacrimal ducts.

Among the more common disorders of vision are astigmatism, farsightedness, and nearsightedness, all of which can be corrected by prescribed lenses. Cataracts and glaucoma, the two main causes of blindness in this country, can be treated surgically. A cornea damaged by disease or accident can now be replaced by a transplant.

Foreign objects in the eye should be dealt with by an eye doctor. Except for washing the eye with an irrigating solution contained in a dropper or an eye cup, no untrained person should attempt to treat any eye discomfort. Eye makeup and especially the brushes used to apply it should never be borrowed or lent as a precaution against the spread of infection.

eye examinations Any variation of vision, no matter how minor, should be evaluated. An ophthalmologist, a physician specializing in the eye, can diagnose or treat any disorder that might be affecting vision. Optometrists can check visual acuity and prescribe corrective lenses, but cannot diagnose organic eye disease. (An optician makes the prescription lens.) Women over forty should schedule a routine checkup for glaucoma once a year.

eyeglasses Lenses ground to individual prescription for the correction of defects in vision, such as nearsightedness, farsightedness, and astigmatism. Bifocals are worn when both short-range and long-range vision require correction. If vision is impaired at the middle distance as well, a second pair of glasses or trifocals may be necessary. For women whose distance vision is normal but who need reading glasses, half-lenses are often a satisfactory solution. Tinted glasses or sunglasses ground to individual prescription are both practical and useful for outdoor purposes. Women engaged in active sports should wear shatterproof glasses, and those who travel should carry an extra pair of glasses or the prescription for their corrective lenses. As changes in vision occur, the eyes should be checked for a new prescription. In order to decide whether to wear conventional glasses or contact lenses it is wise to consult an ophthalmologist.

eyestrain A feeling of tiredness in the eyes often accompanied by headache. The problem may exist with no apparent impairment of vision and is commonly the result of using one's eyes under poor lighting conditions.

It is important that the illumination come from the side and the rear in such a way that no shadow is cast on the object on which the eye is focused. It is also recommended that 60 or 75 watt light bulbs be used for reading. Office workers who suffer from chronic eyestrain due to poor lighting should make every effort to see that the condition is corrected. If the eyes tire before the completion of a task, they can be rested by closing the lids or by gazing into the distance. Television will not cause eyestrain if the set is properly adjusted and the viewer at a distance of approximately 6 feet from the picture. While it is advisable to have light in the room, it is important that it does not bounce off the TV screen into the viewer's eyes.

facial tic *See* TIC.

fainting A brief loss of consciousness caused by a temporary lack of oxygen to the brain; technically called syncope. (Fainting should not be confused with shock which is an emergency situation resulting from a critical loss of body fluids.) Fainting is usually preceded by lightheadedness, weakness, pallor, and a cold sweat. Circumstances that may reduce the brain's oxygen supply are a sudden emotional trauma, an excess intake of alcohol, and standing up for the first time after an illness. Standing still increases the chances of fainting because the blood supply to the brain is temporarily diminished. When one feels faint it is best to lie down or sit down with one's head lowered between the knees until the dizziness subsides. To help someone who has fainted, loosen all clothing and make certain that there is an adequate amount of fresh air to be breathed. Alcohol should not be administered as a means of reviving someone who has fainted. If consciousness is not regained within a minute or two, a doctor should be summoned.

Recurrent fainting spells should be reported to a physician to determine the cause. Heart disease, anemia, or diabetes may be a contributing factor.

fallopian tubes Two tubes, each approximately 4 inches long, extending from the ovaries to the uterus. *See* "The Healthy Woman," "Pregnancy and Childbirth," and "Infertility."

false pregnancy A condition in which overt signs of pregnancy exist, such as swelling of the breasts and the cessation of menstruation, but conception has not occurred; also known as pseudocyesis.

family history Facts concerning the health conditions, both mental and physical, of a patient's blood relatives. Some diseases are clearly inherited; others that do not necessarily have a genetic foundation may run in the family. With the increasing recognition of inheritance and predisposition as determinants of many diseases, every woman should be aware of her family's past and present medical history and should give this information to her doctor in detail. In describing a grandfather's diabetes or another relative's Duchenne muscular dystrophy, for example, the patient is providing the doctor with information that may be a clue for the early diagnosis of a condition.

family practitioner *See* DOCTOR.

farsightedness A disorder of vision in which only distant objects are seen clearly; technically called hyperopia. Farsightedness occurs when the lens of the eye focuses the image behind the retina rather than directly on it because the eyeball is shorter than normal from front to back. This disorder is corrected by wearing a convex lens that bends the light rays to the center of the retina.

fats An essential nutrient, found in both plant and animal food, composed of fatty acids (organic compounds of chains of carbon atoms with many hydrogen and some oxygen atoms added on). *See* "Nutrition and Weight."

feet The underlying cause of most foot problems is often improperly fitted shoes. Shoes and hosiery should be selected carefully in regard to proper fit, comfort, and support. Natural leather is preferred over other shoe materials since it allows the feet to "breathe" and has flexibility. Extremely high heels are inadvisable for those who walk a great deal since they place a strain on the foot and calf muscles and often cause problems with posture. Support hosiery is helpful in cases where constant standing places extra pressure on the blood vessels of the feet and legs. Any blister that does occur must be given prompt attention to avoid the possibility of infection.

Feet can be pampered by elevating them for a short period of time; circulation problems can be helped by immersing the feet in hot water and then rinsing with cold water. Exercises may keep feet limber and counteract the effects of poor circulation. These exercises may be simple ones such as wriggling the toes or picking up small objects with the toes. Walking barefoot on lawns or beaches is also helpful in keeping feet in good condition.

For chronic foot problems, consult a podiatrist (formerly called a chiropodist).

fertility The ability to conceive offspring. *See* "Infertility."

fetus The organism in the uterus after the eighth week of pregnancy. Prior to that time it is called an embryo. Some time around the eighteenth week the fetal heartbeat can be detected by placing an ear or a stethoscope against the mother's abdomen, and "quickening" or fetal movement also begins at about this time. By the twenty-fourth to twenty-seventh week a fetus is considered viable and, if born, may be kept alive with special hospital equipment and intensive care.

fever Body temperature that rises significantly above 98.6°F or 37°C, presumably due to a change in metabolic processes. A 1-degree variation is well within the normal range, since temperature rises this much after exercise, after a heavy meal, during hot weather when the body must work harder to rid itself of heat, or during ovulation when the increase in the secretion of progesterone affects the body processes.

A high fever usually results from a bacterial or viral infection; other causes may be heat stroke, brain injury, shock, or any occurrence affecting the brain center that regulates the balance between heat loss and heat production. Chills often precede or alternate with a high fever. As the temperature rises, the patient feels achy and thirsty, skin becomes hot and dry, urine is scant, and, depending on the cause, vomiting may take place. Until a doctor is consulted, a person with a high fever should stay in bed, drink lots of liquids, and take 10 grains of aspirin every four hours while awake. It should be kept in mind that the temperature reading on a rectal thermometer is usually 1 degree higher than the reading on a mouth thermometer. It should also be kept in mind that the seriousness of an illness cannot be judged by the presence or absence of fever.

fever sores   *See* HERPES SIMPLEX.

fiber   Cellulose or roughage in food. Fiber cannot be digested by humans. However, in small amounts it has a stimulating effect on the peristaltic action of the intestines and thus is useful in preventing sluggish digestive action and constipation. In larger amounts it acts as an irritant and can lead to unpleasant gastrointestinal disturbances. A balanced diet containing whole grain breads and cereals and cooked and raw vegetables provides sufficient fiber. *See* "Nutrition and Weight."

fibrillation   A condition in which the fibers of a muscle contract in groups or singly, rather than in unison, thus causing parts of the muscle to twitch in rapid succession. When fibrillation occurs in the ventricles of the heart, the muscle cannot contract in a coordinated way, and the heart stops beating. A patient in the intensive coronary care unit of a hospital who experiences ventricular fibrillation after a heart attack has a 90 percent chance of survival if treatment begins within one minute. Treatment consists of the use of a machine called a defibrillator, which attempts to jolt the heart back into its proper rhythmic pattern by means of electric current. Monitoring equipment in coronary care units can anticipate the onset of fibrillation by the characteristic EKG pattern of skipped ventricular beats. This monitoring system enables the doctor to prescribe medication that helps to prevent impending danger.

fibroadenoma   A benign tumor composed of fibrous tissue. *See* "Breast Care."

fibroadenosis   *See* "Breast Care."

fibrocystic disease   *See* "Breast Care."

fibroid tumor   *See* TUMOR.

first aid   Emergency treatment administered to the victim of an accident or unexpected illness prior to the arrival of medical assistance. Instruction in the fundamentals of first aid are available under the auspices of local Red Cross chapters, hospitals, or community organizations. Such instruction enables the potential rescuer to provide emergency treatment in the event of a crisis. First aid can be effectively and promptly administered if the proper supplies are on hand. Every home should have the following first aid supplies available:

roll of 2-inch wide sterile gauze
individually packaged gauze squares
cotton-tipped swabs
aspirin tablets
antihistamine tablets
oral and rectal thermometers
adhesive strip bandages, assorted sizes
sterile absorbent cotton
roll of adhesive tape
baking soda (bicarbonate of soda)
rubbing alcohol
surgical scissors and tweezers

fissure A crack in a mucous membrane. Fissures at the corner of the mouth are called cheilosis and result from a riboflavin (vitamin) deficiency. An anal fissure caused by chronic constipation may lead to the further inhibition of bowel movements due to the severity of pain accompanying the passage of stools. Another type of fissure, cracked nipples, is often found in nursing mothers. It can best be prevented by the use of lubricating cream. Since fissures may be a source of infection, a doctor should be consulted for proper treatment.

fistula An abnormal opening leading from a cavity or a hollow organ within the body to an adjacent part of the body or to the skin surface. Anal fistulas that occur because of a lesion or abscess in the anal canal or the rectum eventually become painful enough to require surgical removal. A fistula between the urethra and the vagina that results from damage to the organs during childbirth or during surgery may cause incomplete bladder control and urinary incontinence. A fistula between the vagina and the rectum may also occur after an operation. Both conditions should be evaluated for surgical correction.

flat feet A condition in which there is no arch between the toes and the heel; the imprint of the sole on a level surface is seen to rest flat. Flat feet may be hereditary, a consequence of obesity, a fractured heel bone, or arthritis, or the result of having worn archless or no shoes throughout childhood. Many women who walk long distances on hard surfaces or spend a great deal of time standing may develop flat feet because of stretched ligaments that cause bones to lose their normal position. Since flat feet can lead to fatigue and backaches, an orthopedist should be consulted in regard to special shoes and therapeutic exercises.

flu *See* INFLUENZA.

fluids The maintenance of proper fluid balance within the body is essential. An excessive loss through diarrhea, vomiting, hemorrhage, or perspiration leads to dehydration. The presence of salt and potassium and other electrolytes is essential for normal cellular use of fluids. People using diuretics must have regular tests to determine whether the salt and potassium level is sufficent. The condition of edema, or the abnormal fluid retention manifested in puffiness or swelling of the eyelids, ankles, or other parts of the body, is a symptom of an underlying condition that should be diagnosed by a doctor and corrected.

fluoridation The addition of a fluoride (a chemical salt containing fluorine) to public drinking water. There is still controversy over this practice, but health authorities, including the U.S. Public Health Service, the American Dental Association, the American Medical Association, and the World Health Organization, have not found significant evidence of harmful effects and have found that fluoridation is related to a decrease in dental decay among children. There is no question that the incidence of cavities is much lower where fluorides occur naturally in the water supply than elsewhere.

fluoroscope An X-ray machine that projects images of various organs of the body in motion, as well as bones, when the patient is placed between the X-ray tube and a fluorescent screen. Fluoroscopy can provide the doctor with an immediate picture of a functional disturbance of the heart, an incipient sign of respiratory distress (as the patient breathes), the exact location of a foreign object lodged in the windpipe, and other information that increases the possibility of achieving an accurate diagnosis.

folic acid One of the B-complex vitamins. *See* "Nutrition and Weight."

food additives Various chemicals combined with foods when they are being processed for distribution and consumption. Among the earliest additives were preservatives that kept bread fresh. When it was discovered in the 1920s that iodine was the essential trace element in the diet for the prevention of goiter, iodized salt began to appear on grocery shelves. Many deficiency diseases such as rickets, anemia, and pellagra, once endemic in parts of the United States and among the urban and rural poor, have all but disappeared thanks to the addition of such nutrients as vitamin D to milk, vitamin A to margarine, and niacin, riboflavin, thiamine, and iron to bread. Under the regulations of the FDA intentional additives are permissible if: they upgrade the nutritional value of food, improve its quality, prolong its freshness, or make it more readily available and more easily prepared.

The subject of food additives is somewhat controversial due to the 1958 Delaney amendment which states in part that no additive is permissible in any amount if tests have shown it to be cancer-producing. Women who are concerned about the chemicals that are added to foods for the purpose of artificial coloring, artificial flavoring (monosodium glutamate), or to prevent spoilage (sodium nitrite) should read the labels of processed foods as a means of determining whether certain products contain potentially hazardous ingredients. It is also helpful to scan newspapers and magazines for any results of food tests conducted by the FDA. Local libraries often provide consumer action pamphlets and reference material on this subject.

food poisoning (food-borne illness) The general term for any acute illness, usually gastrointestinal, which is caused by the ingestion of contaminated food or of uncontaminated food which is poisonous in and of itself. The term "ptomaine poisoning" is incorrect. The most common symptoms include nausea, vomiting, abdominal cramps, and diarrhea. Food can be contaminated by bacteria (salmonella, staphylococci, *Clostridium botulinum* which causes botulism, among others), viruses (hepatitis), chemicals (such as sodium fluoride, monosodium gluconate), parasites, plankton, and poisonous plants eaten by milk-producing cows. Salmonella and staphylococci are the most common contaminants. Salmonella are not unusual contaminants of meat, but are killed by proper cooking. When not killed and if present in sufficient numbers, they infect the eater and cause abdominal cramps and diarrhea some ten or more hours after ingestion. Staphylococci, if present, multiply in foods such as salads containing mayonnaise which are left at warm temperatures for several hours. They produce a toxin which causes nausea and vomiting three to six hours after being eaten. Proper cooking and refrigeration are the best ways to prevent disease from these two bacteria. Fortunately, most victims recover quickly and spontaneously from illnesses caused by both of these bacteria, although infants and elderly people can become extremely ill and die.

Poisonous foods include certain mushrooms, fish, berries, and nuts.

Food poisoning can produce serious illness and death especially if the central nervous system is affected as happens in botulism and mushroom poisoning. Any one believed to be ill from food poisoning (usually recognized because several people become ill simultaneously), who has symptoms other than mild nausea, vomiting, abdominal cramps, and diarrhea, should seek medical attention promptly as should those who possibly have been exposed to botulism or poisonous plants. *See also* BOTULISM, WORMS.

fracture A crack or complete break in a bone. A closed or simple fracture is one in which the skin remains intact. An open or compound fracture is one in which the skin is ruptured because the broken bone has penetrated it or because whatever caused the fracture also opened the skin. A complex or comminuted fracture is one in which the bone has been broken into many pieces or part of it has been shattered. Fractures often involve damage to surrounding ligaments and blood vessels. Immobilization, preferably by splinting, is the safest way to manage a fracture until professional treatment is available. In many cases a simple fracture may be indistinguishable from a sprain except by X-ray.

frigidity The term used to describe sexual dysfunction in the sense of inability to derive erotic pleasure from physical sexual activity and absence of any sexual feelings; although the term generally has been applied primarily to women, the condition exists among men as well. Frigidity is called primary when the condition has always been present and secondary if it is of sudden onset. The term was used in the past to describe a nonorgasmic woman, but such women are now said to be suffering from orgasmic dysfunction. While the two conditions are considered separate entities, frigid women are often nonorgasmic. Where clinical frigidity exists, whether because of some physical aberration or for psychological reasons, it should be investigated. A woman or a couple considering a program of sex therapy should consult a doctor about reputable and qualified therapists. In the absence of local professional practitioners, sex manuals may be helpful in guiding couples who are concerned about the woman's inability to achieve an orgasm.

frostbite Injury to a part of the body resulting from exposure to subfreezing temperature or wind-chill factor. Since the affected tissue can be irreversibly destroyed, frostbite is an emergency situation. The parts of the body normally exposed to extreme cold are the ears, nose, hands, and feet. When the blood vessels in these parts become so constricted that the blood supply is cut off, there is no longer sufficient internal warmth to prevent the exposed tissue from freezing and eventually becoming gangrenous. The first signs of frostbite are a tingling sensation and then numbness and a bluish-red appearance of the skin. If countermeasures are not taken at this stage, the affected areas begin to burn and itch as in chilblains, there is a total loss of sensation, and the skin turns dead white. Since the frostbitten area is extremely vulnerable to further injury, any clothing that may be an additional constraint to circulation, such as boots, socks, or tight gloves, should be removed as gently as possible. If circumstances permit, the injured parts of the body should be immersed quickly in warm—not hot—water. If this is not practical, the patient should be wrapped in blankets. If the feet are involved, walking should be forbidden. If an arm or a leg is involved, the victim should be encouraged to elevate it. Absolutely no attempt should be made to massage the affected parts, rub them with snow, or apply heat. Keep the victim comfortable by offering hot beverages and a sedative and painkiller. Smoking is forbidden since the nicotine will constrict the already impaired circulation. A dry sterile dressing should be used to prevent infection. If there is no visible return of circulation after these measures have been taken and the person's condition appears to be deteriorating, medical care should be obtained.

fungus infections Diseases caused by fungi and their spores that invade the skin, mucous membranes, and lungs and may even attack the bones and the brain. These diseases are known as mycoses. Fungi are parasites that may feed on dead organic matter or on live organisms. Fungi and their airborne spores or seeds are everywhere. Of the countless varieties, some cause mold and mildew, some are indispensable in the formation of alcohol and yeast, and a small number cause infection.

The more common fungus disorders are those confined to the skin, such as ringworm which results in red, scaly patches that itch and may form into blisters. Ringworm is highly contagious and can be passed on by household pets as well as by contaminated articles such as towels and bed linens. To prevent its spread from person to person and from one part of the body to another, ringworm should be treated promptly with suitable antifungicides. Athlete's foot (tinea pedis) is a form of ringworm that can be difficult to cure once it takes hold. The fungus usually lodges between the toes, multiplying rapidly in the warm, damp, dark environment and eventually causing the skin to crack and blister. To control a chronic case, feet should be kept meticulously clean and as dry as possible, a fungicidal powder should be sprinkled in the shoes, and a medicated ointment should be spread between the toes. If athlete's foot persists despite these measures, professional attention should be sought. The same fungus sometimes affects the nails (onychomycosis) and usually requires professional care.

Thrush is an oral fungus infection that attacks the mucous membranes of the mouth and tongue, and where resistance to infection is low, especially where the diet is deficient in vitamin B, it may spread into the pharynx. It is characterized by the formation of white patches that feel highly sensitive. Similar patches may also appear in the vagina and rectum (moniliasis or candidiasis). Where only the mouth is involved, mouthwashes containing gentian violet may be recommended. In cases of moniliasis medicated suppositories are usually prescribed.

It is thought that a regimen of certain antibiotics increases vulnerability to various fungus infections, since the medicines kill off not only the bacteria causing a particular disease, but also the benign ones whose presence guards against the growth of fungi. In recent years the medical profession and public health authorities have been concerned with a group of fungus infections that attack the lungs and can eventually invade other organs. Of these, histoplasmosis and "cocci" or coccidioidomycosis (also known as desert fever) are the result of breathing in certain spores that float freely in clouds of dust. The spores are harmless, if swallowed, but those that find their way into the air sacs of the lungs begin to grow and multiply, spreading inflammation through the respiratory system and eventually into other parts of the body. Typical symptoms include a chronic cough, fever, and other manifestations that may be confused with pneumonia or tuberculosis. When tests produce the correct diagnosis, hospitalization may be required for the administration of a specific medication called Amphotericin-B.

gallbladder A membranous sac, approximately 3 inches long, situated below the liver. The gallbladder drains bile from the liver, stores and concentrates it, and eventually sends it on to the duodenum. The alkalinity of the bile is essential for neutralizing the acidity of the digested material leaving the stomach. Its component juices transform fatty compounds into simpler nutrients that can be absorbed by the intestines. A system of ducts controlled by sphincters releases bile when it is needed and forces the excess back into the gallbladder for storage.

In some cases the concentrated bile forms into gallstones. Inflammation of the gallbladder, technically called cholecystitis, may be acute or chronic. In its acute form it usually follows

bacterial infection or a sudden blockage of one of the ducts by a tumor or a large stone. Symptoms of an attack are nausea, vomiting, sweating, and sharp pain in the upper right part of the abdomen under the ribs, possibly extending to the shoulder. Jaundice may also be present. If the acute phase of the attack does not subside, emergency surgery may be necessary to prevent the danger of a rupture. The gallbladder is not usually removed unless X-rays indicate that the condition cannot be cured by routine medical treatment. Chronic gallbladder disease may cause gassiness and discomfort following a meal containing fatty foods. Abdominal pain may be brief but recurrent. In many cases the condition can be alleviated by a low-fat diet. When a low-grade infection of the bile ducts is the source of

GALLBLADDER

Liver
Cystic duct
Hepatic duct
Gallbladder
Duodenum
Bile duct

POSSIBLE SITES OF OBSTRUCTION BY GALLSTONES

the discomfort, antibiotics may be prescribed.

gallstones Solid masses that form within the gallbladder or bile ducts. The lithogenicity or stone-forming tendency of bile results in three different types of stones: those composed of a combination of calcium, bile pigments, and cholesterol, those that are pure cholesterol, and those rare formations that are made of bile pigments only. Gallstones of the first two types are especially prevalent following pregnancy and are most common in both men and women after the age of 40. Cholesterol gallstones can be dissolved medically with a chemical compound similar in composition to natural human bile acid, thus eliminating the necessity for surgery to remove them if they cause an acute gallbladder attack.

gamma globulin The portion of the blood richest in antibodies. It is produced mainly by the lymphocytes in the lymphoid tissues and is one of the body's strongest defenses against infectious disease. Gamma globulin in one of two forms may be injected to confer passive (temporary) immunity to certain diseases. Immune serum globulin is derived from blood taken from donors who have an immunity to a specific disease either naturally or subsequent to active immunization. A specific preparation, such as measles immune globulin, is derived from donors who are convalescing from the disease or who have been recently immunized against it.

gangrene A condition in which tissue dies primarily due to loss of blood supply. Gangrene usually involves the extremities, but may occur in any part of the body where circulation has been cut off or in which massive infection has caused the affected tissue to putrefy. Among the circumstances leading to most gangrene are severe burns, frostbite, accidents involving contact with corrosive chemicals, untreated ulcerated bedsores, a carelessly applied and improperly attended tourniquet, or any other condition that cuts off circulation. When blood supply fails, infection by gas gangrene bacteria sets in. These bacteria live on dead tissue and produce toxins that poison surrounding live tissue. The dry gangrenous condition that occurs due to atherosclerosis, whether or not diabetes is present, most commonly affects the extremities. In such cases a toe or finger will shrink and turn black, and there will be a distinct line of demarcation between the healthy and gangrenous tissues. It is now possible to prevent the spread of gangrene with antibiotics and surgery. Should circumstances indicate the possibility of tissue death, particularly if numbness and discoloration of the extremities are apparent in a diabetic, it is the sign that emergency treatment is necessary.

gastrointestinal disorders Any number of conditions affecting the normal functions of digestion and elimination of food as it passes through the alimentary canal. Disorders may result from an infection caused by bacteria, viruses, or parasites, an obstruction due to a tumor, ulcers, hernias, allergies, food-borne illnesses, metabolic defects, or emotional stress. Symptoms may include mild to severe abdominal pain, constipation, diarrhea, rectal bleeding, jaundice, weight loss, nausea, vomiting, loss of appetite. Diagnosis of many disorders of the esophagus, stomach, small intestines, lower bowel, and rectum is based on X-rays. The diagnosis of other gastrointestinal disorders may require laboratory tests of blood and stools. Depending on the findings, treatment may involve a specific medication, a special diet, or surgery.

general practitioner *See* DOCTOR.

generic drugs *See* "Commonly Prescribed Brand Name Drugs and Generic Equivalents" Table 5, Appendixes.

genetic counseling The National Institute of General Medical Sciences estimates that some 12 million Americans bear the risk of transmitting hereditary disorders. For this group of people genetic counseling has become an important medical service. Counseling involves educating the parents-to-be about the factors associated with genetic diseases, including diagnosis, the usual course of the disorder, and the risk of its occurrence or recurrence. Counseling also explores alternatives that take these factors into account and at the same time conform with the individuals' ethical principles and religious convictions.

Any woman who is interested in finding out whether she is a potential carrier of a genetic illness or how to prevent a genetic illness should ask her doctor for the name of an appropriate counseling agency or write to the National Genetics Foundation, Inc., 555 West 57th Street, New York, New York 10019, which acts as a clearinghouse for information concerning genetic counseling centers located at leading medical institutions throughout the United States. This ad-

visory and referral service is free. Another source of information is the National Foundation–March of Dimes, Box 2000, White Plains, New York 10602.

geriatrics The branch of medical science that deals with the diseases and the health maintenance of the aged. It is related to gerontology which studies not just medical problems, but all aspects of aging—biological processes, environmental factors, and social problems. *See* "Aging Healthfully."

German measles *See* RUBELLA.

gingivitis Inflammation of the gums due to a tissue-destroying enzyme that stems from bacteria that cause the formation of cavities. Inflammation usually starts in the gingival crevice, a groove between the gum and tooth. Since untreated gingivitis may result in the destruction of bone tissue and the loosening or loss of teeth, prompt efforts should be made to control gum inflammation. The dental specialist who treats gingivitis is a periodontist. The form of treatment varies from scraping away the accumulation of plaque and calculus deposits at and below the gumline to oral surgery for the removal of pocket formations in which food and bacteria have collected. Gingivitis is most prevalent in women who smoke, whose diet is deficient in a particular nutrient, and who have been negligent in the dental care of their gums and teeth. Proper oral hygiene is the most effective way to prevent gingivitis or to limit its recurrence. A dentist should be consulted as to the correct way to brush and floss teeth.

gland Any organ that produces and

secretes a specific chemical substance. There are two categories of glands: the ductless or endocrine glands, whose secretions are delivered directly into the bloodstream, and the exocrine glands, whose ducts transport their secretions to a precise location. The major endocrine glands are listed in the chapter "The Healthy Woman."

The most important exocrines are the following. The salivary glands produce the saliva that moisturizes the food in the mouth at the beginning of the digestive process. The sebaceous glands, found under the skin, produce an oil essential for its health. The sweat glands maintain the body's temperature and are part of the excretory system. The pancreas, liver, stomach, and small intestines secrete vital digestive juices. The lachrymal or tear glands are closely involved with emotional response and essential for the cleansing and lubrication of the eyes. The female exocrine glands include the vestibular glands (Bartholin's glands) located on either side of the vaginal opening, and Skene's glands, located on either side of the urethral opening. The mammary glands in the breasts supply milk for offspring. The prostate gland in men produces a secretion related to the reproductive process.

The structures sometimes referred to as lymph glands are not glands and are properly called lymph nodes. *See* LYMPH NODES.

glaucoma An eye disease that leads to progressive impairment of vision due to increased fluid pressure against the retina. Glaucoma is a leading cause of blindness in the United States, affecting approximately 2 million people. While there is no known means of preventing glaucoma, there is a test that can diagnose the disease

in its earliest stages. The test should be done on a regular basis after age 40 and at an earlier age if there is a family history of glaucoma or diabetes.

The onset of glaucoma may be insidious and usually occurs in middle age. Symptoms, which persist even after many changes in eyeglass prescriptions, are blurring of vision, difficulty in focusing, loss of peripheral sight, and slow adaptation to darkness. The machine used for testing glaucoma is called a tonometer. It is a noncontact instrument that measures the pressure within the eyes. Marginal cases may require intermittent tests to establish whether the disease actually exists, since pressure within the eye can be affected by various chemicals found in food and alcoholic beverages or by other circum-

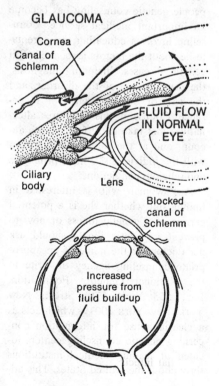

GLAUCOMA

Cornea
Canal of Schlemm
FLUID FLOW IN NORMAL EYE
Ciliary body
Lens
Blocked canal of Schlemm
Increased pressure from fluid build-up

stances. The disease can also be precipitated or aggravated by medications, especially by antihypertensive drugs and cortisone.

While the glaucoma test can be administered by an optometrist, only an ophthalmologist can treat the symptoms. Irreversible damage to vision may be prevented by medication or surgery. The medication usually prescribed is eyedrops that reduce the pressure within the eye or that facilitate the draining away of the fluid before it accumulates in sufficient quantity to damage the optic nerve. In a minority of cases drainage can be accomplished only by surgery.

The National Society to Prevent Blindness, with chapters in many parts of the United States, provides information about the disease. If there is no local chapter, inquiries may be directed to the Society's national office, 79 Madison Avenue, New York, New York 10016.

globus A lump or mass, commonly associated with the term globus hystericus, the sensation often known as "a lump in the throat" that makes it difficult to swallow. The feeling is a manifestation of anxiety neurosis.

glomerulonephritis A kidney disease that affects the coiled clusters of capillary vessels, the glomeruli, through which the fluid content of the blood is partially filtered before it turns into urine. Each kidney consists of approximately a million of these filters. The capillaries may become inflamed following several varieties of bacterial infection, especially following a strep infection in the throat or elsewhere. Since acute nephritis may develop if the initial infection is not successfully

treated with antibiotics, it is extremely important to consult a doctor immediately about any painful sore throat accompanied by a high fever. When glomerulonephritis occurs, the body retains fluid due to a collapse in the kidney's filtering capacity. Typical symptoms of the condition are puffy eyelids, swollen ankles, headaches, and decrease in urinary output. Once the correct diagnosis is made on the basis of red blood cells present in the urine, a regimen of bed rest, special diet, and fluid restriction is the usual procedure.

glucose A sugar that occurs naturally in honey and in most fruit, and the one into which starches and polysaccharide (complex) sugars are converted by the digestive process. Glucose is a major source of body fuel. Because it can be absorbed from the stomach, it is one of the quickest sources of energy. Glucose, or its variant dextrose, is also the nutrient usually administered intravenously when a patient cannot eat normally.

Glucose is present in human blood (blood sugar) at concentrations of 70 to 120 milligrams per 100 cubic centimeters of blood. Higher or much lower concentrations may indicate the presence, respectively, of diabetes or hypoglycemia. Glucose is normally not present in the urine; its presence there may indicate diabetes. The glucose tolerance test (GTT) measures the rate at which the body removes glucose from the blood. After the patient drinks a sugar solution or glucose is given intravenously, a series of blood and urine sugar tests are made during the next three to four hours. The GTT is a more refined screening technique than a single test for glucose in urine or blood and is used to identify disease when these tests provide ambiguous or inconclusive results.

glycogen A starchlike substance derived largely from glucose and stored in various organs of the body. It is converted back to glucose by various enzymes under hormonal influence, including insulin, when needed for body fuel.

goiter An enlargement of the thyroid gland. This endocrine gland, located at the base of the neck, extracts the iodine absorbed by the blood from food and drinking water and uses it for the production of the hormone thyroxin. Thyroxin is stored in the glandular follicles and released into the bloodstream as needed for the regulation of the metabolic rate. The body's iodine requirements are no more than a few millionths of an ounce, and since iodine is generally present in the soil, in most areas the requisite amounts occur naturally in food and water. Certain regions of the United States, mainly inland, are deficient in iodine and these areas have become known as the goiter belt. People living in these areas often have an enlargement of the thyroid gland, unless the deficiency is compensated for by the use of iodized salt. The enlargement occurs because the thyroid's cells increase in number in order to satisfy the body's demand for thyroxin. Eventually the gland may develop nodules or lumps. The danger of goiter is that it may press on the surrounding organs, leading to difficulty in swallowing or breathing. When properly treated with iodine or with thyroxin itself, the goiter usually subsides. Goiter is much more common among women than men because their bodies require considerably more thyroxin during puberty, the menstrual cycle, and pregnancy. A pregnant woman must be sure that her diet contains the iodine essential for the baby's healthy prenatal development.

A goiter is often accompanied by an overactive thyroid gland (hyperthyroidism). In cases where treatment of the hyperthyroidism and the goiter by medication or radioactive iodine is unsuccessful, surgery may be necessary. The scar resulting from such an operation usually fades almost completely.

A less common type of goiter is characterized by an oversized thyroid gland incapable of manufacturing enough thyroxin (hypothyroidism). A baby born to a hypothyroid mother is likely to suffer from the permanent impairment of mental and

GOITER

Swollen
thyroid gland

physical development known as cretinism if the baby is not treated immediately. Successful treatment of hypothyroidism is accomplished easily by taking thyroid hormone extract by mouth. This corrects the underactive thyroid and usually the goiter as well.

Occasionally the thyroid gland enlarges because it becomes inflamed or infected (thyroiditis). Specific treatment is sometimes necessary and recovery usually complete.

gonads *See* OVARY, TESTICLE.

gonorrhea A sexually transmissible disease caused by the bacterium *Neisseria gonococcus,* which thrives in the warm moist linings of the genitourinary tract. *See* "Sexually Transmissible Diseases."

GONORRHEA

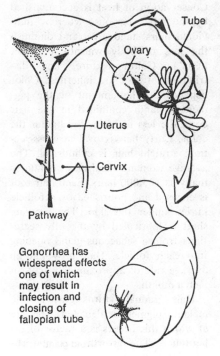

Tube

Ovary

Uterus

Cervix

Pathway

Gonorrhea has widespread effects one of which may result in infection and closing of fallopian tube

gout A form of arthritis resulting from a change in uric acid metabolism. This metabolic aberration may be inherited or may arise from the use of diuretics. It causes the uric acid naturally produced by the body to accumulate in the joints in the form of crystals, leading to acute inflammation and swelling. Joints affected by gout include those in the big toe and fingers and the ankle, elbow, and wrist. Pain in the big toe is most common because of the pressure of body weight on the foot. In chronic gouty arthritis the uric crystals spread and all the joints may be sore and stiff. There is also a possibility that the spreading crystalline deposits will accumulate in the kidneys in the form of stones.

Medicines have recently been developed for the effective treatment of gout. The treatment, which controls rather than cures the disease, consists of two types of drugs: those that stimulate the elimination of uric acid and those that reduce its production. While the victims of gout are usually men, the disease sometimes attacks women, typically after the menopause. Women who feel "aches in the joints" or discomfort in the big toe or observe the beginnings of swellings of the finger joints, especially after dieting or using diuretics, should consult their doctor about the possible onset of gout. A simple blood test for uric acid content can diagnose the presence of the condition.

granuloma   inguinale A sexually transmissible disease most commonly found in southern or tropical regions and caused by a specific organism, the bacillus *Donovania granulomatis. See* "Sexually Transmissible Diseases."

group therapy A psychotherapeutic technique in which interaction among several patients, supervised by a trained person, is used as a means of clarifying certain behavior patterns.

gums The fleshy fibrous tissue that covers the areas of the upper and lower jaw in which teeth are anchored. The mucous membrane that covers the gums forms a network of vessels that carry blood and lymph from the jaws to the face. Healthy gums are pink, firm, somewhat stippled, and form a collar around the neck of each tooth.

Practically all gum inflammation, or gingivitis, starts between the gum and the tooth in a shallow groove called the gingival crevice. It must be treated promptly by a dentist. A gum disease, commonly known as trench mouth and technically called Vincent's angina, is an infection of the mucous membrane. If permitted to spread, it may reach the lips and tongue. It is caused by a particular strain of bacteria, *Borrelia vincentii,* normally present in the mouth. When general health is good the bacteria are usually inactive, but when resistance is low and dental hygiene poor, these organisms, combined with other bacteria, often cause the disease. Its symptoms are inflamed gums, foul breath, and painful ulcers that not only bleed easily but may interfere with swallowing. It may be accompanied by swollen glands, sore throat, and fever. The disease usually clears up when treated with an antibiotic and can best be prevented from recurring by maintaining good health and proper oral hygiene.

The gums can be kept in good condition by brushing the teeth slowly from the gumline upward for the bottom teeth and from the gumline downward for the top teeth. Brushing the teeth horizontally is not correct since it does not stimulate the gums. Food particles lodged between the teeth and at the gumline should be dislodged by unwaxed floss, and tartar deposits should be scraped off by a dentist twice a year. Since improperly fitted dentures may affect gums adversely, dentures should be checked for necessary adjustments from time to time.

gynecologist *See* DOCTOR.

hair A specialized body growth consisting of dead skin cells that are filled with a tough protein material called keratin which is also the main constituent of the nails. Aside from the palms of the hand and the soles of the feet, hair covers almost the entire body surface to protect various areas of the body and to help to retain heat. Conservation of heat is accomplished by the reflex response whereby individual hairs stand erect and diminish the loss of body warmth ("gooseflesh"). Color, texture, and distribution of hair are inherited. Color depends on the amount of the pigment melanin contained in the hair core; the less melanin, the lighter the color. Curly hair is oval in cross-section; straight hair is cylindrical. The average woman's head may contain as many as 125,000 hairs. Each hair root is encased and nourished by a follicle buried under the skin. The growing shaft is lubricated by the oily secretions from a sebaceous gland opening into each follicle. Hair grows at an average rate of approximately half an inch a month.

Hair gradually turns gray as the melanin pigment is depleted. The age at which this occurs is a factor of inheritance. The growth and nourishment of hair are controlled by hormone secretions and the general state of one's health. The application of creams, lotions, vitamins or minerals does not affect the growth and thickness of hair in a healthy individual.

Hair should be shampooed on a regular basis, the frequency depending on a number of factors such as climate or whether the hair is dry or oily. Thorough rinsing is essential to remove all surface matter. Brushing the hair between shampoos eliminates surface dirt and also distributes the natural oils. A brush made with natural bristles is not apt to cause damage to the hair. It should be kept scrupulously clean in order to prevent an infection of the scalp.

Products used on the hair should be selected carefully to avoid any which irritate the skin, contain chemicals that might damage hair or skin, or might clog the pores of the scalp. Hair sprays should not be inhaled. Chemical hair dyes have been subjected to increasingly close scrutiny because of their potentially carcinogenic contents. Warnings in beauty shops and on home products should be evaluated carefully before deciding whether to dye one's hair. The decision may also be affected by consumer advocate reports and medical recommendations.

Women who wear wigs should select them for proper fit and porousness to allow the scalp to "breathe" and to avoid profuse sweating. Hair covered by a wig should be washed often enough to eliminate the inevitable accumulation of sweat. The wigs themselves should be kept scrupulously clean.

hair loss *See* BALDNESS.

hair removal Temporary or permanent elimination of unwanted hair; technically called depilation. The method used depends on the area and amounts involved, whether the removal is to be temporary or permanent, the amount of time and money required, and whether the hair is to be removed at home or by a trained technician. The simplest and least expensive method for removal of unwanted hair from the legs and underarms is shaving after applying cream or a lather of soap. This method does not cause the hair to grow back in increasing amounts, as the number of hair follicles one is born with remains constant unless the hairs are removed by electrolysis. Sparse face hair or unwanted hair between the breasts can be removed with tweezers. While somewhat painful, waxing has become increasingly popular as a hair removal method and with proper training can be done at home. Hot wax is applied to the skin and covered with cloth strips; when the wax has hardened, the strips are yanked off, removing both the wax and the embedded hairs. Prior to application, the wax should be tested on the back of the hand to make certain it will not burn the skin. Any skin irritation following the removal of the strips should be soothed with calamine lotion. Hair may also be removed by a depilatory containing chemicals that dissolve the hair at the surface of the skin. A patch test should precede the use of a depilatory to rule out the possibility of an allergic response to the product. Depilatories should be used with caution on the face and never applied immediately after a bath or shower while skin pores are still open. For the same reason they should be removed with cool rather than warm water.

Permanent hair removal is achieved when each hair bulb is destroyed electrically. The procedure is expensive and time-consuming and must be performed by a trained operator. Electrolysis is the older and more conventional method of permanent hair removal. A more recent version, based on the same principle, is called Depilatron. It supposedly eliminates pain, thus enabling the operator to cover a greater area of skin at each session.

halitosis The technical term for bad breath. The most common cause is poor oral hygiene and health; abscessed teeth, gingivitis, dirty dentures. Food particles trapped between the teeth, and fungus infections of the mouth are sources of decaying matter in the mouth in which microorganisms that cause the odor can grow. Bad breath on arising is characteristic in people who drink or smoke excessively. Halitosis may also be a symptom of certain respiratory, digestive, or kidney disorders, so it is important to determine whether the cause is of dental or medical origin. In the absence of a physical disorder and with normal attention to dental cleanliness and health, the breath of most people is quite acceptable. Mouthwashes and other preparations are helpful in temporarily masking bad breath.

hallucination The perception of a sound, sight, smell, or other sensory experience without the presence of an external physical stimulus. Hallucinations are produced by certain drugs. Hallucinatory episodes may be associated with such organic conditions as hardening of the arteries of the brain (cerebral arteriosclerosis) or brain tumor and with exhaustion, sleep deprivation, or prolonged solitary confinement or isolation from normal stimuli. Such experiences are also characteristic of delirium tremens, some forms of mental illness, and psychotic interludes following sudden withdrawal from barbiturates.

hallucinogens A category of consciousness-altering substances chemically related to each other; more popularly known as psychedelic drugs. *See* "Drugs, Alcohol, and Tobacco."

hand care *See* SKIN CARE.

hangover Symptoms of headache, queasiness, thirst, or nausea occurring the morning after drinking alcohol; also feelings of disorientation and befuddlement following the use of sleeping pills containing barbiturates. The amount of alcohol that will create a hangover varies from person to person and from time to time for the same person. It may result from having had very little to drink while one was tense, angry, or tired, or hungry. Some experts believe that the miseries of a hangover are a self-punitive mechanism caused by guilt feelings after excessive drinking. Many moderate drinkers have discovered that they are more likely to have hangovers after drinking scotch, gin, or bourbon than after drinking vodka and that wine or brandy can be deadly even in small amounts. This may be because of all alcoholic drinks, vodka contains the fewest of the complicated chemicals known as congeners. Since the circumstances that cause the malaise are so varied, each woman must figure out for herself how to prevent its occurrence.

The physiological mechanisms that cause the symptoms originate in the disruptive effects of alcohol on body chemistry. Its diuretic properties result in thirst, irritation of the lining of the gastrointestinal tract causes nausea, and dilation of blood vessels leads to throbbing headache. If a remedy is necessary, aspirin will help a headache and an alkalizer may soothe the queasiness.

hay fever *See* ALLERGIES.

headache Any pain or discomfort in the head; one of the most common complaints and a symptom for which medical science has itemized upwards of 200 possible causes. While it may be difficult to pinpoint a cause in a particular case, it should be comforting to know that 90 percent of all headaches are not caused by structural defects.

Some familiarity with the structures of the head is helpful in understanding why headaches occur. The bony structure of the skull contains the orbits of the eyes, the nasal cavities, the eight nasal accessory cavities, known as sinuses, and the teeth. Two of the sinuses are in the cheekbone (the antra), two above the eyebrows (the frontal sinuses), and four more at the base of the skull. Within the skull and protected by its rigid bony surface is the brain which itself has no pain receptors, but is surrounded by extremely sensitive tissues. It is covered by membranes known as meninges; the cerebrospinal fluid that acts as a cushion between the brain and the skull and also circulates between the brain and its membranous layers as well as around and within the spinal cord. A network of blood vessels interlace the coverings of the brain to supply oxygen and other essential nutrients to the brain and to transport the depleted blood back to the heart. It is not difficult to imagine how many chemical, physical, psychological, neurological, bacteriological, viral, and other variables can lead to changes, usually temporary, in the structures just described, most of which are sensitive to pain. For example, swelling of the blood vessels, inflammation of the nerve endings, or muscular contractions at the base of the skull, will cause the head to pound, throb, or ache.

Headaches can be classified as simple recurring, nonsimple recurring, or acute nonrecurring. Simple headaches occur at varying intervals and may be annoying or mildly disabling. Most simple recurring headaches are generally known as tension headaches. The immediate cause of the pain is the stiffening of the muscles at the base of the skull which sets up a cycle of contraction in response to pain and causes further pain because of the contractions. The usual reason for the stiffening of the muscles is emotional stress. In some cases, a muscle con-

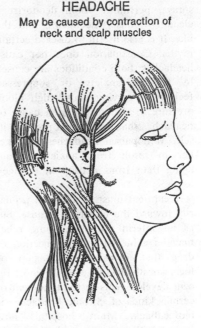

HEADACHE
May be caused by contraction of neck and scalp muscles

May be caused by constriction, edema and dilation of head arteries

traction headache may originate in a simple physical circumstance: a draft from a fan or airconditioner, straining to see or hear, or a response to pain elsewhere in the body. Such headaches may be mild or severe. When they respond favorably to over-the-counter analgesics and occur rarely, they can be viewed as one of life's nuisances.

When the headaches recur with debilitating frequency, further exploration into their cause is essential. They may be caused by injuries to the head or neck, reactions to certain pharmacologic agents, including alcohol, incorrect refraction of vision, or a variety of diseases such as high blood pressure, diabetes mellitus, and hyper- or hypothyroidism. In trying to identify the cause of these headaches, women should not overlook the possibility that they might be triggered by a response to the chemicals in hairsprays, perfumes, room deodorizers, cleaning fluids, insecticides, and the like. It is also useful to discard certain myths. Constipation does not cause headaches; both conditions are caused by tension, anxiety, or suppressed feelings. Worrying about high blood pressure is a more common cause of headaches than high blood pressure itself. Menopausal headaches are likelier to result from anxieties about aging than from a drop in estrogen levels.

Treatment must be directed primarily toward the underlying cause, but as an interim measure, some relief may be achieved by the injection of drugs that act as muscle-relaxants or local anesthetics. One of the most recent developments in the treatment of certain kinds of chronic headaches is biofeedback. Many hospitals now have established centers that use biofeedback techniques based on the pa-

tients' awareness of tension and relaxation mechanisms and how to control them.

Nonsimple recurring headaches differ from simple ones in several ways. They cause more severe symptoms, and they generally are caused by dilation of the blood vessels in the brain for which there is no explanation, as well as by contraction. The most widely known of these vascular headaches are the classic migraine headache and the common migraine headache. The classic migraine tends to be familial, is pulsating in nature, affects only one side of the head at a time, may be preceded more or less immediately by loss of vision, flashing lights, or varying neurological symptoms, and is often accompanied by nausea and vomiting. The pain is most severe during the first hour and then subsides. Frequency tends to increase during stress and to decrease with age. Treatment varies and is varyingly successful. The common migraine headache is more common. Symptoms are less specific than those of classic migraine. Mood changes usually precede it and may last several hours or days before the headache starts. The headache, also on one side of the head, may last several days. Again treatment varies and is varyingly successful. A third type of vascular headache is called the cluster headache. It is a series of closely spaced headaches, each of 20 to 90 minutes duration, continuing for several days, and then often followed by months or years of no such attacks. It may be triggered by certain foods and chemicals, such as caffeine in coffee, tea, and cola drinks; nicotine in cigarettes; monosodium glutamate in various cooked and processed foods; nitrites added to smoked meats; congeners in certain alcoholic beverages; and estrogen in certain contraceptive pills. Treatment for vascular headaches includes drugs such as ergotamine, various analgesics, including narcotics, and biofeedback techniques.

The acute nonrecurring headache usually has a sudden onset. It may be caused by a specific disease or condition which may or may not be serious or it may represent a change in the individual's pattern of simple recurring headaches. It may accompany a generalized infection, such as influenza, infectious mononucleosis, gastritis, sinusitis, otitis media (middle ear), or abscessed tooth, or it may be part of an infection of the central nervous system, such as meningitis, encephalitis, poliomyelitis, or brain abscess. It may also be caused by a brain tumor, aneurysm, or hemorrhage. The hemorrhage may be caused by an injury (contusion, concussion, or skull fracture) or be unrelated to injury. One particular type of headache is associated with a medical procedure called a lumbar puncture or spinal tap. It can be extremely severe, is usually worse when standing or sitting up and subsides in several days. Unless the headache subsides in a few hours a medical diagnosis should be sought so that the proper therapy can be initiated.

hearing aids Electronic instruments that amplify sounds. The instrument may be built into the temple piece of eyeglasses, fit inside the ear, or have a microphone behind the ear or worn on the clothing and a receiver inside the ear. A hearing aid must be fitted and regularly adjusted by a trained specialist (audiologist) after an ear specialist (otologist) has determined that some of the hearing loss can be restored in this way. Under no circumstances should a hearing aid be bought directly from a retail dealer. Community health centers or a doctor can supply the address of a nonprofit hearing aid clinic where the degree and type of deafness is accurately determined, recommendations are made for the type of instrument, if any, best suited to individual needs, and instruction is given in the most effective way to use the aid, including courses in lipreading if that skill might contribute to optimum results.

hearing loss Interruption at any point along the path traveled by sound vibrations before the information can reach the brain for processing. Hearing loss may be partial or total, temporary or permanent, congenital or acquired. The two major causes are disorders of conduction, which generally result in a loss of low-pitched sounds, and nerve defects, which generally result in a loss of high-pitched sounds. When both conditions are present, the disability is called mixed deafness. Conduction deafness may be a consequence of any of the following: obstruction by wax accumulation, inflammation of the middle ear, fluid accumulation, damaged eardrum, infection of the eustachian tube, and otosclerosis. Otosclerosis, most common among the elderly, is a progressive disease that freezes one of the three bones of hearing (the stapes) into immobility by imbedding it in a bony growth, thus preventing the soundwaves from being transmitted to the inner ear.

Nerve deafness may be caused by severe head injury, chronic infection that disables the auditory nerve, tumor, prolonged exposure to damaging noise levels ("boilermaker's deafness"), or drugs taken for some other condition.

Ringing in the ears (tinnitus) that interferes with hearing may be caused by arteriosclerosis, hypertension, or medicines containing quinine. It may also be a symptom of Menière's disease.

Since one of the causes of congenital deafness is presumed to be the mother's exposure to rubella (German measles) during the early months of pregnancy, such exposure should be reported promptly to the doctor in charge of prenatal care to determine what course of action to take.

Any indications of the onset of hearing loss should be investigated by an ear specialist. Conductive hearing loss is more susceptible to correction than nerve impairment and may be treated medically and surgically. New techniques of microsurgery have enabled specialists to restore hearing by a procedure called fenestration which opens up a new path at the inner end of the middle ear along which sound waves can travel when the normal one is obstructed. Another ingenious operation is the stapedectomy in which the otosclerotic growth and the immobilized stapes are removed and replaced by plastic and wire that conduct the sound vibrations.

hearing tests The determination of hearing acuity by the use of diagnostic instruments and procedures. Anyone who suspects a hearing loss, no matter how slight, should arrange to have her hearing tested by a physician. One of the oldest and most accurate tests measures the subject's responses to the vibrations of the stem and prongs of a tuning fork. The test can reveal whether the patient is suffering from nerve deafness or conduction deafness. A more accurate record of deviation from normal hearing is achieved by examination with

an audiometer. The machine tests each ear for sensitivity to different frequencies and intensities of sounds and plots the subject's responses on an audiogram. With the results of other examinations, the audiogram is evaluated by the specialist to determine whether the hearing loss can best be corrected medically, surgically, or by a particular type of hearing aid.

heart The muscular organ that controls the circulation of the blood. It is approximately the size and shape of a fist, weighs about three-quarters of a pound, and lies in the mid-left section of the chest near the breastbone. The heart is actually two pumps lying side by side: the right side collects the venous blood and sends it to the lungs for the removal of carbon dioxide and addition of oxygen. The freshly oxygenated blood then enters the left side of the heart and is pumped out through the aorta for recirculation. The heart is nourished by its own vessels, the coronary arteries. The muscular pumping action consists of a rhythmic contraction (systole) followed by relaxation (diastole). The heart is protected by a tough membrane known as the pericardium. Its inner chambers are lined with endocardium. There are four chambers within the heart; the two upper chambers are the atria, the two lower ones, the ventricles. The atrium and ventricle on each side of the heart form a self-contained unit; there is no connection between the two so that pulmonary and systemic blood flows cannot be mingled. The upper and lower portions of each side are separated by valves, and the blood leaves the heart through two other valves: the pulmonary valve that opens into the pulmonary artery from the right ventricle and the aortic valve that opens into

BLOOD FLOW IN THE HEART

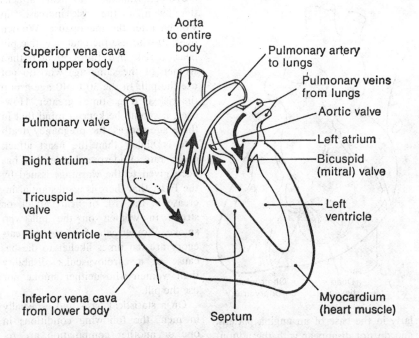

Superior vena cava from upper body

Aorta to entire body

Pulmonary artery to lungs

Pulmonary veins from lungs

Pulmonary valve

Aortic valve

Right atrium

Left atrium

Bicuspid (mitral) valve

Tricuspid valve

Left ventricle

Right ventricle

Inferior vena cava from lower body

Septum

Myocardium (heart muscle)

the aorta from the left ventricle. When the doctor listens to the heart with a stethoscope, the sounds made by the valves as they open and close are indications of health or impairment. The normal sound is heard as "lub-dup." Variations in this sound, some of which are called murmurs, are caused by leaks that occur because the valves do not open and close as they should, usually because of a congenital defect or because of damage during rheumatic fever.

Within the muscle tissue of the heart is a dense network of interwoven fibers which include a part known as the pacemaker because it is responsible for transmitting the electrical impulses that initiate the rhythmic contractions of the heartbeat throughout the network. These impulses, normally transmitted 70 to 80 times a minute, and the contractions are portrayed in an electrocardiogram. One

of the greatest medical advances of modern times is the development of an artificial pacemaker which can be embedded in the chest wall and attached to the heart when the natural one can no longer work efficiently.

heart attack A condition ranging from mild to severe in which one or more of the arteries that supply blood to the heart are blocked or occluded by a clot; also called myocardial infarction, coronary occlusion, or coronary thrombosis. The chief cause of a heart attack is the cardiovascular condition known as atherosclerosis. The deprivation of blood supply results in a sudden and severe pain in the center of the chest. In some cases the chest pain radiates into the shoulders, back, and arms and is accompanied by pallor, nausea, and sweating, followed by shortness of breath. When these symptoms occur, particu-

HEART ATTACK

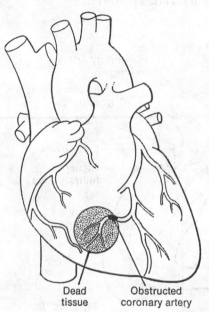

Dead tissue   Obstructed coronary artery

larly in the case of an angina patient, and do not disappear with the administration of nitroglycerin or other prescribed medication, an ambulance should be summoned immediately since the first hour after the attack is the period of greatest danger. Most doctors feel that if a heart attack victim reaches a hospital quickly, the therapeutic measures taken in the intensive coronary care unit can be effective. These measures combine the use of electronic monitoring and nuclear scanning with chemotherapy to reduce pain, decrease clotting, and strengthen the heart muscle. Whether or not coronary bypass surgery should be undertaken, should the cause be atherosclerosis of the coronary artery, is decided later on the basis of the patient's age, general health, and other individual factors.

A heart attack may occur at any time under a variety of physical or emotional circumstances. While men are more vulnerable to heart attacks than women, the risk increases in women after the menopause. Women over 40 who use the contraceptive pill bear a risk five times greater than women of the same age who do not use the pill. In the 30 to 40 age group the risk is three times greater. However, it should be kept in mind that in these age ranges, the pregnancy death rate is higher than the heart attack death rate. Widespread attention has been given to the warnings issued by the FDA that there is a substantial increase in the risk of heart attack or stroke in women on the pill who smoke. Women who fall into this category are ten times likelier to die because of a cardiovascular disability than women who neither smoke nor use the pill.

On a statistical basis and especially in men, the following conditions in one or another combination are responsible for most coronary attacks: obesity, diabetes, high blood-cholesterol, hypertension, sedentary life style, smoking, and emotional stress in the form of suppressed anger, perfectionism, and anxiety. One of the variables that acts as a powerful counterforce against heart attacks is a blood component known as HDL (high density lipoprotein) which appears to remove cholesterol from the arteries and transmit it to the liver for excretion. This component is likely to be higher in women than in men. It is also higher in nonsmokers than in smokers and in those who weigh too little rather than too much. The role of heredity is uncertain.

heart disease, hypertensive A heart muscle condition in which chronic hypertension impairs the functioning of the heart by causing it to pump with increased force. The abnormal demands cause the heart muscle to enlarge and increase the likelihood of heart failure.

heart failure Weakening of the heart muscle to the point where it is unable to pump efficiently enough to maintain a normal circulation of the blood; also called cardiac insufficiency or congestive heart failure. This does not mean that the heart has stopped beating. Heart failure causes the blood reentering the heart to slow down and back up into the veins. The consequent congestion in the blood vessels results in the expulsion of some of the fluid through the vessels' walls into the tissues. This seepage produces edema, which in turn leads to swollen ankles, fluid in the lungs, and other signs of excess fluid retention. Many women who have had heart failure can recover and lead relatively normal lives with proper medical supervision, a salt-restricted diet, the use of diuretics supplemented with potassium where necessary, and suitable amounts of digitalis. Where obesity, diabetes, or hypertension exist as an underlying cause, they must be treated simultaneously.

heart-lung machine A device that takes over the job of circulating and oxygenating the blood so that the heart can be bypassed and opened for surgical repair while it is relatively bloodless. The machine also facilitates operations on the lungs and major blood vessels as well as other types of surgery for high-risk patients.

heartburn A burning sensation in the lower esophagus. The discomfort, which may be concentrated below the breastbone, has nothing to do with the heart. It is the consequence of regur-

gitation by the stomach of a part of its contents upward into the esophagus. Since this partially digested matter contains gastric acid, it acts as an irritant. Heartburn may be associated with eating spicy foods, a hangover, a hiatus hernia, or emotional stress. It is not uncommon during the late stages of pregnancy. The catchall explanation of "hyperacidity" is far from correct and has caused many women to consume vast amounts of alkalizers in self-treatment. Where a hernia is the underlying cause and the heartburn is accompanied by spitting up food, surgical correction may be advisable. Most cases of occasional heartburn can be minimized by a sodium bicarbonate tablet and avoided by cutting down on rich, highly seasoned food, alcohol consumption, and tension-producing circumstances during and after mealtime.

heat exhaustion The accumulation of abnormally large amounts of blood close to the skin in an attempt to cool the surface of the body during exposure to high temperature and humidity. This disturbance of normal circulation deprives the vital organs of their necessary blood supply. The smaller vessels constrict, causing the victim to become pale and eventually to perspire heavily. Pulse and breathing may be rapid, and dizziness and vomiting may follow, but the body temperature remains normal. Fainting may be forestalled by lowering the head to increase blood circulation to the brain. First aid consists of placing the victim in the shade if possible and providing sips of salt water in the amount of half a cup every quarter of an hour for an hour (the solution should consist of 1 teaspoon of salt per 1 cup of water, or 0.25 grams salt per 8 ounces water). Feet should be elevated, clothing loosened, and as soon as it is practical to do so, cool wet compresses should be applied. If the condition does not improve or if the victim is elderly, has diabetes, or has a heart condition, emergency hospital treatment is necessary.

heat stroke A grave emergency in which there is a blockage of the sweating mechanism that results in extremely high body temperature; also known (mistakenly) as sunstroke and not to be confused with heat exhaustion. The victim of heat stroke is more likely to be male than female, old rather than young, and, not infrequently, an alcoholic. The condition is often precipitated by high humidity and may follow unusual physical exertion. Since fever may go as high as 106°F, irreversible damage may be done to the brain, kidneys, and other organs if treatment is not initiated immediately. The skin will be hot, red, and dry. If the face turns ashen, circulatory collapse is imminent. An ambulance must be summoned and in the meantime efforts must be made to bring the victim's temperature down. All clothes should be removed, and the bare skin sponged with cool water. If possible, the victim should be placed in a tub of cold (not iced) water until there are indications of recovery. No stimulants of any kind should be given. Drying off and further cooling with fans should follow the immersion. Since return to normal is likely to be slow and require close medical supervision, hospitalization after emergency treatment is usually recommended.

height The growth hormone of the pituitary gland controls growth during childhood and adolescence. When maximum adult height is reached during adolescence, at about age 16 for girls and 18 for boys, this mechanism stops. Although heredity and hormones determine body build, eventual height may be influenced to a degree by environmental factors such as diet, disease, and activity. With improvements in diet and immunization against many childhood diseases, the average height of Americans increased steadily for about 100 years until around 1914 and since then has remained relatively stable. According to the National Center for Health Statistics, the average stature for a young woman of 18 is 5 feet 4½ inches.

Heimlich maneuver A lifesaving technique used in cases of choking to dislodge whatever is blocking the air passages. An obstruction that cannot

HEIMLICH MANEUVER

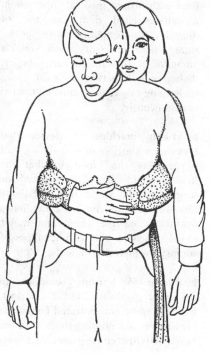

be loosened and coughed up following a few sharp blows on the back is likely to be ejected by the Heimlich maneuver. This is accomplished by squeezing the victim's body in such a way that the volume of air trapped in the lungs acts as a propulsive force against the obstruction, causing it to pop out of the throat. The rescuer stands behind the victim and places both hands just above the victim's abdomen. A fist made with one hand is grasped by the other hand and quickly and firmly pressed inward and upward against the victim's diaphragm. The pressure on the diaphragm compresses the lungs and expels the air. If you are choking and no one else is present, you may perform the maneuver on yourself by making a quick upward jab at the diaphragm with your fist.

hemangioma   *See* BIRTHMARKS.

hematoma   A collection of blood that has escaped from the blood vessels into the tissues, forming a local swelling. Hematomas are often associated with ruptured blood vessels that result from a blow. They are likely to accompany a fracture and frequently occur beneath the skull following a serious head injury. Bleeding that occurs after a minor mishap is usually reabsorbed into the blood vessels without forming a hematoma and without further consequences.

hematuria   The presence of blood in the urine. The bleeding may originate in any portion of the urinary tract, and depending on the cause, may be trivial and temporary or may indicate the need for prompt medical treatment. The cause of hematuria is usually diagnosed by X-rays and cystoscopy. Among the more common causes are cystitis, a stone in the kid-

ney, ureter, or bladder, inflammation of the urethra, or a type of tumor often found in the bladder known as a papilloma. Urine samples taken during a gynecological checkup will reveal the presence of hematuria. Any change in the appearance of urine from a clear, pale yellow liquid to one that is brownish or cloudy should be discussed with a doctor.

hemigastrectomy   Surgical removal of a large portion (possibly as much as half) of the stomach. This operation may be necessitated by chronic peptic ulceration, by the presence of scar tissue causing an obstruction, or by stomach cancer.

hemochromotosis   A rare metabolic disturbance of unknown origin in which large deposits of iron pigments accumulate in the liver, pancreas, or other vital organs, leading to their deterioration. The condition is almost exclusively found in men and is usually accompanied by cirrhosis of the liver and diabetes. Hemochromotosis may be controlled by the periodic withdrawal of whole blood combined with plasma replacement. Due to the characteristic skin color produced by the disorder, it is sometimes referred to as "bronzed diabetes."

hemoglobin   The red pigment in red blood cells; a combination of the iron-containing *heme* and the protein-containing *globin*. This substance carries oxygen to the tissues and removes carbon dioxide from them. The amount of hemoglobin in the blood can be determined by a simple test. A less than normal amount indicates anemia; excess indicates polycythemia.

hemophilia   An inherited blood disorder characterized by a deficiency of those chemical factors in blood plasma involved in the clotting mechanism; also known as bleeders' disease. It is a sex-linked genetic disorder; the gene is carried by the female, but only male offspring have the disease. The sons of hemophiliacs are normal (assuming marriage is with a noncarrying female). Transmission occurs through one of the mother's two sex chromosomes: 50 percent of her sons will be hemophiliacs and 50 percent of her daughters will be carriers. Thus, while the disease runs in families, the pattern of transmission may cause it to skip several generations. Hemophilia varies in severity. It is not curable, but when bleeding occurs, it can be treated by the infusion of clotting components that are separated out from normal blood plasma. Such transfusions may also be used prior to surgery and may be administered regularly as a preventive measure against hemorrhaging. Carrier screening and genetic counseling are available to those women who wish to be checked for the chromosomal defect.

hemorrhage Abnormal bleeding following the rupture of a blood vessel. Hemorrhage may be internal or external; it may come from a vein, artery, or capillary. Subcutaneous hemorrhage follows a bruise or a fracture; blood may appear in the sputum, urine, stools, or vomit. When its source is arterial, it is bright red and spurts forth with the heartbeat; when it is venous, it is wine-colored and oozes out in a steady stream. Any untoward bleeding or signs of blood in the body's discharges should be called to a doctor's attention. Other than the bleeding that results from an accident, hemorrhaging may also follow surgery, even a simple tooth extraction; it

may occur during childbirth; it may also be a sign of a disorder that ruptured a blood vessel, such as an ulcer, tumor, kidney stone, or tuberculosis. Any diseases which affect the clotting mechanism, especially leukemia or hemophilia, are characterized by hemorrhage.

hemorrhoids Varicose veins in the area of the anus and the rectum; also called piles. External hemorrhoids are located outside the anus and are covered with skin; internal hemorrhoids develop at the junction of the rectum and the anal canal and are covered with mucous membrane. Among the causes are chronic constipation, obesity, pregnancy, and, less commonly, a rectal tumor. There is some evidence that the disorder may be hereditary. Typical symptoms are inter-

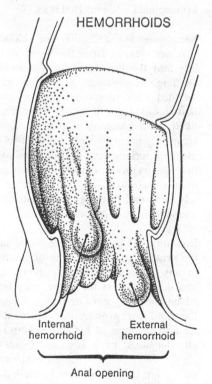

HEMORRHOIDS

Internal hemorrhoid

External hemorrhoid

Anal opening

mittent bleeding during the passage of stools, itching, and when thrombosis (clotting) occurs, acute pain. The hemorrhoids that develop during pregnancy are caused by the increased pressure on the veins of the lower part of the body; and are likely to diminish and disappear soon after delivery if other causative factors, such as overweight and constipation, are not also present. Treatment depends on severity: warm sitz baths are soothing, medication can reduce itching, injections of chemicals can control bleeding and shrink the swollen veins, and, if necessary, an operation can remove the diseased veins by cryosurgery. Any frequent discharge of bright red blood from the anus, even when unaccompanied by pain, should be brought to a doctor's attention.

heparin An anticoagulant found in the mucosal linings of the liver and other tissues. In synthetic form it is used medically and surgically to prevent clotting and to treat clotting disorders.

hepatitis Inflammation of the liver; generally designates a viral infection of the liver caused by one of two related but somewhat different viruses, A (infectious hepatitis) and B (serum hepatitis). Recently a third type of viral hepatitis (non-A–non-B) has been identified. Victims excrete the virus in their saliva, feces, and urine and also carry it in their blood for various periods of time. Thus they can transmit it, directly or indirectly, to others. The virus enters the victim via the gastrointestinal tract (mouth) with contaminated food, water, or saliva or via the bloodstream when a contaminated needle is used to inject medicine or street drugs or when contaminated fluids, usually blood, are injected.

The incubation period for hepatitis A is about a month; for hepatitis B, about three months. Hepatitis A is twice as common as hepatitis B and occurs in about 15 per 100,000 people in the United States each year. It is more common in countries with poor sanitary facilities. Some victims are never ill clinically and have only abnormal blood tests indicative of impaired liver function for a few weeks. Most, however, are sick in varying degrees for several weeks or months and then recover completely. A few become life-time carriers of the virus and, although well, cannot donate their blood. The signs and symptoms of the disease are jaundice, dark urine and light-colored stools, fever, loss of appetite, and fatigue. A few people develop chronic hepatitis with varying degrees of liver involvement. About 1 percent of patients under 45 years of age and 3 percent of those 45 and over die during the acute phase.

Other forms of hepatitis can occur without direct infection of the liver. Diffuse bacterial infections (septicemia) can cause a toxic hepatitis. Certain chemicals, such as carbon tetrachloride, can cause hepatitis in anyone who is exposed sufficiently, and certain medications, such as phenylbutazone, cincophen, and halothane, can cause hepatitis in those who, for unknown reasons, are sensitive to them.

There is no specific treatment. However, when gamma globulin is given to a victim soon after exposure, it is effective in preventing or minimizing the disease by creating a temporary (passive) immunity. Immunization to provide permanent (active) immunity to hepatitis B may soon be available. Those who have had hepatitis develop permanent immunity to hepatitis caused by the same virus.

heredity The transmission of characteristics from one generation to another, from parents to offspring, through the genetic information carried in the chromosomes. Geneticists are providing medical researchers with the tools for exploring the role of heredity in sickness and in resistance to disease. It is hoped that the dissemination of information about genetic disorders and the availability of genetic counseling will bring about a dramatic reduction in the medical, psychological, and economic problems created by hereditary diseases.

Among the more prevalent inherited diseases are: Tay-Sachs, Niemann-Pick, and Gaucher's disease, all three caused by faulty enzyme function and commonly associated with families of middle European Jewish ancestry; sickle-cell anemia, a blood disorder most common among blacks; Cooley's anemia, a more acute blood disease formerly called thalassemia; Huntington's chorea, a degenerative disorder of the central nervous system; hemophilia; several types of muscular dystrophy; galactosemia; phenylketonuria (PKU); cystic fibrosis, the most common genetic disease among Anglo-Saxons, carried by 1 in 20 whites or approximately 10 million Americans. Research on inherited immunities that seem to make some families immune to certain diseases is expected to yield information about resistance to disease in general. This research is still in an early stage of development. *See also* GENETIC COUNSELING.

hernia The protrusion of all or part of an organ, most commonly, an intestinal loop or abdominal organ, through a weak spot in the wall of the surrounding structure; also called a rupture. A hernia, which may be acquired or congenital, is classified according to the part of the body in which it occurs. The inguinal hernia, occurring in the groin, accounts for about 75 percent of all hernias and is much more common among men than women. The umbilical hernia is more common among infants than among adults; some cases are self-correcting and some require surgery. Incisional or ventral hernias may develop after abdominal surgery in cases of unsatisfactory healing or because a chronic cough or obesity subjects the weakened tissue to extra strain. The esophageal or hiatus hernia is more common among the middle-aged than the young. In this condition a portion of the stomach protrudes through the

THREE COMMON TYPES OF HERNIAS IN WOMEN

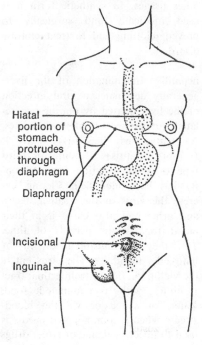

Hiatal portion of stomach protrudes through diaphragm

Diaphragm

Incisional

Inguinal

opening for the esophagus in the diaphragm, producing symptoms that range from mild indigestion and heartburn to serious breathing difficulties and regurgitation of food after each meal. In less severe cases the discomfort can be eased by eating small and frequent meals of bland food and sleeping with the body propped up by extra pillows. Most hernias can be corrected by surgical repair of the weakened tissue.

heroin A narcotic drug derived from opium by altering the chemical formula of morphine. See "Drugs, Alcohol, and Tobacco."

herpes simplex One of several diseases caused by a particular virus or variants of it. The seriousness of the disease depends on the area of infection and the particular strain of the virus. In all cases the symptom is an eruption of painful blisters. When the eruption occurs around the mouth, the cause is usually herpes simplex virus type I (HSV-1) and the disease is often referred to as "cold sores" or "fever blisters." This virus is also responsible for ulceration of the cornea (herpetic keratitis) that can result in scarring of the tissue and loss of vision unless treated promptly. The disorder seems to be activated by exposure to extremes of temperature or by another infection. No cure exists, but the discomfort can be eased by medicated creams or salves.

Type II of the herpes simplex virus (HSV-2) is usually responsible for an infection of the mucous membranes of the genital or anal area and may or may not be spread by sexual contact. See "Sexually Transmissible Diseases."

herpes zoster A painful virus infection of the sensory nerves causing inflammation of the skin along the nerve pathway (herpes zoster means "blister girdle"); commonly called shingles and very closely related to the virus which causes chickenpox. Herpes zoster is far less contagious than herpes simplex. What activates the virus is not clearly understood. Inflammation typically occurs above the abdomen and less often along the path of the cranial nerve on the face and near the eye, with a potential for damage to the cornea. Sensitivity of the involved nerves (neuritis) and blisters may take several weeks to disappear, and in stubborn cases the patient may be left with acute neuralgia. There is no specific cure, but various medicines are available to reduce pain.

hiccups (hiccoughs) Involuntary spasmodic contractions of the diaphragm that force the glottis to close at the same time that a breath is taken in, thus producing the characteristic clicking sound. The common cause is a minor irritation of the diaphragm itself or of some part of the digestive or respiratory system. In more serious cases hiccups may be associated with uremia or encephalitis. Although the typical attack of hiccups is self-limiting, there are remedies for quick relief: sipping water slowly, holding the breath, or breathing into a paper bag. If hiccups persist, a doctor should be called. In all but the most extreme cases, a tranquilizer or a sedative will end the discomfort.

high altitude sickness A condition associated with the ascent to altitudes of 8,000 feet above sea level or higher, where the reduced concentration of oxygen in the air (rarefied air) leads to oxygen deprivation in the blood.

When the red blood cells are unable to absorb a full supply of oxygen as they pass through the lungs, breathing becomes increasingly quick and labored. Giddiness, headache, nausea, and disorientation are among the warning signals of high altitude sickness. Tourists who plan to visit high altitudes and mountain climbers or skiers who intend to reach higher altitudes than customary should have a medical checkup to make sure that their heart and lungs can tolerate the stress. Tourists in high altitudes should eliminate smoking and drinking for the first two days and keep physical exertion to a minimum until the body has adjusted to the environment.

high blood pressure *See* HYPERTENSION.

histamine A chemical compound found in all body tissues, normally released as a stimulant for the production of the gastric juices during digestion and for the dilation of the smaller blood vessels in response to the body's adaptive needs. Under certain conditions some people produce excessive amounts of histamine as an allergic reaction, causing the surrounding tissues to become swollen and inflamed. For such allergic responses, antihistamine medicines are available. Antihistamines should not be used indiscriminately since they cause drowsiness.

hives Irregularly shaped red or white elevations of the skin accompanied by itching and burning, usually caused by an allergic response involving the release of histamine; technically called urticaria. Hives may occur on any part of the body or in the gastrointestinal tract, and in some cases the weals may be as large as an inch in diameter. A topical anesthetic ointment or lotion may provide relief, but an antihistamine drug is usually prescribed to prevent additional eruptions. When hives occur for the first time, an effort should be made to identify the cause, especially if some medication is suspected, to avoid a more serious recurrence.

Hodgkin's disease A disorder of the lymphatic system characterized by the progressive enlargement of the lymph nodes throughout the body, especially of the spleen. It is a type of cancer that typically attacks young adults; men are twice as vulnerable as women. If the disease is localized, a 95 percent cure rate can be achieved by radiation treatment. If the disease spreads to the point where vital organs are endangered, various types of chemotherapy have proved effective. Hodgkin's disease may be caused by a virus. Since it seems to have a family pattern, there may be a hereditary lack of immunity.

holistic medicine An approach to health and healing that views each patient as a psychobiological unit in a particular physical and psychosocial environment. The term holistic conveys the sense that each individual has a reality that is more important than and independent of the sum of his or her parts. Similar views have been propounded in the past, especially by doctors who focus on psychosomatic medicine on the assumption that the mental and physical aspects of a patient are inextricably bound together. The holistic attitude also takes into account the role played by the person's environment, family history, interpersonal situation, occupational factors, exposure to potential carcinogens, and the like.

Practitioners of holistic medicine stress the importance of patient involvement in the healing process, pointing out that passivity on the part of the patient encourages the view that "medicine is magic." The form that this involvement takes includes self-help wherever possible, self-awareness in recognizing messages from one's feelings and one's body, and open-mindedness about the validity of types of therapy other than those that are part of conventional medical practice in the Western world.

homosexuality Sexual and emotional attraction to a member of one's own sex; called lesbianism among women. Extensive research on the subject of homosexuality still has not provided a concrete explanation of its cause. Today, many people consider homosexuality to be as natural to some people as heterosexuality is to most people.

hormone Chemical product mainly of endocrine glands, but also of other organs such as the placenta, secreted directly into the bloodstream for transport to various organs for the regulation of life processes. Hormones normally control growth and sexual maturation and affect emotional response, digestion, metabolism, and other vital functions. Many hormones have been synthesized or extracted from other mammals. Their availability has made replacement treatment possible for certain types of hormone deficiencies. Doctors who specialize in this branch of medicine are called endocrinologists. *See also* ENDOCRINE SYSTEM.

hospital Hospitalization is necessary when specialized treatment or diagnostic procedures require equipment, personnel, or full-time services not available in a doctor's office or on an outpatient basis. In a medical emergency it is usually more practical to get to a hospital than to go to a local doctor. Emergencies may require oxygen, transfusions, intensive care, and on-the-spot laboratory tests as well as other lifesaving services.

If you have a choice among hospitals, a teaching hospital (one associated with a university medical school) is to be preferred. If there is none in your area, every effort should be made to choose an institution that is accredited by the Joint Commission on the Accreditation of Hospitals. This independent nongovernmental organization conducts regular inspections to see that hospitals conform to federal standards for cleanliness, fire protection, competence of nursing services, adequacy of equipment, and professional record-keeping. Also, unaccredited hospitals are ineligible for Medicare and Medicaid funds.

In hospitalization, as in all aspects of health care, every woman should take the time to know her rights. Various consumer-advocate publications of the rights of patients, including the Hospital Bill of Rights, are usually available at a local library. *See also* "You, Your Doctors, and the Health Care System."

hot flash The most commonly reported symptom of the menopause; a disturbance of temperature regulation connected with the decrease in the body's supply of estrogen. *See* "Midlife Transitions."

UNBROKEN HYMEN

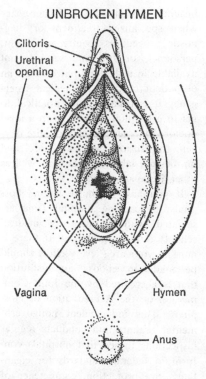

Clitoris

Urethral opening

Vagina

Hymen

Anus

hymen The membrane that partially closes the entry to the vagina; also known as the maidenhead. The hymen varies in size, shape, and toughness. The opening in the hymen allows for the discharge of menstrual flow. While it may remain intact until penetration during the first sexual intercourse, it is by no means unusual for it to be stretched or ruptured by athletic activities or by tampons before any intercourse. In cases where the membrane is so thick or tough that intercourse cannot be accomplished without severe pain or in rare cases in which it completely seals the vaginal opening, it can be cut under a local anesthetic in the gynecologist's office.

hyperglycemia Excess amounts of sugar in the blood. This condition is one of the chief signs of diabetes. Milder cases that develop after the age of 50 may be treated by one of the oral hyperglycemic drugs. *See also* DIABETES.

hypertension High blood pressure. Hypertension occurs more frequently among women, but it is more deadly to the male. Where hypertension exists, the smallest arteries (arterioles) constrict, causing the heart to have to pump harder in order to distribute blood throughout the body. Since the heart is a muscle, the harder it works, the bigger it gets. An enlarged heart in a hypertensive person is therefore a result, not a cause, of high blood pressure.

The causes of what is technically called organic hypertension are detectable, and if they are corrected, hypertension is reduced. Common causes are arteriosclerosis and atherosclerosis, glomerulonephritis, and hyperthyroidism. The more widespread and insidious type of high blood pressure, which typically affects people in their early thirties, is called essential hypertension and is of unknown origin. While the organic type is generally acquired, the essential type is presumed to be inherited. The genetic factor appears to explain why large numbers of infants and children are now known to have high blood pressure. Organic hypertension tends to progress unless treated, eventually attacking a vulnerable organ: the blood vessels of the brain (stroke), the kidneys (uremia), the coronary arteries (heart attack), the organs of vision (eye hemorrhage). Essential hypertension may have no noticeable symptoms, but the increasing blood pressure can gradually damage the heart, blood vessels, and kidneys.

When hypertension of either type is

mild or borderline, it is usually treated without medication unless its cause can be treated. Recommendations include weight loss if necessary, low-salt low-sugar diet, stopping or restricted smoking, moderate alcohol intake (any more than two drinks on a regular basis will increase risks), and a contraceptive other than the pill. It is considered normal for blood pressure to rise somewhat during the menopause and with advancing age, probably due to increased stress, increased weight, hormonal changes, and increased atherosclerosis. There is no indication that estrogen replacement therapy helps hypertension as much as do weight reduction and lowered salt intake.

When the cause of the hypertension cannot be eliminated and treatment is necessary, several types of medication are available. The antihypertensive drugs can produce undesirable long-range side effects: depression, immobilizing headaches, chronic constipation, liver damage, parkinsonism, and diabetes. It is therefore essential that any woman embarking on drug therapy remain in close touch with a physician for the adjustment of doses and changes in type of medication when necessary. For some patients surgical correction of an atherosclerotic obstruction is the most effective treatment.

Any woman whose family history includes hypertension should have an annual blood pressure check. This can conveniently be done at the same time that she has the pap test. Prompt detection and proper treatment help avoid unnecessary complications.

hyperthyroidism Overactivity of the thyroid gland. Typical symptoms include restlessness and weight loss in spite of overeating. In some cases goiter is present. Diagnosis of the condition is based on blood tests and other clinical procedures. Treatment usually consists of medicine or radioactive iodine that reduces the gland's excess secretion of thyroxin and its size or, less frequently, surgery.

hyperventilation Loss of carbon dioxide from the blood caused by abnormally rapid or deep breathing. Hyperventilation produces symptoms of dizziness, muscle spasms, and chest pains and is one of the most common signs of an anxiety attack. Since the symptoms are an additional cause of anxiety, the condition may worsen to the point where it appears to be an emergency. Effective treatment consists of breathing into and out of a paper or plastic bag so that the exhaled carbon dioxide is reinhaled until the proper blood level is achieved, at which point the symptoms vanish.

hypnosis A trancelike state psychically induced by another person or by concentration on an object, during which the subject's consciousness is altered for purposes of responding to the suggestions of the hypnotist. The trance may be so shallow that the subject is scarcely aware of a change in mental state, or it may be so deep as to have all the appearances of sleep. Approximately one person in five may be successfully hypnotized, and practically no one can be a successful subject without prior consent and trust in the hypnotist. The mechanism by which the hypnotic state is achieved is not precisely understood, but the technique has accepted medical applications when used by trained and reputable practitioners. Freud's theory of the unconscious evolved from the successful use of hypnosis for the treatment of hysteria. Hypnosis is now used instead of or together with mild anesthesia to facilitate childbirth; it is being taught to pediatric dentists (hypnodontia); and it has been used with some success by psychiatrists to get patients to stop smoking or nail-biting.

hypochondria An obsessive preoccupation with the symptoms of illness and supposed ill health. Any suggestion that physical checkups indicate normal organic health is greeted with resentment and disbelief. It is a malady in itself, since it is usually an expression of psychic distress. Hypochondria can sometimes be relieved by psychotherapy.

hypoglycemia An abnormally low level of sugar in the blood; a clinical condition of sudden onset characteristic of pre-diabetes and other diseases. It also occurs in diabetics when they have too much insulin or too large a dose of a hypoglycemic agent. Untreated, it can lead to confusion, sleepiness, or in extreme cases unconsciousness. "Low blood sugar" is not a common condition, and no one should embark on a special diet before consulting a doctor and arranging for blood tests. The confusion about hypoglycemia is partially due to the fact that its symptoms—sweating, palpitations, trembling hands—are similar to those produced by an anxiety attack.

hypothalamus The master gland of endocrine activity located in the base of the brain directly above the pituitary gland.

hypothermia Abnormally low body temperature. Hypothermia may occur naturally as a consequence of prolonged exposure to extreme cold, es-pecially when temperature regulation is affected by aging, disease such as pneumonia, or the ingestion of certain drugs and alcohol. The symptoms of hypothermia in such cases are slow breathing, weak pulse, and semiconsciousness. Body heat can be slowly restored by covering the patient. No other treatment should be administered without instructions from a doctor.

Hypothermia can also be artificially induced in order to reduce the tissues' oxygen needs and to slow down the circulation of the blood, thus making certain types of operations possible. Hypothermia allows the surgeon to reach parts of the body that might otherwise be inaccessible in the performance of delicate operations on the brain and heart.

hysterectomy Surgical removal of the uterus. *See* "Gynecologic Diseases and Treatment."

hysteria In the psychiatric sense, a condition of uncontrolled excitability, intense anxiety sometimes accompanied by sensory disturbances (such as hallucinations) and general disorientation. Conversion hysteria is the unconscious simulation of organic disability, such as blindness, deafness, loss of the faculty of speech or locomotion.

hysterotomy Surgical opening of the uterus, similar to a cesarean section. A hysterotomy is done to remove foreign bodies, such as IUDs; occasionally to remove a mole; and for abortion only when other methods are contraindicated because of the age of the fetus.

iatrogenic disease Any disorder or disease caused by a physician's medical treatment. Among the less serious examples of iatrogenic disturbances due to side effects of medication are rashes, cramps, dizziness, itching; among the more serious are birth defects (Thalidomide), cancer (DES), shock (penicillin), hemolytic anemia (chloramphenicol), liver damage (Thorazine). It has been estimated that approximately 300,000 people are hospitalized each year in the United States because of an adverse drug reaction. Iatrogenic conditions are therefore one of the ten leading causes of hospitalization in this country. Women can partially protect themselves by questioning the doctor about the possible side effects of any prescribed medication; by keeping records of any unusual responses (such as allergic reactions) to particular drugs so that drug can be avoided, if possible; and by avoiding the use of any antibiotic for a virus infection except under special conditions. In cases where a particular treatment carries with it a risk potentially equal to the condition being treated, the patient has a right to have this explained so that she can make a responsible choice.

ileitis Inflammation of the lower portion of the small intestine (ileum); also known as Crohn's disease. The typical victim of this disorder is a young adult with a low threshold for psychic stress. Ileitis seems to run in families, and some specialists believe that its underlying cause is an inherited antibody-antigen reaction. The symptoms are similar to those of colitis: diarrhea and abdominal pain. A strict regimen of combined medications and a high-protein diet may be prescribed. When the inflammation cannot be controlled by medication or when intestinal obstruc-

tion persists, surgical removal of the diseased part of the intestine may be the only alternative.

ileostomy A surgical procedure to create an artificial anus to bypass the colon by bringing the ileum (the lowest part of the small intestine) through an opening made in the abdominal wall. An ileostomy is performed when ulcerative colitis, cancer, or other disease requires the removal of the colon (large intestine). It may also be performed as a temporary measure so that an obstruction in the colon can be removed without removing the colon itself.

immunity and immunization Immunity is a biologic state of being resistant to or not susceptible to a disease or condition, usually, and here specifically, due to the presence

IMMUNOLOGY

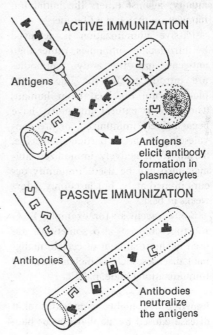

ACTIVE IMMUNIZATION

Antigens

Antigens elicit antibody formation in plasmacytes

PASSIVE IMMUNIZATION

Antibodies

Antibodies neutralize the antigens

of antibodies against the causative agent (antigen). The immunity may be congenital (acquired from the mother and present at birth but not long lasting), natural (resulting from an infectious disease which produces antibodies), or induced by immunization (inoculation).

It was proved that immunity could be induced by artificial means almost 200 years ago when Edward Jenner immunized (vaccinated) people against smallpox. Active immunization is a long-term resistance to an antigen induced by introducing a controlled amount of the antigen into the body in order to stimulate antibody formation. The antigens may be dead viruses (Salk polio vaccine), modified live viruses (Sabin polio vaccine and mumps vaccine), or chemically altered toxins produced by bacteria (tetanus toxoid). Active immunization against some diseases may require periodic boosters to maintain the immunity; against others the initial immunization may last a lifetime.

Passive immunization is achieved by introducing antibodies, rather than antigens, into the body. Antibodies are introduced by the injection of blood serum obtained from humans who have a natural immunity, have been actively immunized, or are convalescing from a particular disease. Serum from actively immunized animals also can be used. Immunity occurs immediately, but lasts only a few weeks at best.

Some vaccines (for example, BCG for tuberculosis) also sometimes are used in the treatment of certain malignant diseases such as melanomas. *See* Immunization Guide, p. 738.

impetigo A highly contagious skin disease caused by staphylococcus bacteria and characterized by blisters that rupture and form yellow crusts. The areas most frequently affected are the face, neck, and scalp and less frequently the arms and legs. Impetigo may be secondary to another skin condition that causes lesions, especially a fungus infection. The disease is spread from one person to another and from one part of the body to another through contact with the liquid discharged by the sores. Care should be exercised to prevent reinfection of the patient and infection of other members of the household through contamination of towels or bed linens. Household pets may also transmit the disease and if infected should receive treatment to curtail its spread. Antibiotic ointments are usually effective in treating impetigo.

impotence Inability of the male to achieve and maintain an erection (erectile impotence); also, inability to achieve orgasm following erection (ejaculating impotence). Almost all men experience impotence at some time in their lives. It may be occasional and temporary or it may be chronic. The cause in over 90 percent of cases is psychological, resulting from conflicts that may arise from guilt, unacknowledged homosexuality, anxiety, distrust of women, or self-punishment. It may also be related to physical causes of fatigue, general poor health, and organic conditions such as diabetes, hormonal aberration, or inherited disorders of the genitals. Alcoholism, drug addiction, and certain prescribed drugs and tranquilizers are other causes. When impotence exists, psychiatric counseling or a sex therapy clinic should be considered only after a complete medical checkup has been conducted.

incest Sexual intercourse between a male and female who are not permitted by their society to marry; the proscription may be based on consanguinity (close blood relationship) or affinity (relationship by marriage). Incest is a punishable offense (with varying legal definitions) in the United States.

indigestion Any disturbance in the digestive process that results in discomfort; also called dyspepsia. An acute attack of indigestion may be sufficiently severe and disabling to require treatment by a doctor. Alkalizers are often ineffective and potentially damaging, particularly if the condition is caused by emotional stress. In most cases of indigestion the cause is not organic and can be corrected without medication. Digestive complaints are often due to eating too much too quickly, failure to chew food properly, poorly prepared food, excessive drinking of iced or carbonated beverages including beer, eating while one is upset or angry, overuse of such medications as aspirin or tranquilizers, eating too much raw food, or changing to a new diet. When indigestion persists in spite of corrective measures, a gastrointestinal study known as a barium X-ray or blood tests should be administered to determine the underlying cause.

induced labor Artificial stimulation of the birth process; often referred to as programmed labor or elective induction. Labor may be induced either by the injection of a synthetic hormone (oxytocin) that stimulates, speeds up, and intensifies uterine contractions or by a surgical procedure called amniotomy, the artificial rupture of the amniotic sac below the fetus. Except in the case of life-threat-

ening emergencies, such as eclampsia or hemorrhage, no woman should agree to induced labor before weighing the advantages and disadvantages of such a procedure. Most doctors feel that induced labor for the purpose of a planned delivery does not warrant the potential risks involved. *See also* "Pregnancy and Childbirth."

infantile paralysis *See* POLIOMYE-LITIS.

infertility The inability to conceive or beget children. *See* "Infertility."

influenza A contagious respiratory disease caused by a virus; generally known as the flu and previously called the grippe. All strains of the flu virus are airborne, and the infection is spread in the coughs, sneezes, and exhaled breath of the affected person. The disease may reach epidemic proportions rapidly, especially since natural or artificially acquired immunity against one particular strain of the virus provides no guaranteed protection against another strain.

Symptoms may range from mild to severe. Typical manifestations are inflammation of the membranes that line the respiratory tract causing a running nose, scratchy throat, and mucous congestion that causes coughing. Fever may not be present or temperature may go as high as 104°F. Aching joints, appetite loss, and general malaise characterize even the mildest cases. Even when symptoms clear up, usually within ten days, the flu patient may feel weak and tired for some time. The cough may be persistent, and relapses may occur as a result of lowered resistance and premature resumption of normal activities. Lowered resistance to bacterial infection is the most serious complication of the flu. When a healthy adult has the illness, the usual treatment is bed rest, aspirin, lots of fluids, and as much sleep as possible. A cough medicine containing an expectorant may be prescribed to facilitate the hawking up of the accumulated phlegm. For flu patients who may be vulnerable to complications, such as people over 65, diabetics, very young children, or anyone with a heart, lung, or kidney disorder, antibiotics may be prescribed.

Many doctors believe that people who are highly susceptible to serious complications should be vaccinated each year with a vaccine made from the killed viruses of the current strains responsible for the disease. Adverse responses to this form of immunization range from a slightly sore and swollen spot in the area of the vaccination, to a low fever and headache of several days' duration, to an uncomfortable response presumed to be allergic, to a 1 in 100,000 risk of severe reaction that affects the nervous system. Anyone contemplating a flu vaccination should ask the advice of his or her doctor.

inguinal glands A group of lymph nodes located in the groin. Any painful swelling or persistent soreness in this area should be brought to a doctor's attention.

inner ear *See* EAR.

insect stings and bites While usually no more than a nuisance, the bite of an insect can at times cause disease or life-threatening emergencies. The stinging insects—hornets, wasps, yellow jackets, and bees—do not transmit disease, but the venom they inject may cause a severe allergic response known as anaphylactic shock. Or-

dinarily, however, the sting results in no more than swelling, redness, and localized pain. In the case of a bee sting the skin should never be squeezed in order to extricate the stinger, since this only forces the venom farther into the tissues. Instead, the stinger should be removed with a pair of tweezers held flat against the skin. Any sign of a systemic response to a sting, such as body swelling or respiratory distress, indicates the need of immediate professional attention. Women who are extremely hypersensitive to the venom should be desensitized by an allergist and continue the maintenance treatments usually necessary four or five times a year. Even after desensitization emergency adrenalin should be carried when there is the threat of a sting.

Biting and bloodsucking flies and mosquitos can transmit serious diseases. The common housefly does not bite, but may be a carrier of infection. Aside from diseases endemic to the tropics, such as yellow fever and malaria, encephalitis can be transmitted by certain local mosquitos. Horseflies are also harmful since they can transmit rabbit fever (tularemia). Among dangerous parasites which are found in several parts of the world are fleas that transmit bubonic plague and typhus. It should be noted that the ticks that cause Rocky Mountain spotted fever are not indigenous to the West and may be found in other parts of the country. Immunization is available against all the above infections and should be taken into consideration by anyone planning a trip to an area of high-risk exposure. A parasite common in the rural South, known as the chigger, is the larval stage of the mite that causes scabies. While chiggers are not disease-bearing, their bite irritates the skin thereby leading the way toward a secondary infection. Once bitten, the victim can be relieved of the itching by the application of a paste of baking soda and water or calamine lotion.

While most spiders and other arachnids are harmless, there are three or four that inflict bites that must receive prompt attention: the scorpion found in the Southwest, the black widow spider (identifiable by its shiny black body whose underside is marked with a red hourglass shape), and a species of hairy tarantula found near the Mexican border. The aggressive fire ant is a more recent menace that is spreading its way through the Southern states. Its attack can be easily identified since it inflicts multiple stings around the original bite. The bite of a fire ant can cause severe systemic response in certain people. Anyone living in an area where fire ants exist should consider the advisability of desensitization.

Certain practical measures can reduce the hazards and discomforts of bites and stings without the use of insecticides that pollute the environment with dangerous chemicals. A few suggestions are the application of insect-repellent lotions containing such effective chemicals as diethyl-meta-toluamide, dimethyl phthalate, or butopyronoxyl on exposed parts of the body several times a day; wearing protective clothing during walks in the country; avoiding the use of perfumes, lotions, sprays, and jewelry since scents and colors attract stinging insects; burning insect-repellent candles or incense sticks at picnics when food is exposed; keeping foods covered; and using screens for indoor protection. Women who own or rent vacation houses in the country should heed the warnings of local health authorities as to insect-borne diseases and the precautions one can take to combat them.

insomnia Sleeplessness, either chronic or occasional. Judging from the many millions of sleeping pill prescriptions filled each year, the overuse of habit-forming barbiturates appears to be prevalent in the United States. Since it is generally believed that dependence on sleeping pills will only intensify insomnia, anyone trying to cope with the situation should try to find another solution for sleeplessness. It is perfectly normal to spend sleepless hours due to a worrisome problem, but when loss of sleep becomes a chronic condition, a person should try to deal with the underlying cause before resorting to sleeping pills. It is interesting to note that medical researchers who monitor sleep patterns have discovered that people who describe themselves as insomniacs actually sleep a good deal more than they think they do.

Sleeplessness may be caused by any one of many factors that are easily corrected, such as eating rich food or drinking beverages containing caffeine within two hours of bedtime, watching overly exciting television programs, sleeping in a poorly ventilated room or on an uncomfortable mattress. When snoring and other noises interfere with sleep, ear plugs can often relieve the problem. Daytime exercise, a hot bath in the evening, and a glass of warm milk before retiring require little effort, but are helpful. Scientists have found that an amino acid, L-triptophane, contained in certain foods, including milk, seems to act as a sedative. When insomnia is a result of depression or anxiety, the cause of the emotional distress should be explored before resorting to medication.

insulin A hormone secreted by the groups of cells in the pancreas called the islets of Langerhans. Insulin performs several vital functions and is especially critical in stabilizing the body's metabolism of sugars and starches. The isolation of insulin by Canadian scientists in 1921–22 inaugurated the successful treatment of diabetes.

insulin shock therapy The earliest and most widely used shock treatment for mentally ill patients unresponsive to other forms of therapy. Treatment consisted of producing a hypoglycemic coma by injecting insulin into the muscles. While electroshock has largely replaced insulin shock, both treatments generally have been superseded by tranquilizing and antidepressant drugs.

intelligence quotient (IQ) A number indicating an individual's relative intelligence. The figure is calculated by dividing mental age by chronological age and multiplying by 100. The mental age is determined by comparing the individual's score on standardized tests with statistical average scores at different chronological age levels. Many people question the accuracy of this form of testing since it is generally agreed that intelligence takes many forms that cannot be measured by a single test or represented by a single number and that many current test instruments measure culturally determined acquired knowledge rather than inborn intellectual or creative ability.

intercourse *See* SEXUAL INTERCOURSE.

interferon A cellular protein produced by white blood cells and fibroblasts which suppresses viral DNA reproduction. It is available as a drug, but only for investigational purposes at this time. It may prove to be effective in treating certain viral diseases such as herpes and possibly some cancers.

internal examination *See* "Gynecologic Diseases and Treatment."

internist *See* DOCTOR.

intestines The section of the alimentary canal from the stomach to the anus. The small intestine, which begins where the stomach ends, is approximately 20 feet of coiled tube. The large intestine, which is about 5½ feet long, consists of the cecum to which the appendix is attached, the colon, and the rectum. *See* "The Healthy Woman."

intrauterine device *See* "Contraception and Abortion."

iritis Inflammation of the iris, the ciliary body, or the choroid, the three structures that comprise the middle layer of the eyeball. The onset of iritis may be sudden, acute, and accompanied by intense pain, blurred vision, and extreme sensitivity to light. Iritis may also be chronic, with less dramatic, but persistent symptoms. In either case the eye reddens and the pupil contracts into an irregular shape. Unless the cause is obvious, as it is when there is an injury to the eye, it may be difficult to isolate. Iritis may be associated with diabetes, syphilis, abscessed teeth, or sudden systemic infections. It must be treated promptly by a doctor to prevent scarring of the eyeball tissues and irreversible damage to vision. The problem of recurring iritis can be solved only by discovering and dealing with the underlying cause.

iron One of the minerals that is an essential micronutrient. *See* "Nutrition and Weight."

A deficiency of iron in the diet is the direct cause of the most common type of anemia, iron-deficiency anemia. There is no such thing as a tendency to anemia; it is a clinical condition measurable by laboratory examination of a blood sample. An iron deficiency may occur temporarily if surgery or other conditions make a restricted diet necessary or during pregnancy when iron stored in the body is depleted by the demands of fetal development. To supply supplemental iron in such cases the preparation known as ferrous sulfate is considered therapeutically superior to tonics advertised for "tired blood"; it is also less expensive. Iron pills or tonics should never be taken unless prescribed by a doctor after a blood test, since excessive amounts may be damaging in the absence of anemia. Only where there is a need to obtain a rapid response or where oral preparations cause gastric upset is iron given by injection.

irritability Impatience, crankiness, oversensitivity to annoyances and frictions of daily life. No one is even-tempered all the time, but anyone who is irritable most of the time should try to find out why. Temporary crankiness may result from a variety of reasons such as a determined effort to stop a bad habit, apprehension connected with an illness, the effects of the contraceptive pill, an unbalanced diet, premenstrual tension, or overwork; such problems usually diminish with time. Assuming physical reasons for the emotional edginess have been ruled out, chronic irritability is usually due to a dissatisfaction with one's self. Since irritability can place a strain on relationships with friends and family, counseling is often advisable.

itching An irritation of the skin; technically called pruritus. Among the most common causes are insect bites, fungus infections, allergies, or contact dermatitis. Itching in the anal region may be caused by worms or hemorrhoids; in the vaginal area it may occur spontaneously or follow the use of certain antibiotics. Severe itching around the pubic hair may indicate the presence of crabs. Among other causes are an accumulation of dried body secretions under the arms, in the crotch, on the scalp, or between the toes; vaginal discharges; the drying out of the vaginal mucous membranes that occurs during menopause; exposure to cold temperatures; new skin growth following sunburn or scar healing; chafing by one body surface against another (e.g., under the breasts) or by tight clothing; emotional stress. A doctor may refer to local or generalized itching as neurodermatitis if no specific cause can be found. Certain serious disorders are accompanied by itching: diabetes, anemia, leukemia, jaundice, gout, liver malfunction, and cancer. Diseases in which an itching rash is a characteristic symptom include chickenpox, measles, and rubella.

The impulse to relieve itching by energetic scratching should be controlled since the irritation will only become more intense and the nails may cause breaks in the skin leading to secondary bacterial infection. Sometimes it is necessary to wear gloves. If topical medication provides no relief, medication taken orally or by injection may be necessary to relieve the itching until the underlying cause can be diagnosed and eliminated. The disorder that has the distinction of being called "the itch" is discussed under scabies.

IUD Intrauterine device. *See* "Contraception and Abortion."

jaundice A yellowish appearance of the skin and the whites of the eyes resulting from an excessive amount of bile in the blood. As a sign of a disorder of the liver or the biliary tract, jaundice may be accompanied by diarrhea, abdominal pain caused by liver enlargement, bitter-tasting greenish vomit, and itching in various parts of the body. Among the usual underlying causes, the most common is infectious hepatitis; others are gallstones, cirrhosis, hemolytic anemia, and tumors that obstruct the normal circulation of bile. The treatment of jaundice depends on the diagnosis of the condition.

joint diseases *See* ARTHRITIS, BURSITIS, etc.

kidneys and kidney disorders The kidneys are twin organs, each about 4 inches long, located on either side of the spinal column at the back wall of the abdomen approximately at waist level. As the lungs expand and contract during respiration, the kidneys move up and down. Examined in cross-section under a microscope, the functional units of the organ—the nephrons—are seen to consist of clusters of blood vessels, the glomeruli, which act as filters. The vital process in which the kidneys are indispensable is the continuous filtering of the blood

to remove wastes and excess fluid while retaining or reabsorbing other materials. The kidneys also secrete hormones involved in the regulation of blood pressure and the red blood cell count. In order to understand how certain disorders originate, it is helpful to have some idea of how the kidneys work. As arterial blood enters the kidneys from the heart, it passes through the millions of nephrons. The waste materials go by way of the ureter into the bladder for eventual elimination through the urethra in the form of urine. The cleansed and filtered blood goes back into circulation through the veins, returning to the heart for recirculation. With a combined weight of only about ⅔ of a pound, the kidneys process more than 18 gallons of blood every hour and filter about 60 percent of all the

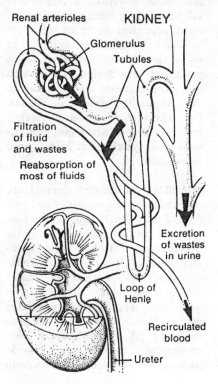

Renal arterioles   **KIDNEY**
Glomerulus
Tubules
Filtration
of fluid
and wastes
Reabsorption of
most of fluids
Excretion
of wastes
in urine
Loop of
Henle
Recirculated
blood
Ureter

fluid taken into the body, excreting as much as 2 quarts of urine each day.

The kidneys are subject to a number of disorders, some merely temporary, others potentially fatal. The most common problem is infection and the most common infection is pyelonephritis, an infection of the kidney's urine collecting ducts. It may occur with no significant symptoms, or it may be accompanied by back pain, fever, and chills. An acute attack of pyelonephritis occurs in about 1 in 500 pregnancies and usually requires antibiotic treatment to prevent recurrences. Kidney obstructions in the form of stones, cysts, or other abnormalities can lead to improper drainage, inflammation, and damage to surrounding tissues. The disease commonly called nephritis, but accurately known as glomerulonephritis, is an inflammation of the filtering vessels. Nephrosis, also known as the nephrotic syndrome, is a group of symptoms frequently accompanying some other condition. It is characterized by the leakage of large amounts of protein into the urine and leads to generalized swelling, especially a marked puffiness under the eyes. Kidney disease may also result from untreated hypertension, gout, and diabetes or as a consequence of chemical poisoning or prolonged shock. When any disorder reaches the point where the kidneys can no longer function, uremia (accumulation of urea nitrogen in the blood) occurs. Acute kidney failure may be helped by short-term dialysis. When irreversible damage to both kidneys has occurred, long-term dialysis or tissue transplant can prevent fatal consequences.

Any signs of kidney disease should be taken seriously, especially during pregnancy. Symptoms may include back pain below the rib cage; a change in the color or composition of urine or discomfort during urination; puffiness of any part of the body, especially the area around the eye. Treatment depends on the results of blood tests and X-rays and may only require changes in the diet and the use of diuretics. Antibiotics are often prescribed for bacterial infection. In the case of an obstruction, surgery may be necessary. *See also* GLOMERULONEPHRITIS.

knee disorders The knee is one of the largest and strongest joints in the body, formed by the junction of the tibia (shinbone), the femur (thighbone), and the patella (kneecap). The bones are bound by ligaments and tendons and cushioned by cartilage and fluid-filled sacs called bursas. "Housemaid's knee," so called because it usually results from frequent kneeling on hard surfaces, is a form

KNEE DISORDERS

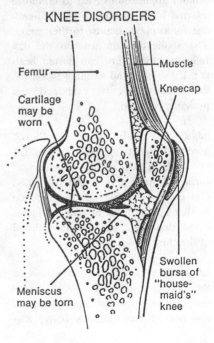

Femur

Cartilage may be worn

Muscle

Kneecap

Swollen bursa of "housemaid's" knee

Meniscus may be torn

of bursitis. "Water on the knee" is a condition in which there is an excessive accumulation of the lubricating fluid secreted by the membranous lining of the ligaments that bind the knee joints together. This oversecretion, which may follow an injury or infection or may accompany arthritis, causes the kneecap to be raised and the surrounding tissue to become painful. Keeping the knee raised and rested is usually sufficient treatment. Chronic inflammation of the joint may occur during arthritis and can be relieved by medication and other forms of therapy. Because of the exposure of the knee and the stresses to which it is subject, it is especially vulnerable to injury. Scrapes, minor bruises, or superficial cuts which do not damage anything except the skin around the knee are not usually a problem of any magnitude. A fall or athletic injury that results in soreness and swelling will benefit from the prompt application of ice to minimize internal bleeding and an elastic bandage for support against further strain. The application of heat on the day following the injury can hasten healing. If the pain and swelling increases, the knee should be examined and probably X-rayed.

labia The Latin word for "lips," used to designate the labia majora, the two folds of skin and fatty tissue that form the outer part of the vulva and that cover the labia minora, the two smaller lips or folds of mucous membrane that form the protective hood of the clitoris.

labor The rhythmic contractions of the muscles in the uterus which transport the baby through the birth canal and out of the mother's body; also called parturition. *See* "Pregnancy and Childbirth."

lacrimal ducts Three sets of ducts involved in the flow of tears: 6 to 12 tiny openings that lead from the lacrimal (tear) gland at the upper, outside rim of the eye to the conjunctival sac; the lacrimal duct that leads from the inner corner of the eye to the lacrimal sac; and the nasolacrimal duct that leads from the lacrimal sac to the nose. When these ducts are overloaded by an abnormally heavy flow of tears, caused by strong feelings or by chemical or mechanical irritants, the excess liquid runs down the cheeks or through the nose. When the duct in the nose is blocked or swollen by allergy or inflammation during a respiratory infection, the eyes become watery. The dry, itchy eyes that may afflict the elderly result from a partial drying up of the lacrimal glands and a consequent decrease in the fluid that keeps the eye surface moist.

EXTERNAL EYE

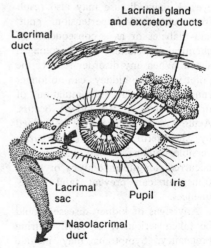

Lacrimal gland and excretory ducts

Lacrimal duct

Lacrimal sac

Pupil

Iris

Nasolacrimal duct

lactation The production of milk in the mother's breasts, beginning about three days following childbirth; also, the period of weeks or months during which the baby is breast-fed.

Lamaze method A system of preparation for childbirth named after its originator, Dr. Ferdinand Lamaze. The method consists in educating both parents-to-be about the birth process, teaching the pregnant woman breathing, relaxation, and concentration exercises, and training the father (or a close friend or relative) to act as a coach who will be present during labor and delivery. Increasing numbers of obstetricians are trained in the Lamaze method, and more and more hospitals are inviting the father to participate in his baby's birth. *See* "Pregnancy and Childbirth."

laryngitis Inflammation of the mucous lining of the larynx, affecting both breathing and voice production. The condition may be chronic or acute, occurring because of a virus or bacterial infection, an allergic response, an irritation of the membrane by chemicals, dusts, or pollens, or recurrent misuse of the voice. The symptoms of milder cases usually include a dry cough, a tickling sensation in the throat, and hoarseness or a complete loss of voice, all of which result from swelling of the vocal cords. Fever may be present when laryngitis is produced by the flu or by a heavy chest cold. The most effective treatment is silence. The condition is also helped by a day or so of bed rest in a room where the temperature is warm and even and the humidity is high enough to prevent irritating dryness, if necessary through the use of a humidifier or a vaporizer. Spicy foods, hot soups, smoking, or any other irri-

tants should be eliminated. Chronic laryngitis may be the result of long-time exposure to such irritants as alcohol, smoking, or industrial fumes. Since hoarseness may also accompany the development of tuberculosis or cancer, it should be investigated by a doctor if it persists for more than a few weeks.

larynx A cartilaginous structure which contains the vocal cords and is held together by ligaments and moved by attached muscles; also called the voice box. It is located in front of the throat and is lined with mucous membrane continuous with the pharynx and the trachea. The larynx is the source of sound that emanates in speech and is also part of the respiratory system, being the passageway for air between the pharynx and the lungs. The largest ring of laryngeal cartilage characteristically

CROSS-SECTION OF MOUTH AND LARYNX

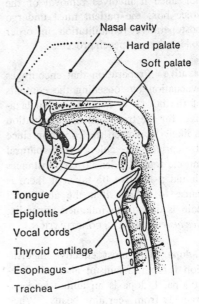

Nasal cavity
Hard palate
Soft palate
Tongue
Epiglottis
Vocal cords
Thyroid cartilage
Esophagus
Trachea

protrudes in the male throat as the Adam's apple. The epiglottis at the base of the tongue forms the lid that closes the larynx during swallowing, thus preventing food and drink from going down "the wrong way" and causing choking. Obstruction of the larynx may occur because of an abscess in the cartilage lining or because of an injury. Tumors are not uncommon and are removed surgically, even if benign. Singers and politicians, due to the professional use of their voices, are more likely to develop nodes on their vocal cords than other people. Such growths may also be eliminated by surgery. Cancer of the larynx, which is more common in men than women, is associated with heavy smoking. If examination with a laryngoscope and various laboratory tests including a biopsy verify the presence of an obstructive malignancy unresponsive to radiation treatment, a laryngectomy, the surgical removal of part or all of the larynx, is performed. The surgery itself is not complicated, but since it involves removal of the voice box, the patient must undergo postoperative rehabilitation in order to learn a new speech process.

laxative Preparation that encourages evacuation by loosening the contents of the bowel. A dependence on laxatives for the treatment of constipation is likely to worsen the condition since it deprives the colon of its natural muscle tone. Under no circumstances should a laxative be taken if there is cause to believe that the abdominal pain is due to an inflamed appendix. *See also* CATHARTIC, CONSTIPATION.

L-dopa The most effective medication for parkinsonism; also called levodopa. L-dopa is an amino acid extracted from certain beans. When taken orally in carefully supervised doses, it increases the brain's amount of dopamine, the natural substance essential for the normal transmission of nerve messages. The loss of this substance causes the tremors and rigidity characteristic of the disease. L-dopa compensates for this loss in approximately 75 percent of all cases.

Leboyer The French obstetrician, Dr. Frederic Leboyer, author of the book *Birth Without Violence* and proponent of a method of delivery that supposedly eases the birth trauma by creating a comforting environment from the instant the newborn baby emerges into the world.

lesbian Woman whose emotional and sexual needs are directed toward other members of her own sex. *See* "Sexual Health."

leukemia A group of neoplastic diseases characterized by a proliferation in the bone marrow and lymphoid tissue of white blood cells whereby their excessive production interferes with the manufacturing of normal red cells. Different types of white cells are involved in the various forms taken by the disease. Acute lymphocytic leukemia, the most common form of childhood cancer and at one time almost always fatal, is now being controlled by a combination of radiation and chemotherapy. One type of acute granulocytic leukemia can occur at any age; the chronic leukemias (myeloid and lymphocytic among others) are unlikely to occur before middle age, with men contracting the disease more frequently than women. While there is no accepted theory about the cause of leukemia, it is assumed that its rising incidence results from increased exposure to radioactivity in its many manifestations: industrial pollution, food contamination, too many diagnostic X-rays over too short a period, or radiation therapy for some other disease. Whatever the age and circumstances of the victim, leukemic symptoms are generally the same: unexplained weight loss, low energy, fever, subcutaneous hemorrhaging, various signs of anemia, and lowered resistance to infection because of the destruction of normal cells. As the disease progresses, especially in its myeloid form, the spleen becomes visibly enlarged and in chronic lymphatic leukemia the lymph nodes swell and become sore. Diagnosis of all leukemias is based on microscopic examination of blood samples, bone marrow, or lymph tissue. Treatment consists of a combination of anticancer drugs, corticosteroids, radiation, antibiotics, and transfusions of hemoglobin and platelets. Several of the leukemias, which were formerly fatal, have gone into remission as a result of the effectiveness of the new drugs, the use of generalized radiation, and the transplanting of healthy bone marrow.

leukorrhea An abnormal vaginal discharge. When the discharge is heavy, when it contains pus and has an unpleasant odor, or when it causes itching or burning of the vagina or the vulva, a diagnosis of the underlying condition should be made. Among the circumstances leading to leukorrhea are: mechanical irritation by a diaphragm, tampon, or IUD; chemical irritation by excessive douching or the use of vaginal deodorant sprays; vaginal infection by bacteria or fungi, especially candidiasis or trichomoniasis; venereal disease, especially gonorrhea; benign growths such as polyps

or fibroid tumors. Heavy discharge may also be a sign of diabetes or cervical cancer. In most cases it can be cleared up by finding the cause and initiating proper treatment.

libido The sexual drive; in psychoanalytic terms, a form of psychic energy that expresses erotic instincts and feelings in different ways at various stages of life.

Librium Brand name of one of the tranquilizing drugs (chlordiazepoxide) that induces a feeling of calm without causing sleepiness. Librium should never be taken in combination with alcohol and prolonged use can create a psychological dependence. *See* "Drugs, Alcohol, and Tobacco."

life expectancy The number of years a person of a given age may be expected to live, based on statistical averages. Current calculations for the life expectancy in the United States of white females at birth is placed between 75 and 76 years. This is 23 years longer than life expectancy for the same group born in 1900. However, there has been little change in the life expectancy of women over 60, that is, an adult woman of 65 in 1900 had a life expectancy of 13 more years and a woman of 65 today can expect to live 15 more years. This lack of improvement is balanced by the fact that more and more women live to be 60, thanks to progress in the prevention of death during childbirth, the control of infectious diseases, and improvements in public health. These advances also account in some measure for the fact that while the average length of life for women born in 1900 exceeded that of males by only two years, in our own time women live at least eight years longer than men on the average. Studies by the World Health Organization on this differential indicate that urban life lowers life expectancy for men and raises it for women. In underdeveloped countries, where women are often overworked, underfed, and frequently pregnant and where there is an age-old prejudice against female children typical of agrarian societies, the death rates for women are much higher than they are for men.

ligament   Band of tough fibrous tissue that connects and stabilizes bones at the joints. An injury resulting in the stretching or tearing of ligaments is called a sprain.

lipoma   A benign tumor composed of fat cells. This type of growth usually occurs close to the skin surface, and while it may reach the size of a golf ball, removal, if necessary or desired, is rarely complicated.

lithium carbonate   A chemical compound of the element lithium, used in the treatment of manic-depressive illness; not to be confused with lithium chloride, another of the salts of lithium and no longer available for patients on low-sodium diets because of its dangerous side effects. Lithium carbonate is considered by specialists to be the first drug effective against a major psychosis. It is also being used increasingly for patients whose lives are disrupted by unaccountable mood swings originating in one of the depressive illnesses. Properly administered in supervised doses, it results in the emotional stabilization of many patients who have not responded well to treatments combining heavy seda-tion with tranquilizers, electroshock, and antidepressants.

liver   The body's largest internal organ, dark red, wedge-shaped, weighing from 3 to 4 pounds, and located underneath the lower right side of the rib cage. Among its many vital functions are: the production of bile essential for fat digestion; the production and storage of glycogen for conversion to glucose; the synthesis of protein and the formation of urea; the storage of vitamins A, D, E, and K; the production of several blood components including the clotting factors; the neutralization of poisons such as carbon tetrachloride, arsenic, and others that may enter the body from without as well as of those created from within. Inflammation of the liver (hepatitis) may be caused by chemi-

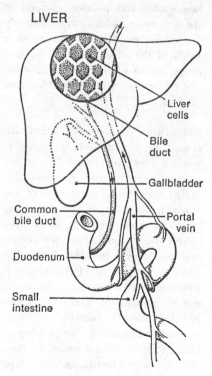

LIVER

Liver cells

Bile duct

Gallbladder

Common bile duct

Portal vein

Duodenum

Small intestine

cal poisons, by sensitivity to drugs such as Thorazine and Chloromycetin, and by disease agents, especially the viruses that cause the several types of hepatitis. If the infection is severe, the cells that are affected may be replaced by scar tissue, causing cirrhosis of the liver. A nourished liver that contains stored amounts of vitamins, proteins, and other nutrients is less likely to suffer irreversible harm from alcohol than a liver that is undernourished. The liver may also be adversely affected by disorders of the gallbladder, especially by gallstones. The signs and symptoms of liver disorder may include the following depending on the severity of the disease: a gradual swelling of the abdomen and sensitivity to pressure below the rib cage, clay colored stools, dark urine, and vomiting of blood. When disorders are treated promptly and a wholesome regimen is followed, recovery is usually complete.

liver spots Irregularly shaped reddish brown skin blemishes once mistakenly attributed to malfunctioning of the liver. The spots, which are concentrations of melanin pigment similar to but larger than freckles, are not due to aging as such, but rather to long exposure to sun and wind, to minor metabolic disturbances, and in some women to systemic changes that occur during pregnancy. The spots are generally harmless and can either be covered with a special cosmetic preparation or caused to fade by the use of an ointment that inhibits melanin production. If such a blemish suddenly thickens and hardens or if the surrounding tissue feels sore, a dermatologist should be consulted.

lobotomy A psychosurgical operation which severs the nerve fibers that connect the frontal lobe of the cerebrum to the rest of the brain, thereby producing a profound personality change that approaches a form of docility. Frontal lobotomies were once performed as a last resort in controlling violent patients or in handling psychoses unresponsive to any other treatment. Today lobotomies have been almost universally replaced by drug therapy in the form of tranquilizers and antidepressants.

longevity *See* LIFE EXPECTANCY.

low blood sugar *See* HYPOGLYCEMIA.

lower back pain *See* BACKACHE.

LSD Lysergic acid diethylamide, a hallucinogenic drug. *See* "Drugs, Alcohol, and Tobacco."

lung One of two spongelike structures, each enclosed in a pleural sac, which together with the bronchial tree, make up the lower respiratory system. Each lung is divided into lobes—three in the right lung and two in the left. Each lobe is divided into segments that have their own segmental bronchi and their own blood supply. The lungs are the organs in which the respiratory exchange of gases takes place. Under normal circumstances a signal reaches the brain approximately 16 to 20 times a minute indicating the need for an adjustment of the oxygen—carbon monoxide balance within the body. At this signal the diaphragm is thrust downward, increasing the chest capacity, making negative pressure and causing air to rush in to fill the pressure void, leading to the expansion of the lungs. This oxygen-laden atmospheric air travels through the airway passages until it reaches the alveoli. It is through the delicate membranes of the alveoli that the carbon dioxide in the blood of the pulmonary capillaries is exchanged for oxygen. The freshened blood then recirculates; a signal from the brain causes the diaphragm to relax, the negative pressure is reduced, the carbon dioxide is exhaled and the lungs compress.

While some lung disorders can be diagnosed accurately by listening to the breathing sounds through a stethoscope or by sounding the chest wall by tapping one finger against it and hearing the effects of the percussion, the state of the lungs can best be assessed by more refined techniques. Ordinary X-rays and those taken after radiopaque materials have been instilled in the bronchial tree can disclose many different types of lung tissue damage. With the use of a bronchoscope, foreign bodies, parts of tumors, or even an entire growth can be localized and removed. Other laboratory procedures for defining lung disorders involve sputum examinations that can identify a bacterial invader, fungus, or dust that may be causing progressive lung damage and examination of pleural fluid. Collapse of a lung (pneumothorax) may be partial, as may occur because of bronchial obstruction by a blood clot, tumor, or plug of mucus, or it may be complete, affecting a lobe or an entire lung damaged by a bullet wound, tuberculosis, or cancer. Spontaneous pneumothorax is a comparatively rare condition that occurs when there is a sudden air leak from the lung into the chest cavity without apparent cause. This spontaneous collapse is accompanied by the onset of chest pain and breathlessness. When the air that has collected in the space between the thorax and the lung is removed by suction, the affected lung expands to its normal capacity. The disorder is rarely serious, but when recurrences are a problem, surgical correction is recommended.

lupus erythematosus An inflammatory disease that may involve various parts of the body and cause permanent tissue damage. Typical victims are women of childbearing age. In its milder discoid form it affects the skin only, producing a butterfly-shaped rash that spreads across the nose to both sides of the face. The rash may be accompanied by fever and weight loss, as well as by arthritic pains in the joints. In its more serious form systemic lupus erythematosus involves the kidneys and the blood vessels. The cause is unknown and the disease may flare up unexpectedly, leaving the patient exhausted and weak. Recent research indicates that the disorder may occur or worsen when a latent virus is activated by overexposure to sunlight, emotional stress, or an unrelated infection. The symptoms have been explained as an aberration in the body's autoimmune system during which disease-fighting cells go awry and devour healthy tissue.

Lupus is a condition requiring long-term supervision. Special medications that control the disorder, especially heavy therapeutic doses of anti-inflammatory drugs, corticosteroids, and other drugs, may produce adverse side effects. The prescribed regimen must be carefully followed and readjusted from time to time depending on individual reactions. Patients with this disease should use a contraceptive other than the pill; if they do become pregnant, special management is needed. In all cases including the mildest, exposure to extreme sunlight should be avoided.

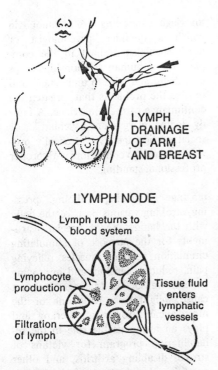

LYMPH DRAINAGE OF ARM AND BREAST

LYMPH NODE

Lymph returns to blood system

Lymphocyte production

Filtration of lymph

Tissue fluid enters lymphatic vessels

lymph nodes Glandlike organs located throughout the body that manufacture the disease-fighting cells known as lymphocytes. These cells are collected in the lymphatic vessels and delivered to the circulatory system in the fluid called lymph. Lymph is part of the blood's plasma. Among the most important lymph nodes and the ones that are superficially located are those found behind the ears, at the angle of the jaw in the neck, in the armpit, and in the groin. When reference is made to "swollen glands," it is the nodes that are involved, since in addition to their providing the system with protective lymphocytes, they also filter foreign bodies and bacteria out of the lymphatic fluid. Other masses of lymphatic tissue that produce specialized white cells for counteracting infection are the tonsils, thymus gland, and spleen. The general term for inflammation of lymphatic tissue, of which tonsillitis is an example, is lymphadenitis; a tumor of this tissue is a lymphoma, and a malignancy of the lymph nodes is a lymphosarcoma.

lymphogranuloma venereum A sexually transmissible disease caused by a viruslike organism. *See* "Sexually Transmissible Diseases."

macrobiotic diet A food regimen, supposedly derived from Zen Buddhism. The basis of the diet is brown rice and tea. The macrobiotic diet may cause a number of serious deficiency diseases and is not recommended.

malaria An infectious disease caused by several species of protozoa (parasites) which are transmitted by a mosquito which has bitten a diseased person, become infected, and then bitten another person. Occasionally it is transmitted by a blood transfusion. The natural disease occurs almost exclusively in underdeveloped tropical areas where mosquitos are prevalent and people are readily exposed to them. It destroys red blood cells and causes bouts of severe chills, fever, and sweating daily, on alternate days, or at two day intervals, depending on the particular parasite involved. Medications are available to prevent it and to treat it, but the most important approach is to eliminate the mosquito population in tropical areas. Malaria is probably the most prevalent disease in the world and certainly is the most serious parasitic disease.

malignant A term used to describe a tumor or growth which spreads to surrounding tissues or migrates through the lymphatics or bloodstream to more distant tissues and whose natural course is usually fatal.

malnutrition Inadequate nourishment resulting from a substandard diet or a metabolic defect. Among common causes unrelated to the availability of adequate food are alcoholism, unnecessary vitamins substituted for essential foods, and crash dieting. Symptoms of malnutrition depend on the missing nutrients. In rare cases where a metabolic aberration, such as abnormal enzyme production or glandular malfunction, is the underlying cause, replacement therapy is usually effective. *See* DEFICIENCY DISEASES, ANEMIA, etc.; *see also* "Nutrition and Weight."

mammography Specialized X-ray examination of the breasts to detect abnormal growths, especially cancer, at an early stage. *See* "Breast Care."

manic-depressive illness A mental disturbance characterized by periods of overenergized and overconfident elation followed by profound depression; also known as bipolar depression. Attacks may be severe and cyclic, with varying periods of normalcy occurring between onsets of the illness. Lithium carbonate administered at the beginning of the manic phase has a stabilizing effect on many people suffering from this disorder.

marijuana A mild hallucinogenic drug derived from the hemp plant (*Cannabis sativa*). Following the discovery that the active chemical ingredient in marijuana, tetrahydrocannabinol, known as THC, dramatically reduces the nausea caused by chemotherapy in most cancer patients, many states have passed laws legalizing the use of the drug for therapeutic purposes. *See* "Drugs, Alcohol, and Tobacco."

marriage counseling A technique in which a qualified psychologist or other specialist trained in the complexities of human relationships helps a husband and wife to understand and resolve the problems that threaten the continuance of their marriage. A family doctor, clergyman, psychiatrist, or social service agency can usually provide referrals to counselors with proper professional standing.

massage Kneading, rubbing, pressing, stroking various parts of the body with the hands or with special instruments for the purpose of stimulating circulation, relaxing muscles, relieving pain, reducing tension, and improving general well-being. Massage does not cause weight loss. It is one of the most ancient forms of therapy and plays an indispensable role in the rehabilitation program for victims of stroke, disabling arthritis, and other conditions in which muscle health has been impaired by disuse. In such cases a trained physical therapist works under the supervision of a doctor. While massage is most commonly done with the hands, electric vibrators and whirlpool baths (hydrotherapy) may be recommended for certain purposes. Family members can learn how to be helpful in relieving a tension headache or an aching shoulder by kneading the affected area rhythmically. An alcohol rubdown or massage can provide comfort following prolonged athletic exertion. Women who wish a body massage should locate a licensed masseuse through their doctor or a nurse.

mastectomy The surgical removal of breast tissue. *See* "Breast Care."

mastitis Inflammation of the breast. Mastitis may be mild or severe, chronic or acute, and is usually the result of infection or of a hormonal change. One of the most common types of mastitis is called fibroadenosis. It is often referred to as having a "lumpy" breast due to the way the tissue feels when touched. The disorder may also produce cysts which tend to enlarge before the onset of menstruation. Any accompanying soreness usually can be relieved by wearing a properly fitted brassiere for support. Since the lumps produced by fibroadenosis are hard to distinguish from tumors during self-examination of the breasts, routine checkups by a physician knowledgeable in diseases of the breast is important. Acute mastitis may occur after delivery and during nursing when it is called puerperal mastitis. This is usually caused by bacterial infection introduced by way of the cracked skin of the nipples. Antibiotics normally cure this condition. If nursing is not to be continued, the breast must be emptied manually and lactation reduced by other medication. In rare instances chronic mastitis may follow an acute inflammation, and in still rarer cases the condition is caused by tuberculosis. *See* "Breast Care."

mastoid Relating to the cells in the temporal bone that forms the part of the skull situated directly behind the ear. Inflammation of these cells, known as mastoiditis, usually results from an untreated infection of the middle ear. An ear infection can usually be halted before it reaches the mastoid area by administering an antibiotic.

masturbation Manipulation of the genitals exclusive of intercourse for the achievement of sexual gratification. Children masturbate as a means of exploring their bodies and sexual responses. Neither physical nor psychological harm results from masturbation, although guilt and anxiety are sometimes associated with the act. Mutual masturbation is commonly practiced as a form of foreplay preceding sexual intercourse. *See also* "Sexual Health."

measles A childhood disease, also called rubeola, against which there is an effective immunizing vaccine. It should not be confused with German measles, called rubella, and discussed under that heading.

Medic Alert A three-part system for emergency medical protection consisting of a metal emblem worn on the wrist or around the neck which identifies otherwise hidden medical problems, a wallet card with addi-

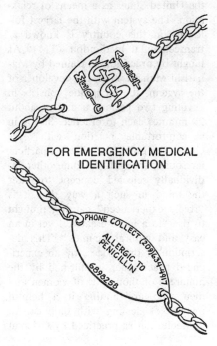

MEDIC ALERT

FOR EMERGENCY MEDICAL IDENTIFICATION

tional information, and an emergency toll-free telephone answering service to provide still further information. Lifetime membership is provided for $15 by the Medic Alert Foundation International (a voluntary, nonprofit organization), Turlock, Calif. 95380.

medical records Personal data; information compiled during visits to the doctor, dentist, hospital, and clinics. Immunization shots, known allergies, X-ray and electrocardiogram reports, blood test results, and other pertinent information should be recorded by the doctor and filed away for future reference. Women should keep their own personal records for use in the event of a change in doctors.

meditation A discipline of concentration or contemplation practiced in the East by yogis and Zen Buddhists and becoming increasingly popular in the United States as a means of relaxation. The system with the largest following in this country is known as transcendental meditation (TM). As taught by practitioners trained by Maharishi Mahesh Yogi, the developer of the system, the technique consists in devoting two periods a day of about 20 minutes each to practice. Sitting in a comfortable position with eyes closed, the individual allows a particular sound, thought, or some other individually selected concept to enter the mind in such a way that it is "freely experienced" causing thought to rise "to a more creative level in an easy and natural manner." This description of the process by an experienced practitioner is affirmed by the hundreds of thousands of women and men who are finding it a helpful method of dealing with daily stress.

Meditation as practiced by Oriental experts has long been known to produce physiological effects involving control of breath, pulse, and other body processes. It now appears that even among newcomers to the technique, brain waves are modified during meditation. Subjects monitored by an electroencephalograph demonstrate a sustained production of alpha waves, the brain waves that occur during the relaxed state. According to an extensive study of meditating subjects, the technique induces what is technically called a wakeful hypometabolic state (slowed-down metabolism). This state, not to be confused with sleep or hypnosis, may have applications in those medical circumstances where the patient would benefit from self-induced relaxation without the use of drugs.

melanin The pigment that determines the color of a person's skin, hair, and eyes. Melanin is produced by specialized cells called melanocytes whose number is the same in all races. Color differences are caused by the quantity of melanin produced and how it is distributed.

melanoma A tumor composed of cells heavily pigmented with melanin. A malignant melanoma, also known as black cancer, is the most treacherous and the rarest type of skin cancer since the diseased cells invade other parts of the body through the circulatory system. Melanomas rarely develop before middle age, typically in women rather than men. Any changes in the size or appearance of a mole or any bleeding or itching in the tissues that surround it should be diagnosed by a doctor immediately.

menarche The first menstrual period.

Menière's disease A disturbance of the labyrinth of the inner ear resulting in vertigo, nausea, hearing loss, and tinnitus (ringing in the ears). The basic cause is not known. The symptoms may recur frequently or as seldom as every three months. An attack may be mild and last for only a few minutes, or it may be severe, with disabling vomiting and dizziness lasting for several hours. Menière's disease, which characteristically affects one ear, is more common among men than among women, especially after the age of 40. Since the immediate cause of the symptoms is a distention of the endolymphatic system of the inner ear, and since there are many causes for this, treatment is varied and includes the use of diuretics, antihistamines, drugs that dilate the blood vessels and speed up the circulatory flow, dietary changes that reduce cholesterol blood levels, lithium carbonate, and various tranquilizers. When all else fails and the condition seriously interferes with normal functioning, an operation on the labyrinth of the inner ear may be the only way to provide relief. Since this operation may result in a degree of permanent hearing loss, all other combinations of treatment are usually tried first.

meningitis Inflammation of the meninges, the membranes that surround the brain and spinal cord; also known as cerebrospinal meningitis. The inflammation may be caused by a virus or bacteria. Children are more susceptible than adults, but both sexes and all ages are vulnerable; epidemics are more likely to occur in temperate than in tropical climates. The most common, the most acute, and the most contagious form of the disease is meningococcal meningitis. It is caused by meningococci bacteria transmitted by contact with an infected person or in the expelled breath of a person carrying the bacteria. Viral meningitis, also called aseptic, may accompany other virus infections, especially mumps, measles, herpes simplex, and the milder forms of polio. Whatever the source of the inflammation, the symptoms are the same: severe and persistent headaches accompanied by vomiting; where the swelling of the meninges causes critical pressure on the brain, delirium and convulsions may also occur. It is characteristic for the patient to hold the neck stiff, since movements of the head intensify the already acute pain. Any signs that indicate the onset of meningitis should be checked immediately by a doctor who can make a definitive diagnosis following laboratory examination of a sample of cerebrospinal fluid. Prompt treatment with antibiotics and other suitable medications usually brings about an early recovery in bacterial meningitis. In the case of tubercular meningitis a longer course of therapy is necessary using the newer antitubercular drugs. The outcome of viral meningitis is varied.

menopause The span of time during which the menstrual cycle gradually wanes and finally ceases; also called the female climacteric or change of life. *See* "Midlife Transitions."

menorrhagia The excessive loss of blood during menstruation. Among the causes are local or general infection, benign or malignant tumors of the uterus, hormonal imbalance, emotional stress, and hematologic disease. The condition may be said to exist when the amount of blood is excessive compared to usual periods. A thorough gynecological examination should be scheduled so that any abnormalities may be ruled out or treated. If menorrhagia goes untreated for several months, it is likely to be the direct cause of anemia.

menstruation The periodic discharge through the vagina of blood and sloughed off tissue from the uterus; the discharged matter is technically known as the menses. *See* "The Healthy Woman."

mental illness Any of a group of psychobiological disturbances, generally categorized as psychoses (as distinct from neuroses) and characterized by such symptoms as severe and pervasive mood alterations, disorganization of thought, withdrawal from social interaction into fantasy, personality deterioration, hallucinations and delusions, bizarre behavior often without a loss of intellectual competence. While there is disagreement about the basic causes and mechanisms of severe mental disorders, one of the greatest advances in treating them has been the use of drugs that make seriously disturbed patients more accessible to other forms of therapy. In evolving current chemotherapy, basic research in the biochemistry of the brain has yielded important evidence to support the theory that psychotic disorders have a physiological foundation in errors of brain metabolism. There is also accumulating evidence that some mental illnesses, especially the syndrome known as schizophrenia, has a genetic basis. *See* DEPRESSION, MANIC-DEPRESSIVE ILLNESS, PSYCHOSIS, SCHIZOPHRENIA, SENILITY, etc.

mercury A silver-white metallic element that remains fluid at ordinary temperatures; also called quicksilver. It is used as the medium of measurement in fever thermometers because of its response to heat and in sphygmomanometers, the instruments that measure blood pressure, because of its weight. Mercury was once the only treatment for syphilis, and until its dangerous side effects became obvious, it was widely used in combination with other drugs as a cathartic, a diuretic, and a pesticide. It is still one of the ingredients in certain contraceptive jellies and creams and may be the source of vaginal irritation.

The dumping of industrial wastes containing mercury has irreversibly polluted many bodies of water in the United States and has so contaminated the fish in them that they are dangerous to eat. Poisoning caused by eating meat that came from animals whose feed was contaminated by pesticides containing mercury became such a health hazard that in 1976 the Environmental Protection Agency outlawed this particular use. Mercury poisoning continues to be a potential danger to anyone exposed to industrial fumes containing the chemical.

metabolism The combined processes involved in the production and maintenance of the substances essential for carrying on the activities of life. Metabolism occurs within each cell where groups of enzymes catalyze and control the chemical reactions that must occur during the normal absorption of oxygen and nutrients. The metabolic activity depends on the performance of specific functional tasks by specialized enzymes. Many diseases, previously mysterious, are now known to be caused by genetically determined enzymatic aberrations in the metabolic process. Metabolism is also adversely affected by diabetes and disorders of the thyroid gland.

metastasis The spreading of a cancerous growth by extension to surrounding tissue (direct metastasis) or by the breaking away of clumps of diseased cells which invade other parts of the body (blood borne or lymphatic metastasis) where they settle and form secondary tumors. The invasive tumors are called metastatic growths.

methadone A synthetic narcotic used as a substitute for morphine and in the United States as a substitute for heroin in supervised centers for the treatment of heroin addiction. Methadone, which is also addictive, but in a less debilitating way than heroin, is theoretically the bridge to the achievement of a drug-free condition. The purpose of the therapy is to diminish the doses of methadone until there is no longer a need for the drug. The brand name of methadone is Dolophine which accounts for its being known as "Dolly."

Methedrine Brand name of methamphetamine hydrochloride.

middle ear *See* EAR.

midwife *See* NURSE-MIDWIFE.

migraine *See* HEADACHE.

milk An essential food containing a good balance of fats, carbohydrates, and proteins, as well as a major source of essential minerals and vitamins A and B_2. Since pasteurization destroys the vitamin C content, other sources for this nutrient, such as citrus fruits and juices, are recommended. Practically all processed milk is enriched with vitamin D and is homogenized for uniform fat distribution. An adult woman should include the equivalent of two cups of milk in her daily diet (this amount may take the form of yogurt or cottage cheese). It is inadvisable for any person to drink raw unpasteurized milk since it may cause undulant fever (brucellosis). When taking antibiotic medication containing tetracycline, milk should not be ingested at the same time since the calcium in the milk interferes with the proper absorption of the medicine.

Miltown Brand name of meprobamate, one of the most widely prescribed tranquilizing chemicals. Another brand name for the same chemical is Equanil. Both these drugs suppress anxiety without causing drowsiness.

miscarriage *See* ABORTION, SPONTANEOUS.

mole A raised pigmented spot on the upper layers of the skin, usually brown and sometimes hairy. Moles may also have a blue appearance when buried more deeply, although the pigmentation is still brown. Yellowish rough-textured bumps produced by an abnormally active oil-secreting gland are called sebaceous moles. Any of these may be present from birth or they may appear early and disappear spontaneously. When such a blemish suddenly begins to itch, to grow, or especially to bleed, it should be examined by a dermatologist. While almost all moles are harmless, a few are malignant and should be removed promptly. The technical name for such skin tumors is melanomas.

moniliasis Infection caused by a yeastlike fungus, *Candida albicans;* also known as monilia, candidiasis.

See "Sexually Transmissible Diseases."

mononucleosis, infectious A virus infection that causes an abnormality of and increase in the number of white blood cells containing a single nucleus; also called glandular fever. The symptoms are somewhat similar to those of the flu: fever, very sore throat, general malaise, and swollen lymph nodes. The infection is diagnosed by simple blood tests. Since the infectious agent, known as the EB virus (Epstein-Barr), is present in the throat and saliva, it is transmitted by mouth-to-mouth contact, explaining why younger people call mononucleosis the "kissing disease." The swelling of the lymph nodes is caused by the fact that the virus stimulates the number and size of the white blood cells known as lymphocytes which then become ineffective in carrying out their disease-fighting function. While the patient may suffer from extreme fatigue and complications such as a jaundiced liver, enlargement of the spleen, or a secondary infection of the throat, hospitalization generally is not necessary. The chief dangers of mononucleosis are possible rupture of the spleen and involvement of the brain.

The treatment is usually no more than bed rest, but it is important that a doctor be in charge of the patient so that any appropriate therapy can be introduced and progress monitored in general. Limited activity is advised until all symptoms disappear. Sometimes cortisone medication is used. Other medications are prescribed for secondary conditions. Since anyone who has had mononucleosis develops EB virus antibodies, it is presumed that one attack confers lifetime immunity.

mons veneris The mount of Venus; the triangular pad of fatty tissue and skin that covers the pubic bone; also known as the mons pubis or pubic mount. It is covered with hair from puberty onward.

morning sickness A feeling of queasiness and nausea often experienced upon arising during the first few months of pregnancy. Vomiting may or may not occur. The cause is assumed to be the increase in estrogen supply to which the body adjusts in time. While more than half of pregnant women suffer from morning sickness, it rarely continues beyond the twelfth week. Starting the day with an unsalted biscuit or dry toast, eliminating fried and highly seasoned food, and having smaller meals at frequent intervals will usually minimize the discomfort.

morphine The active constituent in opium and the basis of the painkilling effects of all opiates, of which codeine (methyl morphine) is the weakest. The application of morphine in current practice is largely restricted to terminal patients and severe accident cases, but the use in these cases may eventually be superseded by other drugs. *See* "Drugs, Alcohol, and Tobacco."

motion sickness Nausea and vomiting resulting from a disturbance in the balancing mechanism of the inner ear. The discomfort may occur in a car, train, airplane, or elevator, but it is most common on a ship that is simultaneously pitching and rolling. Anyone who has ever been seasick is familiar with the symptoms of dizziness, headache, pallor, and cold sweating followed by vomiting. There are various antinauseant medications that can be taken in advance of a trip. A doctor can advise on which medicine might be most suitable for the particular circumstance and what the possible side effects might be. Antihistamines combined with sedatives can be helpful when taken at the first sign of discomfort. The effects of airsickness can be minimized by closing the eyes and lying almost prone in one's seat. Car sickness is rarely experienced by the driver and is less likely to occur to a passenger sitting in the front seat with the window open.

mucous membrane Thin layers of tissue that line a body cavity, separate adjacent cavities, or envelop an organ and contain glands that secrete mucus. The membrane is actually a mixture of epithelial tissue and its underlying connective tissue. The mucus, a watery exudate or slimy secretion, keeps the tissue moist. The discharge of mucus which may occur during infections of the nose, throat, and other parts of the body helps to rid the inflamed area of some of the infectious materials. Sexually transmissible diseases are spread through direct contact with infected mucous membrane.

multiple sclerosis A chronic degenerative disease of the central nervous system and the brain. The cause is not known, although evidence indicates that a factor such as an allergy or a virus triggers an autoimmune response in which the body's defense system turns against its own tissues. There is a progressive destruction of the fatty material known as myelin that sheathes the nerves. The designation "multiple" is used because, while the disease attacks mainly the nerves of the spinal cord and the brain, there is no special order or pattern to the destruction. In some people the first symptom may be eye dysfunction, in others a coronary disorder or a locomotion problem. When the nerve endings of the brain are attacked, symptoms include speech changes and emotional swings.

Multiple sclerosis is prevalent mainly in temperate climates; an estimated 1 in 5,000 persons living in northern United States and 1 in 20,000 living in southern United States are affected by it. The disease commonly appears between the ages of 20 and 40, with women twice as susceptible as men. Because the symptoms are easily confused with other disorders, multiple sclerosis is often very difficult to diagnose. Research has therefore been directed not only toward finding the specific cause, but to developing an accurate blood test that would unequivocally identify the disease and rule out all other possibilities. Treatment must be adjusted to individual cases and continually supervised, since one of the characteristics of multiple sclerosis is that it may subside for months or even years and then flare up suddenly with serious effects. Relief is usually provided by anti-inflammatory medication, corticosteroids, antispasmodics, and muscle relaxant drugs. Physical therapy, bed rest, and special diets are other forms of treatment.

mumps A contagious disease generally occurring in childhood. It is caused by a virus which affects the salivary glands, primarily the parotids (in front of and under each ear) and often the submaxillary (at the lower jaw) and the sublingual (under the tongue) glands. It may also affect the gonads. In a typical case the glands swell and become painful; in many instances, however, symptoms are so mild as to go undetected. Mumps is a serious matter only when secondary complications develop. These are primarily meningoencephalitis in children, a viral infection of the nervous system, and mumps orchitis in postpubescent males, an inflammation of the testicles that is rarely serious and rarely results in sterility. The involvement of the ovaries in adult women who contract mumps is extremely rare. However, when a pregnant woman with no acquired immunity is exposed to this infection and contracts the disease, there is a possibility of miscarriage, premature labor, or congenital defects. The doctor in charge of prenatal care should be informed at once so that proper precautionary measures can be taken. Long-term immunization of children, especially prepubescent boys, is now considered standard procedure.

muscles Bundles of fibers that have the ability to contract. *See* "The Healthy Woman."

Common disorders are muscle fatigue, which results when fibers exhaust their supply of glycogen and other productive substances; spasms and cramps, which occur when a muscle is deprived of sufficient oxygen because of some failure in circulation; strains caused by overstretching; twitching or tic resulting from fatigue or tension. Muscles may also be impaired or immobilized by one or another type of muscular dystrophy and by diseases such as poliomyelitis, multiple sclerosis, or cerebral palsy.

muscular dystrophy Any of a group of chronic genetic diseases characterized by the progressive deterioration of the muscles. The particular designation of the dystrophy is based on the muscle groups first affected,

the age of the patient at the onset of symptoms, and the rate at which the degeneration proceeds. While a dystrophic disease may affect anyone at any time, it occurs five times more often among males than females. No form of the disorder is contagious, and while no cure has yet been found, various types of treatment, including special orthopedic devices, can relieve the debilitating symptoms.

The most common and most crippling of the dystrophic diseases is Duchenne muscular dystrophy. It is named for the French neurologist who categorized it in 1861 as a disease characterized by the apparent enlargement (pseudohypertrophy) of the various muscles, beginning with those in the calf of the leg. The enlargement is caused by the abnormal increase in the fatty and connective tissues that replace the wasting muscles. Of all the dystrophies, the Duchenne is the only one known to be transmitted entirely by female carriers, the sons with a 50 percent likelihood of being affected by the disease and the daughters a 50 percent chance of becoming carriers. Fortunately for women who are aware of the presence of the disease in their family, there is a blood test for the detection of carriers of Duchenne MD. The test is available free of charge at any of the Muscular Dystrophy Association, Inc. clinics. If such a facility is not listed in the local telephone directory, referral information may be requested by mail from the national office, located at 810 Seventh Avenue, New York, New York 10019.

myasthenia gravis A comparatively rare neuromuscular disease characterized by abnormal weakness and fatigue following normal exertion. Depending on the muscles affected, symptoms include drooping eyelids, double vision, difficulty in locomotion, incapacity in chewing and swallowing, and, in the most threatening cases, inability of the muscles controlling respiration to function. Myasthenia gravis may occur spontaneously in anyone at any time (there are approximately 11,000 cases in the United States). The disease may be triggered by an infection, pregnancy, or a tumor of the thymus gland or it may be due to an inherited fault in the body's autoimmune system. Whatever the basic reason for the disturbance, the immediate cause appears to be an aberration in the neuromuscular production of the chemical acetylcholine, essential for stimulating the muscle fibers to contract. Successful treatment for some patients has consisted of medicines that help transmit nerve impulses to the muscles; others have been helped by surgical removal of the thymus gland (thymectomy); and most recently still others have been treated with an effective procedure called plasmapheresis. This involves the pumping out of the patient's blood so that it can be cleansed of destructive antibodies (such as would exist in cases of faulty immunologic response). While this procedure is expensive, a course of about six treatments on an outpatient basis seems to return many myasthenia gravis patients to normalcy for long periods of time without the further use of medication.

mycoses *See* FUNGUS INFECTIONS.

Mycostatin Brand name of the fungicidal chemical mystatin; frequently prescribed in vaginal tablet form for candida vaginal infections.

myocardial infarction A type of heart attack in which a portion of the heart muscle dies because its blood supply has been cut off by an obstruction in a coronary artery.

myomectomy Surgical removal of a fibromyoma, a usually benign tumor consisting of muscle fibers. *See* "Gynecologic Diseases and Treatment."

myopia *See* NEARSIGHTEDNESS.

nail Extension of the outermost skin layer of the fingers and toes. Nails are formed from the fibrous protein substance called keratin that also forms the hair that grows outward from the scalp. This elastic horny tissue (actually made up of dead cells) is pushed upward from the softer living matrix of the nail below the cuticle. It takes about six months for a nail to be replaced from the base of the cuticle to the tip of the finger. The general well-being of nails is best maintained by good hygiene and diet.

Healthy nails should be pale pink, smooth, and shiny. Variations in their appearance may be indications not only of local disorders, but of serious diseases. When nails are bluish and the fingertips clubbed, they are a sign of a circulatory or respiratory disorder; spoon-shaped nails are a sign of anemia; split or deformed nails may occur when there is arthritic inflammation of the finger joints; bitten nails indicate a response to emotional stress or simply a habit. White spots on the nails may develop after a nail has been bruised or injured or when too much pressure is exerted at the cuticle during manicuring. A more serious injury may lead to severe pain and the loss of the nail. Unless the nail bed from which the nail grows has been crushed, the new nail that grows back will be normal in all ways.

Fingernails and toenails are vulnerable to fungus infections, particularly to ringworm which can spread quickly into the nails from their free edge, causing discoloration and deformity. The most effective treatment consists in keeping the fingers and toes as clean and dry as possible and using the antibiotic griseofulvin over a period of many months or until the diseased nail has been replaced by a healthy one. Peeling or splitting may be a sign of poor nutrition or a reaction to a particular brand of detergent or nail polish; the use of nail-hardening preparations may have an adverse effect, especially in chronic or extreme cases, and it may be advisable to consult a dermatologist.

Ingrown toenails are common among women whose shoes are too tight. It is usually the nail of the big toe that is forced to grow forward into the toe's nail bed at one or both corners. This distorted growth can be extremely painful, and it can also lead to infection. Self-treatment is possible, if undertaken early, by inserting a tiny cotton swab under the nail edge, thus lifting up the nail so that it is less painful and can grow forward more easily. During treatment comfortable low-heeled shoes should be worn, since high heels throw body weight against the toes. If there is any sign of redness or pain in the area, a podiatrist or medical doctor should be consulted without further delay. Ingrown toenails are best prevented by cutting the nails straight across rather than in an oval arch and by wearing shoes that fit properly.

Manicuring and pedicuring too often is likely to be damaging, and if nail lacquer is regularly used, it should not extend to the base of the nail since the live tissue there should be exposed rather than constantly covered.

Among the more common diseases associated with the nails are infections of the fingers or toes resulting from cuts, hangnails, or any lesions that permit bacterial invasion. The application of a softening cream will decrease the likelihood of cracked cuticles and hangnails. Such infections, called paronychia, can be extremely painful because of the pus and inflammation at the side of the nail. When soaking does not lead to drainage, it may be necessary to have the infected area lanced. Antibiotics are usually prescribed, especially if there is any danger of the spread of the infection.

narcolepsy A neurological abnormality of the brain that leads to a disruption of sleep and the various components of sleep. The disorder is characterized by four symptoms which may occur singly or in any combination. The most common symptom is constant fatigue combined with attacks of sleep at inappropriate times. The second is a loss of muscle tone (catalepsy) triggered by a strong emotional response such as anger, laughter, or astonishment. The onset of catalepsy causes total body paralysis even though the mind is alert and awake. Such an attack may occur many times in one day or only once or twice a year. The other symptoms are the occurrence of frighteningly real hallucinations immediately before falling asleep or immediately after arising and the experience of complete momentary paralysis at the same times. Narcolepsy was first described over a century ago, but until recently it had been assumed to be a psychological rather than a physical abnormality. It is still so often diagnosed incorrectly that anyone who suspects he or she has the illness should arrange for a simple and accurate laboratory test, in which brain wave patterns and eye movements are monitored during sleep. While narcolepsy is not yet curable, various treatments are available for the different symptoms. The disease is under continuing study at the increasing number of sleep disorder clinics that are a part of hospital research centers. The organization that serves as a clearing house for information about such clinics and about other aspects of this particular disorder is the American Narcolepsy Association, Box 5846, Stanford, Calif. 94305.

narcotic A drug characterized by its ability to alleviate pain, calm anxiety, and induce sleep, such as opium and its derivatives or synthesized chemicals. *See* "Drugs, Alcohol, and Tobacco."

natural childbirth Any one of several methods of delivery in which the mother is a conscious and cooperative participant in the birth of her child. Some of these methods are based on preparation for labor by a schedule of breathing and relaxing exercises in which the father-to-be or some other family member participates as a coach. Systems of natural childbirth usually eliminate all general anesthesia and provide sedation only when requested. Many hospitals are now encouraging this type of delivery and are giving the father-to-be the option of being present at the birth of his baby. *See also* LAMAZE METHOD.

nausea The feeling that signals the possible onset of vomiting. Nausea occurs when the nerve endings in the stomach and in various other parts of the body are irritated. This irritation is transmitted to the part of the brain that controls the vomiting reflex, and when the signals are strong enough, vomiting does occur. Nausea may be triggered by psychological as well as physical conditions. Many people are nauseated by the sight of blood, unattractive sights and smells, strong feelings of fear or excitement, severe pain, or nervous tension. Nausea may be due to physical problems such as infectious disease, gallbladder inflammation, ulcer, appendicitis, and, most typically, indigestion, motion sickness, and irritation of the inner ear. In some women nausea is a side effect of contraceptive pills. The symptom may be relieved by taking the pill at bed time rather than in the morning. When nausea is a chronic condition unrelated to any specific cause, emotional stress is a likely explanation. For the queasiness associated with the early months of pregnancy, *see* MORNING SICKNESS.

nearsightedness A structural defect of the eye in which the lens brings the image into focus in front of rather than directly on the retina so that objects at a distance are not seen clearly; also called myopia. This aberration of vision is usually inherited and occurs when the eyeball is deeper than normal from front to back. Nearsightedness manifests itself at an early age, becomes increasingly worse until adulthood, then remains stable until it is likely to be compensated for by the changes in vision that occur during the aging process. It can be corrected by glasses prescribed by an ophthalmologist or an optometrist; the prescription should be checked regularly for necessary adjustments. There is no conclusive evidence that eye exercises can cure nearsightedness, nor is there any reason to presume that the condition is aggravated by reading, watching television, or any other activity that would not affect the normal eye.

neck, stiff Absolute or relative inability to move one's head without experiencing neck pain. The immediate cause in severe cases is inflammation of the nerve endings related to the spinal vertebrae. In less acute cases it may be muscle fatigue, tension, or intermittent exposure to blasts of cold air. It may follow a whiplash injury or it may be an early symptom of a bacterial or viral infection of the meninges such as polio, meningitis, and other diseases affecting the nervous system. It also can be a symptom of cervical osteoarthritis. When the pain is no more than a "crick" in the neck, it usually can be alleviated by aspirin and a heating pad.

Nembutal Brand name of sodium pentobarbital, a barbiturate drug that induces sleep. In addition to its addictive aspects, Nembutal and other drugs in the same category may be dangerous to the fetus when administered to the mother during labor. It can cause death when combined with alcohol.

neomycin An antibiotic obtained from the streptomyces group of bacteria and especially effective in treating ear and eye infections. It is also the active ingredient in creams, ointments, and powders prescribed for certain skin disorders.

neoplasm The general term for any new and abnormal tissue growth; a tumor, either malignant or benign.

nephritis *See* GLOMERULONEPHRITIS.

nephrosis *See* KIDNEY DISORDERS.

nerve The basic unit of the nervous system; any one of the cordlike structures carrying messages between the brain, the spinal cord, and all parts of the body. Each nerve is composed of bundles of fibers along which messages are transmitted by electrochemical processes. These signals control all the body's activities. *See* "The Healthy Woman."

nervous breakdown *See* DEPRESSION.

nervous system The brain, spinal cord, and nerves—the parts of the body that control and coordinate all activities of the body. *See* "The Healthy Woman."

neuralgia Pain in the form of a sharp intermittent spasm along the path of a nerve, usually associated with neuritis. The term is considered imprecise except when it designates the disorder trigeminal neuralgia.

neuritis Inflammation of a nerve or a group of nerves. The symptoms vary widely from decreased sensitivity or paralysis of a particular part of the body to excruciating pain. Treatment varies with the cause of the inflammation. Generalized neuritis may result from toxic levels of lead, arsenic, or alcohol, from particular deficiency diseases, from bacterial infections such as syphilis, or from a severe allergy response. Among the disorders that are caused by neuritis in a particular group of nerves are Bell's palsy, herpes zoster, sciatica, and trigeminal neuralgia.

neurologist *See* DOCTOR.

neuromuscular diseases A category of disorders affecting those parts of the nervous system that control muscle function. Among these disorders are cerebral palsy, parkinsonism, Bell's palsy, multiple sclerosis, and myasthenia gravis.

neurosis A form of maladjustment in relationship to oneself and to others; usually a manifestation of anxiety which may or may not be expressed in chronic or occasional physical symptoms; also called psychoneurosis.

neurosurgeon *See* DOCTOR.

nipples The round or cone-shaped protuberances normally located in the lower outer quadrant of the breasts near the center, and surrounded by an area of darker tissue called the areola. During puberty, when the female sex hormones stimulate the development of the secondary sex characteristics, the breasts increase in size and the milk ducts branch out from the nipple through the rest of the tissue. From this time onward, the nipples also become a prime area of sexual excitation, being densely supplied with nerve endings. During pregnancy the nipples may require special care. They should be gently cleansed of any accumulation of secretions, and if they are tender or the skin is dry, the doctor may recommend the use of emollient creams to prevent cracking. In many women, inversion of the nipples is a normal condition. However, if this happens suddenly and in one breast only, it is a sign that requires prompt attention. The best way to discover nipple retraction is by raising the arms during self-examination of the breasts. Any itching or ulceration of the nipples should be called to a doctor's attention. *See* "Breast Care."

nitrate, nitrite *See* "Nutrition and Weight."

nodule A localized swelling or protuberance; also called a node. Fibrous nodules develop on the finger joints as one of the characteristics of osteoarthritis and are usually painless. Nodules at the elbow and along the surface of the long bones are typical of rheumatoid arthritis and rheumatic fever and are likely to be painful when touched. Verrucous dermatitis, a fungus infection more prevalent among men than among women, takes the form of warty nodules that grow into ulcerating clusters. This disorder is usually treated surgically in its early stages. Multiple nodes sometimes develop on the thyroid gland, especially among women over 30. Such growths are rarely malignant and are likely to disappear with medical treatment. A single thyroid node that increases in size or resists medical therapy may need to be removed surgically because of possible malignancy. Any nodules that develop on the skin surface, especially those that itch or bleed, should be checked by a doctor.

noise Strictly speaking, any unwanted sound. The unit that expresses the relative intensity of sound is the decibel. On the decibel scale 0 represents absolute silence and 130 is the sound level that causes physical pain to the ear. A civilized two-way conversation measures about 50 decibels. The background noises in major American cities measure more than 70 decibels. Rock and disco music are usually played at about 110 decibels.

High intensity sounds cause physiological damage. The cells that make up the organ of Corti in the cochlea, which transmits sound vibrations to the auditory nerve, are hairlike structures that break down either partially or totally when subjected to abnormally strong sound vibrations. In the cochlea of retired steelworkers, for example, these hair cells are almost totally collapsed, and it is estimated that 60 percent of workers exposed to high intensity on-the-job noise will have suffered significant hearing loss by age 65 in spite of such safety precautions as ear plugs, ear muffs, "soundproofed" enclosures, and the like.

The Environmental Protection Agency estimates that more than 16 million people in the United States suffer from hearing loss caused by sonic pollution and another 40 million are exposed to potential health hazards without knowing it. The dangers to the emotional and physical well-being of individuals, families, and communities are in many cases obvious, but in even more instances they are insidious and cumulative. Here are some facts that trouble environmentalists and health experts. According to the National Institute for Occupational Health and Safety, two or three years of daily exposure to 90 decibel sounds will result in some loss of hearing. Constant exposure to moderately loud noise (over 75 decibels) increases the pulse rate and respiration and may eventually cause tinnitus, ulcers, high blood pressure, and mental problems associated with stress. A daylong ride in a snowmobile can irreversibly damage the organ of hearing. Many young people who wear earphones when they listen to loud music have already sustained some permanent hearing loss; according to an extensive survey of students entering college, 60 percent have some impairment of hearing. Steady, moderately loud noise (power mowers, dishwashers, washing machines, vacuum cleaners, power tools, garbage disposal units) can cause the equivalent in housewives of battle fatigue in soldiers: constricted blood vessels, in-

creased activity of the adrenal glands, irritability, dizziness, and distorted vision. People who are subjected to or subject themselves to high intensity sound are nastier and more aggressive than those who live and work in quiet surroundings. Children who live within earshot of the acoustical overload produced by the traffic on a superhighway are found to have more learning problems than a similar sampling of children whose nervous systems do not have to cope with constant background noise.

If exposure to noise is occasionally unavoidable, the use of ear plugs is recommended. If these are not available in an unexpected situation imperiling one's hearing, the ears should be covered with one's hands or fingers. Elements in the immediate environment that make unnecessary noise should be eliminated or toned down wherever possible. In addition, the Environmental Protection Agency encourages local community groups to establish noise complaint centers empowered to investigate and eliminate all sources of unnecessary noise.

nonspecific urethritis　*See* URETHRA.

nosebleed　Bleeding, either mild or profuse, from the rupture of blood vessels inside the nose; technically called epistaxis. Nosebleeds may be caused by injury, disease, blowing one's nose too energetically, strenuous exercise, or sudden ascent to high altitudes. Other causes are tumors and hypertension. Many women experience nosebleeds during pregnancy. They may also occur for no discernible reason and with no ill effect. Bleeding can usually be controlled by holding the head back and pressing the soft flesh directly above the nostril against the bone for a few minutes. If this method is ineffective, the nostril may be packed with sterile cotton gauze which should remain in place for several hours. If the bleeding cannot be stopped promptly, emergency hospital treatment is advisable. It may be necessary to tie or coagulate the bleeding vessel. Any bleeding from the nose or mouth following an accident or a bad fall requires immediate medical attention.

nuclear medicine A special branch of radiology that applies the advances in nuclear physics to the diagnosis and treatment of disease. One of the most important applications is the use of radioactive isotopes to irradiate abnormalities within the body so that they become visible on scanning machines. Radioactive chemicals are widely used in treating certain cancers and hyperthyroidism, and radioactive needles have made delicate nerve surgery possible.

nurse-midwife Registered nurses who have completed an organized program of study and clinical experience recognized by the American College of Nurse-Midwives. This advanced study qualifies them to extend their practice to the care of pregnant women, to the supervision of labor and delivery, and to postnatal progress in cases where no abnormalities are present. *See* "Pregnancy and Childbirth."

nutrition *See* "Nutrition and Weight."

obesity Overweight in excess of 20 percent more than the average for one's age, height, and skeletal structure. *See* "Nutrition and Weight."

obsession A recurrent, repetitive, and persistent theme that takes control of the conscious mind. It frequently is combined with compulsive behavior, that is, the recurrent, repetitive, ritualistic performance of certain acts. Obsessions are considered to be an expression of anxiety originating in an unconscious desire unacceptable to the conscious self. Obsessive-compulsive behavior may take a form that seems bizarre (the woman who can never throw anything away and is finally imprisoned by old newspapers, bottles, rags, etc.) or it may take a form that is so completely in accord with cultural standards that it escapes detection (the woman obsessed with keeping her house spotlessly neat and clean or with buying "bargains" that she neither needs nor wants).

obstetrician *See* DOCTOR.

Oedipus complex The Freudian designation for the suppressed hostility that a son feels toward his father in competing with him for his mother and the continuance into adulthood of sexual desire for his mother if the conflict is unresolved. The term is derived from the Greek legend about the prince Oedipus who, abandoned in infancy and unaware of his true identity, murders his father and marries his mother. The parallel Freudian designation for the unresolved female attachment to the father is the Electra complex.

onychia Inflammation of the tissue surrounding the fingernails and toenails; also called onychitis.

oophorectomy An operation for the removal of one or both ovaries. *See* "Gynecologic Diseases and Treatment."

ophthalmologist *See* DOCTOR.

opiate Any drug derived from opium, the dried juice of the unripened seed pods of the poppy known as *Papaver somniferium*. All opiates have the effect of depressing the central nervous system to a greater or lesser degree, acting as a pain-killer, producing euphoria, and inducing sleep. Morphine is the strongest of the naturally derived opiates; heroin is one of its semisynthetic derivatives; codeine, the weakest of the opiates, is derived from morphine or may be produced directly from gum opium. Paregoric, once widely used as a tranquilizer for babies, is an anise-flavored tincture of opium similar to laudanum, another opiate more widely used in the nineteenth century than aspirin is now. All opium derivatives are addictive and their use is strictly controlled by law.

optician A person trained to measure and grind optical lenses as prescribed by an ophthalmologist or an optometrist. An optician does not examine eyes or write prescriptions for corrective lenses.

optometrist A professional trained to measure the eye for the purpose of prescribing lenses to correct visual irregularities. Many optometrists are now equipped to test their patients for glaucoma and for the early signs of cataracts, but since they are not medical doctors, they must refer people with such disorders and other diseases affecting the eyes to an ophthalmologist for treatment. Some states have accorded this profession the right to use certain medications to facilitate lens prescription. All optometrists must be licensed by the state in which they practice.

oral contraceptives *See* "Contraception and Abortion."

oral sex Sexual stimulation by mouth and tongue of the female genitals, called cunnilingus, and sexual stimulation by mouth and tongue of the male genitals, called fellatio. Oral-genital contact is widely practiced as part of sexual foreplay and as a way of achieving orgasm. While it is a guaranteed method of avoiding pregnancy, it by no means eliminates the possibility of communicating sexually transmissible diseases.

orgasm The climax of sexual excitement, accompanied in women by vaginal contractions and in men by the ejaculation of semen. *See* "Sexual Health."

Orinase Brand name of an oral antidiabetic medicine containing the chemical tolbutamide, which stimulates insulin production by the pancreas. Orinase is one of the hypoglycemic medications for diabetics whose symptoms are not severe enough to require insulin shots.

orthodontia The branch of dentistry that specializes in the correction of malocclusion, irregularities in the way upper and lower teeth come together when the jaw is closed. Although orthodontia is often undertaken for cosmetic reasons, dentists agree that gross malocclusions should be corrected for reasons of health: chewing is improved, cleaning is simplified, and gum disease is less likely to occur. Corrections in adults are slower and more painful to achieve than in children and adolescents, but in some cases they may be worthwhile to improve the health of the mouth.

The orthodontist takes a series of

X-rays of the mouth and jaw and studies them to determine the extent and nature of the correction advisable. Plaster casts are made, and then various appliances for repositioning the teeth are selected to achieve the correction. These include braces, wires, plastic or metal brackets, neckbraces, rubber bands, and retainer plates. The appliances are readjusted regularly to keep pace with the slow shifting of the teeth.

Before embarking on extensive orthodontia, a prospective patient should, in discussion with the family dentist and the orthodontist, compare the relative benefits of the treatment with any disadvantages, such as adverse effects on teeth, discomfort, time, and expense.

orthopedist *See* DOCTOR.

osteoarthritis A chronic degenerative disease affecting the joints of men and women equally, in most cases after the age of 40; also called degenerative joint disease. *See* ARTHRITIS.

osteopathy A type of therapy practiced by osteopaths (Doctors of Osteopathy) which utilizes generally accepted principles of medicine and surgery, but which emphasizes the importance of normal body mechanics and manipulation of the body to correct faulty body structure. In the United States today there actually is little difference between the way doctors of osteopathy and of medicine diagnose and treat disease.

osteoporosis Degenerative porousness of the bones, causing them to fracture more easily and to heal more slowly. Osteoporosis is a more common ailment of aging women than of aging men and is assumed to be related to the decrease in estrogen production following the menopause. In some cases it may be the result of a diet deficient in calcium salts. When osteoporosis affects the spinal vertebrae, they weaken and collapse, leading to the spinal curvature and decrease in stature characteristic of some older women. Estrogen replacement therapy over a strictly limited and medically supervised period can sometimes slow the progress of this disorder. Another treatment that may be effective is additional calcium intake in tablets or in milk consumption.

otolaryngologist *See* DOCTOR.

otosclerosis A condition in which one of the three bones of hearing, the stirrup, becomes immobilized by abnormal bony deposits. Otosclerosis, a more common cause of deafness among women than among men, can sometimes be corrected by surgery. *See* HEARING LOSS.

ovarian cysts and tumors *See* "Gynecologic Diseases and Treatment."

ovary The female sex organ whose function is the production of eggs and the female sex hormones estrogen and progesterone. *See* "The Healthy Woman."

For disorders which may affect the ovaries, *see* "Gynecologic Diseases and Treatment."

overweight *See* OBESITY; *see also* "Nutrition and Weight."

ovulation The process by which an egg cell or ovum is released from the surface of the ovary to travel through the fallopian tube for possible fertilization. *See* "The Healthy Woman."

ovum The female germ cell which when fertilized by the male sperm develops into the human embryo; the Latin word for "egg"; the plural is ova. The ovum is the largest cell produced by the human body. All the ova released by the female throughout her life are present in her ovaries at the time of her birth. At birth the ovaries contain several hundred thousand immature ova of which only several hundred come to maturity from the onset of puberty to the cessation of menstruation. Each ovum contains the genetic information to be inherited by the offspring from the matrilineal line.

oxygen A colorless, odorless gas that makes up about 20 percent of the air and is essential for the maintenance of life. Combined with two parts hydrogen (H_2O) it forms water. When carbon is added to hydrogen and oxygen, the three elements in various molecular combinations become the chemical foundation for most organic matter. In the respiratory process, air is brought into the lungs where the oxygen is withdrawn for passage into the bloodstream and delivered to the cells throughout the body as fuel for essential metabolic activities. By the time the blood supply has circulated back to the lungs, it is carrying the carbon dioxide and wastes to be expelled in the exhalation of breath. The rapid breathing that accompanies unaccustomed physical exertion is the body's mechanism for keeping the oxygen demand and supply in working balance and eliminating CO_2.

In circumstances when sustained high energy expenditure is required, as in running away from danger or in athletic competition, more oxygen may be demanded than the lungs can supply to the muscles. At this point, an "oxygen debt" occurs in which the muscles borrow oxygen from the other tissues. The "debt" is repaid by the continued panting for air during the rest that follows overexertion. Any tissue deprived of oxygen because of circulatory failure, as occurs in a heart attack caused by a coronary artery occlusion, is irreversibly damaged. Tissue death or gangrene occurs because of oxygen deprivation when the blood supply is cut off altogether by disease or by such conditions as frostbite. Deficiency of oxygen, technically called anoxia, may occur in high altitudes or in certain diseases of the heart and lungs that produce cyanosis, a condition in which the lips and the extremities turn blue. Various chemicals—carbon monoxide and cyanide in small amounts and barbiturates in overdoses—are fatal because they interfere with the body's normal use of oxygen.

To prevent respiratory collapse following surgery under anesthesia oxygen is administered by an oxygen mask so that the air sacs of the lungs are expanded to their normal capacity. Oxygen at high pressure, provided by the device known as a hyperbaric oxygen chamber, is used in the emergency treatment of victims of carbon monoxide poisoning, gas gangrene, or accidents that have caused potentially fatal damage to arteries. Another procedure for oxygen administration is the oxygen tent, an enclosure or transparent plastic that surrounds the bed and the patient. The release of a continuous and controlled oxygen supply into the enclosure facilitates respiration in cases of lung damage.

oxytocin A pituitary hormone naturally secreted under the normal circumstances of delivery for the stimulation of uterine contractions and of the secretion of milk. Synthetic oxytocin (Pitocin) may be given by injection or in pills to induce labor or to speed up contractions in a prolonged and painful labor.

pacemaker, artificial A transistorized device implanted under the skin in the area of the shoulder and connected by wires to electrodes implanted in heart tissue for the purpose of supplying a normal beat when the natural pacemaker has been irreversibly damaged or destroyed by disease. The effectiveness of artificial pacemakers is based on the fact that the heart naturally generates electrical impulses which cause the normal contractions of the blood-pumping mechanism. The implantation operation is safe and simple. The device with all its components weighs less than half a pound, and recent models last for about five years. It is tested regularly by telemetry so that operational defects can be corrected. Experimental pacemakers powered by nuclear energy are expected to last 20 years; however, their use will be limited until there is definitive proof that they do not affect the wearer adversely in some secondary way after several years.

Paget's disease Two unrelated disorders named after the British surgeon who first identified them. In the first, Paget's disease of the bone, also called osteitis deformans, various parts of the skeleton become softer and larger through a loss of calcium and eventually become lumpy and deformed. The bones most commonly affected are those of the pelvis, the legs, and the skull. The disease is rare, occurring mostly in elderly men, although it is not entirely unknown in postmenopausal women. In a number of cases symptoms are so mild as to remain undetected until an X-ray taken for some other purpose reveals the skeletal deterioration. The cause is unknown and there is no specific cure, but X-ray treatments, physical therapy, and one of the newer antibiotics can halt some of the disabling effects. The second disorder, Paget's disease of the nipple, is a type of breast cancer the onset of which is characterized by ulceration and soreness of the nipple and areola.

pain A distress signal from some part of the body, usually of brief duration and originating in the largest number of cases in a traceable disorder. Pain—throbbing, aching, pulsating, stabbing—arises in two different ways. Peripheral pain resulting from a cut finger or an abscessed tooth begins in nerve fibers located in the extremities or around the body organs; central pain, usually caused by injuries or disorders affecting the brain or central nervous system such as a tumor, stroke, or slipped disk, originates in the spinal cord or the brain itself. When this type of pain is chronic, it is the most difficult to assuage. Both types of impulses eventually reach the brain stem and thalamus where pain perception takes place.

It is now known that the brain produces chemical substances that are the body's own opiates against pain perception. These are known as endorphins and include the recently isolated dynorphin which is 200 times more powerful than morphine in its action, and 50 times more powerful than any previously known substance of its kind. It is hoped that with greater understanding of how these chemicals work, they will be used as powerful nonaddictive drugs for the control of pain as well as to produce other important effects on the brain for those suffering from mental illness and seizure disorders.

In the meantime, where pain is chronic and severe, medical science continues to explore other methods that provide relief: acupuncture, electrical stimulation, biofeedback, hypnosis. The chief dangers connected with the use of chemicals for minimizing severe or persistent pain are serious adverse effects of a particular chemical itself or in combination with other drugs and the possibility of drug addiction.

palpitations A condition in which the heartbeat is so strong, irregular, or rapid that it calls attention to its abnormal behavior. This occurrence is almost always associated with anxiety and is rarely associated with any disability of the heart itself. In a few instances rapid heartbeat may be caused by a disease or may be a side effect of a strong dose of certain chemicals, such as caffeine or medication containing amphetamines. Where palpitations occur with intrusive frequency, they should be discussed with a doctor, and if anxiety is indeed the cause, alternatives to tranquilizers should be explored as treatment.

pancreas The large, mixed gland situated below and in back of the stomach and the liver. The pancreas is about 6 inches long. Its function is two-fold. One is the secretion of pancreatic juice which contains the enzymes that flow into the digestive tract and are essential for the continuing breakdown in the duodenum and small intestine of fats, carbohydrates, and proteins. The second function is the secretion of insulin, produced by almost a million clusters of specialized cells called the islands of Langerhans.

When these cells produce insufficient insulin for the body's needs, the result is diabetes. Other disorders of the pancreas include the formation of stones and of benign and malignant tumors, both treated surgically. Inflammation of the pancreas, pancreatitis, may be acute or chronic. Acute pancreatitis is a grave condition in which one of the enzymes begins to devour the tissue itself, leading to hemorrhage, vomiting, severe abdominal pain, and collapse. It may be associated with overdrinking, gallbladder infection, gallstones, or trauma. Chronic pancreatitis may be the result of recurrent acute pancreatitis. It is characterized by abdominal and back pain, diarrhea, and jaundice. When these symptoms exist, exploratory surgery is usually recommended to rule out the possibility of cancer.

pantothenic acid One of the B complex vitamins. *See* "Nutrition and Weight."

pap test A diagnostic procedure used chiefly for detecting the first signs of cancer of the cervix and sometimes the uterus. The test is named for Dr. George Papanicolaou, the American anatomist who discovered that cancerous cells are shed by uterine tumors into the surrounding vaginal fluid and can therefore be detected when a sample is examined microscopically. The procedure is simple and painless: while the speculum dilates the vagina, the doctor inserts a flat stick and scrapes some cells from the cervical canal, the outer cervix, and the pooled secretions in the vagina. These "smears" are transferred to three glass slides and stained. They are then inspected under a microscope for the presence of any abnormal cells. The value of the test is that it can reveal the presence of cervical cancer long before any symptoms appear, thus making effective treatment possible at the earliest moment. However, the test in and of itself is not definitive. In many cases where cellular anomalies are found in the sample, further examination in a biopsy may indicate that the existing condition is cervical erosion, cervical inflammation, or some other benign condition rather than cancer. This test occasionally reveals cancer of the uterus, but cell washings from the uterus obtained by another technique are better.

Medical opinions vary concerning how often a woman should have a pap test. *See also* Suggested Health Examinations, p. 737; "Gynecologic Diseases and Treatment."

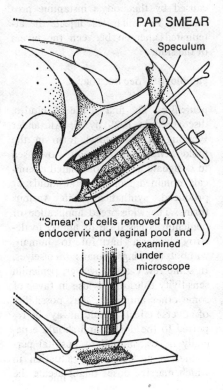

PAP SMEAR

Speculum

"Smear" of cells removed from endocervix and vaginal pool and examined under microscope

paralysis Permanent or temporary impairment of muscle power caused by damage through disease or injury of a part of the nervous system. The extent and nature of paralysis depend on what part of the nervous system has been affected. If the brain and spinal cord are involved, central paralysis occurs, that is, the limb as a whole is immobilized rather than any individual muscle. This involvement may cause hemiplegia (paralysis of one side of the body), paraplegia (paralysis of both legs and the trunk), or quadriplegia (paralysis of all four limbs). The most common cause of central paralysis other than an injury is a cerebrovascular stroke in which the blood supply to a part of the brain is cut off. Other causes are brain tumors, the ingestion of certain poisons, and infectious diseases, especially poliomyelitis, late syphilis, and tuberculosis.

Impairment of any part of the peripheral nervous system (the nerves that connect the central nervous system with various parts of the body) can cause dysfunction of individual muscles, the reception of sensation on the skin surface, vision, and the normal behavior of various organs. Peripheral paralysis may be caused by nerve inflammation or neuritis as occurs in Bell's palsy or sciatica. It may result from such neuromuscular diseases, as myasthenia gravis, or from infectious diseases, chiefly polio. One of the results of birth injury can be paralysis associated with cerebral palsy.

Hysterical paralysis is a condition in which deeply buried emotional conflict takes a physical form, such as the inability to swallow or to walk. Such episodes may be no more than a fleeting psychogenic conversion, as in the inability to move the fingers when taking a written examination, but when conversion hysteria is chronic, some type of psychotherapy is advisable.

Many types of paralysis can be overcome partially or totally by prompt treatment. Physical therapy in its many aspects can rehabilitate disabled muscles, and supportive efforts in other areas can restore confidence and competence to victims of a paralyzing accident or illness.

paranoia A mental disturbance characterized by delusions of persecution and sometimes accompanied by feelings of power and grandeur. A clinically paranoiac person may not suffer from personality disintegration and may appear to be living a normal life, but it is not unusual for the disturbance to erupt into psychotic behavior. The term paranoid may be used to describe a general mental state that is not psychotic, but is characterized by distrustfulness, suspiciousness, and a tendency toward persecution of others.

parkinsonism A mild or severe disorder of body movement characterized by slow mobility, stiffness, and tremor; also known as Parkinson's disease. Most of the estimated million and a half victims of the disorder are over 60. Symptoms similar to those of Parkinson's disease may set in after encephalitis lethargica (once called "sleeping sickness"), may result from a stroke or a brain tumor, or may be a reversible side effect of tranquilizers such as Thorazine or antihypertensives such as Serpasil. True parkinsonism is a disorder of a particular group of brain cells that normally release a substance called dopamine which is essential to the regulation of normal body movement. In most cases the debilitating aspects of the disease

are now controlled by dopamine medications in combination with other drugs. Surgery, physical therapy, and supportive psychotherapy are additional forms of treatment that can reduce the damaging effects on the body as well as on the personality of victims. Since patients over 60 are likely to be on medication for some other condition, the supervising doctor should be expected to make a regular check of all prescriptions being filled so that a dangerous combination of drugs can be avoided.

patch test A diagnostic procedure for determining hypersensitivity to a particular allergen by applying it to the surface of the skin in a diluted solution or suspension. A positive allergic response is indicated by the appearance of a raised welt or hive caused by the body's histamine production. A similar test injects the attenuated allergen between the layers of the skin.

pathologist *See* DOCTOR.

penicillin The first of the antibiotics, discovered in 1929 by Sir Alexander Fleming in its natural form in the mold *Penicillium notatum;* now used to designate a group of related chemicals obtained from several molds or produced synthetically in various forms. The widespread application of penicillin is based on its ability to destroy bacteria harmful to humans without harming humans themselves. In some few cases, however, penicillin sensitivity rules out its use in favor of some other antibiotic. Any possibility of adverse effects should always be reported to the doctor and should especially be transmitted to hospital personnel in an emergency situation in which massive doses might create the greater emergency of anaphylactic shock.

pediatrician *See* DOCTOR.

penis The external male organ through which semen is ejaculated and urine is passed.

pep pills *See* amphetamines, in "Drugs, Alcohol, and Tobacco."

peptic ulcer *See* ULCER.

perineum The triangular layer of skin between the vulva and the anus in the female and between the scrotum and the anus in the male. Beneath the perineum in the female are the muscles and fibrous tissues that must stretch sufficiently to accommodate the passage of the baby during childbirth. To prevent the danger of tearing, a simple surgical incision called a perineal episiotomy is often performed.

peritonitis Inflammation of the peritoneum, the membrane that lines the abdominal cavity and covers the organs within it. Peritonitis may be chronic or acute. Chronic peritonitis is a comparatively rare condition associated with tuberculosis. The cause of acute peritonitis is usually the perforation or rupture of the appendix with a consequent spread of bacteria and interference of circulation. Symptoms are immobilizing abdominal pain, shallow breathing, and clammy skin. The condition is an emergency requiring prompt hospitalization and a more precise diagnosis on the basis of X-rays, blood tests, and physical exploration. Surgery is almost always inevitable: the peritoneal cavity is opened and drained of infectious material, and the cause of the problem,

for example, a diseased appendix, is removed. Postoperative care involves intravenous feeding, antibiotics, and in some cases blood transfusions. When the stomach and intestines become dilated by the accumulation of gas, relief may be provided by a procedure called nasogastric suction.

perspiration The process by which the salty fluid (99 percent water and 1 percent urea and other wastes) is excreted by the sweat glands of the skin; also the fluid itself. The body has approximately 2 million sweat glands located in the lowest layers of the skin. They are connected with the outer skin layer, the epidermis, by tiny spiral-shaped tubes. The largest sweat glands are located in the groin and the armpit. The sweat glands normally produce about 1½ pints of sweat a day in a temperate climate. The chief function of perspiration is to maintain constant body temperature despite variation in environmental conditions or energy output. Thus, when the internal or external temperature goes up, sweat can be seen on the skin surface where it cools the body by evaporation. At the same time the blood in the superficial capillaries is cooled before it recirculates within the body. The sweating process is controlled by the hypothalamus at the base of the brain. Since this gland is also responsive to emotional stress, fear and excitement will cause an increase in perspiration. "Breaking out in a cold sweat" is a common phenomenon.

Any disturbance in the functioning of the sweat glands is likely to be a symptom of some other disorder. Excessive perspiration may be due to a disease that also produces a high fever such as malaria or one that produces a chronic rise in temperature such as tuberculosis. Excessive sweating and urinating are possible symptoms of untreated diabetes. The hot flashes of the menopause are often accompanied by heavy sweating. Excessive sweating of the palms or soles of the feet is usually psychogenic in origin. While perspiration contains certain antibacterial chemicals that protect the skin surface, it can also be an irritant to tender skin. Prickly heat rash occurs when the sweat glands become blocked and the ducts leading to the skin surface rupture. The condition is usually a consequence of unaccustomed and profuse perspiration that keeps the skin damp. While prickly heat is more common among babies than among adults, clothing that chafes can cause it in adults as well. Fresh perspiration does not have an unpleasant odor.

pessary A device, often in the shape of a ring, worn inside the vagina to support a prolapsed uterus; also a vaginal suppository and sometimes another term for a contraceptive diaphragm.

PET Positron emission tomography. *See* SCANNING MACHINES.

pH A measure of the degree of alkalinity or acidity of a given solution; the letters derive from *pouvoir Hydrogène* ("hydrogen power" in French), since the concentration of the hydrogen ion determines the pH number. Acidity is indicated by pH values from 0 to 7; pH 7.0 is neutral, and pH values above 7 indicate alkalinity.

pharyngitis Inflammation, either acute or chronic, of the pharynx, the tube of muscles and membranes that forms the throat cavity extending from the back of the mouth to the esophagus. Infection is most commonly viral, occurring as a minor sore throat. In more serious cases the cause is bacterial, as in streptococcus or strep throat, and results in high fever, severe discomfort when swallowing, and a stiff neck. It is extremely important that a sore throat or tonsillitis accompanied by fever over 100°F be checked by a doctor to prevent serious complications. Chronic pharyngitis and hoarseness is usually the result of the misuse of the voice, regular exposure to irritating vapors or fumes, or heavy intake of alcohol. Even mild pharyngitis is aggravated by smoking.

phenobarbital A mild, slow-acting barbiturate prescribed as an anticonvulsant for some cases of epilepsy and as a sedative to relieve anxiety and induce sleep. Like all barbiturates, it is habit-forming and dangerous when abused. Evidence has accumulated to indicate that it is one of the tranquilizing medicines that may cause birth defects when taken during the early months of pregnancy.

phlebitis Inflammation of the vein walls, most commonly of the legs, and especially where varicosities exist. Phlebitis in a superficially located vein is usually accompanied by tenderness, redness, and swelling. The inflammation is potentially more serious when it develops in a deep vein. Clotting may occur on the damaged wall, a condition known as thrombophlebitis, and it may impede circulation or may break away from the wall and circulate as an embolism. Simple phlebitis may be caused by overweight or by progressive arterio- or atherosclerosis; it may follow an illness such as pneumonia or a long convalescence in bed.

A phlebitis that affects the large vein of the thigh may occur about a week after childbirth. The condition is familiarly called "milk leg" and like most inflammations of this type can be counted on to heal if the leg is raised for part of the day and support hosiery is worn. When phlebitis is so severe as to be disabling, or if there is a strong possibility of clot formation, surgery may be recommended.

phobia An irrational and exaggerated fear of an object or condition, usually related to an anxiety neurosis. Everyone experiences fear as a response to what each perceives as present or impending danger, but phobic response may be so encompassing as to be immobilizing. In severe anxiety attacks the victim may experience dizziness, palpitations, profuse sweating, and in some cases a tendency toward suicide. Although almost any object or situation may elicit phobia in different individuals, several have been identified as common sources of phobic response, for example, agoraphobia, the fear of being in open places; acrophobia, the fear of heights; ailurophobia, the fear of cats; and claustrophobia, the fear of being confined in small areas.

Neurotic fear is a form of mental illness that is difficult to cure. In some cases the phobia may decrease as a result of life experiences that resolve the underlying conflict; in other cases psychotherapy can be helpful in diminishing a particular phobia.

physical examination A part of a medical evaluation, the results of which provide information as to the general and specific condition of a person's health. In order to perform a comprehensive medical evaluation, the doctor must obtain the medical history, perform routine diagnostic tests, and do a careful physical examination of the various parts of the body, including an internal pelvic examination. It is extremely important to have periodic examinations so that any changes from previous evaluations can be recognized and treated if necessary. *See* Suggested Health Examinations, p. 737.

physical therapy Treatment of disease or injury by physical rather than by medicinal or surgical means. The chief goals of physical therapy are the achievement of normal mobility through the relief of pain and the rehabilitation of impaired muscle function. Where irreversible disablement is present, treatment also consists in training the patient to accomplish essential tasks in alternative ways to achieve the greatest possible degree of autonomy in the participation of normal life. Techniques and means depend on the patient's needs. Exercises designed to strengthen specific muscles or to coordinate the movements of a group of muscles may be active or passive. In passive exercise the therapist moves the affected parts until the patient is able to do so alone. In hydrotherapy the patient exercises in water which, because of its buoyancy, requires a smaller expenditure of energy. When patients are entirely immobilized as may occur in a stroke, physical therapy is begun in bed with massaging and applying heat. Physiotherapists, who are trained in schools approved by the American Medical Association, usually work under the supervision of doctors in hospitals and clinics that have rehabilitation programs for both inpatients and outpatients.

physician *See* DOCTOR.

pilonidal cyst A fluid-filled sac that develops under the skin at the base of the spine. *See* CYST.

pituitary gland The pituitary gland, no larger than a pea, is situated at the base of the brain directly above the back of the nose. It is controlled in part by the hypothalamus and in part by the hormones from the various endocrine glands (biofeedback), and it in turn controls the hormone production of all the other endocrine glands. *See* "The Healthy Woman."

placebo A preparation or procedure without pharmacologic or physiologic properties, which is administered for psychological benefit; literally, Latin for "I shall please." While usually no more than water with sugar flavoring, placebos are known to cause a measurable difference in how patients feel. They are also used as a control in testing the efficacy of a new therapeutic drug.

placenta The organ that attaches to the wall of the uterus during pregnancy and through which the developing fetus is nourished by the mother because it serves as an exchange between the mother's and the fetus's vascular systems; also known as afterbirth. *See* "Pregnancy and Childbirth."

plantar wart A wart that develops in the sole of the foot. Such growths often are especially painful because they grow inward and thus interfere with walking. All such warts are technically called verrucae and are assumed to be caused by virus infection. Treatment is often surgical. Postoperative care involves several days of immobility to permit the tissue to heal before pressure is put on it by walking.

plaque A flat patch; most commonly, dental plaque, which refers to an accumulation of food and other organic material on the surface of a tooth. This accumulation inevitably provides a medium for the bacterial growth that leads to the destruction of tooth enamel and cavity formation. Dental plaque should be routinely removed by brushing the teeth, using unwaxed floss according to the dentist's instructions, and having a professional cleaning twice a year.

plastic surgery Operations in which damaged or abnormal tissue is repaired and rebuilt. Such damages or abnormalities may be congenital, as a hare lip, or they may be acquired, as disfiguring scars caused by burns or other injuries. Growths that are extensive enough to require skin grafting once they have been removed are also the province of the plastic surgeon. Another aspect of this specialty is the reconstruction of missing tissue with a prosthesis, a substitute manufactured of metals and plastics rather than of organic materials taken from another part of the body. Artificial limbs, jaws, breasts, and ears are some of the more customary prosthetic replacements. Change in appearance for esthetic reasons where no striking malformation exists, such as a face lift or nose reshaping, is called cosmetic surgery. The benefits of such elective surgery should be carefully weighed against the inconvenience and risks of surgery. *See* "Cosmetic Surgery."

platelets Round or oval disks in the blood that contain no hemoglobin and are essential to the clotting process; also called thrombocytes. Platelet deficiencies occur in a number of diseases (leukemia, myeloma, lymphoma), as a result of certain drugs, and spontaneously (idiopathic thrombocytopenic purpura). This latter mainly affects women and children. Platelets can be transferred fresh or frozen.

pleurisy Inflammation of the pleura, the double membrane that lines the chest cavity and encloses the lungs. The membrane consists of two layers of pleurae separated only by a lubricating fluid. Under normal conditions this double membranous structure permits the lungs to expand freely within the chest. However, under certain adverse circumstances two different disorders can occur: wet pleurisy, in which because of an inflammation of the pleura, abnormal fluid accumulates between the pleural layers; and dry pleurisy, in which the pleura is inflamed, but there is no abnormal fluid. Pleurisy may or may not be acutely painful, but it always requires prompt treatment. Any chest pains, especially a stabbing sensation accompanying the intake of breath or a persistent cough accompanied by weakness and loss of appetite should be investigated by a doctor. Dry pleurisy (pleurodynia) is caused by several viruses and is usually self-limiting. Wet pleurisy is caused by direct infection, cancer, congestive heart failure, or the spread of infection from another respiratory disturbance, such as pneumonia, bronchitis, lung abscess, or tuberculosis. Pus accumulation is called empyema (not emphysema) and usually needs surgical drainage. *See* EMPYEMA.

pneumonia An acute infection or inflammation of one or both lungs, causing the lung tissues and spaces to be filled with liquid matter. Pneumonia, which may be a primary infection or a complication of another disorder, has three main causes: bacteria, viruses, and mycoplasmas. Inflammation may also be caused by fungus infections or by the aspiration of certain chemicals, of irritant dusts, or of food or liquids while unconscious due to anesthesia, intoxication, or other causes. The latter type is called aspiration pneumonia. Among the bacteria, the pneumococci are by far the most common cause; there are over 80 different types responsible for approximately 500,000 cases of the disease each year. Streptococcal pneumonia is less common; staphylococcal pneumonia usually is contracted in a hospital and has a high mortality rate; victims of pneumonia caused by the klebsiella bacteria also have poor chances of recovery. The pneumonias that are viral in origin account for about half of all cases. While in some cases recovery may be spontaneous without treatment or special precautions (many people have had "walking pneumonia" without realizing it), the disease known as primary influenza virus pneumonia is extremely serious, especially because the infectious organism multiplies with practically no accompanying sign of disease in the lung. Mycoplasmas, which were identified during World War II, are microorganisms smaller than bacteria, larger than viruses, and sharing characteristics of both. Mycoplasma pneumonia typically involves older children and young adults and is usually mild in its symptoms and brief in duration. Pneumonia that involves a major part or an entire lobe of a lung is known as lobar pneumonia, and when both lungs are involved, double pneumonia. Bronchopneumonia, which affects a smaller area, is slower to develop and is localized in the bronchial tubes, with patches of infection reaching the lungs. While rarely fatal, bronchopneumonia is insidious because it may recur and resist conventional treatment.

In all cases of bacterial pneumonia, but especially in cases where resistance is low because of age, debility, or alcoholism, treatment with antibiotics must be initiated at once. In general, at the first sign of any of the following manifestations, a doctor's evaluation is mandatory: shaking chills, high fever, chest pains, dry cough, breathlessness, bluish cast to the lips and nail beds, expectoration of rust-colored or greenish sputum when coughing. Some cases may require hospitalization, while others may be supervised at home. According to the American Lung Association, prompt treatment with antibiotics almost always cures bacterial and mycoplasma pneumonia. While there is as yet no effective treatment for viral pneumonia, adequate rest, proper diet, and sufficient time devoted to convalescence usually result in full recovery. Since 1977 an immunizing vaccine has been available that offers protection against some types of pneumococci. It is administered on an individual basis to those considered especially vulnerable to infection—people over 50, anyone in a nursing home, and anyone of any age suffering from chronic diseases of the heart, lungs, and kidneys and from diabetes and other metabolic disorders. One injection of the vaccine is supposed to provide immunity for three years. The use of the vaccine is especially important since many strains of pneumococci have developed a resistance to previously effective antibiotics.

podiatrist A practitioner who specializes in the care and treatment of the feet; formerly called a chiropodist. While not a physician, a podiatrist is entitled to be called "Doctor" as the recipient of the degree of Doctor of Podiatric Medicine (D.P.M.), conferred by independent, state-accredited podiatric colleges. Holders of the degree are licensed by the state to prescribe medications and to perform minor surgery. A medical doctor might refer a patient to a podiatrist for the treatment of flat feet, ingrown toenails, bunions, or disorders resulting from daily running in the wrong shoes. When foot disorders are the result of such systemic problems as circulatory failure, the podiatrist usually refers the patient to a physician.

poison Any substance which can severely damage or destroy living tissue. Certain substances are harmful in any amount, while others, which are harmless or even beneficial in supervised doses, are poisonous in excessive amounts. Poisons can be absorbed through the skin, injected into the bloodstream, or inhaled, but the largest number of poisonings result from swallowing dangerous substances in small amounts or taking medications in overdoses. The most frequent victims are children under 5, and of these, more than half the fatalities occur following an overdose of a medicine (usually aspirin), often disguised as "candy." Among adults the greatest numbers of poisonings are also caused by an overdose of medicine, either swallowed accidentally or in a suicide attempt.

Poisons are usually classified by their destructive effects within the body. Blood toxins, such as carbon monoxide and rattlesnake venom, deprive the blood of the oxygen essential for nourishing the brain and other tissues or cause other blood problems like hemolysis. Nerve toxins, especially alcohol, barbiturates, and various opiates, destroy the nerves and interfere with normal cell processes. Corrosives, such as lye, ammonia, phenol, destroy the tissues directly. Irritants, such as arsenic, lead salts, copper sulfate, and zinc, cause inflammation of the mucous membranes. The most effective action to take in the event of poisoning is to call the nearest poison control center at once for emergency instructions. Since prompt action can make the difference between life and death, every member of the family, including children from the earliest possible age, should know that the number of this agency is posted next to the telephone with other emergency numbers. Local telephone directories usually list the number under poison control. When no such listing appears, efforts should be made *before* a crisis occurs to locate the closest agency by consulting the telephone operator, the nearest hospital, or the Red Cross chapter or by writing to the Division of Poison Control, U.S. Department of Health and Human Services, 5600 Fishers Lane, Rockville, Md. 20852.

poison control center A service organization on the community level that can be consulted 24 hours a day for information about the toxicity of a particular substance and the most effective countermeasures to take against it. The FDA provides these centers with up-to-date information on all potentially dangerous products. The centers are listed in telephone directories under Poison Control. The number of the nearest one should be immediately accessible at the home phone for quick use in a crisis.

poison ivy, oak, and sumac Plants containing a poisonous chemical, urushiol, to which a majority of people in the United States eventually become sensitive. It is extremely unwise to assume that insensitivity to these plants is permanent. The chemical, which is contained in all parts of the plants—leaves, berries, roots, and bark—produces contact dermatitis in those allergic to it. In cases of hypersensitivity the itching and blistering rash may develop not only when the skin has touched the plant directly, but also when a part of the body touches a piece of contaminated clothing or a dog or cat whose coat is contaminated by the allergen. Since the chemical can be spread by smoke from burning the plant, it should never be burned, but destroyed by a suitable herbicide. When exposure does occur, contaminated clothing should be removed at once and the potentially affected parts of the body washed with a strong, alkaline laundry soap. These preventive measures should be undertaken as soon as possible to limit the spread of the poison. When the rash appears, the discomfort can be reduced by the application of preparations recommended by a pharmacist or a doctor. In severe cases cortisone may be recommended as well as antihistamines to reduce the itching. The best way to prevent contact is to make a serious effort to learn what the plants look like so that they can be scrupulously avoided.

poliomyelitis An acute infectious disease caused by a virus that attacks the central nervous system and causes partial and temporary muscular paralysis when the nerve cells are injured and complete permanent paralysis when the nerve cells are totally destroyed; also known as polio and infantile paralysis. While any part of the body (except the brain) may be damaged, the muscles most often affected are those of the legs. Milder cases may produce symptoms so slight they go undetected. A severe attack causes stiffness in the neck accompanied by pain and tenderness in the leg muscles which begin to deteriorate in a few weeks. In its gravest form, bulbar polio, the disease attacks the spinal cord and cranial nerves. The disease invades the body through the mouth; the viruses enter the bloodstream and, after they produce symptoms of varying degrees of severity, are eventually excreted. Infection is spread by contaminated sewage or human excrement that in turn contaminates the drinking water supply, the community swimming pool, or food or by indirect transfer from the soiled fingers of a previous patient to the food of a potential victim. While polio has always been more widespread among children than among adults because adults have had time to develop natural immunity through asymptomatic infection, it can attack anyone at any age. In asymptomatic cases no serious signs of the disease are observable, but in fact antibodies have been formed. Symptomatic cases may or may not produce paralysis.

The disease has practically been eliminated in the United States as a result of immunization of most children when the vaccines were first introduced in 1954. It is important that children born since then be immunized. Since polio epidemics are not uncommon in areas with primitive sanitation, anyone planning a trip to such a place should be immunized or re-immunized. *See* Immunization Guide, p. 738.

polyp A smooth, tubelike growth, almost always benign, that projects from mucous membrane. Such growths are of two main types: pedunculate polyps, that are attached to the membrane by a thin stalk, and sessile polyps, that have a broad base.

While polyps may occur in any body cavity with a membranous lining, they are most commonly found in the nose, uterus, and cervix. Those that develop in the nasal canal or sinuses may result from such irritations as frequent colds or allergies. While rarely dangerous, they can interfere with breathing and with the sense of smell; they may also be the cause of chronic headaches. Surgical removal is recommended in such cases, but there is no guarantee that the underlying irritation will not produce them again. Uterine polyps may cause irregular or excessive menstrual flow and may also be one of the causes of sterility. They can usually be removed without the need for hospitalization. The presence of cervical polyps may be manifested by bleeding between menstrual periods, after menopause, or with intercourse or they may be "silent," only discovered during a routine gynecological checkup. Removal is considered advisable, with a biopsy to rule out the possibility of cancer. When polyps form anywhere along the alimentary canal, they are usually benign, but since there is always an outside possibility of their becoming malignant, they should be removed surgically as soon as their presence is discovered, either through an X-ray for some other reason or because of the symptoms they produce. A stomach polyp, for example, may be painless, but if the stalk is long enough so that if it is drawn into the duodenum, it will make its presence known. Intestinal polyps may cause no symptoms unless they become ulcerated and eventually bleed. Such growths, as well as polyps in the colon or the rectum, are likely to cause discomfort in the lower abdomen, diarrhea, as well as blood and mucus in the stools.

posture The natural position or carriage of the body when sitting or standing. Good posture is the unconscious result of mental and physical health. While a rigidly held neck or a sunken chest may be second nature by the time adulthood arrives, poor posture can be improved by suitable exercise. Women who sit at a desk or typewriter for a large part of the day should have a posture chair that discourages slouching and supports the spine. For women who are on their feet a great deal, poor posture and attendant backaches may result from wearing ill-fitting shoes or shoes with heels that are too high or too low for comfort and healthy carriage. A critical review of footwear, office furniture, and posture when doing household chores may go a long way to eliminating back pain. Good posture during pregnancy is especially important, since the growth of the fetus and the enlarged abdomen place an extra strain on the spine. Standing against a wall several times a day with head up, shoulders back, belly sucked in, and buttocks tucked under can develop posture that will eliminate back discomfort before and after delivery.

potassium A chemical element which, in combination with other minerals, is essential for the body's acid-base balance and muscle function. Most foods contain a supply of potassium adequate for the body's needs. However, vomiting or diarrhea may create a temporary deficiency. Interference with potassium metabolism may also result from corticosteroid medication, diuretic medication, or a disorder of the adrenal glands known as Cushing's syndrome. Since all cells, but especially those that form muscle tissue, require a high blood-potassium level, a critical deficiency results in weakness (even paralysis), lethargy, rapid pulse, and a tingling sensation. Following a diagnosis based on blood tests, the condition is corrected by oral medication containing potassium salts.

pre-eclampsia A condition of pregnancy characterized by abnormal retention of water, elevated blood pressure, and large amounts of protein in the urine, signaling the possible onset of convulsions (eclampsia). *See* "Pregnancy and Childbirth."

pregnancy test *See* "Pregnancy and Childbirth."

premature ejaculation *See* EJACULATION.

proctologist *See* DOCTOR.

progesterone The hormone secreted by the corpus luteum each month at the time of ovulation to prepare the lining of the uterus for embedding and nourishing of the fertilized egg. It is produced by the placenta during pregnancy and is important for the maintenance of pregnancy. Diminishing progesterone secretions is one of the changes that occurs during menopause. In its synthetic form this hormone is the sole ingredient of a type of contraceptive pill, and it is also released in tiny amounts into the uterus by one of the newer, medicated IUDs. The long-term effect of the progesterone IUD, which must be replaced each year, is not yet known.

Progesterone may also be prescribed in replacement therapy when a deficiency is responsible for certain menstrual disorders connected with infertility.

progestin Umbrella term for various types of progesterone.

prolactin A hormone secreted by the pituitary gland which initiates and maintains lactation after pregnancy.

prolapse The downward or forward displacement of a part of the body; most commonly, the dropping of the uterus. A prolapsed womb is a consequence of impaired muscle support, which most often results from the stress of childbirth, but is not unknown among women who have never had children. Dropping of the uterus may occur after menopause when muscle tone diminishes or when the cumulative effect of a lifetime of hard physical work takes its toll. The symptoms of uterine prolapse are frequent and painful urination, low backache, vaginal discharge, and a feeling of pressure on the vagina. Lying down

provides relief from this last discomfort. When the prolapse is severe enough to cause the cervix to protrude through the vagina, special support in the form of a pessary may be a satisfactory alternative to surgery.

prostaglandin A hormonelike substance composed of unsaturated fatty acids and found in almost every tissue and body fluid. Prostaglandins are being identified in increasing numbers as indispensable for normalizing blood pressure, kidney processes, the reproductive system, gastrointestinal activity, and the release of sex hormones. Of those specifically isolated, the prostaglandins manufactured by the endometrium increase considerably just before the onset of the menstrual period. Since they cause strong uterine contractions, they are responsible perhaps for the premenstrual cramps suffered by some women. This stimulating action on the uterus can induce menstrual flow and may be the cause of some spontaneous abortions. Prostaglandin is now available in solution and as a suppository for inducing abortion. Continu-

PROLAPSE OF UTERUS

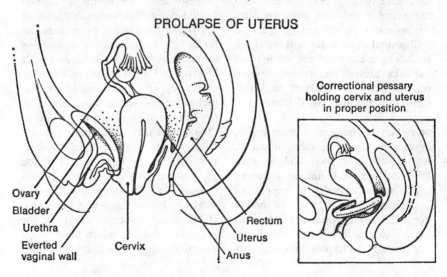

Correctional pessary
holding cervix and uterus
in proper position

Ovary
Bladder
Urethra
Everted   Cervix
vaginal wall

Rectum
Uterus
Anus

ing studies of this group of prostaglandins may result in a pill that will bring about abortion.

prostate gland In the male genitourinary system, the gland surrounding the neck of the bladder and the beginning of the urethra. As a sexual organ, its function is the manufacture of prostatic fluid, a component of seminal fluid in which the sperm cells are mixed to create semen.

protein One of several complex substances composed of combinations of amino acids; the basic substance of which living cells are composed; essential nutrient in the diet of all animal life. *See* "Nutrition and Weight."

The symptoms of protein deficiency are physical weakness, poor resistance to disease, and fluid accumulation in the legs and abdomen. Liver disease and certain other disorders may interfere with normal protein metabolism. Over-the-counter medications for "tired blood" will not correct protein deficiencies.

The classification of *serum proteins* includes globulin and albumin. Globulin, which is divided into alpha, beta, and gamma globulin, is an essential component of the blood. Since gamma globulin is the richest in antibodies, it is often used to provide passive immunity to such infectious diseases as hepatitis. Albumins are serum proteins found in all living matter. Among the most important ones are egg albumin found in eggwhite; fibrinogen and hemoglobin in blood; myosin in meat; caseinogen in milk; casein in cheese, and gluten in flour. *See also* LIPOPROTEIN.

pruritis *See* ITCHING.

psoriasis A common skin disease of unknown cause, characterized by excessive production of cells of the outermost skin layer which produces scaly red patches. As the new cells proliferate, they cover the patches with a silvery scale, and as the scales drop off, the area below is revealed as tiny red dots. Psoriasis is neither contagious nor dangerous. Symptoms may appear for the first time in early childhood, in adolescence, or not until later in life. The condition may be chronic or intermittent; it may be triggered by injury, illness, emotional stress, or exposure to excessive cold. The red patches may or may not be accompanied by itching. The parts of the body most often affected are the scalp, chest, elbows, knees, abdomen, palms, and soles of the feet. About 10 percent of patients have an associated arthritis.

In spite of advertising claims to the contrary, there is no cure for psoriasis. Professionally prescribed treatments which have been somewhat effective have had unfortunate side effects in many instances or have required weeks of hospitalization. The most recent treatment to show promising results is known as photochemotherapy. It combines oral medication with a photoactive drug followed by exposure to ultraviolet radiation.

psychiatry The medical specialty that deals with the diagnosis and treatment of disorders of the mind and the emotions. *See* DOCTOR. *See also* "Your Mind and Feelings."

psychoanalysis A method originated by Dr. Sigmund Freud for treating mental illness and emotional disturbances. The method is based on certain assumptions about the development from infancy onward of the human psyche or the mind as an entity with a life of its own that governs the total organism in all its relationships with others and with the environment. Psychoanalysts may be psychiatrists as Freud himself was, or they may be lay practitioners.

psychoneurosis *See* NEUROSIS.

psychosis Any mental illness characterized by disorganization of personality and a disordered contact with reality, combined with bizarre behavior consisting of unpredictable mood swings and garbled speech, and accompanied by hallucinations, delusions, and disconnected thoughts. *See* "Your Mind and Feelings."

psychosomatic illness Any disorder that is functional in nature and that may be ascribed wholly or partly to emotional stress. *See* "Your Mind and Feelings."

psychotherapy The treatment of mental disorder. *See* "Your Mind and Feelings."

puberty The period of development during which sex organs begin to function, that is, become capable of reproduction, and secondary sex characteristics develop. In females it is marked by the onset of menstruation (menarche), commonly any time from age 11 to 14.

puerperal Relating to childbirth. Puerperal fever is an obsolete term for a formerly widespread and often fatal infection of the vagina and uterus just after delivery. Such infections are rare nowadays thanks to aseptic medical procedures. When there is any sign of such infection, it is usually controllable by antibiotics.

pulse The beat of the heart as felt through the expansion and contraction of an artery, especially through the radial artery at the wrist below the fleshy mound of the thumb. The best way to take the pulse is to place the three middle fingers on this artery with sufficient pressure to detect the beat, but not so heavily as to suppress it. Pulse rate is the term for the number of beats felt in 60 seconds. The normal adult rate ranges from 60 to 100 beats a minute. An abnormally slow pulse (brachycardia) may be caused by an overdose of digitalis, abnormal pressure within the skull, the onset of thyroid deficiency, or a crisis involving heart malfunction. An abnormally fast pulse (tachycardia) may result from high altitude sickness, congestive heart failure, hyperthyroidism, fever, excitement, or too much caffeine, alcohol, smoking, amphetamines, thyroid extract, or antispasmodics. The rhythm of the pulse in a normally healthy person is regular. Where perceptible irregularity exists, it may be associated with thyroid disease or it may be caused by auricular fibrillation, a symptom of chronic heart failure. If the pulse is not perceptible at the wrist, it may be felt through the carotid artery at the side of the neck.

pus The thick yellowish or greenish liquid that develops during certain infections. Pus is composed of white blood cells, tissue decomposed by bacteria or other microorganism, and the destroyed organism that caused the infection. It is often contained in an inflamed swelling called an abscess.

pyorrhea The discharge of pus; especially pyorrhea alveolaris, a condition in which the chronic discharge of pus from diseased gums causes deterioration of the bone and the eventual loss of teeth. *See* GINGIVITIS.

Q fever An acute infectious disease with symptoms similar to those of influenza and caused by microorganisms known as rickettsiae. The disease normally infects cattle and sheep and is passed from animal to animal and from animals to humans by tick bites, contaminated milk, and contaminated dust which may be inhaled or ingested in food. Mild cases last for less than a week, with fever, chills, headache, muscle pains, and some respiratory symptoms. Recovery is usually complete following bed rest, aspirin, and light diet. Antibiotics may be given when the fever stays dangerously high and there is the possibility of heart and lung involvement.

quarantine The isolation of people who might be incubating a communicable disease. The word itself derives from the Latin "forty," which was the number of days that a ship with contaminated passengers, crew, or livestock was kept in port before debarkation was permitted. Nowadays the quarantine period is as long as the incubation period of the particular disease in question. This public health measure, less frequent in modern times, is usually enforced to protect the general public from infection by members of a group returning by plane, ship, or other conveyance from places where they or the conveyances were in contact with yellow fever, cholera, and the like.

quickening The stage of pregnancy in which the mother becomes aware of fetal movements within the womb; also, the fetal movements themselves. Quickening usually occurs some time around the eighteenth week of pregnancy, at which time the fetal heartbeat is first detectable.

rabies An almost always fatal disease of the central nervous system caused by the rabies virus. It occurs in warm-blooded mammals such as humans, foxes, dogs, bats, and skunks. It is transmitted by the bite of an infected animal because the virus is present in saliva. The virus is occasionally transmitted to humans by intimate contact with an infected human or animal and by inhalation of air in caves housing infected bats.

The wound from any animal bite should be allowed to bleed and be scrubbed and flushed with soap and water; then, if possible, it should be washed with zephiran chloride or some other substance (alcohol) of proven lethal effect on the virus. Suturing the wound is not advised. Whether the victim of the bite has been exposed to rabies depends, of course, on whether the biting animal is infected. This is more likely if the bite was not provoked and if the animal was wild. Further, the more severe the wound, especially if the bite was on bare skin, the more likely the victim is to get rabies if the animal was infected. The animal should be observed, caged if necessary, for approximately 10 days to see if it is sick, gets sick, or dies. If it has to be killed to be captured, care should be taken not to shoot it in the head because an examination of the brain is essential to determine if it is rabid. If the victim has been exposed or probably exposed to rabies, it is essential that rabies vaccine and probably antirabies serum be administered. Judgment must be used in deciding about the use of vaccine and serum since there are hazards associated with both.

The incubation period of rabies in

humans varies from 10 days to 12 months, the average is about 42 days, and is characterized initially by fever, headache, and general malaise and then by a variety of central nervous system signs such as spasms of the muscles of the mouth, pharynx, and larynx on drinking. This symptom explains another name for rabies, hydrophobia (the fear of water). Death usually is caused by paralysis of the respiratory muscles. There is no specific treatment for the disease.

radiologist *See* DOCTOR.

radiotherapy The treatment of disease with X-rays and with rays from such radioactive substances as cobalt, iodine, and radium; also called radiation therapy or irradiation. The effectiveness of radiotherapy, which is the special province of the radiologist, is constantly being increased by the invention of new machines and techniques that minimize the dangers of radiation exposure to healthy tissues at the same time that enough irradiation can be provided to benefit tissue already diseased. Radiotherapy is used in the treatment of inoperable cancers and localized skin malignancies and in combination with chemotherapy or alone as a postoperative means of halting the progress of metastasis or of cancer recurrence.

radium A highly radioactive metal that spontaneously gives off rays affecting the growth of organic tissue. Radium was isolated from pitchblende ore by Marie Curie in 1898, and since that time has been used to halt the progress of certain types of cancer, especially those that are inoperable. In the form of needles or tiny glass tubes, radium is embedded within the diseased tissues where the emanation of gamma rays may have a therapeutic effect. Body exposure, inhalation, or ingestion of radium may produce burns as well as several kinds of cancer, especially of the lungs, blood, and bones.

rale Any abnormal sound that accompanies the normal sound of breathing when perceived through a stethoscope or by the ear placed against the chest; pronounced *rahl*. Rales are said to be either moist or dry depending on the lung disorder or disease that produces them.

rape *See* "Rape and Spouse Abuse."

rapid eye movement (REM) A phenomenon that accompanies a particular phase of sleep during which there is also an intensification of body processes. During this phase, known as REM sleep, sleep is deep, blood pressure rises, heartbeat quickens, and there is an increase in the rate of electrical impulses produced by the brain. When perceptible rapid eye movements during sleep were reported by researchers in 1953, they were assumed to be an accompaniment of dreaming. It is now known that one process does not inevitably involve the other.

rash A skin eruption often accompanied by discoloration and itching and in most cases a temporary symptom of a particular infectious disease, allergy, or parasitic infestation. Rashes may be flat or raised, some run together into large blotches, and others turn into blisters. Many of the diseases of which rashes are a symptom, such as measles and rubella, are on the wane because of widespread immunization. Prickly heat, contact dermatitis, hives, and allergic responses to poison ivy, oak, and sumac are common causes of rashes. Rashlike symptoms usually accompany infections caused by funguses, parasites, and rickettsial organisms such as ticks. Virus diseases (mononucleosis) and sexually transmissible diseases, especially secondary stage syphilis, are characterized by rashes. Any skin eruption accompanied by fever or other acute symptoms such as a sore throat or tender swollen glands should be examined by a doctor.

Raynaud's disease A condition in which spasms in the blood vessels of the fingers and toes, triggered by exposure to cold, cause the extremities to become white, numb, and in extreme cases, acutely painful and ulcerated. Women are five times more vulnerable than men to this disorder for which no specific cause has yet been found. Factors contributing to attacks include emotional stress, smoking, and atherosclerosis. Onset of symptoms can often be prevented by wearing protective socks and gloves of suitable weight both outdoors and during sleep. Some cases have been successfully treated through special exercises and training in biofeedback techniques through which patients learn to control their own finger temperature.

rectocele The protrusion of the rectum into the vagina. This type of hernia causes difficulty in emptying the bowel and leads to constipation. It can be corrected by surgery.

rectum The lowest portion of the large intestine before the anal opening to the exterior of the body. It consists of the rectal canal, 5 to 6 inches long in crescent-shaped folds, and the anal canal, 1 to 1½ inches long. When the rectum is filled with feces as the solid

wastes of digestion are pushed downward by intestinal action, nerve impulses send messages to the brain signaling the need to defecate. The rectum may be affected by various disorders, most commonly hemorrhoids, polyps, prolapse, pruritis, and cancer. Proctitis (inflammation of the rectum) can be one of the consequences of gonorrhea. A rectal examination, called a proctoscopy, is usually considered advisable for diagnosis of such symptoms as constipation alternating with diarrhea, rectal bleeding, and a constant feeling of pressure in the lower bowel.

REM *See* RAPID EYE MOVEMENT.

remission The decrease or disappearance of signs and symptoms during the course of a disease or a chronic disorder. The term spontaneous remission is used when there appears to be no therapeutic explanation for the abatement of the symptoms.

repression In Freudian terms the refusal of the conscious mind to acknowledge unacceptable impulses, thoughts, and feelings and their relegation to the unconscious where they find expression in dreams, anxiety, and various mechanisms such as sublimation and transference. If an individual fails to develop effective ways of dealing with the repressed feelings, they may be expressed in anxiety neurosis or physical illness. The purpose of a Freudian analysis is to uncover the repressed desires which stand in the way of normal functioning. Many other types of psychotherapy also attempt to help the patient get in touch with her feelings so that she can deal with them without anxiety and guilt.

reproductive system The organs and processes involved in the generation of reproductive cells, conception, gestation, and childbirth. For a description of the female reproductive system, *see* "The Healthy Woman."

reserpine An alkaloid extracted from the Southeast Asian plant *Rauwolfia serpentina*. The substance known as rauwolfia was extracted from the root of the plant and used as a tranquilizer for centuries in India. Its active chemical component, reserpine, was later isolated. After World War II it was widely used in the treatment of schizophrenia and manic-depressive illness, but it has since been superseded by drugs with fewer negative side effects. Reserpine has also been one of the standard medicines for reducing hypertension. Since it has been suggested that it is associated with the development of breast cancer, its prescription as an antihypertensive is open to question.

resistance The body's ability to ward off or minimize disease either through genetic capability, the presence of antibodies produced by immunization or environmental exposure, or a high enough level of physical and psychological health to combat infection without succumbing to it. An example of inherited resistance is the fact that the darker a woman's skin, the less likely she is to develop skin cancer because of overexposure to the sun. Resistance to many of the infectious diseases caused by various organisms, especially viruses, in a particular environment may result from the presence of antibodies developed against one or another strain of the disease-bearing agent. However, should a different strain be brought into the environment from some other part of the world, as has occurred over and over again with various types of flu, epidemics are likely to result. Resistance is also a variable capacity at different times of one's life. When the body is young, it operates with considerably more efficiency and rallies its protective forces more quickly than when it is aged. Thus for the elderly, whose metabolism is inevitably slower and whose cardiovascular system has deteriorated somewhat, loss of resistance to hot weather and resultant heat stroke is more common than in younger persons. Some people find it difficult to grasp the concept that many illnesses are contracted not from other people but from themselves. Many people have been infected by the virus that causes cold sores (herpes labialis) which remain dormant after the cold sore heals. When resistance is lowered by malnutrition, too little sleep, too much stress, or a generally debilitated physical condition, the virus can become activated and the cold sore reappears. The most efficient way to produce resistance to an increasing number of infectious diseases is by immunization.

respiratory disorders *See* ASTHMA, BRONCHITIS, etc.

retina The innermost layer of cells at the rear of the eyeball; a membrane consisting of the light-sensitive rods and cones that receive the image formed by the lens and transmit it through the optic nerve to the brain. Retinal disease of one kind or another is the chief cause of blindness in the United States. With the extension in the life span of diabetics through the use of insulin a disease called diabetic retinopathy has come to the attention of medical science. According to the National Eye Institute, it threatens the vision of more than 300,000 people.

This impairment of the retina through spontaneous bleeding from retinal vessels affects, to some degree, 95 percent of the diabetics who have been on insulin therapy for 25 years or more. Many cases are successfully treated with the technique called photocoagulation in which finely focused beams of intense light are directed into the eye in such a way that miniscule burns are caused on the retina. These burns destroy the abnormal blood vessels, and the minute scars that result do much less harm to vision than the disease.

Photocoagulation may also be used to treat some patients with macular degeneration. This is a disorder of unknown cause which affects the macula, the tiny orange-yellow portions in the center of the retina through which the color and detail of daytime vision are received. While this is chiefly a disease of the elderly, it may occur at any time, depriving the victim of reading vision. When a hole or tear develops in the retina or when an eye infection or tumor forces an excess of the vitreous fluid to seep between the retinal layers, the result can be a retinal detachment which can result in a permanent loss of eyesight. There is an increased risk that this condition may occur in people with severe myopia. Thanks to photocoagulation and new microsurgical techniques, restoration of vision is accomplished in a large number of cases.

Rh factor A group of genetically determined antigens found in the red blood cells of most people. The designation comes from the rhesus monkey involved in the original experiments. About 15 percent of the Caucasian population lacks this inherited blood

Rh FACTOR

If mother lacks Rh antigen present on father's·cells and on fetal cells

Mother's blood vessel

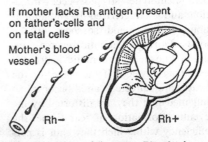

Rh−   Rh+

During delivery of first baby Rh+ fetal blood may enter maternal bloodstream and mother's Rh− blood will produce Rh antibodies

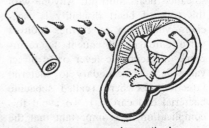

In subsequent pregnancies mother's antibodies may destroy fetal blood cells

substance, and this group is therefore known as Rh negative. Its absence in other races is much rarer. When the substance is missing, the blood is described as Rh negative, regardless of whether the major blood type is A, B, AB, or O. It is vitally important that Rh compatibility be established before a transfusion, especially when the recipient is a woman who may want children in future years. The reason for checking the Rh factor during pregnancy is to avoid the complications that ensue when the woman is Rh negative and the man is Rh positive. The mixing of the two bloods can have serious consequences so it is imperative to determine early in pregnancy if the Rh negative problem exists. *See* "Pregnancy and Childbirth."

rheumatic fever A disease of the growing years triggered by a group A beta hemolytic streptococcus infection and characterized by inflammation, swelling, and soreness of the joints. During rheumatic fever a condition known as rheumatic heart disease may develop. If the valves of the heart are affected and become so inflamed that they are distorted by the eventual formation of scar tissue, the efficiency with which they shut is permanently impaired. The impairment results in a backspill of blood that can be heard through a stethoscope as the so-called heart murmur. Anyone with this type of heart disability is especially vulnerable to further indirect valve damage subsequent to recurrence of rheumatic fever or to direct valve damage secondary to bacterial infection elsewhere (called subacute bacterial endocarditis). To avoid this complication, it is important that the proper precautions be taken against bacterial invasion of the bloodstream that may occur when a tooth is extracted, during urinary tract surgery, etc. Fortunately, antibiotics started prior to such procedures have eliminated this grave complication in most cases.

rheumatism A nonscientific designation for any painful disorder or disease of the joints, muscles, bones, ligaments, or nerves. *See* ARTHRITIS, BURSITIS, etc.

rheumatoid arthritis *See* ARTHRITIS.

rhinitis Inflammation of the mucous membranes that line the nasal passages, caused by viral or bacterial infection, allergy, or inhalation of irritants. Acute rhinitis, the technical medical term for the nasal disturbance of the common cold, is its most common form. In some cases viral rhinitis is complicated by bacterial invasion which may reach the ears and the throat. When streptococcus, staphylococcus, or pneumococcus bacteria are involved, the nasal discharge will be thick and yellowish with pus instead of being practically colorless, loose, and runny. Another form of inflammation is caused by an allergic reaction to grass, trees, dog hair, or other substances.

Rhinitis may become prolonged or chronic because of constant inhalation of noxious dusts, heavy smoking, constant exposure to excessively dry air, low resistance to infection by cold viruses, or constant bouts of sinusitis. Under these circumstances, the nasal membranes may thicken and swell to the point where breathing is impaired, headaches and postnasal drip are chronic, and the sense of smell is damaged. Also associated with chronic rhinitis is the development of polyps and of a separate disorder known as ozena in which the erosion of the mucous membrane results in a thick malodorous discharge that creates heavy crusts impeding proper breathing and attempts at nose-blowing.

Obvious symptoms of chronic rhinitis should be treated by a doctor. When rhinitis is associated with fever or other manifestation of bacterial infection, antibiotic therapy may be advisable. However, the typical stuffed or runny nose characteristic of an ordinary cold is likely to clear up as the cold runs its course. It has recently been observed that thousands of Americans abuse nasal sprays, especially those containing long-lasting vasoconstrictors that shrink the blood vessels in the nose, those eliminating the symptom of "stuffed nose" associated with colds, allergies, and some sinus conditions. This dependence produces a "rebound" phenomenon in which the "cure" causes the symptoms to return in more acute form, so that more and stronger nasal decongestants are needed. Specialists therefore advise a careful reading of label warnings about dosage and continued application of all such medications.

rhythm method *See* "Contraception and Abortion."

riboflavin A component of the vitamin B complex; also known as vitamin B_2. When a deficiency exists, as may occur in liver disease, alcoholism, or an improperly balanced diet, the early signs are a reddening and soreness of the tongue, painful cracks in the skin at the side of the mouth, and eye inflammation that affects vision. Therapeutic doses, usually combined with other vitamins, will correct these disorders. *See* "Nutrition and Weight."

ribonucleic acid *See* RNA.

rickettsial diseases A category of infectious diseases caused by microorganisms larger than viruses, smaller than bacteria but with characteristics of both, called rickettsiae after their discoverer, the pathologist H. T. Ricketts (1871–1910). Rickettsiae inhabit certain rodents as parasites and are transmitted to humans and animals by the bites of ticks, mites, fleas, and lice. The rickettsial diseases, which range from mild to extremely serious, commonly produce a rash and a fever. While they are comparatively rare in places where public health practices keep rodents and carrier insects at a minimum, epidemic outbreaks of Rocky Mountain spotted fever and Q fever have occurred in various parts of the United States. The incidence of these diseases as well as of typhus fever, the most serious of the rickettsial

infections, has been considerably reduced by the availability of effective immunization. When a particular rickettsial disease is accurately diagnosed on the basis of laboratory findings, it is usually treated with antibiotics. (This group of diseases should not be confused with rickets, a vitamin D deficiency disease.) *See* Q FEVER, ROCKY MOUNTAIN SPOTTED FEVER, TYPHUS.

ringworm *See* FUNGUS INFECTIONS.

RNA Ribonucleic acid, the chemical compound contained in the cytoplasm of all cells and the carrier of genetic information provided by DNA to the ribosomes, the structures that synthesize amino acids into proteins. Through the information transmitted by RNA, inherited characteristics make their way from one generation to the next.

Rocky Mountain spotted fever An infectious disease transmitted to humans by the bite of the American dog tick in the Eastern states and from rodents to humans by the wood tick in Western states; also called tick fever or Eastern spotted fever. This is one of the rickettsial diseases that produces fever, headache, aching muscles, and a rash. One of the distinguishing characteristics of the disease is that the rash begins on the palms of the hands and the soles of the feet, spreading upward during the course of the illness, which, if untreated, may lead to serious respiratory complications. Other symptoms include sensitivity to light, abdominal cramps, and vomiting. Tetracycline halts the progress of the infection. Vacationers should find out if warnings of tick infestation have been issued in their location. Dogs should not be permitted to roam in tick-infested surroundings; where, in an attempt to eliminate ticks, areas have been sprayed with chemicals harmful to people and their pets, precautions should be taken against potentially dangerous contact. Another precaution against tick bites is suitable clothing: long pants in a light color and sturdy shoes.

root canal The passageway through the root of a tooth for the nerve. When tooth decay has proceeded unchecked from the enamel into the dentin that surrounds the pulp chamber and the root canal, the only treatment that can prevent the loss of the tooth by extraction is known as root canal therapy. This consists in removing the nerve and the diseased pulp, sterilizing the chamber, and filling the area with an inert substance. The specialist who performs this type of treatment is called an endodontist.

rubella An acute virus infection accompanied by fever and a rash, a common contagious disease of childhood; also known as German measles. In spite of the fact that long-lasting immunization against this disease is available, many young women reach childbearing age without vaccination against it and without natural immunization from infection during childhood. Rubella immunity precludes the potentially harmful fetal consequences from exposure to the disease during the early months of pregnancy. Such consequences include brain damage, blindness, and other deformities in as many as 50 percent of the affected offspring. It is therefore of the utmost importance that a woman who is planning a pregnancy or who thinks that she is pregnant already be tested for rubella immunity. Vaccination against rubella is strongly recommended in any case. Pregnant women without

immunization should avoid exposure to rubella.

Rubin test A diagnostic procedure used in cases of infertility to discover whether the fallopian tubes are obstructed; also known as tubal insufflation. Carbon dioxide gas is carefully blown through the cervix into the uterus. If the passage is normal, the gas will escape through the fallopian tubes into the abdominal cavity. In cases in which mucous congestion or minor scar tissue has blocked the tubes, the pressure of the gas may open them sufficiently to make conception possible. When the pressure gauge indicates insurmountable blockage, other procedures are used to solve the problem.

rupture A popular term for a hernia. *See* HERNIA.

saccharin A chemical coal tar derivative, used as a sugar substitute and approximately 500 times sweeter than cane sugar by weight. Saccharin had been used routinely by diabetics and by people on low calorie diets, until recent scientifically controlled experiments conducted with laboratory animals pointed to carcinogenic properties in saccharin. However, debate continues about the validity of these tests when applied to human consumption since no such controlled experiments can be duplicated with humans. A sugar substitute is by no means necessary for weight reduction; women concerned about controlling their weight might use sugar in small quantities or use no sweeteners at all.

sacroiliac The cartilaginous joint that connects the sacrum at the base of the spinal column to the ilium, the open section on either side of the hipbone.

Low back pain can sometimes be ascribed to arthritis in this joint.

sadism In the clinical sense, a perversion in which sexual gratification can be achieved only through inflicting pain on the partner. The term, derived from the perversities described in the writings of the Marquis de Sade, has come to be used loosely to characterize excessive cruelty or pleasure derived from inflicting physical or mental pain. Sadomasochism is a condition in which sexual or more generalized pleasure is achieved either by inflicting or receiving physical or mental pain.

saline abortion A procedure, performed under local anesthesia, in which a pregnancy is terminated by the withdrawal of amniotic fluid from the uterus and the injection of a concentrated salt solution into the amniotic fluid space. *See* "Contraception and Abortion."

saliva The secretion of the salivary glands in the mouth. The largest of these, the parotids, are situated in front of and below each ear and discharge saliva through openings in the cheeks opposite the lower back teeth. The saliva secreted into the floor of the mouth comes from the sublingual glands below the tongue and from the submaxillar glands inside the lower jaw. Saliva not only keeps the mouth and tongue moist to facilitate speech and swallowing, it also softens food and through its enzymes initiates the digestive process by chemically changing the carbohydrates in the mouth into simpler sugars. Since the flow of saliva is activated by the nervous system, stimuli of sight, smell, taste, and even mental images of food will increase salivation. For the same rea-

son, fear and anxiety will inhibit the flow, leading to the "dry mouth" sensation that accompanies some types of stress situations. Nutritional deficiencies and some medicines may also result in an uncomfortable decrease of saliva.

salmonella A group of rod-shaped bacteria especially irritating to the intestinal tract and responsible for most cases of acute food poisoning as well as for paratyphoid and typhoid fever. Abdominal cramps and diarrhea are the typical symptoms of salmonella infection.

salpingectomy The surgical removal of one or both of the fallopian tubes. This operation is usually necessary when surgery is done for a tubal ectopic pregnancy.

salpingitis Inflammation of the fallopian tubes. It is usually caused by gonococci or other bacteria that ascend from the cervix, but may also be caused by tuberculosis. Acute salpingitis, especially when it is recurrent, can result in scar tissue that obstructs the tubes (chronic salpingitis), thereby becoming a possible cause of sterility. Any acute pain on both sides of the lower abdomen accompanied by a vaginal discharge and frequent and uncomfortable urination should be diagnosed promptly for treatment with antibiotics.

salt The chemical compound sodium chloride (NaCl); also called table salt. The average daily U.S. diet contains 7 to 13 grams of sodium. While a certain amount is essential for maintaining the body's chemical balance, it is advisable for people suffering from hypertension and certain types of heart or kidney disease to restrict their salt intake, since too much sodium may cause fluid retention. Modern food processing makes this difficult, since practically all processed foods, including frozen vegetables, contain salt; all baked goods, cake mixes, breads, and soft drinks contain salt, and the nitritex used to preserve cold cuts and smoked meat is sodium nitrite which has the same water-retention effect as sodium chloride. Anyone who must restrict sodium intake might find some help in cookbooks that specialize in low-salt recipes and menu planning. When the body loses too much fluid, as in a long siege of diarrhea or heavy sweating, a salt deficiency may occur, manifested in muscle cramps, nausea, fatigue, and in extreme cases collapse. Prompt replenishment can be accomplished by eating salted crackers or nuts or by swallowing a sodium chloride tablet with some orange juice. However, salt tablets should not be taken routinely during hot and humid weather unless the recommendation is made by a doctor. How much salt, if any, a pregnant woman should eliminate from her diet to reduce the likelihood of edema is a matter to be discussed with the physician in charge of her prenatal regimen.

sarcoma A malignant tumor composed of connective tissue such as bone or of muscle, lymph, or blood vessel tissue; one of the two main groups of cancer, the more common being carcinoma (cancer of epithelial or gland cells). A sarcoma usually metastasizes rapidly, either through the bloodstream or through the lymphatics. While treatment is difficult, a combination of chemotherapy, radiation, and surgery can be effective in halting the progress of different types of sarcoma.

scabies An infestation of the skin by insectlike parasites; also known as "the itch." The scabies mites burrow under the skin, usually between the fingers, in the groin, under the breasts, or in the armpits, to lay their eggs. When the eggs hatch, they produce new adult parasites that work their way to the skin surface and begin the cycle again. The severe itching accompanied by a rash begins about a week after the initial infestation and is especially acute at night. Constant scratching during sleep may result in lesions that are vulnerable to bacterial infection. Scabies may spread quickly through an entire family and may also be contracted during sexual contact. Treatment should therefore be simultaneously undertaken by all those who have been exposed to contamination. A doctor usually identifies the itch mite by microscopic examination. A daily change of underclothing, towels, and bed linens is advisable until the eggs and the parasites have been eliminated by laundering from anything that might be in contact with the skin. Topical medicines are usually prescribed to kill the eggs under the skin and to minimize the itching. Hot baths before bedtime may also be helpful.

scanning machines Diagnostic equipment by means of which parts of the body that cannot be examined by conventional X-ray can be seen and analyzed. Scanners use radioactive materials, special cameras, and new techniques made available by nuclear medicine. One of the most widely used of these machines is called a CAT (computerized axial tomography) scanner, also known as a brain scanner. While being rotated around the patient's head, it records information about layers of the brain and feeds the information into a computer that creates a composite picture in which it is possible to locate a tumor or some other disorder previously invisible in an X-ray picture. A more recent scanner, known as PET (positron emission tomography), detects changes in the biochemistry of the brain, and by revealing areas of abnormal glucose metabolism, provides heretofore unavailable information about brain activity of mentally ill patients. The accumulation of PET data on normal and abnormal brain function is expected to lead to epilepsy control by destroying those cells responsible for inducing the seizures.

schizophrenia A general term for mental disorders classified as psychotic rather than neurotic, in which the victim suffers from severely disturbed patterns of thinking and feeling that lead to bizarre behavior. The schizophrenic syndrome, for which there is no known direct cause and no specific cure, is most likely to occur in early adulthood, although no age is immune. Common parlance has given the term the sense of a split personality, but this popular definition actually has very little to do with the psychiatric diagnosis of mental illness. As with the manic-depressive psychosis, schizophrenic symptoms may be periodic, sometimes so immobilizing the victim that hospitalization is necessary, at other times mild enough to liberate the patient for a comparatively normal life. Among the most striking symptoms of the condition are auditory hallucinations; delusions, usually of grandeur or of persecution (paranoia); obsessive-compulsive behavior; distinct personality changes and mood swings without visible cause; and, above all, loss of control over fantasies. While there are many theories about the cause of the illness, circum-

stances that trigger its onset, and reasons for its remission, no single explanation is definitively convincing. Among the areas of current research are constitutional predisposition in the form of an inherited recessive gene or a combination of genes; constitutional predisposition associated with oxygen deprivation of the brain during birth, triggered by a metabolic aberration, or related to a prenatal protein deficiency; environmental circumstances that create an atmosphere of anxiety and hostility and especially a conflict between parents or extreme parental disapproval and criticism.

When the disease is suspected, diagnosis is usually based on a complete physical examination, a series of psychiatric interviews, an electroencephalogram, and standard psychological tests. Conventional treatment may begin with chemotherapy combined with psychotherapy which may involve the family. Environmental therapy, involving residence in a halfway house rather than a hospital, is used in many cases. This form of therapy conditions or reconditions the schizophrenic for participation in the normal world even though some symptoms are ineradicable. Megavitamin therapy is used by some doctors, but since conclusive evidence of its effectiveness has not yet been provided, this approach is not sanctioned by the profession as a whole. In cases where the more immobilizing symptoms cannot be alleviated in any other way, electroshock may be used as a last resort.

sciatica Pain extending along the sciatic nerve which is the largest nerve in the body and which supplies sensation from the back of the thigh, along the outer side of the leg, and into the foot and toes. The most common cause of sciatica is a slipped or herniated disk of the lower spine. Osteoarthritis is another cause. In some cases the pain is accompanied by a paralysis of some of the associated muscles of the thigh and leg. Inflammation of the sciatic nerve (sciatic neuritis), while rare, may be a consequence of diseases such as alcoholism or diabetes or of vitamin deficiencies. Sciatica may vanish unaccountably as it arrives, but in cases where it is persistently painful and immobilizing, efforts should be made to discover the underlying cause. Until the cause can be treated, relief may be provided by physical therapy, a surgical girdle, or support tights.

scopolamine A chemical similar to belladonna, derived from a plant of the nightshade family and used medically as a sedative and painkiller; also known as "twilight sleep." It induces stupor, forgetfulness (pain is experienced but not remembered on awakening), and in some cases physical agitation. When given with barbiturates and tranquilizers in the early stages of labor, it may produce respiratory suppression in the newborn baby and transitory postpartum depression in the mother.

scrotum *See* SEX ORGANS, MALE.

scurvy A deficiency disease resulting from an insufficiency of vitamin C in the diet. Vitamin C requirements are between 10 and 20 milligrams daily. Considerably more than that amount is provided by a conventional diet that contains citrus fruits and juices and various green vegetables both raw and gently cooked. While scurvy is now a rare disease, it may occur from an improperly balanced diet; infants who are not given supplementary ascorbic acid may also suffer from scurvy. Signs of the disorder are bleeding gums, rup-tured blood vessels, and eventual anemia and bone changes. Treatment consists of therapeutic doses of vitamin C in the form of ascorbic acid tablets or, in extreme cases of metabolic disorder, by injection.

sebaceous glands The oil-secreting glands situated in the epidermal layer of the skin, lubricating the surface and protecting it from the harmful effects of absorbing too much or too little moisture. The number of these glands, which may be as many as 12 to the square inch, varies from person to person and from one part of the body to another. The sebaceous glands secrete sebum which constantly seeps upward through the pores. Too little sebum production results in dry skin, too much in oily skin. During adolescence and pregnancy hormonal changes may affect the activity of the glands, leading to acne. Another condition resulting from sebaceous disorder is dandruff.

Seconal Brand name of a drug in the barbiturate family. Seconal is a central nervous system depressant prescribed in small doses as a sedative and in larger doses to induce sleep. Like other barbiturates, it creates a dependency. There are strong indications that Seconal and similar medications should not be administered during labor since they may have a depressant effect on the fetal brain and respiration.

sedative A category of drugs that in small doses reduce excitability, irritability, and nervousness by depressing the central nervous system and in larger doses induce sleep. This category includes barbiturates, tranquilizers, and bromides, as well as chloral hydrate and alcohol. If used regularly or abused even over short periods, practically all sedatives produce dependencies of one kind or another that can lead to addiction. *See* "Drugs, Alcohol, and Tobacco."

semen The thick, whitish fluid produced and secreted by the male organs of reproduction and containing the sperm cells. A single ejaculation of semen contains 300 to 500 million spermatazoa in a little less than a teaspoon of fluid. One of the diagnostic procedures in infertility cases is analysis of semen to determine the shape, number, and motility of the sperm.

seminal vesicles *See* SEX ORGANS, MALE.

senescence The normal process of growing old. *See* "Aging Healthfully."

senility A manifest and abnormal deterioration of mental function associated with aging and caused by physical or mental disease or a combination of both. While damage to brain function by arteriosclerosis and stroke are among the conspicuous causes of senility, psychological and social factors that lead to personality deterioration may be equally responsible. Among the most prominent of these factors are withdrawal from normal life, lack of interpersonal relationships, feelings of worthlessness aggravated by familial and social neglect, unrelieved anxieties about disease and death. *Senile* is a clinical term and should never be used to describe anyone who is going through the normal aging process which may involve a slower rate of activity and response. *See* "Aging Healthfully."

serum *See* BLOOD SERUM.

sex-linked abnormalities Inherited disorders transmitted by a genetic de-

fect in the X chromosome. Women have two X chromosomes and men have one X chromosome paired with a Y chromosome. Since the presence of a Y chromosome determines maleness, fathers always transmit their X chromosome to their daughters and their Y chromosome to their sons. Because of these factors, defective genes in the X chromosome follow a particular pattern of heredity. If in a female an inherited disordered X chromosome is balanced by a normal X chromosome, she will carry the disease trait without having the disease itself. If a male offspring of the female carrier inherits her genetically abnormal X chromosome, since it is his only X chromosome, he will have the disease. When a mother is a carrier, there is therefore a fifty-fifty chance that her male offspring will inherit her abnor-

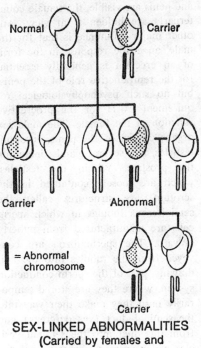

= Abnormal chromosome

SEX-LINKED ABNORMALITIES
(Carried by females and appear in males)

mal X chromosome and have the disease. Female offspring have a fifty-fifty chance of inheriting the abnormal chromosome and therefore a fifty-fifty chance of being carriers. Among the sex-linked abnormalities are such diseases as hemophilia, Duchenne muscular dystrophy, and the metabolic disorder known as the Lesch-Nyhan syndrome. The relatively new field of genetic counseling seeks to inform a couple of the likelihood of having a genetically defective child so that they can make educated decisions.

sex organs, female *See* "The Healthy Woman."

sex organs, male The male reproductive organs. One of the most obvious differences between the reproductive organs of the male and the female is that whereas the scrotum and penis are visible, the female counterparts are hidden from view. Another major difference is that for the male, an erotic response in the form of an erection is generally essential for the reproductive role of the penis, but no such psychophysiological requirement exists for the procreative function of the female. The male sex organs consist of the penis, scrotum, testicles, and several glands, including the prostate. Within the testicles, which are loosely contained in the scrotum, are structures called the seminiferous tubules in which sperm cells are manufactured from puberty onward. The spermatozoa are conveyed from the tubules into the epididymis, part of the sperm conduction system, where they are stored temporarily until they make their way into the seminal duct (vas deferens) and from this duct into the seminal vesicles which secrete a viscous material

that keeps them viable. The urethra, which also carries urine from the bladder, is enveloped by the prostate gland. The prostate manufactures another fluid that mixes with the sperm and the seminal fluid to form the combination known as semen. The urethra passes through the length of the penis. When the penis is in a state of erection, muscular spasms send the semen through the urethra in the act of ejaculation that immediately follows the male orgasm. Any traces of urine that might be present in the urethra are neutralized during sexual excitation by an alkaline secretion from two tiny organs known as Cowper's glands. This chemical process is critical since spermatozoa cannot remain viable in an acid environment. Because of the dual role of the urethra and its location, the male reproductive channel is also called the genitourinary tract.

sexual intercourse The entry of the penis into the vagina, usually preceded by sufficiently stimulating foreplay to cause an erection in the male and the flow of lubricating secretions in both partners; also called coitus. Extravaginal intercourse is also a common practice, involving anal entry and oral sex (fellatio and cunnilingus) that give satisfaction as foreplay or may be another means of achieving orgasm. Painful sexual intercourse for the female (dyspareunia) may result from inflammation of any part of the genitourinary system, prolapsed uterus, abnormal vaginal contractions, or psychogenic causes.

shingles *See* HERPES ZOSTER.

shock A disruption of circulation which may be fatal if not promptly treated; not to be confused with electrical shock or insulin shock. The immediate cause of circulatory shock is the sudden drop in blood pressure to the point where the blood can no longer be effectively pumped through the vital organs and tissues. Among the circumstances leading up to this crisis are: low-volume shock following severe hemorrhage as occurs in multiple fractures, bleeding ulcers, major burns, or any accidents in which so much blood and plasma are lost that there is an insufficiency for satisfying vital needs; neurogenic shock in which the nervous system is traumatized by acute pain, fear, or other strong stimulus that deprives the brain of oxygen and results in a temporary loss of consciousness; allergic shock, also called anaphylactic shock, following the injection into the bloodstream of a substance to which the recipient may be fatally hypersensitive; cardiac shock in which the pumping action of the heart is impeded by an infarction or by fibrillation; septic shock resulting from the toxins introduced into the circulatory system by various harmful bacteria. Whatever the circumstances, shock produces similar symptoms in different degrees of swiftness: extreme pallor, profuse sweating combined with a feeling of chill, thirst, faint speedy pulse, and, as the condition intensifies, increasing weakness and labored breathing. Immediate hospitalization is mandatory. If shock is the result of a serious accident or of a heart attack, the patient should not be moved except by people professionally trained to do so.

shock treatment *See* ELECTROSHOCK TREATMENT.

sickle cell disease An inherited disease characterized by the substitution

of 90 to 100 percent of normal hemoglobin by an abnormal hemoglobin, called hemoglobin S. When exposed to normal but low oxygen tension, red blood cells containing this much hemoglobin S acquire the shape of a sickle. These red blood cells are destroyed more rapidly than normal red blood cells and a hemolytic anemia results. In addition, the sickled red blood cells occlude blood vessels, thus depriving various body cells of their oxygen supply, causing them to die and producing rather widespread disease. There is as yet no cure.

A variant of sickle cell disease is sickle cell trait in which only 25 to 45 percent of normal hemoglobin is replaced by hemoglobin S. Persons with sickle cell trait may have a mild anemia, but only rarely have other problems. A simple blood test identifies the

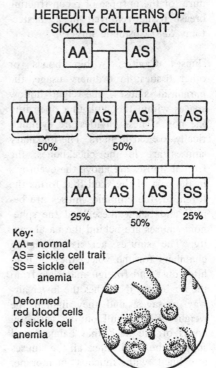

HEREDITY PATTERNS OF
SICKLE CELL TRAIT

AA — AS

AA AA AS AS — AS
50%   50%

AA AS AS SS
25%   50%   25%

Key:
AA = normal
AS = sickle cell trait
SS = sickle cell
        anemia

Deformed
red blood cells
of sickle cell
anemia

presence and quantity of hemoglobin S. Hemoglobin S is found almost exclusively in black persons of African origin. In the United States about 8 percent of Afro-Americans have the trait and about 0.2 percent have the disease. Because hemoglobin S is transmitted genetically both parents must have either the disease or the trait for any of their children to have the disease. If only one parent has the disease or the trait, none of their children will have the disease, though some will have the trait. *See* GENETIC COUNSELING.

silicone implantation A surgical procedure in which one of the silicone compounds in the form of a gel or a saline solution enclosed in a bag is inserted into the breasts in order to augment their size; also a similar procedure for the purpose of reconstructing breast tissue removed in a mastectomy. *See* "Cosmetic Surgery."

sinuses Cavities within bones or other tissues; in ordinary usage, the paranasal sinuses, the eight hollow spaces within the skull that open into the nose. These cavities are symmetrically located in pairs. The maxillary sinuses are in the cheekbones, the frontal sinuses are above the eyebrows in the part of the skull that forms the forehead, the ethmoid sinuses are behind and below these, and the sphenoid sinuses are behind the nasal cavity. The sinuses act as resonating chambers for the voice; they help to filter dust and foreign materials from the air before it reaches the lower airway passages; and they lighten the weight of the skull on the vertebral bones of the neck that balance and support the head. Since all the sinuses are lined with mucous membrane,

they are vulnerable to infection, to inflammation by allergens, and to the formation of polyps.

sinusitis Inflammation of the mucous membranes that line the sinuses. The passageway that connects the sinuses to the nasal cavity is narrow and therefore susceptible to obstruction because of colds, allergies, or the presence of polyps. Such obstruction prevents free drainage of the sinuses, causes an entrapment of air that cannot escape through the nostrils, and leads to an accumulation of mucus which can become a locus of viral or bacterial infection. Infectious organisms may be transported into the sinuses through the nose when an individual is swimming in contaminated water or may invade the maxillary sinuses by way of an abscessed tooth in the upper jaw. The characteristic symptom of sinusitis is a severe headache and face pain in the location of the affected sinus. Fever, swelling, discomfort in the neck, earache, and a stuffed nose are other symptoms.

Acute sinusitis usually clears up in a few days of bed rest; aspirin or other analgesic, limited use of nosedrops, steam inhalation, and air filters can make the recovery period more comfortable. If secondary bacterial infection develops in the sinuses the doctor may prescribe antibiotics.

When sinusitis becomes chronic, every effort should be made to find out the cause. If it can be traced to nasal polyps, consideration should be given to having them removed. When an allergy is responsible, precautions may require the use of an antihistamine combined with other medications that will keep the nasal passages clear. Heavy smoking is another cause as well as a contributing factor when other causes already exist. Irritation by the chlorinated water in swimming pools is yet another cause. Aside from the pain that accompanies chronic sinusitis, there is the remote danger of eventual complication in the form of osteomyelitis or meningitis. Since surgical drainage is advisable only in extreme cases, chronic sufferers should do what they can for themselves: smoking should be minimized, air conditioners and humidifiers installed, and the environment indoors kept as free of dusts and pollens as possible by using air filters.

skin The body's outer surface and its largest organ, covering an area of approximately 25 square feet and weighing about 6 pounds. The skin envelops the body completely and is also a continuation of the mucous membranes of the mouth, nose, urethra, vagina, and anus. Among its many vital functions are the following: It provides a barrier against invasion by infectious agents; offers the delicate tissues beneath it a large measure of protection against injury from the outside; regulates body temperature by the expansion and contraction of its supply of capillaries and by the activities of the sweat glands; and participates in the excretion of some of the body's wastes. Through its production of melanin, it wards off some of the damage of the sun's ultraviolet rays, and it also helps transform sunshine into essential vitamin D. In addition, the skin is one of the body's most delicate sense organs: through its vast network of nerve fibers, it transmits messages of pain,

CROSS-SECTION OF SKIN

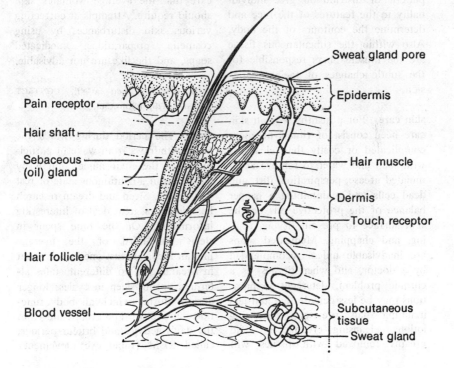

Sweat gland pore

Epidermis

Pain receptor

Hair shaft

Sebaceous (oil) gland

Hair muscle

Dermis

Touch receptor

Hair follicle

Blood vessel

Subcutaneous tissue

Sweat gland

pleasure, pressure, and temperature.

What is commonly identified as "the skin" is merely its visible portion or the outermost layer of the epidermis. The epidermis is made of several layers of living cells and an outer horny layer of dead cells constantly being shed and requiring no nourishing blood supply from below. This is the comparatively tough layer that provides a shield against germs as long as it remains unbroken. The same nonliving skin cells form the hair and nails. Beneath the epidermis lies the dermis or true skin, bright red in appearance and containing the nerve endings and nerve fibers, sweat and sebaceous glands, and hair follicles. Beneath the dermis is a layer of fatty tissue, called subcutaneous tissue, which helps to insulate the body against heat and cold and which contains the fat globules which through a pattern of distribution give individuality to the features of the face and determine the contours of the body. Also within the subcutaneous tissue are the muscle fibers responsible for the subtle changes of facial expression.

skin care For a healthy woman skin care need consist of rituals no more complicated or costly than cleansing with soap and water to remove accumulated grease, perspiration, dirt, and dead cells and maintaining a proper balance of the protective oils on the skin surface to prevent drying, scaling, and chapping. Medicated soaps are inadvisable unless recommended by a doctor, and when dryness is a chronic problem, detergent preparations may be less dehydrating and less irritating than true soap. Cleansing lotions, cleansing creams, or cold creams removed with tissues will never leave the skin as clean as rubbing a lather over it with a soft washcloth and removing the suds with warm water. All makeup should be removed before going to bed. The cheapest cleansing cream will do, followed by washing with soap and water.

Whether or not the skin is naturally oily or dry is an inherited factor. A vaporizer or humidifier is the best aid to counteracting the drying effects of central heating or air conditioning. Animal fat, especially lanolin which comes from sheep wool, is the oil closest to human sebum and is therefore the best thing to use when skin begins to flake or crack at the knees, elbows, or fingers. It is to be preferred to mineral oil or vegetable oil for the purpose of lubrication. A sensible regimen of diet, rest, exercise, and good habits of personal hygiene are all the care that the average woman's skin should require. Attempts at correcting various skin disturbances by using cosmetic preparations, medicated soaps, and the like are not advisable.

skin diseases *See* ACNE, CONTACT DERMATITIS, PSORIASIS, etc.

sleep The period during which the body withdraws from wakeful participation in the environment, but is by no means in a continuous state of rest and repose. Sleep and dream research has yielded a great deal of interesting information. Of the time spent in sleep (one-third of the average human life), at least one-fifth is spent in dreaming. Two different states alternate during sleep in cycles: longer periods during which all body functions slow down and recuperate from the day's activity and briefer periods, called REM (rapid eye movement) sleep, when the heartbeat quickens, pulse rises, and all processes speed up as if to be at the alert. It is during REM sleep that most dreaming occurs, but they do not always occur together. For reasons which are unclear, both types of sleep are essential for wakeful well-being. One of the dangers of barbiturate and alcohol addiction is that these drugs suppress REM sleep and also suppress dreaming.

A normal state of health is characterized by as well as promoted by good sleeping patterns, and when sleeping problems exist over a considerable period or when they arise suddenly without visible explanation, they should be investigated; the solution to the problems cannot be found in immediate recourse to hypnotics or barbiturates. Unaccustomed sleepiness or drowsiness may be a temporary phenomenon resulting from a wide variety of causes: overexposure to the sun; too much alcohol, especially in an overheated room; poor ventilation; too many tranquilizers; antihistamines; hangover effects of sedatives, tranquilizers, or sleeping pills; and low-grade infection. Chronic sleepiness may be due to thyroid deficiency, anemia, hardening of the arteries of the brain, or in rare cases the disorder known as narcolepsy. Escape into sleep rather than sleeplessness may be a sign of the onset of depression.

sleeping pills *See* BARBITURATES; "Drugs, Alcohol, and Tobacco."

slipped disc *See* DISC, SLIPPED.

smallpox An acute, severe, highly infectious virus disease, characterized by multiple blisters appearing first on the face, neck, and upper extremities. Enforced vaccination throughout the world has led to the extinction of this disease. Since there are no silent carriers and no source of infection other than human carriers, and since the last human case, other than a laboratory infection, was reported in 1977, it is assumed by the World Health Organization that the virus has been eliminated everywhere. This is the only communicable disease over which immunization can record apparent total success. While vaccination against smallpox is no longer relevant as a health measure, the federal government's Communicable Disease Center, together with similar laboratories in other countries, maintains a stockpile of smallpox virus to make smallpox vaccine in the event of some future outbreak of the disease.

smegma A sebaceous secretion of a cheeselike consistency that accumulates near the clitoris and under the foreskin of the penis. Unless scrupulously washed off, it is likely to be retained and cause irritation under the foreskin of the uncircumcised male, leading to inflammation and pain.

smoking Among the health hazards unequivocally connected with inhaled tobacco smoke are increased vulnerability to lung cancer, chronic respiratory infection, heart attack (especially when combined with the use of the contraceptive pill), emphysema, and fetal damage leading to stillbirth, miscarriage, or chronic respiratory illness during infancy and early childhood. Recent research indicates that if parents smoke, it is likely that their children will, too. There are also indications that day-in-day-out exposure to "second-hand" smoke may produce a significant increase in lung disease risk for the nonsmoker. The American

Medical Association estimates that at least 35 million Americans have respiratory ailments that are made worse by tobacco smoke. Increasing efforts by the lobbying group ASH (Action on Smoking and Health) and other concerned organizations have resulted in laws protecting the rights of non-smokers in public places, on the job, on airplanes, etc. *See also* "Drugs, Alcohol, and Tobacco."

snoring The sound made during sleep by the vibration of the soft palate when air is inhaled through the open mouth. Snoring is a likely consequence of breathing through one's mouth when sleeping flat on one's back. The sound itself becomes louder with advancing age because of the sagging of the muscle tissue at the back of the mouth. Unless it is merely the temporary result of a stuffed nose or an allergy that has closed up the nasal passages, snoring is difficult to overcome.

soap A substance compounded of fatty acids and alkali, usually with the addition of a pleasant scent. Although all soaps are antiseptic, some contain stronger chemicals than others and may cause contact dermatitis on sensitive skin. Deodorant soaps can effectively slow down the multiplication of bacteria, even though they do not kill them. Soaps containing lanolin are helpful in lubricating dry skin, and medicated soaps contain ingredients that can promote the healing of cracked skin. The vegetable fat in cocoa butter soap is not as effective a lubricant as lanolin.

sodium chloride *See* SALT.

spasm An involuntary contraction of a muscle or group of muscles, usually the consequence of irritation of a nerve. Spasms in which there is an alternation of muscle contraction and relaxation, as occurs in hiccups, are called clonic spasms. When uncontrollable and repetitive spasms are without apparent cause, they are known as tics. Such tics, accompanied by pain, occur in trigeminal neuralgia. Any spasm that affects the entire body is called convulsive, as in the convulsions that accompany some epileptic seizures or that may occur when a high fever irritates the brain.

speculum A metal or plastic instrument with rounded blades which dilate a body passage or cavity to facilitate examination. *See* "Gynecological Diseases and Treatment."

speech disorders Abnormalities in spoken word formation which may be the result of organic anomalies, medication, disease, or emotional stress. For example, disordered speech may be caused by a cleft palate or severe malocclusion, overmedication with tranquilizers or an addictive use of barbiturates, diseases such as parkinsonism or cerebral palsy, conditions such as cumulative hearing loss, and normal occasions of emotional tension resulting in "stammering with embarrassment" or "sputtering with rage." Mild speech defects, such as a lisp or an inability to articulate the *r* or *l* sound correctly, may be a sufficient source of self-consciousness to require concentrated corrective therapy, especially if the defect causes a curtailment of such activities as speaking in public or produces difficulties during job interviews. A pronounced stutter can be agonizing. New audiovisual biofeedback techniques are being used in some speech therapy clinics with varying success depending on the seriousness of the disability. For adult stutterers corrective procedure may combine psychotherapy, medication, and disciplined reeducation of the tempo of word production as well as counseling for family members in how to help the stutterer. Anyone who wishes to consult an accredited speech pathologist can receive helpful information free of charge by writing to the American Speech-Language-Hearing Association, 10801 Rockville Pike, Rockville, Maryland 20852.

sperm   The male germ cell that must penetrate and fertilize the female ovum in order to accomplish conception. Sperm cells, technically called spermatozoa, are produced by the testicles under the stimulation of gonadotropins from the pituitary gland. The cells are carried in the semen which is ejaculated during the climax of sexual intercourse (orgasm). Each sperm cell resembles a translucent tadpole and is about 1/5000 of an inch long, with a flat elliptical head containing a complete set of chromosomes and an elongated tail by which it propels itself through the cervical canal in the direction of the ovum. Of the millions that move upward into the uterus, only a few live long enough to reach the fallopian tubes. If an ovum is available, fertilization may occur. Only one sperm cell ordinarily penetrates. The single penetration barricades the ovum against further penetration, and the processes of reproduction are initiated. Where male infertility exists, the main cause is poor sperm production, either because of testicular disease, general ill health, radiation exposure, dietary deficiency, alcohol, emotional stress, or overheated testicles.

sperm bank   The storage of spermatozoa for future use in artificial in-

semination. Sperm banks are sometimes used by men who have had vasectomies, but this practice, never widespread to begin with, is on the decline since the increasing success of vasectomy reversal surgery. It is considered unlikely that stored sperm continue to be viable and otherwise biologically normal for more than 18 months.

spinal cord   Tissue of the central nervous system that extends downward through the spinal column from the medulla oblongata of the brain to the second lumbar vertebra. The cord is protected by the bony projection of each vertebra, by the thin membranous meninges, and by the cerebrospinal fluid that serves as a shock absorber. The 31 pairs of nerves that extend from the spinal cord control practically all of the body's muscles and transmit sensory impulses to the brain. Thus the consequences of spinal injury or disease depend on the part of it that has been damaged: total paralysis and loss of sensation may occur because of a broken neck, but crushed lumbar bones may not affect the spinal cord at all.

spinal tap   Withdrawal of a sample of cerebrospinal fluid by the insertion of a sterile hollow needle, usually between the third and fourth lumbar vertebrae; also called a lumbar puncture. The fluid sample is subjected to various laboratory analyses that can provide clues to such disorders of the brain or other parts of the nervous system as tumors, encephalitis, meningitis, or polio. A spinal tap is not usually performed unless other diagnostic measures are inconclusive.

spleen   A flattened, oblong organ located behind the stomach in the lower left area of the rib cage. It is purplish red in color and weighs approximately 6 ounces. The spleen acts as a reservoir for red blood cells which it supplies to the bloodstream in any emergencies that diminish oxygen content. Through a network of white cells called phagocytes, the spleen also cleanses the blood of parasites, foreign substances, and damaged red cells. In its paler lymphatic tissue it manufactures the white cells known as lymphocytes which ward off infection. When removal of the spleen is essential because of hemorrhage following an injury, because it is affected by malaria, tuberculosis, or other diseases, or to control thrombocytopenia (shortage of blood platelets) or other diseases, its functions are taken over by the liver and bone marrow.

spotting Irregular or recurrent nonmenstrual bleeding from the uterus, cervix, or vagina. The most common cause of spotting prior to menopause is hormonal imbalance, either natural or resulting from taking oral contraceptives. Causes after menopause are fibroids, endometrial cancer, excess synthetic estrogen. Spotting that occurs after strenuous exercise or sexual intercourse may indicate the presence of cervical polyps or erosions or small vaginal tears. Spotting should be investigated promptly with a pelvic examination, pap smear, and perhaps a D&C. When it occurs during pregnancy, it may signal the onset of a spontaneous abortion. The occurrence should be called to the doctor's attention at once, since a prompt regimen of bed rest may be all that is necessary to prevent the abortion.

sprain An injury to the soft tissues around a joint. Ligaments can be torn or stretched, with damage to associated tendons, blood vessels, and nerves. The severity of a sprain depends on how badly the joint was twisted or wrenched. In some cases the pain is immobilizing and there is considerable swelling accompanied by a large area of discoloration. Since the symptoms are practically indistinguishable from those of a simple fracture, it is sensible to have the injured part X-rayed. If this procedure must be delayed, the following first aid measures should be observed. The injured joint should be elevated and rested on pillows or on a folded blanket. If the site of the sprain (or possible fracture) is in the wrist or elbow, the arm should be supported by a neck sling improvised from a large scarf or a torn sheet. No attempt should be made to strap the joint except by someone properly trained to do so. Rest, application of cold compresses, and aspirin should provide relief from pain and reduce swelling until the doctor can be consulted. In milder injuries the healing process may be hastened by the application of heat the next day, the intermittent application of heat for short periods of time thereafter, and the use of an elasticized bandage.

staphylococcus infection A category of diseases caused by various strains of staphylococcus bacteria, so named for their tendency to grow in grapelike clusters (staphylo) and their round shape (coccus). They are responsible for some types of food poisoning; they produce skin disorders such as impetigo, boils, and sties; and they are also a cause of osteomyelitis, an inflammation of the bones. Staph infections present a particular problem in hospitals, where they are known to cause epidemics among the newborn. Many of these bacteria are now difficult to eradicate because they have developed strains resistant to penicillin and other antibiotics.

sterility   *See* INFERTILITY.

sterilization   Any process that removes the organs of reproduction or makes them incapable of functioning effectively. *See* "Contraception and Abortion."

steroids   *See* CORTICOSTEROIDS.

stethoscope   A diagnostic instrument which amplifies the sounds produced by the lungs, heart, and other organs; used by doctors during the listening part of an examination known as auscultation.

stillbirth   The delivery after the twentieth week of pregnancy of a baby that shows no sign of life.

stimulant   A category of drugs that temporarily increase the activity of a particular part of the body. *See* "Drugs, Alcohol, and Tobacco."

stomach   The pouchlike digestive organ into which food is emptied from the esophagus. The stomach, which leads directly into the duodenum, lies below the diaphragm in the upper left portion of the abdomen, hanging more or less freely and moving with the intake and exhalation of breath. It is composed of three layers of different types of muscle fibers which respond to the need for expansion as the stomach fills with food and are responsible for the rhythmic contractions of peristalsis during which the digestive juices are mixed with the partially digested food and churned into a semiliquid consistency. The full stomach holds about 2½ quarts; when empty, its walls lie flat against each other. The mucous membrane lining contains the glands that secrete hydrochloric acid and the digestive enzymes. The normal functioning of these glands is controlled by the actual presence of food in the stomach and by the neurological reflexes activated by the expectation or the sight of food. Like all glands, those of the stomach can be adversely affected by strong feelings. Anger especially increases the gastric secretion leading to a "churning" sensation and which, if chronic, may eventually be the cause of an ulcer. A sudden attack of anxiety or of acute fear may actually cause paralysis of the muscular wall of the stomach so that it dilates and drops to a lower part of the abdominal cavity resulting in a sinking sensation. Stomach disorders include mild indigestion, chronic or acute gastritis, and ulcers as well as tumors, both benign and malignant.

strain   A mild injury to a muscle, usually caused by subjecting it to unaccustomed tension, as occurs through overexertion or an accident; also called a pulled muscle. (A sprain is more serious, involving stretched or torn ligaments.) Among the most common are twisted ankles caused by a misstep and strained back muscles caused by lifting a heavy weight incorrectly. Wrist muscles may also be strained in various athletic endeavors. The best treatment is rest of the affected part, heat application, an elasticized bandage for support, and a mild painkiller if necessary. Most strained muscles recover in a day or two without further discomfort.

streptococcus infection   A category of diseases caused by strains of streptococcus bacteria, so named for their chainlike arrangement (strepto) and their round shape (coccus). Among the strep-caused disorders are pharyngitis (strep throat), scarlet fever, puerperal fever, and some pneumonias. Rheumatic fever and glomerulonephritis sometimes follow certain strep infections. The species *Streptococcus viridans,* which is normally present in the mouth and harmless for most people, is a cause of subacute bacterial endocarditis in people who have damaged heart valves. Since this species also surrounds the roots of abscessed teeth and since they may enter the bloodstream following the extraction of the tooth, a prophylactic dose of antibiotic medicine, usually penicillin, before a tooth is pulled is always advisable for those who have damaged heart valves.

streptomycin An antibiotic discovered in the 1940s, widely used in the following decades because of its effectiveness against tuberculosis, and more recently abandoned in favor of other medications because of its negative side effects.

stress Physical, chemical, or emotional factors that constrain or exert pressure on body organs or processes and on mental processes; in contemporary, popular usage, psychological pressures. *See* "Your Mind and Feelings."

stretch marks Subcutaneous red streaks that eventually turn into silvery, slightly sunken lines; technically called striae. These marks are usually the result of ruptured skin fibers caused by an excess of subcutaneous fat, by prolonged use of steroids, or in some cases by the distension of the abdomen in pregnancy. Stretch marks typically appear wherever layers of fat are likely to accumulate: on the thighs, abdomen, breasts, and upper arms. When

goiter is present, they will also appear on the neck.

stroke A discontinuity or interruption of the flow of blood to the brain causing a loss of consciousness and, depending on the severity and length of the circulatory deprivation, resulting in partial or complete paralysis of such functions as speech and movement: also known as a cerebrovascular accident and sometimes still called apoplexy. The processes leading to a stroke are cerebral thrombosis, cerebral embolism, and cerebral hemorrhage. When the blood vessels of the brain have been damaged and constricted by atherosclerosis, the formation of a clot may completely block circulatory flow. A similar blockage may occur because an embolus of air, fat, or other foreign matter impedes blood flow to the brain.

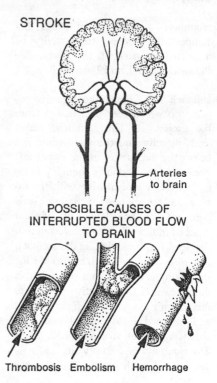

STROKE

Arteries to brain

POSSIBLE CAUSES OF INTERRUPTED BLOOD FLOW TO BRAIN

Thrombosis   Embolism   Hemorrhage

The chief underlying cause of cerebral hemorrhage is a preexisting condition of hypertension, especially in combination with arteriosclerosis or atherosclerosis. The consequences of a stroke, short of being fatal, depend on what part of the brain has been deprived of oxygen and for how long. The deprivation may be so brief as to be inconsequential, an arm or a leg may be paralyzed, speech may be impaired, or the victim may go into a coma. Hospitalization in an intensive care unit must be prompt, since the correct treatment immediately following the stroke and for the first few days afterward is crucial to the amount of recovery achieved by the patient. Physical therapy for the rehabilitation of the affected muscles should begin while the patient is still in bed. A team of medical experts as well as regularly scheduled counseling by the hospital's psychotherapy staff can lead to successful partial rehabilitation.

stuttering *See* SPEECH DISORDERS.

sty An infection of a sebaceous gland at the rim of the eyelid, usually at the root of an eyelash. The infection, which results in inflammation and abscess, is usually caused by staphylococcus bacteria. If it does not respond to home treatment of hot compresses applied for about fifteen minutes every two hours and the use of ophthalmic ointment that can be bought without prescription, a doctor should be consulted. The most likely causes of frequently recurring sties are a generally poor state of health with low resistance to everpresent germs and the careless habit of rubbing the eyes with unwashed hands. Unclean or borrowed articles of eye makeup may also carry infection resulting in sties.

sugar Any of the following sweet carbohydrates found in various foods or chemically derived: sucrose (beets, cane, maple syrup); lactose (milk); maltose (malt products); glucose and dextrose (fruit, honey, corn syrup); fructose (honey, fruit juices); galactose and mannose (do not appear in free form in food); and ribose, xylose, and arabinose (do not appear in free form in foods, but are derived from meat products and seafood). *See also* CARBOHYDRATES, GLUCOSE.

suicide The act of taking one's own life. Since an action intended to result in one's death may be camouflaged as an accident, statistics are incomplete. However, in the United States in 1977 there were 28,681 documented deaths by suicide, making it the ninth leading cause of death. This is an overall rate of 13.3 per 100,000 people, but it ranges from 0.5 for persons aged 5 to 14, to 13.6 for persons 15 to 24, to 21.5 for persons 75 to 84. There are three times as many male suicide deaths as female. In addition to these deaths by suicide there are a large number of suicide attempts, more frequent among women than men, which do not result in death. These are often referred to as "cries for help." Most people who commit suicide are severely depressed for fairly long periods of time prior to taking their lives. Prevention involves recognition of the depression, sometimes by the depressed individual but usually by another, and getting psychiatric help. Anyone who talks seriously about suicide must be considered to be at real risk of suicide and needs help. "Hot lines" for emergency suicide prevention counseling listed in the telephone directory are one source of help. Some people consider activities such as cigarette smoking, high-speed automobile driving, and excessive consumption of alcohol to be self-destructive behavior and therefore related to suicide.

sulfonamides A group of medicines, known as sulfa drugs, that inhibit the growth and reproduction of various bacteria. Because many of these drugs have negative side effects, they have largely been replaced by antibiotics. However, some sulfa drugs, especially sulfadiazine, may be prescribed, often in combination with other sulfa drugs, for meningococcal, *E. Coli,* and other infections.

sunburn Inflammation of the skin caused by overexposure to the ultraviolet rays of the sun or a sunlamp. The lighter the skin, the more quickly it burns. The condition may be limited to a reddening or it may be equivalent to a second-degree burn with blisters and a fever. The best treatment for a mild burn is to avoid the sun for a while and to leave the burned area alone or apply cold, wet dressings to reduce swelling and discomfort. A severe burn may require professional medical attention.

Excessive exposure to sun or a sunlamp does more harm than good for almost everyone. Irrefutable conclusions of medical research indicate that prolonged exposure increases the risks of skin cancer and of wrinkles. For the elderly and anyone with a heart condition, lupus erythematosus, or high blood pressure, the sun can be downright dangerous, especially if there is any possibility of the onset of heat stroke. Women taking certain medicines either for indefinite or short-term therapy should be aware of the fact that overexposure to the sun may produce skin eruptions. While reactions differ in individual cases, the following drugs should be suspected as a possible cause when a rash appears following a period of sitting or lying in the sun: birth-control pills, antihistamines, oral medication for diabetes, diuretics, antibiotics, fungicides, and tranquilizers.

When exposure is unavoidable, sensible precautions should be taken: protective clothing, a brimmed hat, a heavy umbrella, and the use of a cream or lotion containing para-aminobenzoic acid, listed in the contents of over-the-counter sunscreens as PABA in alcohol.

suppositories Medicated substances in solid form, usually conical or cylindrical in shape, to be inserted into the rectum or vagina. The medication is contained in glycerin or fatty material which is melted and diffused by body heat. Suppositories may be recommended as a temporary way of dealing with constipation, especially in order to lubricate feces that have caked within the rectum. Vaginal suppositories containing spermicidal chemicals are available without prescription. They are less reliable contraceptives than creams, jellies, and foams (which are themselves not the last word in reliability), because the effective chemicals in suppositories are not likely to be evenly distributed when they finally diffuse. Vaginitis may be relieved by suitably medicated suppositories; rectal suppositories containing a surface anesthetic may be recommended to relieve the discomfort of pruritis or hemorrhoids.

surgery Operations that repair, remove, remodel, replace, or explore the body's tissues, organs, and cavities using such processes as X-ray, ultrasonics, cautery, and laser beams, as well as such instruments as scissors, knives, and tweezers. Surgery may involve organ transplants (kidneys, corneas, coronary arteries); implants (pacemakers, silicone bags, intraocular lenses), and prosthetic attachments. An operation may be elective, that is, a matter of some degree of choice as in the repair of a hiatus hernia, a tonsillectomy, or the removal of nasal polyps, or it may be a nonelective, often lifesaving or essential, measure as in a crisis dealing with a ruptured appendix, a perforated ulcer, or an ectopic pregnancy. Of the 25 million operations performed in the United States each year, only about 20 percent are considered unequivocally essential. Reasons given for the remaining 80 percent include the prevention of a more complicated problem, pain relief, and improvement of appearance.

Consumer advocates, health insurance companies, and professional medical organizations, including the American College of Surgeons, make the following suggestions about evaluating the need for elective surgery and selecting a surgeon. If the family doctor or an internist suggests a visit to a surgeon based on diagnosis of a particular problem, select, if possible, a surgeon with specialty board credentials. While almost 95,000 doctors perform operations, only about 52,000 have board certification. Also select, if possible, a surgeon who is a Fellow of the American College of Surgeons. While these credentials do not guarantee competence, they do mean that the doctor is (or was) a qualified specialist. The documents are usually highly visible in the consulting office, but if the only way to ascertain credentials is to ask to see them, then do so. When an operation is recommended, get a second opinion from another accredited surgeon unconnected with the first surgeon. Find out if there is a medical alternative to surgery and ask to have all the advantages and disadvantages of

either choice spelled out. If surgery is decided upon, make every effort to have the operation performed by a surgeon on the staff of a teaching hospital. Find out in advance what coverage is provided by your health insurance policy, including the cost of the anesthesiologist's services and of the postoperative visits to the surgeon's office. *See also* ANESTHESIA, HOSPITALIZATION, "You, Your Doctors, and the Health Care System," "Gynecologic Diseases and Treatment," "Cosmetic Surgery."

surrogate mother A woman who contracts to bear a child for another woman who is sterile. The pregnancy is achieved by artificial insemination with sperm, usually from the partner of the sterile woman. The surrogate mother agrees to turn the baby over for adoption right after birth to the couple or sterile woman who pay for all the medical and legal expenses involved. In some cases, surrogate mothers act voluntarily; in others, they receive a large fee for their services. Most of the moral and legal questions raised by this procedure have yet to be resolved.

swelling An abnormal enlargement, inflation, or distension of any part of the body occurring either internally or externally. Swelling of the lymph nodes (mistakenly called swollen glands) accompanies such infections as mononucleosis, parasitic invasions such as filariasis, cancers such as leukemia and Hodgkin's disease, and the condition commonly called blood poisoning and technically known as septicemia. Swellings that follow a bruise are usually minor, resulting from the fact that there is bleeding into the bruised tissues. The puffy swelling that indicates edema typically occurs because of circulatory failure or because of abnormalities in the composition of blood as occurs in the nephrotic syndrome. Internal organs may swell when diseased as occurs in cirrhosis of the liver. A swelling under the skin may be a sebaceous cyst. When bacterial infection is the cause, the condition may be a boil. Allergies and abscesses of any kind result in swelling. The superficial bumps that occur after an insect bite or the hives that erupt because of an allergic response are a consequence of the liberation of histamine into the skin. Any swelling of mysterious origin that persists, especially if it is accompanied by pain, should be diagnosed by a doctor without too much delay.

syndrome A group of signs and symptoms that occur together and characterize a particular disease or abnormal condition.

syphilis *See* "Sexually Transmissible Diseases."

tampon A plug of absorbent cotton or similar material placed within a body cavity in order to soak up secretions and hemorrhagic blood, and especially to contain the menstrual flow. Tampons for this latter purpose are designed for easy insertion into the vaginal opening and for removal by an attached string. Where the hymen is still unruptured, tampons may be difficult and occasionally impossible to insert. Recent attention has focused on tampon use because of its connection with a severe and acute disease known as toxic shock syndrome. Package labeling should therefore be given serious consideration by tampon users of all ages, but especially by younger women. *See* TOXIC SHOCK SYNDROME; "Gynecologic Diseases and Treatment."

Tay-Sachs disease An incurable and usually fatal genetic disease of fat metabolism found almost exclusively among Jews of central and eastern Europe. There is a statistical probability that in 1 of 900 marriages of these Ashkenazic Jews, both partners will be carriers of the gene. Genetic counseling in advance of a pregnancy is considered advisable for those who might be carriers. When the pregnancy already exists, amniocentesis can determine whether the fetus has the disease. Should this be the case, a therapeutic abortion usually is possible.

TB *See* TUBERCULOSIS.

tear glands *See* LACRIMAL DUCTS.

teeth *See* DENTAL CARE, ORTHODONTIA.

telemetry The long-distance transmission by electronic signals of measurement data and other information. Telemetric devices, originally developed for rocketry and space science, have been adapted for attachment to telephones so that, for example, a doctor in a rural hospital can transmit a patient's electrocardiogram or electroencephalogram to medical specialists thousands of miles away for further evaluation. The technique is also widely used for testing artificial pacemaker competence by telephone.

temperature *See* FEVER.

tension Physical and emotional response to stress. *See* "Your Mind and Feelings."

Terramycin Brand name of oxytetracycline, one of the broad spectrum antibiotics. *See* TETRACYCLINE.

test tube baby A birth resulting from the conception of a human embryo outside its mother's body. In cases where infertility is caused by defective or diseased fallopian tubes, a mature ovum is removed surgically from a woman. It is placed in a laboratory dish along with sperm. If conception occurs, the fertilized ovum is implanted into the woman's uterus within a few days of the "in vitro" (in a glass) conception. It is then possible for pregnancy to continue normally. This technique, also known as a tubal bypass, was perfected by two English doctors and resulted in the first "in vitro" conception birth in 1978. On December 28, 1981, the first American test tube baby was born in Richmond, Virginia.

testicles The principal male organs of reproduction; the sex organs; also called testes. The testicles are located within the scrotum and produce the hormone testosterone which determines the secondary sex characteristics of the male at puberty: deep voice, hair distribution, body build, and sexual drive. They also produce sperm cells. Each testis contains about 250 lobules in which tiny tubes produce the spermatozoa which leave the testicles at maturity by way of the convoluted passage called the epididymis. Removal of the testes (castration) before puberty causes male sterility and prevents the development of male sex characteristics. Castration following puberty also causes sterility, but the diminishment of male sexuality can be compensated for by testosterone injections. Castration is done occasionally to treat metastatic cancer of the prostate because the progress of this type of cancer is slowed by the absence of testosterone which is secreted by the testes.

tetanus An acute infectious disease caused by the entrance into the body through a break in the skin of the microorganism *Clostridium tetani*. A tetanus-prone wound is one which is deep, has much tissue damage and necrosis (destruction), is uncleaned for four or more hours, and is contaminated by soil or street dirt. The exotoxin produced by the *C. tetani* bacteria affects the nervous system in such a way as to cause paralyzing muscle spasms, hence the term lockjaw to describe one of the early symptoms. The tetanus bacilli grow in the intestines of all mammals and are found in soil and dust contaminated by the feces of the carriers. Once a widespread and fatal disease, particularly in rural areas and in wars, it affects fewer than 500 people a year in this country, thanks to routine immunization of infants and booster shots for children and adults. Any injury which might be a tetanus-prone wound is sufficient reason for consulting the closest doctor within 24 hours about the proper immunization and other protective measures. All wounds should be cleaned promptly and thoroughly. See Immunization Guide, p. 738.

tetracycline A broad spectrum antibiotic prepared synthetically or derived from several species of the genus of funguslike bacteria (Streptomyces) found in soil. The tetracyclines have no effect on viruses; they are usually prescribed, especially for patients with penicillin sensitivity for such bacterial infections as gonorrhea, pneumonia, bronchitis, meningitis and for the rickettsial diseases. Among their undesirable side effects are skin rashes and gastrointestinal irritation. They may discolor teeth and interfere with the bone development of a child whose mother took tetracycline in the last half of pregnancy, so they are contraindicated after the fourth month of pregnancy. For similar reasons the American Medical Association recommends that other antibiotics be prescribed for children under 8 years of age. Two of the brand names under which tetracyclines are sold are Aureomycin and Achromycin.

thermography A technique for recording variations in skin temperature by the use of photographic film sensitive to the infrared radiation given off by the surface of the body. The result of the test is called a thermogram. Because tumor cells produce somewhat more heat than normal ones, this procedure can be helpful in the detection of incipient breast cancer. Thermography is noninvasive, but for purposes of diagnostic accuracy it is not as definitive as mammography.

thiamin One of the B complex vitamins; also known as vitamin B_1. A deficiency of vitamin B_1 leads to neurological disorders, especially to the psychosis known as Korsakoff's syndrome, characterized by memory impairment and time and place disorientation, to paralysis of the extremities (beriberi), and to heart failure. People who eat substandard diets and those whose food is overcooked (thiamin is destroyed by heat) may not be getting enough B_1 in their food. Signs of deficiency can be detected by a doctor and corrected with a prescribed regimen of thiamin. *See* "Nutrition and Weight."

Thorazine Brand name of chlorpromazine.

throat disorders Any disease or malfunction affecting the pharynx or the larynx. *See* STREP THROAT, TONSILS, GLOBUS HYSTERICUS, etc.

thrombosis The formation of a clot, technically called a thrombus, in a blood vessel, most commonly in a varicose vein in the leg or in any artery in which the interior walls are roughened by atherosclerosis. The blockage of a narrow blood vessel by a thrombus may have grave consequences: when the obstruction occurs in one of the coronary arteries (coronary thrombosis), the result may be a major heart attack; obstructive thrombosis in the brain is a cause of stroke. A complication of thrombosis is thromboembolism in which a part of the clot breaks off to form what is called an embolism, circulates to other parts of the body, and causes obstruction, as in pulmonary thromboembolism. The risks of thrombosis increase not only with age, but with the use of the contraceptive pill, particularly among cigarette smokers. Two drugs used specifically to treat or prevent thrombosis are heparin, which is given intravenously or subcutaneously, and coumarin, which is taken orally. These drugs are called anticoagulants. There are also a number of drugs which have an anticoagulant effect especially when combined with coumarin. Included among these are steroids, salicylates (aspirin), and sulfonamides.

thyroid disorders *See* GOITER, HYPERTHYROIDISM.

tic Involuntary and repeated spasmodic contractions of a muscle or group of muscles; also called habit spasms or nervous tics. Such movements usually develop in childhood in response to emotional stress, and while they may subside from time to time during adulthood, they almost inevitably return during periods of fatigue or tension. Among the more common tics are blinking, clearing the throat, jerking the head, twitching the lips. Psychotherapy and tranquilizers can sometimes eliminate a tic, but the former treatment may be too time-consuming and too expensive and the latter may lead to problems more unpleasant than the tic itself. The specific instance in which involuntary spasms of facial muscles originate in a physical disorder is the symptom known as tic douloureux discussed under TRIGEMINAL NEURALGIA.

ticks Blood-sucking parasites. Some ticks are comparatively harmless, but others transmit disease. *See* RICKETT-SIAL DISEASES, ROCKY MOUNTAIN SPOTTED FEVER, TYPHUS.

tinnitus The sensation of hearing sounds—humming, buzzing, ringing—that originate within the ear rather than as a result of an outside stimulus. Tinnitus should not be confused with the auditory hallucinations of some mental illnesses. The buzzing and ringing may be the temporary result of a blocked eustachian tube such as occurs during an upper respiratory infection or an allergic response. It may also occur after a head injury, following exposure to an extraordinarily loud noise, or as a side effect of certain medications, especially streptomycin. The diseases with which it is associated are Menière's disease, otosclerosis, and brain tumor, but most cases are of mysterious origin. If the noises can be ignored, so much the better. When they are disturbingly intrusive at bedtime, they can be masked by soft music from a nearby radio. In recent years, ultrasonic irradiation of the inner ear has achieved some success. Where a hearing problem is also present, an electronic device that produces a sound that masks

the noise of tinnitus can be fitted inside the casing of the ordinary hearing aid.

Tolinase Brand name of one of the oral diabetic drugs that stimulate the pancreas to produce insulin. Because of their implication in the deaths of diabetics from cardiovascular causes, these drugs are considered to be a less desirable means of controlling the disease than proper diet and weight management alone or, when necessary, combined with insulin.

tonsils Two clumps of spongy lymphoid tissue lying one on each side of the throat, visible behind the back of the tongue between the folded membranes that lead to the soft palate. Together with the adenoids, which are located behind the nose at the opening of the eustachian tube, the tonsils function somewhat like filters, guarding the respiratory tract against foreign invasion. When they become infected, inflamed, or enlarged, they are the source of complications leading to difficulties in swallowing and to the spread of the infectious agent to surrounding tissues. When the infection is streptococcal (strep throat), antibiotic treatment must be prompt to prevent the further complication of kidney infection or heart involvement. When enlarged tonsils are a chronic cause of respiratory difficulties over several years or when the adenoids constantly transmit infection to the sinuses or the middle ear, removal by surgery should be considered. However, a tonsillectomy or adenoidectomy should not be undertaken without substantial indication that the operation is justifiable as a health measure.

toxemia The presence in the bloodstream of poisonous compounds (toxins), especially those produced by various pathogenic microorganisms; popularly called blood poisoning, also called septicemia. The toxemia of pregnancy is different and is discussed under ECLAMPSIA.

toxic shock syndrome A rare condition, fatal in some cases, characterized by high fever, diarrhea, vomiting, a dramatic drop in blood pressure, and a rash. The syndrome is associated in almost all reported instances with the use of menstrual tampons, especially highly absorbent tampons, and is thought to be caused by toxins produced by staphylococcus bacteria. TSS came to public attention in 1980. Since then there appears to have been a decline in the number of cases, perhaps because few women are now using highly absorbent tampons and more women are using only sanitary pads. Whether frequent changing of tampons and using only pads while sleeping is a successful preventive measure remains uncertain.

toxoplasmosis A parasitic infection transmitted to humans usually in the fecal droppings of cats and occasionally by eating infected meat. It usually produces symptoms so mild as to escape detection or to be mistaken for a cold. However, congenital toxoplasmosis, in which the infectious organisms are transmitted by the recently infected and thus previously nonimmune mother to the fetus, may be the cause of miscarriage, stillbirth, or irreversible birth defects. Animals which harbor the parasite usually show no symptoms. However, laboratory analysis of their stools will indicate whether or not this parasite is present. Pregnant women should avoid handling cat feces.

tranquilizers A category of drugs that suppress anxiety symptoms or modify disturbed behavior without effecting a cure. Tranquilizers (also called relaxants) are designated as minor if they have only the effect of allaying stress and as major if they alter such psychotic manifestations as hysteria, hallucinations, extreme aggressiveness, or suicidal tendencies. The minor tranquilizers are the most commonly prescribed drugs in the United States, especially those that are members of the benzodiazepine group (Valium, Librium). The major tranquilizers (Stelazine, Thorazine) can be numbing and, in large doses, fatal. All tranquilizers have the potential of producing mild to extremely adverse side effects. When combined with alcohol, barbiturates, antihypertensive medicines, diuretics, and antihistamines, they can result in death. Tranquilizers of any kind should be avoided especially during the early months of pregnancy, since they can cause irreversible damage to the fetus. *See also* "Drugs, Alcohol, and Tobacco."

transcendental meditation *See* MEDITATION.

transfusion The transfer of blood or any of its components—plasma, serum, platelets—from a specific donor or from a blood bank to a recipient. When the transfusion involves whole blood, correct matching of the blood type, including the Rh factor, is a vital consideration. Plasma, serum, and platelets are compatible among all donors and recipients. Transfusions are common practice not only in life-saving circumstances, but in any situation when replenishment of the blood supply is routine therapy. Among the more frequent causes of varying amounts of blood loss are burns, other injuries, delivery, and surgical complications. In most cases the transfusion is indirect, that is, the blood comes from a blood bank and is not transferred directly from one person to another. The technique of exchange transfusion, in which blood is simultaneously taken from the donor to replace the blood as it is removed from the recipient, is used rarely.

transplant The transfer of an organ or of tissue from one individual to another; the term is also used for the organ itself and for the grafting of skin from one part of the body to the other. Corneal transplants have the fewest complications. Following these, the most frequently and successfully transplanted organs are kidneys. Since the first successful transfer of a human heart in 1967 in South Africa, hundreds of similar operations have been performed throughout the world with varying length of survival. Liver and pancreas transplants are attempted occasionally, usually unsuccessfully. In 1976 the first successful transplant of bone marrow was accomplished. The biggest problem still to be solved in practically all such operations is the rejection by the recipient's immune system of the donor organ as a foreign invasion. This rejection, known as graft-versus-host disease (GVH), can eventually produce fatal liver damage and bone marrow disease. Until the recognition of blood types, transfusions, actually a type of tissue transfer, frequently resulted in the death of the recipient for this reason. Thus, in the case of kidney transplants, whether the organ comes from a close relative or a complete stranger, the recipient must take medicine over a lifetime to prevent rejection. The medicine, which includes various chemicals that suppress the body's immune responses, has to be adjusted in careful amounts: if there is too little immune suppression, the transplanted organ will be destroyed by the recipient's antibodies; if there is too much immune suppression, the recipient becomes vulnerable to fatal bacterial invasion.

If more lives are to be saved by organ transplants, the general public must become aware of the importance of donating organs to transplant banks. Most states now permit residents to register their organs for donation when they renew their driver's license. Community efforts of this kind have as their goal the routine, legally binding donation at the time of brain-death of hearts, kidneys, livers, eyes, and other potentially useful body tissues.

tremor Involuntary shaking or quivering, usually of the hands, but also of the head or other parts of the body. Tremors may be coarse or fine, depending on the amplitude of the oscillation. They may occur when the body is at rest, ceasing when intentional movement occurs, or they may occur only during acts of volition. They may be slow or rapid, intermittent or continuous, and symptomatic of organic diseases that affect the central nervous system or of an emotional disturbance. They may accompany a chill or fever or may be one of the symptoms of withdrawal from alcohol, cocaine, barbiturates, and other drugs. Among the diseases with which tremor is associated are cerebral palsy, multiple sclerosis, parkinsonism, hyperthyroidism, arteriosclerosis of the brain, and late syphilis. The trembling that accompanies an anxiety attack or the onset of hysteria may be controlled by sedatives. When an organic disorder is the cause, the tremor usually diminishes with proper treatment of the disease.

trench mouth *See* GUMS.

trichomonas vaginalis A species of parasite that can cause vaginal inflammation in females and urethral inflammation in males; also called trichomoniasis. *See* "Sexually Transmissible Diseases."

trigeminal neuralgia Intermittent and acute sensitivity of the fifth cranial nerve (the sensory nerve of the face); also known as tic douloureux. The condition is characterized by the sudden and unpredictable onset of paroxysms of extreme pain seemingly unaccompanied by any change in the nerve itself. The disorder is of unknown origin. It is more common among women than men and rarely occurs before middle age. The spasms of pain may be triggered by such random circumstances as a draft of cold air, blowing the nose, or an anxiety attack. Spontaneous remission may occur after a month of attacks, with recurrence months or years later. Drug therapy provides some pain relief; in some cases the most effective treatment is injecting the nerve with alcohol. When these measures fail to produce results and the recurrent attacks become so frequent and so painful that they interfere with eating and interrupt sleep, neurosurgery may be recommended.

triglycerides A group of fats, also called lipids, derived from the fatty content of ingested food. Together with cholesterol, triglycerides are among the essential cell nutrients. In excessive amounts they may accumulate within the walls of the blood vessels and cause atherosclerosis. Triglyceride blood levels are measurable in laboratory tests, and when the levels are considered a threat to health, attempts to lower them are usually recommended. Countermeasures may include weight loss, change in eating habits, and, if hormonal imbalance is thought to be involved, a contraceptive other than the pill.

tubal ligation A method of sterilization in which the fallopian tubes are tied in such a way that the ovum becomes inaccessible for fertilization. *See* "Contraception and Abortion."

tuberculosis A major infectious disease caused by the tubercle bacillus which usually attacks the lungs and less frequently the bones, joints, kidneys, or other parts of the body; once called phthisis and consumption, now commonly referred to as TB. The disease continues to flourish wherever poverty, poor diet, and crowded substandard living conditions prevail. The infectious organisms are spread through the air from person to person on the coughs and sneezes of anyone with the disease in an active stage. Public health authorities know that in the United States and especially in urban areas, many millions have been infected with the bacillus and are carrying it in their bodies in latent form without knowing it. If resistance is high, the bacilli may be killed by white blood cells, or they may be walled up temporarily and immobilized in small masses called tubercles. Many people have gone through an active TB episode, mistaking the symptoms, if any, for those of a heavy cold: a cough, chest pains, and feelings of fatigue. Such an occurrence usually leaves a small area of scar tissue in the affected part of the lungs. It is not at all uncommon for a woman between the ages of 20 and 40 to take a tuberculin skin test as part of a thorough physical checkup and to be told that the results are positive. Under these circumstances a chest X-ray is suggested to find out if the lungs show any active disease. If the patient does not have active disease, prophylactic medication is often prescribed to suppress the possibility of later activation of the dormant disease. Antituberculosis drugs almost always are completely effective in treating the active disease. Witness to their effectiveness is the closing down of practically all TB sanitariums. Treatment for active cases may begin in a hospital, but the patient is sent home as soon as the noninfectious stage is reached to resume all normal activities while continuing to take the prescribed medications. The most important of these for prophylactic purposes is isoniazid. Several drugs exist for treating the disease. Anyone suffering from a chronic cough, chest pains, breathing difficulties, chronic feelings of fatigue, weight loss, heavy sweating at night, and irregularity in the menstrual cycle is advised to have these symptoms checked to rule out the possibility of TB.

tumor A swelling in or on a particular area of the body, usually created by the development of a mass of new tissue cells having no function. Tumors may be benign or malignant; benign tumors may, but usually do not, become malignant. The presence of a tumor within the body may be unsuspected until it grows large enough to produce symptoms of pain or to interfere with the normal function of an adjacent organ or nerve. Diagnosis by biopsy determines whether the growth is cancerous or not. A malignant tumor may be treated surgically or with radiotherapy and chemotherapy. A benign growth may or may not be removed surgically, depending on its location and its potential for becoming cancerous. *See also* SWELLING.

Tylenol Brand name of an analgesic containing no aspirin; the active chemical compound is acetaminophen. It is a useful over-the-counter medication for the reduction of fever and relief of pain for individuals who are hypersensitive to aspirin in any form.

typhoid fever An acute and highly contagious disease caused by the bacterial bacillus *Salmonella typhosa* (related to the bacteria that cause food poisoning); also called enteric fever. Typhoid and paratyphoid infections are endemic wherever the laxity of public health measures results in the contamination of the food and water supplies by urine and feces containing the disease-bearing organisms. Flies may transmit the disease; restaurant workers or food handlers who have had the disease may be carriers who spread the disease unless they are scrupulous in matters of personal hygiene. The infection may also be transmitted by shellfish from contaminated waters. In a case of typhoid fever, the bacteria attack the mucous membranes of the small intestine, producing stools and occasionally urine containing the typhoid bacteria. Symptoms begin after an incubation period of about two weeks and include fever, headache, vomiting, stomach cramps, fatigue and mental disorientation. A rash of a few days' duration may erupt on the chest and abdomen. Milder cases subside spontaneously within a week or so. However, in a severe case the patient may go into delirium as the fever rises. Perforation of the bowel may occur at this stage. Fortunately, antibiotics with or without corticosteroids will effect a complete cure when administered before major complications occur. Immunization against typhoid fever in adulthood is considerably less trouble than the infection and is at least moderately effective. Travelers to those parts of the world where the disease is endemic are therefore advised to get the necessary shots against it. Since three successive inoculations are necessary over a three-week period, the immunization or the booster shots should be planned well in advance of departure.

typhus An infectious rickettsial disease transmitted by the body louse. The disease is endemic in parts of Asia, Africa, and on the shores of the Mediterranean. In another form known as flea typhus it is common in the Far East and the Southwest Pacific. Typhus is not related to typhoid fever in any way. The onset of the disease begins with a headache, acute pains in the legs and back, and sieges of uncontrollable shivering. Within a few days a rash spreads from the torso to the arms and legs, and high fever may cause delirium. Antibiotic treatment is usually effective. Untreated typhus has a death rate of one case in five. The literature of the Western world contains many accounts of typhus epidemics, especially those that occurred during the major wars. While the use of DDT effectively halted the pandemics of typhus following World War II, outbreaks still occur where primitive and overcrowded living conditions prevail. Travelers to places where the disease

is prevalent should have an antityphus vaccination which provides immunity for about one year.

ulcer A chronic lesion in the epithelial tissue either on the visible surface of the body or on the lining of an interior cavity such that the tissues below the skin or mucous membrane may be exposed. Ulcers may occur for many reasons: poor circulation (bedsores, ulcerated varicose veins), infections by microorganisms (ulcerated gums, syphilitic sores), and damage caused by extremes of heat, cold, malignant growths, or chemicals.

Peptic ulcers include gastric ulcers, which occur in the stomach itself, and duodenal ulcers, which occur in the upper portion of the small intestines and are ten times more common than gastric ulcers. The immediate cause of

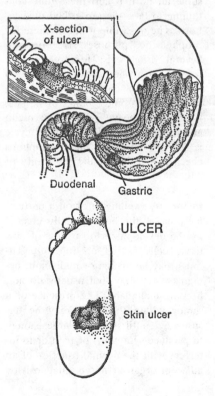

X-section of ulcer

Duodenal   Gastric

ULCER

Skin ulcer

peptic ulcers is the secretion of hydrochloric acid when there is no food in the alimentary canal to neutralize its corrosive effects. The disorder cuts across age, sex, and class. Men used to be the chief victims by far, but now half the patients are women. Children can also suffer from peptic ulcers. Peptic ulcers have long been considered one of the most typical of the psychosomatic illnesses, and there is no doubt that emotional stress is a major contributing cause. Evidence has accumulated to indicate that blood relatives of people with ulcers are likelier to develop them than other people, especially if they share blood type O. When the potential vulnerability exists, there is no doubt that it is exacerbated by tension, alcohol, spicy food, nicotine, and the caffeine in coffee, tea, cola drinks, even in decaffeinated coffee. An ulcer that is diagnosed and treated when the symptoms first appear is more likely to heal quickly and less likely to recur than if it is ignored or treated with home remedies for indigestion. The first indication is a burning pain that recurs a few hours after eating. When the condition worsens to the point where the acid that has been burning a hole in the mucous membrane eventually eats into a blood vessel and causes a hemorrhage, the condition (bleeding ulcer) requires hospitalization and emergency treatment. The presence of an ulcer is visible in an X-ray picture after the patient has swallowed barium. Conventional treatment consists in certain dietary prohibitions and recommendations combined with supervised medication. A comparatively new antihistamine drug that inhibits gastric secretions with no apparent undesirable side effects is the chemical compound known generically as cimetidine and sold under the brand name Tagamet.

umbilical cord The structure that connects the fetus to the placenta of the mother, functioning as a lifeline through which maternal blood is transmitted to the fetus and fetal blood is returned to the mother. At the time of birth the umbilical cord, which is approximately 2 feet long and is attached at what is to become the infant's navel, is tied at two points close to each other and cut in between them. The vestige dries out and falls off naturally within less than a week.

undulant fever A disease caused by drinking unpasteurized milk taken from cows (also from sheep or goats) infected with Brucella microorganisms; also called brucellosis or Malta fever. In rare cases improperly cooked meat contaminated with these microorganisms also can be a source of the disease. Characteristic symptoms are pains in the joints, fatigue, chills, and a fever that may rise and fall at various times of the day or be low in the morning and rise slowly to 104°F by evening. These fluctuations in temperature account for the name of the disorder. If the disease goes untreated, the liver, spleen, and lymph nodes become swollen and sore. Since the symptoms may be confused with those of mononucleosis or rheumatic fever, a blood test should be made so that the nature of the infectious agent can be identified. The disease is curable with antibiotics. It is inadvisable to drink unpasteurized milk (unless instructed to do so by a doctor for some particular condition), even from a herd that has been government-inspected.

uremia *See* KIDNEY DISORDERS.

ureter One of two tubes, each about 12 inches in length, connecting the kidney to the bladder. The urine produced in the kidney is transmitted by the muscular contractions of the ureters into the bladder, where it is stored until it passes through the urethra in the act of urination. Inflammation of the ureter (ureteritis) may result from the presence of a stone or cysts as well as from infection.

urethra The muscular tube, approximately 1½ inches long in women, that carries urine from the bladder to the exterior. Both sexes are vulnerable to urethritis (inflammation of the urethra) caused by gonorrhea infection. Contamination by other infectious organisms during catheterization or as a result of bladder infection is also common. Symptoms of urethritis include painful urination, swelling of the vulva, and a yellowish puslike discharge from the urethra. When untreated, the condition may develop into cystitis. When inflammation over a considerable period causes scar tissue to develop, the urethra may become so constricted that surgical correction is indicated.

urination The excretion through the urethra of liquid wastes stored in the bladder. The fluid secreted by the kidneys travels through the ureters into the bladder where it accumulates. The urine accumulated within the bladder is prevented from flowing into the urethra by the internal sphincter of the urethra (a sphincter is a circular muscle in a state of involuntary contraction). When the stimulus from a full bladder is transformed into a conscious effort to urinate, the bladder muscles are contracted and the sphincter is relaxed. The external sphincter of the urethra is also relaxed. These motor reflexes result in the deliberate discharge of accumulated urine through the urethra to the exterior. The act of passing urine is technically called micturition. Conscious sphincter control may be reduced temporarily in adults by acute fear or some other emotionally charged reaction. It may also be a sign of a neurological disease such as epilepsy or the result of a stroke. Loss or impairment of bladder control, technically called incontinence, may be a consequence of infection of the bladder or other part of the urinary tract, displaced pelvic organs, and, especially in aging men, disease of the prostate gland.

About 1 quart of urine is eliminated each day, somewhat more during cold weather and less during hot weather, since in warmer weather larger amounts of fluid wastes are eliminated through the skin in the form of sweat. On the average women urinate about four times daily, with frequency depending on the amount and type of liquid consumed, state of health, age, and other variables. For example, the consumption of large amounts of tea or coffee may increase frequency of urination not only because of the extra fluid, but also because caffeine is a mild diuretic. Frequency increases during pregnancy not only because the uterus presses on the bladder, but also because nutritional demands require a greater intake of liquids, especially of milk. The need to urinate more frequently occurs in older women as a consequence of a natural loss of muscle tone.

Any persistent abnormal sensations during the act of urination or any sudden changes in frequency or color should be reported to a doctor. Painful urination accompanied by a burning sensation is symptomatic of infections that affect the bladder or urethra. The sudden onset of abnormally frequent urination may be caused by cystitis, diabetes, or incipient kidney failure. An inability to empty the bladder completely is usually related to interference by a stone, a tumor, or partial blockage by pressure from a prolapsed uterus or to neurological disease.

urine tests The examination of a urine specimen by various laboratory procedures; also called urinalysis. Since normal urine is of constant composition within definite limits, changes in the color, consistency, clarity, or specific gravity are usually, but not always, a sign of disorder. Thus, every complete physical checkup, whether during health or illness and especially at frequent intervals during pregnancy, should always include a urine test as well as questions about urination. Any visible changes in the color of urine, which is normally a pale amber, might suggest disease. Laboratory tests check for the following abnormalities. Albuminuria (proteinuria) is the presence in the urine of certain proteins (albumins) indicating the possibility of kidney disease, inflammations such as cystitis or urethritis, or, during pregnancy, pre-eclampsia. Albuminuria may also be a response to certain drugs, and it may exist from time to time without pathological significance in the condition known as postural or orthostatic albuminuria. Glucosuria is the consistent presence in the urine of glucose (not the occasional presence of one of the other sugars) and is usually the indication of diabetes. Hematuria, or blood in the urine, warrants further examination by instruments (cystoscopy) or X-ray if the hematuria persists in order to discover what part of the urinary tract is the source of the bleeding. Among the more common causes are the presence of a kidney

stone, a tumor, or some degree of kidney failure. Pyuria, or white blood cells in the urine, is an indication of an infection of the urinary tract, in most cases cystitis or urethritis. Urine can be cultured to ascertain whether and what bacteria are present.

urologist   *See* DOCTOR.

uterus   The hollow, pear-shaped, muscular organ situated in the pelvis above the bladder; also called the womb. When a woman is not pregnant, the uterus is about 3 inches long, 2 inches wide, and 1 inch thick; it weighs about 2 ounces. As the cradle containing the fully developed fetus, it will weigh as much as 30 ounces and expand greatly in size. The uterus is suspended within the pelvis by the uterine ligaments which are extended like wings. The fal-

**POSSIBLE LOCATIONS OF
UTERINE FIBROIDS**

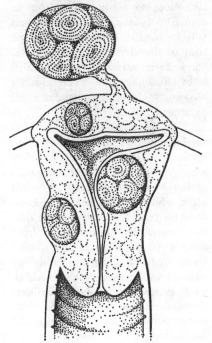

lopian tubes enter the upper part at each side. The broad and flat portion of the uterus is called the body; the lower part which opens downward into the vagina is the neck or narrow tubular cervix. During a gynecological examination the insertion of the speculum as far as the cervix enables the doctor to see many of the abnormal conditions that might affect the uterine area. Any cell changes that might be indicative of malignancy are detected microscopically during a pap test. The muscular walls of the uterus are lined with mucous membrane called endometrium that goes through the monthly changes as part of the menstrual cycle. This cycle is interrupted by pregnancy during which the lining of the uterus in its secretory stage anchors the placenta through which the fertilized egg is nourished. Among the more common disorders of the uterus are benign growths called fibroid tumors, prolapse (the dropping of the uterus from its normal position), and displacement (the forward or backward tilt of the body of the uterus from the cervix). Surgical removal of the uterus is called a hysterectomy. *See* "The Healthy Woman," "Gynecologic Diseases and Treatment."

vaccination Inoculation with a preparation of dead or attenuated live germs for purposes of immunization against a specific disease. The word itself, which derives from the Latin word for cow, was created at the time that Jenner developed vaccine from cowpox as a method of immunizing humans against smallpox. Until very recently, vaccination has been used almost exclusively to mean smallpox vaccination. The word is now used synonymously with inoculation and immunization.

vaccine A preparation of dead or weakened live microorganisms or of other effective agents injected into the body of humans or animals for the purpose of stimulating the production of antibodies against a particular disease without producing disease symptoms.

vacuum curettage *See* DILATATION AND EVACUATION.

vagina The passageway that slopes upward and backward from the external genitals, the vulva, to the cervix; the female organ of sexual intercourse. Within the pelvic cavity the bladder is in front of the vagina and the rectum is behind it. In the normal adult woman the empty vagina is about 3 inches long. It receives the male spermatozoa; it is also the conduit for the menstrual discharge and the final passage through which the fetus travels at birth. The vaginal opening is partially closed by the hymen, until the hymen is stretched or ruptured by intercourse, use of tampons, or physical activity. The mucous membranes that line the vaginal walls normally secrete a fluid that is acidified by normal bacteria, thus creating a chemical environment that protects the tissues from invasion by various harmful microorganisms. This environment is likely to be destroyed by douching with strong chemicals, by the use of vaginal sprays, and by certain antibiotic medicines. Under normal circumstances and especially during sexual excitation, the vaginal discharge is thin and practically odorless. During a pelvic examination, the vagina is inspected for cysts or tumors and the possible development of a fistula. Another standard procedure is the insertion of the doctor's rubber-gloved fingers into the vagina at the same time that the other hand presses down on the outside of the abdomen. In this way the uterus and ovaries are palpated (diagnosed by touch) for any signs of cysts, tumors, or other abnormalities. Aside from the changes in the vaginal walls during pregnancy when hormonal activities affect the muscles, membranes, and discharges, any unusual symptoms should be discussed with the doctor. Symptoms that require professional diagnosis include itching, burning, the onset of pain during intercourse, the formation of ulcers, and the discharge of pus.

vaginal care Since the vagina of a healthy woman is a self-cleansing organ, daily washing of the outer genital area with soap and water normally provides sufficient care. Many doctors feel that habitual douching, for hygiene, contraception, or medical treatment, may be harmful rather than beneficial. Douching and the many vaginal sprays on the market are likely to inhibit the natural secretions of the vaginal tissues, causing dryness and consequent irritation to the membranes. They also destroy the healthy bacterial environment of the area, upsetting the normal acidity that discourages the proliferation of damaging microorganisms. The genitalia of the healthy woman have a characteristic odor which is not unpleasant and which is sexually stimulating. Not only do sprays mask this odor, but they may also mask a malodorous discharge that should be diagnosed, not deodorized. As a method of birth control, douching alone is ineffective since it takes only about 90 seconds for sperm to reach the cervix after they have been ejaculated. When a mild infection does exist, a douche consisting of 2 tablespoons of distilled white vinegar in 1 quart of warm water will increase the acidity of the vaginal environment and

discourage the spread of the infection. In cases of infertility where postcoital tests indicate the necessity for doing so, douching with bicarbonate of soda will alkalize the cervical environment, thus improving the chances of preserving the viability of sperm cells. With increasing age, the mucous secretions of the vagina tend to dry up, and the tissues are therefore more easily irritated. At this time, a mild nonprescription lubricating jelly or cream similar to the one used by the doctor during a pelvic examination should be applied before sexual intercourse.

vaginal discharge Any emission from the vagina, including the menstrual flow, the secretion of a clear, slippery lubricating fluid during sexual intercourse, and between periods a mucoid secretion from the cervix. A vaginal discharge is abnormal if it has a bad odor, is thick and cheesy in consistency, is yellowish or greenish in color, or is tinged with blood between periods or after the menopause. A burning or itching sensation is another indication of abnormal discharge. When the disorder exists, it may be caused by mechanical irritation (IUD), chemical irritation (sprays and douches), or infection by fungi, bacteria, or other microorganisms. Blood-streaked discharge may be a symptom of fibroids, other tumors, or cysts or of some other cervical or uterine disorder. While any abnormal discharge should be diagnosed and treated if it persists, prompt attention is especially indicated if there is any change in vaginal secretions during pregnancy, after an abortion, or during a regimen of estrogen replacement therapy.

vaginal smear A sample of vaginal secretions taken by the doctor during an internal examination for purposes of diagnosing any condition that produces such symptoms as a malodorous discharge, itching, pain during urination, or discomfort during sexual intercourse. The smear is usually transferred to a glass slide and examined under a microscope. It may also be processed in order to begin a laboratory culture that may yield information about the particular microorganisms responsible for the symptoms.

vaginitis Any disorder characterized by inflammation of the vulvo-vaginal membranes accompanied by leukorrhea or burning and itching aggravated by urination. Vaginitis may be classified as specific in cases where the infectious agent is identifiable and as nonspecific in cases where the symptoms are not traceable to a particular cause. Nonspecific vaginitis is usually treated with medicated suppositories, creams, or douches. Since the vaginal membranes are as delicate as those in the mouth, they may be irritated not only by germs, but by the chemicals in deodorant sprays, by tampons, and by contraceptive devices. Mechanical irritation is likely to increase the possibility of infection. See "Sexually Transmissible Diseases," "Gynecologic Diseases and Treatment."

Valium Brand name of a tranquilizing drug in the chemical category benzodiazepine. In the United States it is a frequently prescribed drug which recently has provoked a controversy regarding its undesirable side effects such as impaired intellectual functions and its addictive qualities. See "Drugs, Alcohol, and Tobacco."

varicose veins Veins that are swollen and enlarged; also called varicosities. Varicosities include hemorrhoids (swollen anal veins), but the superficial veins of the legs, especially those located in the back and inner side of the calf, are the ones most frequently affected. Varicosities of smaller veins are visible through the skin as a bluish-red network of delicate lines going off in different directions from a particular source. A larger varicose vein is likely to have the appearance of a bumpy, purplish rope. Varicose veins are more common among women than among men, among people who spend a great deal of time standing in one place, and among the obese; they are a frequent development during pregnancy; most women over 40 develop some varicosities; and there seems to be an inherited predisposition to the condition.

Varicosities result from heavy pressure of the blood against the walls of the veins. The blood that returns to the heart from the legs must do so against gravitational force. The muscles that surround deeply buried veins support the veins and promote the antigravitational movement of the blood, and these veins are therefore less likely to become distended. All veins contain valves set into the walls in pairs. These flaplike projections are open when the blood is flowing correctly toward the heart; the valves close to prevent any reverse movement away from the heart. However, when prolonged standing in one spot or the pressure of pregnancy or excessive weight puts an abnormally heavy strain on the veins with no accompanying support from surrounding muscles, the column of blood constantly bearing down on the closed valves causes the valves to weaken and the walls to dilate. The valves may become incapable of closing. This disability in turn causes the downward flowing blood to collect in the veins, further swelling and weakening the walls. When the condition becomes increasingly serious, the knotty protrusions become vulnerable to ulceration and possible hemorrhage.

Prevention, decreasing the likelihood of occurrence, and therapy for mild cases all involve relieving the pressure on the veins. Feet should be raised whenever possible. Constriction by crossing the legs or wearing tight girdles or garters should be eliminated. Tasks that involve being in one place for a long time should be done sitting instead of standing if possible. If prolonged standing is unavoidable, moving from one spot to another and occasional walking about will provide some relief.

Symptoms such as muscle cramps in the middle of the night, swollen ankles, and a general feeling of soreness in the legs indicate that additional therapeutic measures are necessary to prevent further deterioration of the condition. Individually fitted support stockings are preferable to elasticized partial bandages and should be worn during the waking hours. Swimming, bicycling, and hiking as well as special leg exercises are effective therapy. Somewhat more drastic treatment consists of injections with medications that cause the swollen veins to harden and eventually wither so that the circulation is rerouted to healthier vessels. A more effective and permanent treatment for seriously distended veins is an operation that ties them or removes them completely. The spiderlike varicosities that develop during pregnancy are likely to disappear if proper weight is maintained and beneficial exercise is routine.

vasectomy A surgical procedure which effectively sterilizes the male without impairing his hormone levels or his sexual performance. *See* "Contraception and Abortion."

vegetarianism A dietary regimen which, at its strictest, includes no food of animal, bird, or fish origin and derives essential proteins from plant sources. Less rigid vegetarians may or may not eat eggs, but include all other dairy products. Nutritionists do not believe that irrefutable evidence has yet been presented equating longevity with vegetarianism as such. However, every nutrient necessary for normal growth and continuing health can be obtained from meals based on plant foods plus eggs and dairy products. When eggs and dairy products are also eliminated, there is an inevitable deficiency of the essential nutrient vitamin B_{12} which comes entirely (for all practical purposes) from animal sources. Ongoing studies of the vegetarian discipline indicate the following: adherents in a particular group of young people had lower blood pressure, lower cholesterol, and lower weight than a group comparable in age on a regular meat diet. A religious sect that includes eggs and dairy products in its meals, but eliminates all meat, poultry, and fish is known to have a significantly lower incidence of heart disease and the breast and colon cancers that appear to be traceable to heavy intake of animal fats than the standard rate for Americans on a nonvegetarian diet. Information on various aspects of the vegetarian movement is available from the North American Vegetarian Society, P.O. Box 72, Dodgeville, NY 13329. *See also* "Nutrition and Weight."

vein A blood vessel through which blood is transported back to the heart. Unlike arterial blood which is bright red as a result of being freshly oxygenated, venous blood is dark, the only exception being the blood in the pulmonary veins which is being transported directly from the lungs to the heart. Because veins are less elastic and weaker than arteries they are more vulnerable to such disorders as varicosities and phlebitis. For a description of the circulatory system, *see* "The Healthy Woman."

venereal disease *See* "Sexually Transmissible Diseases."

vertebra Any of the bones of the spine. The spinal column, which supports the body's weight and which provides the bony corridor through which the spinal cord passes, is comprised of 33 vertebrae, some of which are fused together. Depending on their location, they differ somewhat in structure and size: 7 cervical vertebrae are at the back of the neck; 12 thoracic vertebrae support the upper back; 5 lumbar vertebrae are in the lower back; 5 fused vertebrae make up the sacrum near the base of the spine, and 4 fused vertebrae form the coccyx. The vertebrae are separated from each other by fibrous tissue and cartilage discs which act as shock absorbers. When the displacement of one of these discs causes pressure on a nerve, the result may be acute pain. Osteoarthritis of the vertebral bones is one of the chronic diseases of aging responsible for backaches. Back discomfort may also originate in poor posture that affects vertebral position in relation to surrounding musculature. Osteoporosis of the vertebrae causes their collapse and the consequent loss of height seen in many older people. Tuberculosis of the spine is also a cause of vertebral collapse and deformity.

vertigo A sensation of irregular or whirling motion, either of oneself or of nearby objects; also called dizziness, although this latter term often is used incorrectly to describe a sensation of light-headedness or feeling faint. There are many possible causes of vertigo. It can be brought on by rapid, continuous, whirling motion, such as riding a merry-go-round, or by watching objects in apparent rapid motion, such as telephone poles observed from a fast-moving car. It can be caused by various diseases that affect, directly or indirectly, the labyrinthine canals in the middle ear. Included among these diseases are inflammation or infection of the labyrinthine canal, tumors or vascular disorders of the brain, and gastritis.

Vincent's angina *See* GUMS.

virus A submicroscopic disease-causing agent capable of reproducing only in the living cells of plants, animals, and humans. Among humans, viruses are responsible for a long list of otherwise unrelated communicable infections ranging from the common cold to a very rare and fatal brain disease (Creutzfeld-Jakob). When a viral strain responsible for a particular disease can be isolated and transformed into an effective immunizing vaccine, the disease itself can eventually be controlled. This has been the case with smallpox and may eventually be the case with such virus-caused infections as polio, measles, and rubella. Antibiotics are ineffective, and usually inappropriate, therapy for virus diseases except in cases where the patient might be critically vulnerable to secondary bacterial infection. *See* HEPATITIS, INFLUENZA, etc.

vitamins A number of unrelated organic substances essential in minute quantities as catalysts in metabolic processes. *See* "Nutrition and Weight."

vitiligo A harmless, but disfiguring skin condition, especially conspicuous when it occurs among blacks, in which an abnormal loss of melanin pigment results in irregular patches of pale skin. The patches usually appear symmetrically on the face, neck, hands, and torso. The condition, which appears to be hereditary, can be successfully masked to some extent by cosmetics individually blended to match the normal skin color.

vocal cords The two ligaments within the larynx which vibrate to create the extraordinary range of human sounds. Each reedlike cord is attached at one end to the front wall of the larynx (voice box) with the ends placed closely together. The other ends are connected to small rotating cartilage rings near the back wall of the larynx. These rotations cause the cords to sep- arate or to close, thus controlling the amount of air that passes through the larynx. When the cords are open, the air passes through the larynx without producing sounds. When the cords are close together, the air that is forced through them causes them to vibrate like the reeds in a musical instrument. These vibrations create sound waves in the form of a voice, and when the sound waves are articulated and controlled in a particular way, they produce speech and song. The pitch of the voice depends on the tension in the cords, and its depth depends on their length. Men's voices are deeper than women's because their vocal cords are longer. A common occurrence among singers and public speakers is the development of nodes on the vocal cords. These growths are usually removed by surgery. Sometimes they are malignant. *See* LARYNX.

VOCAL CORDS

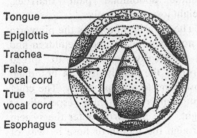

Tongue
Epiglottis
Trachea
False vocal cord
True vocal cord
Esophagus

BREATHING

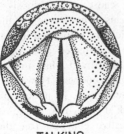

TALKING

vomiting The mechanism whereby the sudden contraction of the muscles of the stomach and the small intestines forces the partially digested contents of these organs upward and out of the mouth; technically called emesis. Vomiting and the feeling of nausea that characteristically precedes it may occur as a reflex response to tickling the inside of the throat, to an overfull stomach, to ingesting an emetic such as mustard or a poison, or to the presence of bacterial toxins acting as an irritant on the gastric membrane. It may also occur because of stimulation of the vomiting center of the brain. Motion sickness, overdoses of certain drugs and anesthetics, and emotional stress, such as strong feelings of revulsion or anxiety, can cause a reaction of vomiting. Medicines such as Dramamine and antiemetics prevent vomiting by depressing the response of this part of the nervous system. Vomiting may also occur because of obstructions in the intestines, uncontrolled paroxysms of coughing, the hormonal changes associated with pregnancy, and migraine headaches. Other less obvious causes are associated with brain injuries and disorders affecting the brain such as tumors, abscesses, or meningitis. Certain forms of mental illness or severe emotional disturbances are characterized by vomiting spells.

Any recurrent or uncontrollable attacks of vomiting should be diagnosed by a doctor. In coming to the aid of someone who is vomiting following an accident, precautionary measures should be taken so that the patient does not inhale the vomitus and fatally obstruct breathing.

vulva   The term for the external genital organs of the female. The vulva surround the vaginal opening. Proceeding from front to back, they consist of the mons veneris, the labia majora and minora, the clitoris which is partially covered by the clitoral hood, the urethra, the vaginal opening, Bartholin's glands on either side of the vaginal entrance (just inside of which is the hymen if it has not been ruptured), the perineum, and the anus. *See also* entries for each organ and "The Healthy Woman."

wart   An abnormal growth on the skin caused by a virus; technically called a verruca. Warts may occur at any age. Since the virus can spread to lesions in the skin caused by scratching, shaving, or other factors, warts may appear in groups or in succession. Because some other skin disorder may be mistaken for a wart or because the wart itself may become infected with bacteria, a doctor should be consulted about the

nature of the growth and the advisability of having it removed. Techniques include cauterization with chemicals or an electric needle or surgical incision. *See also* PLANTAR WART.

water retention   *See* EDEMA, DIURETICS.

weight   *See* "Nutrition and Weight."

withdrawal method   *See* COITUS INTERRUPTUS.

womb   *See* UTERUS.

worms   Parasites that invade the body and multiply within one or another part of it. They are usually transmitted by an intermediate host, and in the United States by far the largest number enter the body through food or water contaminated by the excreta of an already infected person. When intestinal infestation is heavy, symptoms include abdominal pain, diarrhea, weight loss, and anemia.

The parasite known as the pinworm is not uncommon among children and is sufficiently contagious to spread through the family if it is not diagnosed and treated promptly. The chief symptom is anal itching, especially at night. The pinworms enter the system through the mouth or nose by way of contamination on the hands.

Two other varieties common in the United States are *Trichinella spiralis,* the cause of trichinosis, and hookworms. The larvae of the trichinae, which are embedded in the muscle tissue of infected pork or other meat, are destroyed when the meat is thoroughly cooked. However, if the infected meat is undercooked ("pink pork") and the larvae survive, the digestive enzymes free the larvae in the intestines where they come to maturity. The females burrow into the intestinal walls, where they lay their eggs before they die. The larvae are then carried throughout the body, causing inflammation wherever they settle. In most places in the body they are eventually destroyed by the body's defense system, but once they penetrate muscle tissue, they coil into spirals and become encapsulated in cysts. Symptoms of infestation during the early phases include diarrhea and abdominal cramps, followed by edema, fever, chills, and profuse sweating. By the time the larvae become encapsulated in the muscles, these symptoms may have abated and additional symptoms of general fatigue and muscle discomfort appear. Muscle biopsy and serologic testing are helpful in establishing the diagnosis. While there is no specific cure for trichinosis, the disease is more discomfiting than dangerous. Although most pork is inspected for the presence of trichinae, the only foolproof method of avoiding trichinosis is to see that it is always properly cooked, gray in color rather than pink or white. An additional warning: never nibble on raw or uncooked pork products such as link sausages or frankfurters.

Hookworms enter the body primarily through the skin. Thus, anyone who goes barefoot in the country (especially children) is vulnerable to infestation, since hookworm larvae develop in soil that has been fertilized with or otherwise contaminated by human feces carrying the infection. When the larvae enter the body, the bloodstream carries them to the lungs and then to the intestines where they mature into adult worms and lay their eggs in the intestinal walls. A serious infestation causes anemia, with its attendant disabilities, as well as persistent nausea and cramps. Diagnosis is made on the basis of examination of a stool sample, and treatment is simple, safe, and almost always effective. Reinfection can be prevented by wearing shoes especially in those areas where public sanitation and general habits of personal hygiene are minimal.

For the less common forms of worm infestation, and there are many, the most practical measures for prevention include the following. Be careful about personal hygiene, especially when traveling in countries where public health measures are inadequate. Avoid eating raw fish, raw meat, and undercooked pork, no matter where it is served. Avoid swimming in any waters known to be contaminated by dangerous parasites. In countries where human excrement is commonly used for fertilizer, all fruit should be peeled, all vegetables cooked, and those that are to be eaten raw, such as salad greens, should be washed thoroughly to get rid of any worm eggs that might be harbored in the leaves.

wound   A body injury, ranging from superficial to severe, in which the skin or interior tissues may be cut, pierced, or otherwise damaged. Wounds are classified as abrasions (scrapes that remove part of the skin and bleed only slightly), incisions (cuts that may be slight or deep and are caused by a sharp object such as a knife, razor, or broken glass), punctures (deep injuries caused by thin pointed objects such as nails or needles), and lacerations (jagged tears in the skin and underlying tissues). The most important aspects of emergency treatment for wounds are the control of bleeding and the prevention of infection. An abrasion may bleed very little, but since the skin is broken, the danger of infection is always present. Scrapes should therefore be washed thoroughly with soap and running water and covered with a sterile gauze. Until the doctor determines whether a more extensive wound should be stitched (sutured), firm continuous pressure should be applied for about ten minutes with the fingers over a gauze pad, a clean handkerchief, or a piece of brown wrapping paper. The pressure must not be interrupted for wiping and for inspection since interruptions delay the clotting. While a puncture wound may not appear to be serious, its potential for tetanus infection makes it one of the most dangerous types of wound. A laceration in which the skin has been torn may be superficial enough to be treated like an abrasion, or it may be so extensive as to require prompt additional care.

wrinkles The lines and furrows that mark the skin as it ages and loses elasticity. Heredity, hormonal interplay, emotional and physical health, and exposure to sun and wind are the chief factors that determine the age at which skin begins to wrinkle. Also, the skin of women who smoke seems to wrinkle earlier and more than of those who do not. Wrinkles cannot be removed or permanently delayed by creams or lotions; cosmetics can mask them, but those that claim to contain "magic" ingredients may do more harm than good. The technique of dermabrasion can temporarily erase the more superficial lines, but they will inevitably reappear as the sagging skin continues to move away from the supporting structures beneath. Cosmetic surgery can eliminate wrinkles for several years, but the decision to undergo such a procedure should be carefully considered. *See* "Cosmetic Surgery."

xerography A mammography technique (also called xeroradiography or xeromammography) in which the images of breast tissue produced by radiation exposure are made on a Xerox plate instead of on film. The result of this technique is a blue-toned image on opaque Xerox paper rather than a film negative.

X-ray Radiation of extremely short electromagnetic waves capable of penetrating certain matter opaque to ordinary light and producing images on photosensitive surfaces; also the image produced. X-rays have become indispensable in medical study, diagnosis, and treatment. The radiation is created by an electrical apparatus that produces a beam of the desired intensity and scope by bombarding a tungsten target with high-speed electrons in a vacuum tube. X-rays are also called Roentgen rays after their discoverer. The area of specialization dealing with X-ray technology is radiology or roentgenology. Under ordinary circumstances, X-rays are more easily absorbed by bone than by flesh. By placing a fluorescent screen behind the body, the bones are delineated as shadows. This technique is called fluoroscopy. When permanent records are wanted, photographic plates that are sensitive to X-rays are used to produce images that can be dated and preserved as part of a patient's medical history. From its original application to injuries or disorders of the skeletal system, X-ray technology has been broadened by the technique of introducing radiopaque substances into the patient's body to provide information about nonskeletal disorders such as in the gastrointestinal tract.

More recently, computerized scanners have been developed that can take layered pictures of parts of the brain previously inaccessible by ordinary radiological methods.

Whether for diagnostic purposes or, more likely, as treatment (*see* RADIOTHERAPY), the danger of overexposure to X-rays has become a widespread problem. Among the consequences of overexposure are destruction of skin, loss of hair and nails, development of certain cancers, and damage to the genes, the reproductive organs, and fetuses. Pregnant women should avoid exposure to X-rays except in the greatest emergency. Under any circumstances a patient should always ask that a lead sheet cover those parts of her body not intended to show on the film. Because of the serious disabilities created by exposure, experts on radiation hazard advise patients to ask the following types of questions before X-rays are taken. Before having a complete set of 16 to 18 pictures as part of a routine dental checkup, ask the dentist what special problem exists that can be dealt with only in this way and why a whole series has to be taken if trouble is suspected in a particular area of the mouth. When a medical doctor suggests X-rays, ask what their purpose is, whether other tests do the same thing, whether the lowest possible radiation is being used to achieve the necessary result, and when the equipment was last inspected. Many states have no laws requiring that X-ray equipment be checked every year to make sure that it does in fact deliver intended doses rather than perilously higher ones and that it in no way exposes the patient to unnecessary hazards because it is incorrectly operated or outmoded. If X-ray pictures must be taken, it is advisable to have them done by a radiologist. While specialists are more expensive than general practitioners, they are more likely to have the most up-to-date equipment and the best-trained technicians operating it. Anyone who has undergone a series of X-rays and is moving to another city should ask the doctor or dentist for the films so that they can be turned over to whoever will be in charge of medical care in the new location. Unnecessary duplication with its attendant hazards, not to mention expense, is therefore avoided.

yeast infection   *See* "Sexually Transmissible Diseases."

yoga exercises   An ancient Hindu discipline, increasingly popular in the West, for the achievement of physical and mental relaxation. The exercises combine control of consciousness with various specific body positions coordinated with breathing patterns. While self-instruction is possible, beginners are likely to achieve greater proficiency in a group under the tutelage of an experienced teacher. The exercises can then be done at home or even at work at times convenient to one's own schedule.

yogurt   A food of custardlike consistency created by heating milk to produce the beneficial bacillus *Streptococcus thermophilus* and then fermenting the milk with an additional beneficial bacterial strain (*Lactobacillus bulgaricus*). In the process of fermentation the milk sugar lactose is transformed into lactic acid, giving yogurt its characteristically tart flavor. In addition to its nutritional assets, yogurt is more easily digested than milk, and its bacteria have a beneficial effect on the intestinal tract, fighting off infectious bacteria and adding benign ones, especially those that might have been destroyed by antibiotics. It should be kept in mind that yogurt sold as a frozen solid may be a less fattening dessert than ice cream, but its beneficial bacteria are presumed to have been destroyed in the freezing process.

Appendixes

TABLE 1.

Suggested Health Examination Schedules for Women at Normal Risk

Interval Between Examinations (in months) *

	Age 18–40	Age 41–60	Age 61+
General physical examination and life-style counseling	36	12	12
Dental examination	6	6	6
Eye examination including glaucoma test	24	12	12
Breast examination	36	12	12
Breast self-examination	1	1	1
Pap smear	12 (36†)	12 (36†)	12 (36†)
Pelvic examination	36	12	12
Tests for sexually transmissible diseases	6–12‡	6–12‡	6–12‡

	Age 35–49	Age 50+
Mammography	Initial at age 35–40; thereafter as recommended by physician	12
Endometrial tissue sample	At menopause and periodically thereafter for women taking estrogens	

	Age 40+	Age 50+
Finger rectal examination	12	12
Test for blood in stool		12
Proctosigmoidoscopy		36–60

* Different intervals may be recommended for some women by their physicians.
† 36-month interval (after two initial negative pap smears a year apart) recommended by the American Cancer Society, March, 1980. There are differences of opinion among professional groups and individuals regarding the ideal interval.
‡ Intervals depend on individual sexual life styles.

TABLE 2.

Immunization Guide

ACTIVE IMMUNIZATION: Recommended for Routine Use

Disease	Causative Agent	Type of Vaccine	Duration of Protection
Diphtheria	bacterium	toxoid	booster every 10 years and after exposure
Mumps	virus	live	probably lifetime
Pertussis (whooping cough)	bacterium	killed	several years; consider booster after exposure
Poliomyelitis	virus	live (Sabin) killed (Salk)	probably lifetime uncertain, possibly lifetime
Rubella (German measles)	virus	live	probably lifetime
Rubeola (measles)	virus	live	probably lifetime
Tetanus	bacterium	toxoid	booster every 10 years and after exposure

ACTIVE IMMUNIZATION:

Recommended for special use (for persons at high risk because of chronic illness, old age, occupational or natural exposure, or travel to certain foreign countries; duration of protection against each disease varies from a few months to years)

Disease	Causative Agent
Adenovirus infections	virus
Anthrax	bacterium
Botulism	bacterium
Cholera	bacterium
Cytomegalovirus	virus (experimental vaccine under investigation)
Hemophilus influenza	bacterium (experimental vaccine under clinical trials)
Hepatitis B	virus (experimental vaccine under investigation)
Influenza	virus
Meningitis	bacterium
Plague	bacterium

Pneumococcal infection	bacterium
Rabies	virus
Rocky Mountain spotted fever	rickettsiae
Trachoma conjunctivitis	Chlamydiae
Tuberculosis (BCG)	bacterium
Tularemia	bacterium
Typhoid	bacterium
Typhus	rickettsiae
Variola (smallpox)	virus
Yellow fever	virus

PASSIVE IMMUNIZATION:

Recommended for special use (to provide temporary protection, 1 to 6 weeks, for nonimmune persons exposed, possibly exposed, or likely to be exposed to the disease; antitoxins also used to treat the respective diseases)

Disease	*Type of Vaccine*
Botulism	antitoxin (animal)
Clostridial myositis (bacterium)	antitoxin (animal); unproven value
Diphtheria	antitoxin (animal)
Hepatitis A	immune serum globulin (human)
Hepatitis B	Hepatitis B immune globulin (human) immune serum globulin
Herpes zoster (virus)	zoster immune globulin (human)
Mumps	mumps immune globulin (human); unproven value
Pertussis (whooping cough)	pertussis immune globulin (human); unproven value
Rabies	rabies immune globulin (human) antiserum (animal)
Rubella (German measles)	immune serum globulin (human); unproven value
Rubeola (measles)	immune serum globulin (human)
Tetanus	tetanus immune globulin (human) antitoxin (animal)
Varicella (chickenpox)	zoster immune globulin (human) immune serum globulin (human); unproven value
Variola (smallpox)	vaccinia immune globulin (human)

TABLE 3.

Common Medical Terms

Most of the words used by doctors are made up of two or three parts (prefixes, roots, suffixes) that come from Greek or Latin. Knowing the meaning of these word parts makes it easier to understand and use medical terminology.

prefixes

a-, an-	without (anesthesia)	hyper-	excessive (hyperacidity; hypertension)
ad-	toward or near (adhesions; adrenal)	hypo-	under, below (hypothyroid; hypothermia)
anti-	against (antiseptic; antihistamine)		
bi-	two (biceps; bisexual)	leuko-	white (leukocytes; leukorrhea)
co-, con-	with, together (concussion; constipation)	ortho-	straight, correct (orthodontia; orthopedist)
cyano-	blue (cyanosis)	pre-, pro-	before (premenstrual; prophylaxis)
dys-	impaired, abnormal (dysmenorrhea; dysfunction)	re-, retro-	back, again (regression; retroperitoneal)
ecto-	outer, outside (ectopic)	sub-	beneath, under (subconscious; subcutaneous)
endo-	inner, within (endocardium; endometrium)		
epi-	over, among (epiglottis; epidermis)	super-	higher, above (superego)
		sym-, syn-	together (symbiosis; synapse)
eu-	good, well (euphoria; euthanasia)	trans-	across (transfusion)
ex-	out, away from (expectorant)		

roots relating to medicine and the body

aden-	gland (adenoma; adenoid)	angio-	blood vessel (angiography; hemangioma)

arthro-	joint (arthritis)	hepato-	liver (hepatitis)
bronchos-	throat (bronchitis; bronchoscopy)	metro-	uterus (endometritis)
cardi-, coro-	heart (cardiogram; coronary)	myo-	muscle (myocardial; myoma)
cerebro-	brain (cerebral palsy)	narce-	numbness (narcotic; narcolepsy)
chole-	bile (cholesterol; chololith)	nephros	kidney (nephritis)
colo-	colon (colostomy)	osteo-	bone (osteoarthritis)
cyst-	sac; bladder (cystoscope)	ophthalmos-	eye (ophthalmologist)
cyto-	cell (leukocyte)	otos-	ear (otitis)
derma-	skin (dermatitis; epidermis)	pepsis-	digestion (peptic ulcer; dyspepsia)
diaeta-	regimen (diet)	pneuma-	lungs (pneumonia)
emetos-	vomit (emetic)	proctos-	anus (proctoscope)
enterion	intestines, gut (enteritis; dysentery)	rhinos-	nose (rhinitis)
		sarcos-	flesh (sarcoma)
gastro-	stomach (gastric ulcer; gastritis)	sphygmos-	pulse (sphygmomanometer)
haemo-	blood (hemangioma; hemoglobin)	soma-	body (psychosomatic medicine)
		phlebs-	vein (phlebitis)

suffixes related to symptoms, diagnosis, surgery

-algia	pain (neuralgia)	-osis	disease (tuberculosis)
-ectomy	cutting out (appendectomy)	-ostomy	opening (colostomy)
-genic	source (psychogenic)	-otomy	incision (episiotomy)
-graph	record, writing (electrocardiograph)	-pathy	disease (psychopathic)
-itis	inflammation (laryngitis)	-rhagia	overflow (hemorrhage)
-lysis	dissolving, separating (analysis; dialysis)	-rrhea	stream, discharge (dysmenorrhea; rhinorrhea)
-oid	resembling (fibroid)	-scopy	inspection (cystoscopy; microscopy)
-oma	tumor (lymphoma)		

TABLE 4.

How to Read a Prescription

Rx	prescription	mg	milligrams
Sig	label	min	minim, a drop
ac	before meals	od	right eye
ad lib	whenever you want	os	left eye
bid	twice a day	pc	after meals
cc	cubic centimeter	qd	every day
dr	dram	qh	every hour
extr	extract	qid	four times a day
gm	gram	qs	as much as is sufficient
gr	grains	tid	three times a day
gt	drop		

TABLE 5.

**Commonly Prescribed Brand Name Drugs
and Generic Equivalents**

In most states druggist must supply generic drug if doctor signs "substitution permissible" on the prescription.

Proprietary Name	Generic Name	Proprietary Name	Generic Name
Achromycin V	tetracycline	Atarax	hydroxyzine HCL
Actifed	triprolidine and pseudoephedrine	Atromid-S	clofibrate
		Azo-Gantrisin	azo-sulfisoxazole
Aldactazide	spironazide	Benadryl	diphenhydramine
Aldactone	spironolactone	Bendectin	doxylamine and pyridoxine
Aldomet	methyldopa		
Amoxil	amoxicillin	Bentyl	dicyclomine
Antabuse	disulfiram	Butazolidin Alka	phenylbutazone alka
Antivert	meclizine		
Apresoline	hydralazine HCL	Chlortrimeton	chlorpheniramine
Aristocort	triamcinolone	Compazine	prochlorperazine

Proprietary Name	Generic Name	Proprietary Name	Generic Name
Coumadin	sodium warfarin	Librax	clidinium bromide
Dalmane	flurazepam	Librium	chlordiazepoxide
Darvon	propoxyphene	Lomotil	diphenoxylate and atropine
Demerol	meperidine		
Diabinese	chlorpropamide	Lotrimin	clotrimazole
Dilantin	phenytoin	Mycostatin	nystatin
Diuril	chlorothiazide	Nembutal	pentobarbital sodium
Donnatal	hyoscyamine	Neosporin	polymyxin, neomycin and gromicidin
Drixoral	dexbrompheniramine and pseudoephedrine		
		Omnipen	ampicillin
		Orinase	tolbutamide
Elavil	amitriptyline	Pavabid	papavarine time caps
Empirin and Codeine	aspirin, phenacetin, caffeine, and codeine	Pen Vee K	penicillin V(K)
		Percodan	oxycodone, aspirin, phenacetin, and caffeine
Equanil	meprobamate		
Erythrocin	erythromycin	Periactin	cyproheptadine
Esidrix	hydrochlorothiazide	Persantine	dipyridamole
Flagyl	metronidazole	Phenergan	promethazine
Fulvicin	griseofulvin	Premarin	conjugated estrogens
Gantrisin	sulfisoxazole	Provera	medroxyprogesterone
Hydrodiuril	hydrochlorothiazide	Ritalin	methylphenidate
Hydropres	hydroserpine	Robaxin	methocarbamol
Inderal	propranolol hydrochloride	Sudafed	pseudoephedrine
		Talwin	pentazocine
Indocin	indomethacin	Tenuate	diethylpropion
Isordil	isosorbide	Thorazine	chlorpromazine
Kenalog	triamcinolone	Tigan	trimethobenzamide
Kwell Cream	gamma benzene hexachloride	Tylenol	acetaminophen
Lanoxin	digoxin	Valium	diazepam
Larotid	amoxicillin	V-Cillin K	penicillin V(K)
Lasix	furosemide	Vibramycin	doxycycline

TABLE 6.
Directory of Health Services

Abortion

National Abortion Federation
  110 East 59th Street, New York, NY   10022
American Family Planning Services
  149 Lewis Road, Havertown, PA   19083
National Abortion Rights Action League (NARAL)
  825 Fifteenth Street, NW, Washington, D.C.   20005
National Right to Life Committee, Inc.
  341 National Press Building, Washington, D.C.   20045

Aging

National Institute on Aging
  U.S. Department of Health and Human Services
  National Institutes of Health
  9000 Rockville Pike, Bethesda, MD   20205
American Association of Retired Persons
  1909 K Street, NW, Washington, D.C.   20049
National Council on the Aging, Inc.
  1828 L Street, NW, Washington, D.C.   20036

Alcoholism

Al-Anon Family Group Headquarters, Inc.
  P.O. Box 182, Madison Square Station, New York, NY   10010
National Clearing House for Alcohol Information
  P.O. Box 2345, Rockville, MD   20852
A.A. General Service Office
  P.O. Box 459, Grand Central Station, New York, NY   10017
National Council on Alcoholism, Inc.
  733 Third Avenue, New York, NY   10017

Allergy

Asthma & Allergy Foundation of America
  19 West 44th Street, New York, NY   10036
National Institute of Allergy and Infectious Diseases
  U.S. Department of Health and Human Services
  National Institutes of Health
  9000 Rockville Pike, Bethesda, MD   20205

Anorexia Nervosa

National Anorexic Aid Society, Inc.
  P.O. Box 29461, Columbus, OH   43229

Arthritis

The Arthritis Foundation
    3400 Peachtree Road, NE, Suite 1101, Atlanta, GA   30326
National Institute of Arthritis, Metabolism, and Digestive Diseases
    U.S. Department of Health and Human Services
    National Institutes of Health
    9000 Rockville Pike, Bethesda, MD   20205

Birth Control

Planned Parenthood Federation of America, Inc.
    810 Seventh Avenue, New York, NY   10019
Zero Population Growth, Inc.
    1346 Connecticut Avenue, NW, Washington, D.C.   20036

Birth Defects

March of Dimes Birth Defects Foundation
    Box 2000, White Plains, NY   10602
National Genetics Foundation, Inc.
    555 West 57th Street, New York, NY   10019

Blindness

American Foundation for the Blind, Inc.
    15 West 16th Street, New York, NY   10011
The National Society to Prevent Blindness
    79 Madison Avenue, New York, NY   10016
Recording for the Blind, Inc.
    215 East 58th Street, New York, NY   10022

Blood

American Association of Blood Banks
    1828 L Street, NW, Suite 608, Washington, D.C.   20036
American Red Cross
    National Headquarters, Washington, D.C.   20006

Cancer

American Cancer Society
    777 Third Avenue, New York, NY   10017
Office of Cancer Communications
    National Cancer Institute
    Bethesda, MD   20205
Reach to Recovery
    19 West 56th Street, New York, NY   10019
Leukemia Society of America, Inc.
    800 Second Avenue, New York, NY   10017

Cerebral Palsy

United Cerebral Palsy Associations, Inc.
    66 East 34th Street, New York, NY   10016

Cystic Fibrosis

Cystic Fibrosis Foundation
   6000 Executive Boulevard, Suite 309, Rockville, MD   20852

Dental Health

American Dental Association
   Bureau of Health Education & Audiovisual Services
   211 East Chicago Avenue, Chicago, IL   60611
National Institute of Dental Research
   National Institutes of Health
   U.S. Public Health Service
   Building 31, Room 2C34, Bethesda, MD   20205

DES

DES Registry, Inc.
   5426–27th Street, NW, Washington, D.C.   20015
DES Action
   Long Island Jewish–Hillside Medical Center
   New Hyde Park, NY   11040

Diabetes

American Diabetes Association
   600 Fifth Avenue, New York, NY   10020

Digestive Diseases

Digestive Diseases Information Center
   6410 Rockledge Drive, Suite 208, Bethesda, MD   20034
American Digestive Disease Society, Inc.
   420 Lexington Avenue, NewYork, NY   10017
National Foundation for Ileitis and Colitis, Inc.
   295 Madison Avenue, New York, NY   10017

Drug Abuse

Drug Enforcement Administration
   1405 I Street, NW, Washington, D.C.   20537
National Clearinghouse for Drug Abuse Information
   5600 Fishers Lane, Rockville, MD   20857

Epilepsy

The Epilepsy Foundation of America
   1828 L Street, NW, Washington, D.C.   20036

Exercise

American Alliance for Health, Physical Education, Recreation and Dance
   1201 Sixteenth Street, NW, Washington, D.C.   20036

Eye Diseases

National Eye Institute
  National Institutes of Health
  Building 31, Bethesda, MD   20205
American Optometric Association
  243 N. Lindbergh Boulevard, St. Louis, MO   63141
The Eye Bank Association of America
  3195 Maplewood Avenue, Winston-Salem, NC   27103

Genetic Counseling   See BIRTH DEFECTS

Gynecological Disorders

American College of Obstetricians and Gynecologists
  One East Wacker Drive, Suite 2700, Chicago, IL   60601

Handicapped

Federation of the Handicapped, Inc.
  211 West 14th Street, New York, NY   10011
ICD Rehabilitation & Research Center
  340 East 24th Street, New York, NY   10010
American Coalition of Citizens with Disabilities
  1200–15th Street, NW, #201, Washington, D.C.   20036

Health

American Public Health Association
  1015 Fifteenth Street, NW, Washington, D.C.   20005
Council on Family Health
  633 Third Avenue, New York, NY   10017

Hearing

American Speech-Language-Hearing Association
  10801 Rockville Pike, Rockville, MD   20852
The Deafness Research Foundation
  342 Madison Avenue, New York, NY   10017

Heart Disease

American Heart Association
  7320 Greenville Avenue, Dallas, TX   75231
National Heart, Lung, and Blood Institute
  National Institutes of Health
  9000 Rockville Pike, Bethesda, MD   20205
The Mended Hearts, Inc.
  7320 Greenville Avenue, Dallas, TX   75231

Hemophilia

National Hemophilia Foundation
  19 West 34th Street, New York, NY   10001

Hypertension

High Blood Pressure Information Center
   120/80 National Institutes of Health, Bethesda, MD   20205

Infertility

American Fertility Society
   1608 13th Avenue South, Suite 101, Birmingham, AL   35205
Resolve, Inc.
   P.O. Box 474, Belmont, MA   02178

Kidney Disease

National Kidney Foundation
   Two Park Avenue, New York, NY   10016
Kidney, Urologic & Blood Diseases
   National Institute of Arthritis, Metabolism, and Digestive Diseases
   National Institutes of Health, Bethesda, MD   20205
National Association of Patients on Hemodialysis and Transplantation, Inc.
   505 Northern Boulevard, Great Neck, NY   11021

Lung Disease   See RESPIRATORY DISEASES

Marriage Counseling

New York Association of Marriage & Family Therapy
   41 Central Park West, New York, NY   10023
CONTACT Teleministries USA, Inc.
   900 South Arlington Avenue, Harrisburg, PA   17109

Mental Health

Family Service Association of America, Inc.
   44 East 23rd Street, New York, NY   10010
National Mental Health Association
   1800 North Kent Street, Arlington, VA   22209
National Institute of Mental Health
   Alcohol, Drug Abuse and Mental Health Administration
   U.S. Department of Health and Human Services
   5600 Fishers Lane, Rockville, MD   20857

Multiple Sclerosis

National Multiple Sclerosis Society
   205 East 42nd Street, New York, NY   10017

Muscular Dystrophy

Muscular Dystrophy Association, Inc.
   810 Seventh Avenue, New York, NY   10019

Myasthenia Gravis

Myasthenia Gravis Foundation
   15 East 26th Street, New York, NY   10010

Narcolepsy

The American Narcolepsy Association
   Box 5846, Stanford, CA   94305

Nutrition

Community Nutrition Institute
   1146 Nineteenth Street, NW, Washington, D.C.   20036
The American Dietetic Association
   430 North Michigan Avenue, Chicago, IL   60611
Department of Foods and Nutrition
   American Medical Association
   535 North Dearborn Street, Chicago, IL   60610
North American Vegetarian Society
   P.O. Box 72
   Dolgeville, NY   13329

Ostomy

United Ostomy Association
   2001 West Beverly Boulevard, Los Angeles, CA   90057

Parkinson's Disease

American Parkinson Disease Association, Inc.
   116 John Street, New York, NY   10038

Plastic Surgery

American Society of Plastic & Reconstructive Surgeons, Inc.
   29 East Madison Street, Suite 800, Chicago, IL   60602
American Board of Plastic Surgery, Inc.
   1617 J. F. Kennedy Boulevard, Suite 1561, Philadelphia, PA   19103

Pregnancy

American College of Obstetricians and Gynecologists
   One East Wacker Drive, Suite 2700, Chicago, IL   60601
Office of Maternal and Child Health
   U.S. Department of Health and Human Services
   Room 7-39 Parklawn, Rockville, MD   20857
Community Health Services
   Health Service Administration
   Parklawn Building
   5600 Fishers Lane
   Rockville, MD   20857
C/Sec Inc.
   Cesareans/Support Education & Concern
   66 Christopher Road, Waltham, MA   02154
American College of Nurse–Midwives
   1012 Fourteenth Street, NW, Washington, D.C.   20005

Rape

National Center for the Prevention and Control of Rape
   National Rape Information Clearinghouse
   National Institute of Mental Health
   5600 Fishers Lane, Parklawn Building, Room 13A-44
   Rockville, MD   20857
Center for Women Policy Studies
   2000 P Street, NW, Suite 508, Washington, D.C.   20036
Women's Crisis Center, Rape
   211½ North Fourth Avenue, Ann Arbor, MI   48107

Respiratory Diseases

National Heart, Lung, and Blood Institute
   National Institutes of Health
   9000 Rockville Pike, Bethesda, MD   20205
American Lung Association
   1740 Broadway, New York, NY   10019

Retardation

National Association for Retarded Citizens
   P.O. Box 6109, 2709 Avenue E East, Arlington, TX   76011
American Association on Mental Deficiency
   5101 Wisconsin Avenue, NW, Washington, D.C.   20016

Sex Education and Therapy

Sex Information and Education Council of the United States (SIECUS)
   84 Fifth Avenue, New York, NY   10011
American Association of Sex Educators, Counselors & Therapists
   5010 Wisconsin Avenue, Washington, D.C.   20016
American College of Sexologists
   1523 Franklin Street, San Francisco, CA   94109

Sexually Transmissible Diseases

American Social Health Association
   260 Sheridan Avenue, Suite 307, Palo Alto, CA   94306
Center for Disease Control, Venereal Disease Control Division
   Public Health Service
   Atlanta, GA   30333
National VD Hotline
   260 Sheridan Avenue, Palo Alto, CA   94306

Sickle Cell Disease

Sickle Cell Disease Foundation of Greater New York
   209 West 125th Street, Room 108, New York, NY   10027

Skin Care

American Academy of Dermatology
   2250 NW Flanders Street, Portland, OR   97210

Smoking

Office on Smoking and Health
    Park Building 1-58
    Rockville, MD   20857
Smokenders
    Route 22 at Prospect Street, Phillipsburg, NJ   08865

Speech

American Speech-Language-Hearing Association
    10801 Rockville Pike, Rockville, MD   20852
Speech and Hearing Institute
    ICD Rehabilitation and Research Center
    340 East 24th Street, New York, NY   10010

Sterilization

Association for Voluntary Sterilization, Inc.
    708 Third Avenue, New York, NY   10017
Zero Population Growth, Inc.
    1346 Connecticut Avenue, NW, Washington, D.C.   20036

Suicide

The Samaritans
    802 Boylston Street, Boston, MA   02199
CONTACT Teleministries USA, Inc.
    900 South Arlington Avenue, Harrisburg, PA   17109

Tay-Sachs Disease

National Tay-Sachs & Allied Disease Associations, Inc.
    122 East 42nd Street, New York, NY   10017

Weight Control

Overeaters Anonymous
    2190 West 190th Street, Torrance, CA   90504
Weight Watchers International
    800 Community Drive, Manhasset, NY   11030

Index

Page references in italics refer to illustrations. Bold face page references refer to the Encyclopedia in Part II.

Abdominal lift, 87
Abdominal pain, 230, **513**
  menstrual cramps, 228–29
Abortion, induced, 158–62, **514**, 744
  complications, 159–60, 161, 206, 212
  emotional and moral considerations, 162
  legal considerations, 158, 159
  multiple, 158, 162
  techniques, 159
Abortion, spontaneous, 181, 182, **514**
Abscess, **515**
Abuse, *see* Rape; Spouse abuse
Accident and health insurance, 493
Accidents, avoidance of, 463–65
Acetaminophen (Tylenol), 743
Achromycin (tetracycline), **515**, 742
Acidity and alkalinity, **515, 528**
Acne, **516**
Acromegaly, 19
ACTH, *see* Adrenocorticotropic hormone
Actifed (triprolidine and pseudo-ephedrine), 742
Acupuncture, **516**
Acute symptom, **517**
Adaption by elderly, 476
Addiction, **517**
Addison's disease, 21, **517**
Additives, food, 47–50
Adductor longus muscle, *8*
Adenoma, **517**
Adenovirus infections, immunization, 738
Adhesions, 212, 243, **517**
Adolescence, 103, 377
Adoption, **517**
  artificial insemination as alternative, 219
Adrenal glands, 19, 20, 21, **518**
  infertility and, *208, 210*
Adrenalin, 21, **518**
Adrenocorticotropic hormone (ACTH), *20,* **516**

Adultery and Other Private Matters, 131
Afterbirth, *see* Placenta
Agility exercises, 83
Aging persons, 744
  crimes against, 468–69
  diabetes, 456–57
  drug and alcohol problems, 459–62, 474
  educational opportunities for, 477
  emotional problems, 469–78, 482–83
  financial and related problems, 466–68, 476–77
  infection and, 457
  leverage of group, 482
  medical care, 457–58
  nursing homes, 458
  nutrition, 57–58
  Parkinson's disease, 449
  percentage of population, projected, *441*
  physical changes, 442–56, 462–65, 480
  psychotherapy, 475–76
  sexual activity, 105, 471, 478–79
  stroke, 448–49
Agriculture, U.S. Department of, food grading by, 47
Air pollution, *see* Pollution
Air sickness, *see* Motion sickness
Al-Anon, **518**
  Family Group Headquarters, Inc., 744
Alcohol, 118, 320, 325–31, **519**
  aging and, 474
  alcoholism, *see* Alcoholism
  choice as to, 30, 357–58
  cross-tolerance, 322, 328, 330, 342
  depressant, as, 327
  infertility and, 207, 209
  intoxication, 329
  marijuana and, 342
  metabolism, 14, 330–31
  pregnancy, during, 179, 350
  society and, 325–26
  tolerance, 332–33

violence and, 380
Alcoholics Anonymous, 33, 354, 355, 356, **520,** 744
General Service Office, 744
Alcoholism, **520**
associations concerned with, 744
danger signs, 331–33
detoxification, 354
fetal alcohol syndrome, 179, 350
incidence, 321, 331
predisposition, 325, 332
progression, 332
recovery, 354–55
Aldactazide (spironazide), 742
Aldactone (spironolactone), 742
Aldomet (methyldopa), 742
Aldosterone, 21
Allergies, **521,** 744
emotion as factor, 29
infertility and, 207
vaginal irritation, 233
Alternate toe touch, 79
Alveoli, 10, *11,* **522**
Alzheimer's disease, 448
AMA, *see* American Medical Association
Amebiasis, 261
Amenorrhea, 227, 522
American Academy of Dermatology, 750
American Alliance for Health, Physical Education, Recreation, and Dance, 746
American Association of Blood Banks, 745
American Association of Geriatric Psychiatry, 475, 476
American Association of Retired Persons, 744
American Association of Sex Educators, Counselors and Therapists, 751
American Association on Mental Deficiency, 750
American Board of Plastic Surgery, Inc., 749
American Cancer Society, 745
American Coalition of Citizens with Disabilities, 747
American College of Nurse-Midwives, 749
American College of Obstetricians and Gynecologists, 747, 749
American College of Sexologists, 750
American Dental Association, 746
American Diabetes Association, 746
American Dietetic Association, The, 749
American Digestive Disease Society, Inc., 746
American Family Planning Services, 744
American Fertility Society, 748

American Foundation for the Blind, Inc., 445, 745
American Heart Association, 747
American Hospital Association, 499
American Lung Association, 750
American Medical Association, **522**
American Narcolepsy Association, The, 749
American Optometric Association, 747
American Parkinson Disease Association, Inc., 749
American Public Health Association, 747
American Red Cross, 745
American Social Health Association, 750
American Society of Plastic and Reconstructive Surgeons, Inc., 296, 749
American Speech-Language-Hearing Association, 747, 751
American Way of Sex, An Informal Illustrated History, The, 131
Amino acids, 14
Amitriptyline (Elavil), 398, 743
Amnesia, **522**
Amniocentesis, 189, *190, 191,* **523**
Amnion, *170,* **523**
Amniotic cavity, *170*
Amoxicillin (Amoxil, Larotid), 742, 743
Amoxil (amoxicillin), 742
Amphetamines, 63, 322, **523**
action of, 327, 334–35
dangers of, 335–36
list, 334
overdose, 335
social acceptance, 326
Ampicillin (Omnipen), 253, **523,** 743
Amytal, 328
Analgesic, **523**
Analysis, *see* Psychoanalysis
Androgens, 21, 180, 237–38, **524**
Androgynous, **524**
Anemia, 72, 448, **524**
pregnancy, during, 176
Anesthesia, 194–95, **526**
cosmetic surgery, 299, 305
endotracheal, 299
risks, 243
Aneurysm, **526**
Angel dust (PCP), 323–24, 326, 337, 340–41
Angina pectoris, 450, **527**
Angiography, **527**
Animal bites, **528**
Ankles, swollen, **528**
Anorexia, 26
Anorexia nervosa, 64–65, 744
Antabuse (disulfiram), 355, **528,** 742
Antacid, *see* Acidity and alkalinity

Anterior tibial artery, *9*
Anterior tibial vein, *9*
Anthrax immunization, 738
Antibiotics, **528**
   (*see also* individual drugs)
   breast infections, 280–81
   genital, 231–32, 233
   limitations, 237
   pregnancy and, 185
   sexually transmissible disease and, 246, 248
Antibody, **529**
Anticonvulsants, effect on fetus, 180
Antidepressant, **529**
Antidote, **530**
Antigen, **530**
Antihistamines, **530**
Anti-hypertensive drugs, 117
Anti-oxidants, 48
Antiperspirant, **530**
Antiseptic, **530**
Antitoxin, **531**
Antivert (meclizine), 742
Anus, *12, 13,* 14, 15, *23, 24,* **531**
Anxiety, 29, 69, 385–86, **531**
   sexual problems and, 117
Aorta, *9,* **531**
Aortic arch, *9*
Aortic valve, 85
Aphasia, **531**
Aphrodisiac, **531**
Apoplexy, *see* Stroke
Appendectomy, 239
Appendicitis, **531**
Appendix. *12, 13,* 212
Appetite, **532**
Apresoline (hydralazine HCL), 742
Arch Back, 86
Archery, calorie expenditure in, 71
Areola, **533**
Aristocort (triacinolone), 742
Arm Rotator, 88
Arteries, *9*
Arterioles, 10
Arteriosclerosis, **533**
Arthritis, *455,* **533**
   associations concerned with, 745
   emotional factors, 29
Arthritis Foundation, The, 745
Artificial insemination, 219–20, **535**
Artificial respiration, **535**
Art therapy, 398
Ascorbic acid (Vitamin C), 40, 41, 44, 48, **535**
Aspirin, 30, **535**
Assault, rape as, 363
Association for Voluntary Sterilization, Inc., 751
Asthma, 29, 348, **536**

Asthma and Allergy Foundation of America, 744
Astigmatism, **536**
Atarax (hydroxyzine HCL), 742
Atherosclerosis, **536**
Athlete's Foot, *see* Fungus infections
Atkin's Diet, 60
Atria, 8
Atromid-S (clofibrate), 742
Atrophy, **537**
Atropine, 337, 343–44
Atropinic drugs, 337
Aureomycin, **537**
Auscultation, **537**
Austin, Tracy, 66
Auto-immune responses, **537**
Autosomes, *190*
Axillary artery, *9*
Azo-Gantrisin (azo-sulfisoxazole), 742
Azo-sulfisoxazole (Azo-Gantrisin), 742

"Baby blues," 201–2
Backache, **538**
Back Lift, 86
Backpacking, benefits of, 74
Back-Up, 85
Bacteria, **538**
Bacterial endocarditis, **538**
Badminton, 71, 75
Bag of waters, *see* Amnion
Baldness, **538**
Baldwin, Faith, 481
Barbiturates, 328, 356, 398, **538, 676**
Barium test, **539**
Bartholin's gland, *22, 25,* **539**
   abscess, drainage of, 238
   infection, 232
Basal metabolism test, **539**
Baseball, calorie expenditure in, 71
Basilic vein, *9*
Basketball, 71, 75
Bed sore, **540**
Bee stings, **638**
Bell's palsy, **540**
Benadryl (diphenhydramine), **540,** 742
Bendectin (doxylamine and pyridoxine), 742
Benedek, Therese, 430
Bentyl (dicyclomine), 742
Benzedrine, 334, **540**
Beriberi, 42
Biceps, *8*
Bicycling, 71, 74
Bifocals, *see* Eyeglasses
Bile, **540**
Billings method, 154
Biofeedback, **540**
Biopsy, 225, 226, **541**
   breast, 286–87
   cone, 226, 238

Biotin, 40, 41, 44
Birth canal, *see* Vagina
Birth control, *see* Abortion; contraception
Birth defects, **541**, 745
  (*see also* Fetus)
  congenital rubella syndrome, 185–86
  drugs taken by mother, 179–80
  epilepsy of mother, 184
  fetal alcohol syndrome, 179
  hereditary, 185
  infertility caused by, 207
Birth injuries, **541**
Birthmarks, **541**
Bisexuality, 127–29, **542**
Black eye, **542**
Blackheads, **542**
Bladder, *392*, **542**
Bleeding, *see* Hemorrhage
Bleeding, vaginal:
  abortion and, 160, 161
  IUDs and, 146–47
  menstrual, *see* Menstruation
  midcycle, 228
  postpartum, 202
  sexual relations, after, 229–30
Blepharoplasty, 294, 307–8
Blindness, associations concerned with, 745
Blister, **543**
Blood, **543**, 745, 748
  chemical analysis, 72
  clotting, 161, **544**
    oral contraceptives and, 138, 140
  pressure, **544**
    elevation of, *see* Hypertension
    oral contraceptives and, 139
Blood serum, **545**
Blood sugar, 139
Blood tests, **545**
Blood transfusions, 187, **545**
Blood types, **546**
Blood vessels, emotion and, *392*
Blue Cross-Blue Shield, 493
  "sixty-five plus" contract, 493
Body odors, **546**
Boils, **546**
Bones, 4, *6*, *7*, **547** (color insert)
  osteoporosis, 454–55
Boric acid, **547**
Bottle feeding, 204–5
Botulism, 48–49, **547**, 738, 739
Bowling, 71, 74
Brachial artery, *9*
Brachial plexus, *18*
Brachioradialis muscle, *8*
Brain, 17, *18*, *548*
  emotion and, *392*
Brassiere, selection and fitting, 271

Breast, 265, 271, 274, 275, 287–88, **549**
  (color insert)
  areola, 266, *268*, *269*
  cancer, *see* Breast cancer
  cosmetic surgery on, 310, *311*, 312–14
  cysts, 277, *278*, 279, 286
  development, 266, 267, *268*, 275–76
    (color insert)
  examination, *see* Breast examination
  infections, 204, 205, 280–81
  lactation, *see* Breast feeding
  menstrual cycle changes, 28, 266, *268*, 276–77
  menopause, 267, 270, 454
  nipples, 266–67, *268*, *269*, 274, *392*, **665**
    inversion, 275
  oral contraceptives, 140, 141
  reconstruction, 290, 314
  structure, 266, 267, *269*, 271, 274, 275
  table of disorders, 274, 275
  tenderness, 141, 171
  tumors, 280
Breast cancer, 281–90
  chemotherapy, 289
  diagnosis, 284–87
  emotional factors, 290–91
  growth of, *283*
  radiation therapy, 289
  risk factors, table of, 281
  surgery:
    reconstruction after, 290, 314
    types, 288–89
  symptoms, 281, *282*
Breast examination, 30, 33, 454, 737
  screening, 31
  self-examination, 270, *272*, *273*
Breastfeeding, 19, 203–5, **645**
  colostrum, 203
  contraceptive effect, 155
  infections during, 204
  nutrition during, 57, 204
  physical effects, 202
Breathing, *see* Respiratory system
Breech presentation, 199, 200, **549**
Bright's disease, **549**
Bromides, **549**
Bronchioles, 10, *11*
Bronchitis, 348, 452, **549**
Broomstick exercises, 90–91
Bruises, **550**
Bunions, **550**
Burns, 464, **550**
  sunburn, 442, **711**
Bursitis, **551**
Butazolidin Alka (Phenylbutazone alka), 742
Butler, Dr. Robert N., 482
Butylated-hydroxy anisole, 48

Caffeine, 336–37, **551**
  pregnancy and, 350–51
Calcium, 44, **551**
Calculus, **551**
Calendar rhythm family planning, 153, 552
Callus, **552**
Calories, 36, 70–71, **552**
  aging and, 57–58
  lactation, during, 57
  obesity and, *see* Obesity
  weight maintenance and, 53, 54
Cancer, **552, 651,** 745
  breast, *see* Breast cancer
  cervical, 234
  contraception and, 140, 149
  endometrial, 229, 234–35
  fallopian tubes, of, 236
  food additives, 49
  ovarian, 236
  pap smear, 224–25
  screening programs, 30, 31
  smoking and, 348, 452
  therapy, 243
Candidiasis, **553**
Canker sore, **553**
Canoeing and kayaking, 71, 74
Capillaries, *9,* 10
Carbohydrates, 14, 37, **553**
  (*see also* Starches; Sugars)
Carbon monoxide, 347–48
Carcinogen, **553**
Carcinoma, 234, **553**
Cardiac evaluation, 72
Cardiac muscle, *see* Myocardium
Cardiologist, **584**
Cardiopulmonary resuscitation (CPR), 553
Cardiovascular system, oral contraceptives and, 138, 140
Careers, women's, 406–7, 412–15
Carotene, 39, **554**
Carotid, *9*
Carpals, *6*
Car sickness, **658**
Cartilage, 7, **554**
CAT, **696**
Cataract, 444, **554**
Catecholamines, 21
Cathartic, **555**
Catheterization, **555**
Caudal anesthesia, 195
Cauterization, **555**
  molluscum contagiosum, 254
  venereal warts, 237, 238
Cavities, *see* Dental health
Celibacy, 121
Cell, **555**
Cellulose, 45
Center for Disease Control, Venereal

Disease Control Division, 750
Center for Women Policy Studies, 750
Cephalic vein, *9*
Cerebellum, *17, 18*
Cerebral palsy, associations concerned with, 745
Cerebrospinal fluid, 17
Cerebrovascular accident, *see* Stroke
Cervical caps, 152–53
Cervical mucus, 28, 209, 212
Cervix, *23, 25,* 167, *168, 170, 223,* **556**
  cancer of, 234–35
  dilation in labor, 181, 194
  disorders involving, *211*
  polyps, 234
Cesarean section, 192, 198–201, **556**
  placenta previa, 182
  vaginal delivery after, 199, 201
Chafing, **557**
Chancre, 256, **557**
Chancroid, 249
Chapping, **557**
Cheeks, cosmetic surgery involving, 307
Chemosurgery, 306
Chemotherapy, 243, 289, **557**
  marijuana and, 337–38
Chest, 10, 14, **558**
Chicken pox, immunization, 739
Chilblains, **558**
Childbirth, *see* Delivery
Childbirth Without Fear, 193
Child development
  divorce and, 416
  incest, 378
  leaving home, effect on mothers, 433
  lesbian mother, 409
  masturbation by child, 124, 125–26
  molestation, 376–78
  parental sexuality and, 119
  sex education and role expectations, 102–3, 404–5
  working mother, 407, 414–15
Chills, **559**
Chin, cosmetic surgery involving, 307
Chiropodist, 508, **680**
Chiropractors, 508–9, **559**
Chlamydial infections, 250
Chloramphenicol, 185
Chlorine, **559**
Chlordiazepoxide (Librium), 328, 398, **674,** 743
  fetus, effect on, 179
Chloroform, **559**
Chloromycetin, **559**
Chlorpheniramine (Chlortrimeton), 742
Chlorpromazine (Thorazine), 328, 398, **559, 715,** 743
Chlorpropamide (Diabinese), 743
Chlorothiazide (Diuril), 743
Chlortrimeton (Chlorpheniramine), 742

Choking, 560
Cholera immunization, 738
Cholesterol, 38, 560
Choline, 42
Chondromalacia, 73
Chorea, 560
Chorion, 170
Chorionic gonadotropin (HCG), 28
Chromosomes, 560
    amniocentesis, 189, 190, 191
    sperm, carried by, 167
Chronic symptom, 561
Circulatory system, 450–52, 561
    arteries, 9, 10 (color insert)
    heart, see Heart
Circumcision, 24
Cirrhosis, 561
Classes for pregnant women, 176
Claustrophobia, 562
Clavicle, 6
Cleanliness, sexually transmissible
        diseases and, 247–48
Clidinium bromide (Librax), 743
Climacteric, 562
Climbing, 71, 75
Clinics, 494, 562
Clitoris, 21, 22, 23, 25, 562
Clofibrate (Atromid-S), 742
Clomid, see Clomiphene citrate
Clomiphene citrate, 209, 217
Clostridial myositis, 739
Clotrimazole (Lotrimin), 743
Coagulation, see Blood clotting
Cobalamin (Vitamin B$_{12}$), 40–41, 43–44
Cobalt, 562
Cocaine, 324, 333, 334, 336, 562
Coccyx, 6
Codeine, 344, 562, 743
Coffee, 336–37, 350–51, 562
Coitus interruptus, 154, 562
Cold sores, see Herpes simplex
Colic, causes of, 497
Colitis, 29, 563
Collagen injection, 306
Colon, see Intestines
Colostomy, 563
Colostrum, 203, 563
Colposcopy, 226, 564
Colpotomy, 156
Coma, 564
Comaneci, Nadia, 66
Comfort, Dr. Alex, 105
Common cold, 185, 564
Common peroneal nerve, 18
Communal living, 417, 480
Communication as coping mechanism,
        389
Community Health Services, 749
Community Nutrition Institute, 749
Compazine (prochlorperazine), 742

Compulsion, 565
Conception, 565
    fallopian tube, in, 167, 168
Concussion, 565
Condoms, 135, 150, 152, 565
    disease prevention by use of, 247
Condyloma acuminata, 259–60
Cone biopsy, see Biopsy: cone
Congenital abnormalities, see Birth
        defects
Congestive heart failure, 450–51
Conjunctivitis, 565
Consciousness-raising groups, 565
Consent laws, see Informed consent
Constipation, 453, 566
Consumer Movement, medical care and,
        34
Contact dermatitis, 566
Contact lenses, 567
CONTACT Teleministries U.S.A., Inc.,
        748, 751
Contraception, 134, 135, 136, 142, 745
    abortion, see Abortion
    barrier type, 150–53
    coitus interruptus, 154
    diagrams, 135, 151
    information teaching of, 130
    IUDs, see Intrauterine devices
    lactation and, 155
    male hormonal, 143
    natural methods, 153–54
    non-medical considerations, 136, 162–63
    oral, see Oral contraceptives
    sexually transmissible disease, choice
        affecting vulnerability to, 246
    sterilization as, see Sterilization
Contraction, 567
Convalescent care, 501, 567
Convulsions, 19, 183, 567
Cooper's ligaments, 266, 267, 269
Coordination exercises, 83, 86–87
Coping mechanisms, 388
Copper, allergy to, 150
Copper 7, 146
Corneal transplant, 568
Corns, 568
Coronary artery, 9
Coronary artery disease, see Heart attack
Corpus luteum, 27, 28, 169, 569
Corticosteroids, 21, 569
    synthetic, 235
Cortisone, 21, 209
Corynebacterium vaginale, 253
Cosmetics, 443, 569
Cosmetic surgery, 293–317
    (see also individual procedures)
    chemosurgery, 306
    complications, 298, 301
    dermabrasion, 576

economic and social consideration, 293–94, 297
emotional aspect, 294–95, 316–17
foreign substances, insertion of, 298
preliminary consultations, 295–98
scar removal, 305
surgeon, selection of, 296
Coughing, 569
Coumadin (sodium warfarin), 743
Council on Family Health, 747
Counseling, 243, 397
Cowper's gland, 24, 25
Crab lice, 255, 570
Cramps, 570
Cranial nerves, 17
Cranium, 17
Crime against elderly, 468–69
Cross-tolerance defined, 319
Cryosurgery, 570
C/Sec, Inc., 749
Cumming, Anne, 479
Curettage, 570
Cushing's syndrome, 21, 570
Cuts, 602
Cyanosis, 571
Cyproheptadine (Periactin), 743
Cystic disease (breasts), 277, 278
Cystic fibrosis, 572, 746
Cystic Fibrosis Foundation, 746
Cystitis, 231, 542
Cystocele, 572
Cystoscopy, 572
Cysts, 238, 571
Cytology, 225
Cytomegalovirus, 250, 738

D&C, see Dilatation and curettage
D&E, see Dilatation and evacuation
Dairy products, Vitamins added to, 48
Dalkon shield, 146
Dalmane (flurazepam), 328, 743
Danazol, 235
Dancing, 74, 398
Dandruff, 572
Darvon (propoxyphene), 344, 743
Daytop Village, 355
Deafness, see Hearing loss
Deafness Research Foundation, The, 747
Death, 572
de Beauvoir, Simone, 481
Defense mechanisms, types of, 388
Deficiency diseases, 41, 573
anemia, 72, 176, 448, 524
Degenerative disease, 573
Dehydration, 574
Delirium tremens (DTs), 574
Delivery, 196, 198
age of mother, 425–27
breech, see Breech presentation

Cesarean, see Cesarean section
complications, availability of help for, 173, 174
forceps used in, 196
placenta, of, 198
place of, 166, 174–75, 198
professional supervising, choice of, 172–74
recovery, 201–3
Deltoid muscle, 8
Delusions, 574
Demerol (meperidine), 194, 322, 326, 344, 575
Dental health, 447, 508, 575, 746
dentures, 576
frequency of visits, 737
orthodontia, 306, 668
Dentin, 576
Dentures, 576
Deodorants, 576
Deoxyribonucleic acid, 584
Department of Foods and Nutrition, 749
Depilatory, 615
Depo-Provera, 142
Depressants, 327–30, 576
alcohol, see Alcohol
sedatives, see Sedatives
tranquilizers, see Tranquilizers
volatile solvents, 327
Depression, 391, 576
aging and, 448, 472–73
menopausal, 430, 431
Dermabrasion, 576
Dermatitis, 29, 576
contact, 566
DES (diethylstilbestrol), 576, 746
DES Action, 746
Descending lateral circumflex artery, 9
Desensitization, 577
Desirability, age and, 120
Desk exercises, 100
Desoxymethylamphetamine, 326, 338
DES Registry, Inc., 746
Detoxification, 577
Deutsch, Helene, 430
Dexedrine, 322, 334, 577
Dextrose, 577
Diabetes, 58, 72, 456–57, 577, 746
eye care and, 444
infertility, 208, 209, 210, 212
insulin production, 19
pregnancy and, 184
retinopathy, 580
sexual dysfunction and, 117
Diabetic retinopathy, 580
Diabinese (chlorpropamide), 743
Dialysis, 580
Diaphragm (contraceptive), 135, 150, 151, 152, 580
disease prevention, use as, 247

Diaphragm (muscle), *11, 12*, 14, **580**
Diarrhea, **581**
Diazepam, *see* Valium
Dick-Read, Grantly, 193
Dicyclomine (Bentyl), 742
Dietary habits, 30
Diethylpropion (Tenuate), 743
Diethylstilbestrol (DES), 139, 142, 179,
    576, 746
Diet pills, 63
    (*see also* Amphetamines; Diuretics)
Diets, reducing, 60–62
    menstrual periods and, 227
Digestive Information Center, 746
Digestive system, 14, 15, 16, 453, **581,**
    746
    diagrams:
        anatomical, *12* (color insert)
        functional, *13* (color insert)
Digitalis, **582**
Digoxin (Lanoxin), 743
Dilantin (phenytoin), 743
Dilatation and curettage, 159, 238–39,
    582
Dilatation and evacuation, 159, 160,
    238–39, **582**
Dildos, 114
Dimethyltriptamine (DMT), 338
Diphenhydramine (Benadryl), **540,** 742
Diphtheria immunization, 29, 738, 739
Dipyridamole (Persantine), 743
Disability, minimizing, 29, 31
Disc, slipped, **582**
Discharge, **583**
Dislocation, **583**
Disulfiram (Antabuse), 742
Diuretics, 15, 63, **584**
Diuril (chlorothiazide), 743
Diverticulosis, **584**
Divorce, 406, 415–16, 435–36
Dizziness, *see* Vertigo
DMT, *see* Dimethyltriptamine
DNA, **584**
Doctor, **584**
    (*see also* specialists by specialty)
DOM, *see* Desoxymethylamphetamine,
    326
Dopamine, **587**
Donnatal (hyoscyamine), 743
Doriden, 328
Douches, 233, 248, **726**
Down's syndrome, 189, *190,* **587**
Doxycycline (Vibramycin), 743
Dramamine, **587**
Driving, drugs and, 330
Drixoral, 743
Drug abuse, 319, 326, 746
    emergencies, 356–57
    susceptibility, 325, 352–53, 358

treatment for, 353–56
Drug Enforcement Administration, 746
Drugs, 318–25, 327, 742
    (*see also* individual drugs and drug
        groups)
    absorption speed, 14, 323–24
    abuse, *see* Drug abuse
    addiction, definition of, 219
    aging and, 459–62, 474
    alcohol, *see* Alcohol
    consumption statistics, 321
    cost, 461
    definitions concerning, 318–19
    dosage, 324
    generic and brand names, 461–62,
        742–43
    habituation defined, 319
    individual reactions, 324–25, 459–60
    individual responsibility, 320, 357–59
    infertility and, 207–9
    interaction, 461
    pregnancy and, 179, 349–52
    psychotherapy and, 398–99
    quality of, 324
    society's attitude toward, 326
    stress and, 30
    tobacco, *see* Smoking
DTs, *see* Delirium tremens
Duct ectasia, 279–80
Ductless glands, *see* Endocrine system
Dumbbell exercises, 92–94
Duodenal ulcer, **587**
Duodenum, *13,* 14 (color insert)
Dysentery, **587**
Dysmenorrhea, 228–29, **588**
Dyspareunia, 233, **588**
Dyspepsia, *see* Indigestion
Dysplasia, 234, **589**
Dyspnea, **587**
Dwarfism, pituitary, 19

Ears, **589, 590**
    cosmetic surgery on, 309
    wax in, 141
Echogram, **591**
Eclampsia, 183–84, **591**
Ectopic pregnancy, 147, 172, 182–83,
    591
Eczema, **591**
Edema, **592**
    eclampsia and, 183–84
Education for the elderly, 477
Ed-U-Press, 131
EEG, *see* Electroencephalogram
Egg, *see* Ovum
Ejaculation, **592**
EKG, *see* Electrocardiogram
Elastic stockings, **592**
Elavil (amitriptyline), 398, 743
Elbow, *6*

Elderhostel, 477
Elective surgery, *see* Surgery
Electrical injury, **592**
Electrocardiogram (EKG), 72, **592**
Electroencephalogram (EEG), **592**
Electrolysis, *see* Hair removal
Electroshock therapy, **593**
Elephantiasis, **593**
Elimination, 15, 69
    urine, *see* Urine
Embolism, **593**
Embryo, **593**
    (*see also* Fetus)
Emergency care, 497–98
Emetic, **593**
Emotional health, *see* Mental and emotional health
Emphysema, 348, 452, **593**
Empirin and codeine, 743
Empyema, **594**
Encephalitis, **594**
Endocrine system, 19, *20*, 21, 236–37, **594** (color insert)
Endometriosis, 209, 212, 235, **594**
    infertility after, 209, *211*, 212
    therapy, 218, 237–38
Endometritis, **594**
Endometrium, 26, *27*, 28, 235–36, 737
    aspiration, **594**
    biopsy, 213, *215*
    cancer, 229, 235–36
    implantation, 169
Endorphins, **595**
Endoscopy, **595**
Endurance, 68–69, 78, 83
Enema, **595**
Energy, 70, 71, **595**
ENT defined, **595**
Enterocele, **595**
Enuresis, **595**
Enzymes, 14, **595**
Ephedrine, **595**
Epididymis, *24*
Epidural anesthesia, 195
Epiglottis, **596**
Epilepsy, **596**, 746
    birth defects and, 184
Epilepsy Foundation of America, The, 746
Epinephrine, 299, **518**
Episiotomy, 195, 196, 202, **596**
Epithelioma, **597**
Equanil (meprobamate), **597**, 743
Erection, **597**
Erogenous zone, **597**
Erysipelas, **597**
Erythema, **597**
Erythrocin (erythromycin), 743
Erythrocytes, **597**

Erythromycin (Erythrocin), 185, **598**, 743
Esidrix (hydrochlorothiazide), 743
Esophagus, *12, 13,* 14, **598**
Estriol, 192
Estrogen, 21, **598**
    fetus, effect on, 139, 180
    menopausal therapy, 237, 428, 431
    menstruation and, 26, *27*, 28
    smoking and, 348
Estrogen receptor assay, 289
Eunuchism, 21
Eustachian tube, **598**
Excision biopsy, *see* Biopsy: cone
Excretion, *see* Waste removal
Exercise, 68, 70–77, 746
    aging and, 462
    calories burned, table of, 70
    clothing, 72–73
    obesity and, 62–63
Exercises:
    agility, for, 83
    coordination, for, 83, 87
    endurance, for, 78, 83
    flexibility, *see* Flexibility exercises
    job, during, 100
    routines by age group, 97–100
    strength, for, *see* Strength exercises
Experimental sex, society's view of, 105
Extensor tendons, *8*
External iliac artery, *9*
External iliac vein, *9*
External oblique muscle, *8*
Extramarital sex, 121–24
Eye Bank Association of America, The, 747
Eyebrow lift, 308–9
Eyeglasses, **599**
Eyelids, cosmetic surgery on, 307–8
Eyes, **598**, 747
    aging, 444–45
    disorders, 444–45
    eclampsia and, 183–84
    examinations, **599**, 737
    retina, **690**
    strain, **600**

Face lift, *see* Rhytidoplasty
Facial tic, *see* Tic
Fainting, **600**
Fallopian tubes, *22, 23, 25*
    abnormality, 209, *211*
    menstrual cycle and, *27*, 28
    pregnancy in, *see* Ectopic pregnancy
    scarring, *211*, 212
    surgery on, 218, 242
False pregnancy, **600**
Family history, **600**
Family planning, *see* Family size

Family practitioners, **584**
  obstetrical practice by, 173
Family relationships, violence in, 377–81
Family Service Association of America,
    Inc., 748
Family size, 133–34
  limitation:
    abortion, by, *see* Abortion
    contraception, by, *see* Contraception
    natural methods, 153–54
    sterilization, by, *see* Sterilization
Family therapy, 398
Fantasies, sexual, 126
Farsightedness, **601**
Fathers, prospective, attitudes of, 177
Fat necrosis, 280
Fats, 14, 37, 38, **601**
Fear, sexual problems caused by, 117
Federation of the Handicapped, Inc.,
    747
Feet, aging and, 456
Female nucleus, *168*
Feminism, *see* Women, changing roles of
Femoral artery, *9*
Femoral nerve, *18*
Femoral vein, *9*
Femur, *6*
Fencing, calorie expenditure in, 71
Fertility, **601**
  return after childbirth, 202
Fetal alcohol syndrome, 179
Fetus, **601**
  abortion, *see* Abortion, induced
  alcohol and, 179
  amniocentesis, 189, *190,* 191
  death of, 182, 187–88, 514
    (*See also* Abortion, induced)
  development, 169, *170,* 171
  drugs and chemicals affecting, 179–80
  heart rate, 191–92
  monitoring, 188–92
  position at delivery, 196, 199, *200*
  sex determination, 189
  sexually transmitted diseases, 250,
    254
  smoking by mother, 179
  vaccines, effect on, 180
Fever, **601**
Fever sores, *see* Herpes simplex
Fiber, dietary, 45, 58, **602**
Fibrillation, **602**
Fibroadenoma, 277, *278,* **602**
Fibroadenosis, *see* Breasts
Fibrocystic disease, *see* Breasts
Fibroid tumor, *see* Tumor
Fibula, *6*
Fidelity, marital, 121–22, 123–24
Figure 8, 83
Finkel, Dr. Sanford, 475

First aid, **602**
Fissure, **603**
Fistula, **603**
Fitness, 66–69
  exercise, *see* Exercise; Exercises;
    Sports
  nutrition, *see* Nutrients; Nutrition
  physical examination, 72, 76
  program development, 75–77
5–10–15 Agility Drill, 83
Flagyl (metronidazole), 258, 743
Flat feet, **603**
Flexibility, physical, 68
Flexibility exercises:
  Alternate toe touch, 79
  Arm rotator, 88
  Back lift, 86
  Back-up, 85
  Broomstick exercises, 90–91
  Dumbbells, with, 92–94
  Kickover, 84
  Knee lift, 81
  Leg raiser, 86
  Rocker, 86–87
  Shoulder stand, 82
  Side bender, 81
  Sprinter's drive, 82
  Squat bender, 78
  Squat thrust, 80
  Trunk rotator, 89
  Weights, with, 94–96
  Wing stretch, 88
Flexors, *8*
Flu, *see* Influenza
Fluids, 28, **603**
  retention, *see* Edema
Fluoridation of water, 29, 48, **603**
Fluoroscope, **603**
Flurazepam (Dalmane), 328, 743
Flutter Legs, 82
Folacin, *see* Folic acid
Folic acid (folacin), 40, 41, 43, **604**
  pregnancy, during, 56
Follicle stimulating hormone (FSH),
    20, 26, *27,* 216, 217
Food additives, **604**
Food and Drug Administration labeling
    requirements, 47
Food coloring, 48
Food groups, 45–46
Food labels, 47
Food poisoning, **604**
Forceps, use of, 196
Fordham University, College at 60
    Program, 477
Foreskin, *24*
Foster Grandparents, 479–80
Fracture, **605**
Franklin, Benjamin, 479
Fraternal twins, 169

French fries, 50
Frigidity, **605**
Fromm Institute of Lifelong Learning, 477
Frostbite, **605**
Frustration, sexual, 105–6
FSH, *see* Follicle stimulating hormone
Fulvicin (griseofulvin), 743
Fungus infections, **606**
Furosemide (Lasix), 743

Galactorrhea, 280
Gallbladder, *12, 13,* 14, **607**
Gallstones, **608**
    oral contraceptives and, 139
Gamma benzene hexachloride (Kwell), 255
Gamma globulin, **608**
Gangrene, **608**
Gantrisin (sulfisoxazole), 743
Gastrocnemius muscle, *8*
Gastrointestinal disorders, **608**
General practitioner, 173, **584**
Genetic abnormalities, infertility and, 207
Genetic counseling, 185, **609**
Genital tract, male, injuries to, 207
Geriatric psychiatry, 475–76
Geriatrics, 457–63, 479, **609**
German measles, 176, 185–86, **694**
    immunization against, 29, 738, 739
Gerontology, 477
GH, *see* Growth hormone
Gigantism, 19
Gingivitis, **609**
GI tract, *see* Digestive system
Gland, **609**
Glands of Montgomery, 266–67, *269*
Glans, *24*
Glaucoma, 444, **610**
    marijuana and, 337–38
Globus, **611**
Glomerulonephritis, **611**
Glucagon production, 19, *20*
Glucose, **611**
Glue sniffing, 324
Glycogen, 4, **612**
Goiter, 48, **612**
Golf, 71, 75
Gonads, *see* Ovaries; Testicles
Gonorrhea, 251–52, **613**
    dangers of, 207, 212, 245
    pregnancy and, 185, 186
    prophylaxis, 248
    symptoms, 230, 251–52
    treatment, 252
Gordon, Sol, 131
Gout, 455, **613**
Granuloma inguinale, 252–53, **613**
Gray Panthers, 478, 482

Greater saphenous vein, *9*
Grief, 469–70
Griseofulvin (Fulvicin), 743
Group living, 480
Group marriage, 479
Group therapy, 397–98, **614**
    alcoholism, 33, 354–56
    obesity, 63–64
Growth hormone, 19, *20*
Guilt, 117, 119, 162
Gums, 447, **614**
Gymnastics, *see* Exercises
Gynecology, 221, **584,** 747
    biopsy, 238
    cautery, 238
    chemotherapy, 243
    counseling, 243
    hormone therapy, 237–38
    infections, 237
    infertility, 207
    radiation therapy, 243
    self-help groups, 221
    surgery, 238–39, *240, 241,* 242–43
        (*see also* individual procedures)
    training, 172–73

Haeberle, Erwin J., 131
Hair, **614**
    loss of, *see* Baldness
    removal, **615**
Haldol, 328
Halitosis, **616**
Hallucinations, **616**
Hallucinogens, 330, **616**
    action of, 327, 337, 338–39
    atropine, *see* Atropine
    "bad trips," 339
    cross-tolerance, 342
    hashish, *see* Hashish
    LSD, *see* LSD
    marijuana, *see* Marijuana
    PCP, *see* Angel dust
    pregnancy and, 351
    scopolamine, *see* Scopolamine
    types, 337
Hamill, Dorothy, 66
Hammurabi, Code of, 364
Handball, 71
Hand care, *see* Skin care
Handicapped, associations concerned with, 747
Hangover, **616**
Hashish, 323, 337
Haycock, Mervyn, 7
Hay fever, *see* Allergies
HCG, *see* Chorionic gonadotropin
Headaches, 183, 195, **617**
Head injuries, mental capacity and, 448
Healers, 509
Health, 3, 34–35, 67, 747

Health education, 488
Hearing aids, 445–46, **619**
Hearing loss, 445–46, **619, 620,** 747
Heart, **620**
    disorders, 450
    emotion and, 29, *392*
    exercise and, 68, 69, 72
    physiology, 5
Heart attacks, **621**
    oral contraceptives and, 138
    smoking and, 138, 348
Heartburn, **623**
Heart disease, 747
    aging, 448
    exercise and, 72
    hypertensive, **622**
    pregnancy and, 184
Heart failure, **623**
Heart-lung machine, **623**
Heat exhaustion, **623**
Heat stroke, **624**
Height, **624**
Heimlich maneuver, **624**
Hemangioma, *see* Birthmarks
Hematoma, 304, 310, **625**
Hematuria, **625**
Hemigastrectomy, **625**
Hemochromotosis, **625**
Hemoglobin, **625**
Hemophilia, **625,** 747
Hemophilus influenza, immunization,
    738
Hemophilus vaginalis, 253
Hemorrhage, **626**
    hormone therapy, 237
    surgical risk, as, 243
Hemorrhoids, 203, **626**
Heparin, **627**
Hepatitis, 29, 262, **627**
    drug abuse and, 324
    immunization, 29, 738, 739
Herbal teas, 349
Heredity, **628**
Hernia, **628**
Heroin, 344, **629**
    cutting, 324
    tolerance, 346
Herpes simplex virus, 253–54, **629**
    pregnancy and, 185, 186–87
Herpes zoster (shingles), **629,** 739
Hiccups (hiccoughs), **629**
High altitude sickness, **629**
High blood pressure, *see* Hypertension
High Blood Pressure Information Center,
    748
Histamine, **630**
Hives, **630**
Hockey, 75
Hodgkin's disease, **630**
Holistic medicine, **630**

Home delivery, 175
Homosexuality, **631**
    disease transmission, 261–62
Hormones, 19, *20,* **631**
    breast cancer and, 289
    fetus, effect on, 180
    infertility and, 209, 213, 216
    menstrual cycle and, 227, 228
    muscle development, 68
    oral contraceptives, *see* Oral con-
        traceptives
    sexual activity and, 105
    tests, 213, 216
    therapy, 237–38
    types, 21
Horner, Matina, 405
Horseback riding, 71, 74
Horse shoe pitching, 71
Hospices, 470
Hospitalization, 499–501
    patient's bill of rights, 499
    private room, 500
    psychiatric, 399–400
Hospitals, **631**
    complications, for, 174, 175
    costs, 31
    delivery, for, 174
    pregnancy tours, 176
    social service departments, 508
Hot flashes, 229, 429, **631**
Housing for elderly, 468
Howard, Jane, 480
How to Select a Nursing Home, 458–59
HPL, *see* Lactogen, placental
Humerus, *6* (color insert)
Humidity, skin and, 442–43
Hydatidiform mole, 188
Hydralazine HCL (Apresoline), 742
Hydrochloric acid, digestive use of, 14
Hydrochlorothiazide (Esidrix, Hydro-
        diuril), 743
Hydrodiuril (hydrochlorothiazide), 743
Hydropres (hydroserpine), 743
Hydroserpine (Hyropres), 743
Hydroxyzine HCL (Atarax), 742
Hymen, *22, 25,* **632**
Hyoscyamine (Donnatal), 743
Hyperglycemia, **632**
Hypertension, **632**
    aging and, 450, 451
    associations concerned with, 748
    caffeine and, 337
    eclampsia and pre-eclampsia, 183–84
    emotion and, 29
    exercise and, 72
    oral contraceptives and, 139
    pregnancy and, 184
    salt and, 50
Hyperthyroidism, 19, 212, **633**
Hyperventilation, **633**

Hypnosis, **633**
Hypospadias, 219
Hypothalamus, 19, *20*, **634**
    emotion and, 236, 392
    menstruation and, 26, 428
Hypothermia, **634**
Hypothyroidism, 19, 212
Hysterectomy, 156, 239, *240, 241,* 242,
    634
    pregnancy, during, 161–62
Hysteria, **634**
Hysterosalpigram, *215,* 216
Hysteroscopy, 156
Hysterotomy, 161

Iatrogenic disease, **634**
ICD Rehabilitation and Research Center,
    747
Identical twins, 169
Ignorance, sexual problems caused by,
    117
Ileitis, **635**
Iliostomy, **653**
Imipramine, 398
Immunity and immunization, 29, **635,**
    738
Immunotherapy, 289
Impetigo, **636**
Impotence, 115, 207, **636**
Incest, 116, 378, **637**
Income, aging and, 466–68, 476
Inderal (propanolol hydrochloride), **743**
Indigestion, **637**
Indocin (indomethacin), **743**
Indomethacin (Indocin), **743**
Induced labor, **637**
Infant, 252, 254, 258
    sexual health, 102
Infantile paralysis, *see* Poliomyelitis
Infections:
    aging, 448, 457
    breast, 280–81
    drug use, from, 324
    genital, 231–33
    infertility resulting from, *208,* 209,
        210, *211,* 212
    IUD and, 148, 149
    pelvic, 183
    sexually transmitted, *see* Sexually
        transmissible diseases
    treatment, 237
Inferior vena cava, *9*
Infertility, 206–20, **637,** 748
    abortion, after, 206
    artificial insemination, 219–20
    female:
        causes, 209, *210, 211,* 212
        tests, 213, *214, 215,* 216
        treatment, 217–18
    gonorrhea and, 252

incidence, 206
    male, 207, *208,* 209
    medication, 217
    surgery:
        female, 218
        male, 209
    tests, 207, 213, *214, 215,* 216
Influenza, 457, **637,** 738
Information, consumer's right to, 31–32
Informed consent, 499, 503, **566**
Inguinal glands, **638**
Injections, infection risks from, 323
Injuries, sports, 73
Inner ear, *see* Ear
Inositol, 42
Insanity, 394
Insect stings and bites, **638**
Insomnia, **639**
    caffeine and, 337
    sleeping pills, *see* Sleeping pills
Insulin, **640**
    production, 19, *20*
    shock therapy, **640**
Insurance for preventive services, 32
Intelligence quotient (IQ), **640**
Intensive care, 501
Intercostal nerves, *18*
Intercourse, sexual, *see* Sexual inter-
    course
Interferon, **640**
Internal examination, *see* Pelvic examina-
    tion
Internist, **584**
Intestines, *12, 13,* 14, 15, *392,* **640**
Intoxication, 329
Intra-amniotic infusion, 161
Intraductal papilloma, 279
Intra-uterine devices (IUDs), 143–50,
    642
    contraindications, 136, 150
    diagrams, *135, 145*
    expulsion, 148–49
    hazards, 135–36, 148
    infection, 148, 149, 150, 230, 255
    infertility from use of, 212
    insertion, 144, *145*
    oral contraceptives compared, 144
    pain and, 144, 146–47, 229
    pregnancy during use, 147–48
    types, 144, *145,* 146
Introitus, 25
Iodine, 45
Iritis, **640**
Iron, 44–45, 56, 228, **641**
Irritability, **641**
Islets of Langerhans, 19, *20*
Isobutyl nitrite, 324, 349
Isordil (isosorbide), **743**
Isosorbide (Isordil), **743**
Itching, 443, **641**

IUDs, *see* Intra-uterine devices

Jackson Memorial Hospital Rape
    Treatment Center, 366, 371
Jaundice, 262, **642**
Jaws, cosmetic surgery involving, 306–7
Jealousy, 122–23
Jogging, 66, 69
Joints, 4, *7*
    aging, 454, 455
    diseases, *see* Arthritis; Bursitis; etc.
Joy of Sex, 105
Jugular vein, *9*
Jumping Jack, 78

Karate, benefits of, 74
Karmel, Marjorie, 193
Kenalog (triamcinolone), 743
Ketosis, 60–61
Khayyam, Omar, 320
Kickover, 83
Kidneys, *15*, **642**, 748
    dialysis, **580**
    disorders, 231, 448, **642**, 748
    role of, *16*
King, Billie Jean, 66
Klinefelter's syndrome, *190*
Knee disorders, **643**
Knee lift, 81
Kuhn, Maggie, 478
Kwell Cream (gamma benzene hexa-
    chloride), 255

Labia, 21, *22*, *23*, **644**
Labor, 166, 191–98, **644**
    contractions, frequency and duration
        of, 193–94
    delivery, *see* Delivery
    exercises, 193
    fetal monitoring, 191–92
    first stage, 193–94, *197*
    inducing, 194
    rupture of membranes, 194
    second stage, 195–96, *197*, 198
    transition, 194
Lacrimal ducts, **644**
Lactation, *see* Breastfeeding
Lactogen, placental (HPL), 28
Lamaze method, 193, **645**
Lanoxin (digoxin), 743
Laparoscopy, *215*, 217, 226
Laparotomy, 155–56
Larotid (amoxicillin), 743
Laryngitis, **645**
Larynx, *11*, **645**
Laxis (furosemide), 743
Laudanum, 322
Laxative, **646**
L-dopa, **646**

Leboyer, **646**
Leggitt, Hunter, 131
Leg raiser, 86
Lennane, K. J., 497
Lesbianism, 127–29, 409, 479, **646**
Lesser saphenous vein, *9*
Leukemia, **646**
Leukemia Society of America, Inc., 745
Leukorrhea, **647**
Levinson, Daniel, 423–24
LH (luteinizing hormone), 26, *27*, 216
Libido, 117–18, **647**
Librax (clidinium bromide), 743
Librium (chlordiazepoxide), 179, 328,
    398, **647**
Life expectancy, **647**
    average, 403–4
    sex difference chart, *440*
    smoking and, 348
Life review, 481
Ligaments, 4, *7*, **648**
    round, *22*
Lighting, accidents and, 463
Line jump, 83
Lipectomy, 314–16
Lipoma, **648**
Lipoprotein, 38
Lippes loop, 144, *145*
Lithium, 398, **648**
    fetus, effects on, 179
Liver, *12*, *13*, 14, **648**
    disease, infertility and, 209, 212
    oral contraceptives and, 139, 140
Liver spots, **649**
Living Wills, 482
Lobotomy, **649**
Lochia, 202
Lomotil (diphenoxylate and atropine),
    743
Longevity, *see* Life expectancy
Lopez, Nancy, 66
Loss of appetite, *see* Anorexia
Lotrimin (clotrimazole), 743
Love, 107–8
*Love Habit: The Sexual Odyssey of an
    Older Woman, The*, 479
Lower back pain, *see* Backache
Lozoff, Marjorie, 405–6
LSD, 324, 337, 338, **649**
    action, 337–39
    psychotic reactions, 325
Lumbar plexus, *18*
Lumbo-sacral plexus, *18*
Lungs, 5, 10, *11*, **649**
    aging, 452
    diseases, 348, 452
        (*see also*) individual respiratory
        diseases)
    emotions and, 392
Lupus erythematosus, **650**

Luteinizing hormone, 26, *27*, 216
Lymph nodes, **651**
Lymphogranuloma venereum, **651**

McIlvenna, Ted, 131
McKain, Walter, 478
McKinley and Jeffreys, 429
Macrobiotic diet, **651**
Magnesium, 45
Major medical insurance, 493
Makeup, 443, **569**
Malaria, **651**
Malarplasty, 306, 307
Male infertility, 207, *208*, 209
Malignancy, *see* Cancer
Malnutrition, 207, **652**
Mammography, 285–86, 310, **652**, 737
Mammoplasty, 294, 310, *311*, 312–13
Mandibuloplasty, 306, 307
Manic depressive psychosis, 394, **652**
March of Dimes Birth Defects Founda-
    tion, 745
Marijuana, 320, 321–24, **652**
    alcohol and, 342
    effects, 341–43
    legal penalties, 358–59
    medical uses, 337–38
    social acceptance, 326
Marriage, 409–12
    arranged, 364
    open marriage, 417–18
    role changes and, 405–7
Marriage counseling, 398, **652**, 748
Massage, **652**
Mastectomy, **652**
    cosmetic surgery after, 314
    types, 288–89
Mastitis, 280, **652**
Mastoid, **653**
Mastopexy, 313–14
Masturbation, 102, 121, 122, 479, **653**
    children, by, 124–26
Maternity center delivery, 175
Maxilloplasty, 306–7
Mayo Diet, Magic, 60
Mead, Margaret, 481
Measles, 29, **653**, 739
Meat preservatives, 48–49
Meatus, 15, *22, 23, 24, 25*
Meclizine (Antivert), 742
Median nerve, *18*
Medicaid, 493
Medical care costs, 31, 493
Medic-Alert, 498, **653**
Medical history, *214*, 222
Medical insurance, 493
Medical prefixes and suffixes, 740–41
Medical records, **654**
Medicare, 493
Medicines, *see* Drugs

Meditation, **654**
Meditations on the Gift of Sexuality, 131
Medroxyprogesterone (Provera), 743
Medulla oblongata, 17
Melanin, **654**
Melanocyte stimulating hormone
    (MSH), *20*
Melanoma, **654**
Memory, aging and, 449
Menarche, 26, **654**, **686**
Mended Hearts, Inc., The, 747
Menières disease, **655**
Meninges, 17
Meningitis, **655**, 738
Menopause, 229, 427–32, **655**
    age of, 26, 428
    breast changes, 267
    hormones and, 21, 270
    misdiagnoses and, 496–97
    sexual pleasure after, 113
Menorrhagia, **655**
Menstrual extraction, 159
Menstruation, **656**
    amount of flow, 227–28
    commencement, 226, 227
    cycle, 25–28
        changes in, 21, 28
        irregularity, 21, 226–27
        phases of, 26, *27*, 28, 167
    hormone production and, 21
    iron loss, 45
    missing period, 171, 227
    oral contraceptives and, 141
    pain, 228–29
    return after childbirth, 202
Mental activity of elderly, 480–81
Mental and emotional health, 383–401
    associations concerned with, 748
    bodily interaction with, 28, 391–93
        (color insert)
    depression, *see* Depression
    need for help, determining, 395
    nervous breakdown, 394
    neurosis, 393–94
    psychosis, 394–95
    psychotherapy, *see* Psychotherapy
    self-help groups, 400–1
    stress and, 384–85, 389, 390
Mental illness, **656**
Mentoplasty, 306, 307
Meperidine, *see* Demerol
Meprobamate (Equanil), 398, **597**, 743
Mercury, **656**
Mescaline, 338
Metabolism, **656**
Metacarpals, *6*
Metastasis, **657**
Metatarsals, *6*
Methadone, 325, 344, 355, **657**
Methaqualone, 328

Methedrine, 322, 334, **657**
Methocarbamol (Robaxin), 743
Methyldopa (Aldomet), 742
Methylphenidate (Ritalin), 743
Metronidazole (Flagyl), 258, 743
Midcycle bleeding, 228
Middle age, 421–38
    adolescence, comparison with, 437
    evaluation period, as, 423
    menopause, *see* Menopause
Middle ear, *see* Ear
Midwives, 174, 508
    nurse-midwives, *see* Nurse-Midwives
Migraine, *see* Headache
Milk, 48, **657**
Miltown (Meprobamate), 328, 398, **657**
Minerals, 44–45, 48
Miscarriage, *see* Abortion, spontaneous
Mitral valve, *8*
Mole, **657**
Molesting children, 376–78
Molluscum contagiosum, 254
Mongolism, *see* Down's syndrome
Monilia, *see* Yeast infections
Monogamy, 123–24, 247
Mononucleosis, infections, **658**
Mons pubis (mons veneris), 21, *23*,
    658
Moral values
    abortion and, 162
    contraception and, 153
    sexuality and, 104, 119
    sterilization, 158
More Joy, 105
Morning sickness, 171, **658**
Morphine, 322, 344, **658**
Mosaic law, 364
Mother-in-Deed, 80
Motion sickness, **658**
MSH, *see* Melanocyte stimulating
    hormone
MS Society, 507
Mucous membrane, **659**
Multiple sclerosis, **659**, 748
Mumps, **659**
    immunization, 738, 739
    infertility and, 207
Muscles, 4, 5, *8,* **660** (color insert)
    development, 68
    emotions and, *392*
    pectoral, 266
Muscular dystrophy, **660**, 748
Muscular Dystrophy Association, Inc.,
    748
Myasthenia gravis, 6, **660**, 748
Myasthenia Gravis Foundation, 748
Mycoses, *see* Fungus infections
Mycostatin (nystatin), **661**, 743
Myers, Lonny, 131
Myocardial infarction, 450, **661**

Myocardium composition, 4, 5
Myomectomy, 235, 239, **661**
Myometrium, 25
Myopia, **663**
Myxedema, 28

Nail, **661**
Nalloxone, 355–56
Narcolepsy, **662**, 749
Narcotics, 322, 344–46, **663**
    (*see also* individual drugs)
    addiction, 325, 344, 345–46, 355–56
    chemical action, 327, 344
    overdose, 346
    pregnancy and, 351
    withdrawal, 346
National Abortion Federation, 744
National Abortion Rights Action League
    (NARAL), 744
National Anorexic Aid Society, Inc., 744
National Association for Retarded
    Citizens, 750
National Association of Patients on
    Hemodialysis and Transplanta-
    tion, Inc., 748
National Center for the Prevention and
    Control of Rape, 363, 750
National Clearing House for Alcohol
    Information, 744
National Clearinghouse for Drug Abuse
    Information, 746
National Committee on the Aging, Inc.,
    744
National Council on Alcoholism, Inc.,
    744
National Eye Institute, 747
National Foundation for Ileitis and
    Colitis, Inc., 746
National Genetics Foundation, Inc., 745
National Heart, Lung, and Blood Insti-
    tute, 747, 750
National Hemophilia Foundation, 747
National Institute of Allergy and Infec-
    tious Diseases, 744
National Institute of Arthritis, Metabo-
    lism, and Digestive Diseases, 745
National Institute of Dental Research,
    746
National Institute of Mental Health, 748
National Institute on Aging, 482, 744
National Institute on Drug Abuse, 321
National Kidney Foundation, 748
National Mental Health Association, 748
National Multiple Sclerosis Society, 748
National Research Council. Food and
    Nutrition Board, recommenda-
    tions of, 47
National Right to Life Committee, Inc.,
    744

National Society to Prevent Blindness, The, 745
National Tay-Sachs & Allied Disease Associations, Inc., 751
National VD Hotline, 750
Natural childbirth, 193, **663**
Natural family planning, 153–54
Nausea, 171, **663**
Nearsightedness, **663**
Neck, *392,* **664**
Neighbors Helping Neighbors, 81
Nembutal (pentobarbital sodium), 328, **664**
Neomycin, **664**
Neoplasia, 140, **664**
Neosporin, 743
Nephritis, **611**
Nephron, 16
Nephrosis, *see* Kidney disorders
Nerves, 17, *18, 304,* **664**
"Nervous breakdown," 394
Nervous system, 16, 17, *18,* 448–50, **664** (color insert)
Neugarten, Bernice, 423
Neuralgia, **664**
Neuritis, 42, **664**
Neurologists, **584**
Neuromuscular diseases, **664**
Neurons, 15
Neurosis, 393–94, **665**
    male attribution of female symptoms to, 496–97
Neurosurgeon, **584**
New York Association of Marriage & Family Therapy, 748
Niacin (Vitamin B₃), 40–41, 43
Nicotine, 347
Night sweats, 429
Nipples, 266–67, *268, 269,* 274, 275, *392,* **665**
Nitrates, 48, 49
Nitrosamines, 49
Nitrous oxide, 333
Nodule, **665**
Noise, **665**
Norepinephrine, 21
North American Vegetarian Society, 749
Nose:
    bleeding, **666**
    cosmetic surgery, *see* Rhinoplasty
Nuclear medicine, **667**
Nudity, 131
Nurse-Midwives, 173–74, **667**
Nurses, "special duty," 500
Nursing, *see* Breast-feeding
Nursing homes, 458–59, 471
Nutrition, 36–46, 749
    (*see also* individual nutrients)
    balances, 45–46

calories, 54–55
    pregnancy, during, 55–56, 177
    vitamins, *see* Vitamins
Nystatin (Mycostatin), 743

Obesity, 29, 58–60, **667,** 751
    reduction, *see* Weight control
Obsession, **667**
Obstetrician-gynecologists, 172–73, 207, **584**
Occupational therapy, 398
Odyssey House, 355
Oedipus complex, **667**
Office of Cancer Communications, 745
Office of Maternal & Child Health, 749
Office on Smoking and Health, 751
Ohio State University, Program 60, 477
Omnipen (ampicillin), 253, **523,** 743
Oncology, 289
Onychia, **667**
Oophorectomy, 242, **667**
Ophthalmologist, **584**
    (*see also* Eyes)
Opiate, **668**
Opium, 320, 322, 344
Optician, **668**
    (*see also* Eyeglasses)
Optometrist, **668**
    (*see also* Eyeglasses; Eyes)
Oral contraceptives, *135,* 136–41, 180
    menstrual cycle and, 171, 227
Oral hygiene, 30
Oral sex, 114, **668**
Orgasm, 106, 110–12, **668**
Orinase (tolbutamide), **668,** 743
Orthodontia, 306, **668**
Orthopedist, **584**
Osteoarthritis, **669**
Osteopathy, 508, **669**
Osteoporosis, 431, 432, 454–55, **669**
Ostomy, associations concerned with, 749
Otolaryngologist, **584**
Otoplasty, 294, 309
Otosclerosis, **669**
Ovaries, 21, *22, 23, 25,* **669**
    cancer of, 236
    cysts, 242
    follicular ripening, 167, *168*
    hysterectomy and, 239
    infection, 240
    infertility and, 212
    menstrual cycle and, 26, *27*
    oral contraceptives and, 140–41
    ovulation, *see* Ovulation
    tumors, 230, 236
Overdose emergencies, 356–57
Overeaters Anonymous, 33, 63, 751
Overweight, *see* Obesity

Ovulation, 26, 27, 28, 167, *168*, 209, 229, **669**
Ovum, 21, 26, *27*, 167, *168*, 169, **670**
Oxygen, 70, **670**
Oxytocin, 19, 194, **670**

Pacemaker, **671**
    sinoauricular node as, 5
Paget's disease, **671**
Pain, **671**
    IUDs and, 144, 146–47
Palmar artery, *9*
Palpitations, **672**
Pancreas, 12, 13, 14, **672**
    Islets of Langerhans, 19, *20*
Pantothenic acid, 40, 41, 43, **672**
Papanicolaou, Doctor, 224
Papavarine time caps (Pavabid), 743
Pap test, 72, 224–25, **672**, 737
Paracervical block, 195
Paralysis, **673**
Paramedical services, 507–8
Paranoia, **674**
Parasympathetic nervous system, 18
Parathyroid glands, 19, 20
Parathyroid hormone, 19, 20
Parenthood, 129
    avoidance or delay, 406, 411
    single parent, 119
Parents, elderly, 435
Parkinson's disease, 449, **674**, 749
Patch test, **674**
Patella, *6*
Pathologist, **584**
Pavabid (papavarine time caps), 743
PCP (angel dust), 323–24, 326, 337, 340–41
Pectineus muscle, *8*
Pectoralis major, *8*
Pediatrician, **584**
Pelvic examination, *214*, 222, 737
Pelvic inflammatory disease, 230, 254–55
Pelvis, *6*
Penicillin, 185, **674**
    allergy to, 249
    sexually transmissible diseases and, 249, 258
Penicillin V (K) (Pen Vee K; V-Cillin K), 743
Penis, *24*, *25*, **675**
Pentazocine (Talwin), 328, 344, 743
Pentobarbital sodium (Nembutal), 328, **664**
Pen Vee K (penicillin V [K]), 743
Pep pills, *see* Amphetamines
Pepsin, 14
Peptic ulcer, *see* Ulcer
Percodan, 322, 344, 743
Pergonal, 218
Periactin (cyproheptadine), 743

Perineum, *22*, *23*, *24*, *25*, **675**
    episiotomy, 195, 196
Peristalsis, 14
Peritonitis, **675**
Peroneal artery, *9*
Peroneal nerve, *18*
Peroneal vein, *9*
Persantine (Dipyridamole), 743
Perspiration, **675**
Pertussis (whooping cough), 29, 738, 739
Pessary, **676**
Pesticides, effect on fetus of, 180
PET, **697**
Peyote, 338
pH, **676**
Phalanges, *6*
Pharmacists, 460
Pharyngitis, **676**
Pharynx, *11*
Phencyclidine, *see* PCP
Phenergan (promethazine), 743
Phenobarbital, 328, 398, **676**
Phenylbutazone alka (Butazolidin Alka), 742
Phenytoin (Dilantin), 743
Phlebitis, **676**
Phobia, **677**
Phosphorus, 45
Physical examinations, 222, **677**, 737
    infertility workup, *214*
    pelvic, *214*, 222
Physical health, mental health and, 28
Physical therapy, **677**
Physician, 32, 33, **677**
    duty of, 501–4
    group practice, 490
    hospitalization by, 501–2
    patient's duty toward, 504–7
    payment plans, 492–94
    qualifications, 490, **584**
    relationship with, 32, 488–89, 491–92
    second opinion requests, 503
    selection, 32, 489–91, 495
    specialists, 495, **584**
        (*see also* individual specialty)
    women, treatment of, 496
    women physicians, 491
PID, *see* Pelvic inflammatory disease
"Pill, The," *see* Oral contraceptives
Pilonidal cysts, **678**
Pineal gland, *20*, 21
Ping-Pong, 71
Pitocin (Oxytocin), 194
Pituitary gland, 19, *20*, 236, **678**
    infertility and, *208*, *210*
    menstrual cycle and, 26, *27*
Pizza, 50
Placebo, **678**
Placenta, 28, 169, *170*, **678**
    delivery of, 198

detachment of, 182
hydatidiform mole, 188
Placental lactogen, 192
Placenta previa, 181, 182
Plague immunization, 738
Planned Parenthood Federation of
    America, Inc., 130, 745
Plantar wart, 678
Plaque, 678
Plastic surgery, 678, 749
    cosmetic, see Cosmetic surgery
Platelets, 678
Pleurisy, 679
Pneumococcal infection, immunization,
    739
Pneumonia, 679
Podiatrists, 508, 680
Podophyllin, 259–60
Poison, 680
Poison control center, 681
Poison ivy, oak and sumac, 681
Poliomyelitis, 29, 681, 738
Pollution, air, 29
Polpectomy, 234, 238
Polyps, 229, 682
Pornography in sex education, 104
Postcoital test, 215, 217
Postpartum depression, 201–2
Posture, 683
Potassium, 45, 48, 683
Pre-eclampsia, 683
Pregnancy, 165–92, 749
    abortion of, see Abortion, induced
    alcohol use during, 179
    attitudes toward, 117, 166, 176–77
    author's experience, 165–66
    blood pressure and, 183
    complications of, 136, 181–88
    conception, 167, 168
    congenital birth defects and, 185–87
    contraceptive risks compared, 135–36
    death of fetus, 187–88
    delivery, see Delivery
    diabetes and, 184, 192
    diet during, 55–56, 177, 178
    drug and chemical use during, 179–80
    due date, calculation of, 171
    ectopic, 147, 172, 182–83, 591
    exercise during, 72, 180
    falls during, 180
    false, 600
    fetal development, 169–71
    health care during, see Prenatal care
    home tests for, 172
    hormones during, 180
    hydatidiform mole, 188
    hypertension and, 183–84, 192
    implantation of ovum, 169
    infections during, 185–87, 257
    IUD problems, 147–48

labor, see Labor
    menstrual cycle and, 167
    miscarriage, see Abortion, spontaneous
    placenta previa, 182
    pre-eclampsia and eclampsia, 183–84
    prevention, see Contraceptives
    quickening, 687
    rape, after, 374
    sexually transmissible diseases and,
        186–87, 257
    sexual relations during, 180–81
    smoking during, 177, 179
    tests, 139, 158, 171–72, 227
    travel and, 180
    vaccines, 180
    weight gain, 178
Preludin, 322, 334
Premature ejaculation, 115, 592
Premenstrual tension, 28
Prenatal care, 30–31, 72, 176–81
    (see also Pregnancy)
    nutrition, 55–56, 177, 178
"Preparation for childbirth" classes,
    176
Prepayment plans, 492–93
Presbyopia, 444
Prescriptions, see Drugs
Preventive medicine, 29–31, 493
Prochlorperazine (Compazine), 742
Proctologist, 584
Progestasert, 146
Progesterone, 237, 428, 683
    menstruation and, 26, 27, 28, 228
    pregnancy and, 169, 180
Progestin, 684
Prolactin, 19, 20, 216, 684
Prolapse, 684
Promethazine (Phenergan), 743
Propanolol hydrochloride (Inderal), 743
Propoxyphene (Darvon), 344, 743
Prostaglandins 229, 684
Prostate gland, 24, 25, 685
Protein, 14, 37, 685
    pregnancy and nursing, 56, 57
Provera (medroxyprogesterone), 743
Pruritis, see Itching
Pseudoephedrine (Sudafed), 743
Psilocybin, 338
Psoriasis, 685
Psychiatrists, 396, 685
Psychoanalysts, 397, 685
Psychologists, 396–97
Psychoneurosis, see Neurosis
Psychosis, 394–95, 686
    drug induced, 335, 337, 339
Psychosomatic illnesses, 28–29, 391, 393,
    497, 686
Psychotherapy, 396–99, 686
    cosmetic surgery and, 295
    elderly persons and, 475–76

group therapy, 397–98, 476
Psychotropic drugs, 398–99
Puberty, 26, **686**
Pubic hair, 21
Pubic lice, 255, **570**
Public health measures, 29
Pudendal block, 195
Puerperal fever, **686**
Pulmonary artery, *9*
Pulmonary evaluation, 72
Pulmonary vein, *9*
Pulmonic valve, *5*
Pulse, **686**
Pus, **686**
Push-back, 89
Push-up, 84
Push-up, Knee, 84
Pyelonephritis, 231
Pyorrhea, **686**
Pyridoxine (Vitamin B₆), 40–41, 43

Q fever, **687**
Quaalude, 328
Quadriceps femoris, *8*
Quarantine, **687**
Quickening, **687**

Rabies, **687**, 739
Racquetball, 75
Radial artery, *9*
Radial nerve, *18*
Radiation, infertility and, 207
Radiation therapy, 243, 289
Radiologist, **584**
Radioreceptor assay (RRA) for HCG
    (human chorionic gonadotropin)
    test, 172
Radiotherapy, **688**
Radium, **688**
Radius, *6*
Rale, **688**
Rape, 116, 362–76
    anger as motive, 362
    associations concerned with, 750
    definition, 363
    incidence, 365
    myths about, 366–68
    prevention, 368–69
    rapist, prosecution of, 373, 376
    victim
        attitude towards, 363–65
        behavior, 369–71
        psychological recovery, 374–76
        treatment, medical, 371–74
        wife as, 363
Rapid eye movement (REM), **688**
Rashes, **688**
    syphilis, 257
Raynaud's disease, **689**
RDAs, 47

Reach and Lift, 87
Reach for Recovery program, 290, 488,
    507, 745
Recommended Daily Dietary Allow-
    ances, 47
Recording for the Blind, Inc., 745
Rectal examination, frequency, 737
Rectocele, **689**
Rectum, *12, 13,* 15, **689**
    female, *23*
    male, *24*
Rectus abdominus muscle, *8*
Reflexes, 15
Rehabilitation, 31
"Relationships," 417
REM (Rapid eye movements), **688**
Remission, **689**
Renal artery, *9, 16*
Renal vein, *9, 16*
Repression, **689**
Reproductive system, 21, 25, **689**
    female, *22, 23* (color insert)
    male, *24,* **699**
    menstrual cycle, *see* Menstrual cycle
    pregnancy, *see* Pregnancy
Reserpine, 398, **690**
Resistance, **690**
Resolve, Inc., 748
Respiratory diseases, 750
    (*see also* individual condition, e.g.
        Asthma, Bronchitis, etc.)
Respiratory system, 10, *11*
Restlessness, 29
Retardation, associations concerned
    with, 750
Retina, **690**
Retirement Marriage, 478
Rheumatic fever, **691**
Rheumatism, 29, **692**
Rheumatoid arthritis, *see* Arthritis
Rh factor, 187, **691**
    amniocentesis and, 176, 189, 191
Rhinitis, **692**
Rhinoplasty, 294, 299, *300,* 301
Rhythm method, 153–54, **552**
Rhytidoplasty, 294, 301–2, *303,* 304–5
Riboflavin (Vitamin B₂), 40–43, **693**
Ribonucleic acid, *see* RNA
Ribs, *6*
Rickettsial diseases, **693**
Ringworm, **606**
Ritalin (methyl phenidate), 743
RNA, **693**
Robaxin (methocarbamol), 743
Rocker, 86–87
Rocky Mountain spotted fever, **693**, 739
Roman Catholic Church, 153
Rooming in, 201
Root canal, **694**
Round ligament, *22, 23*

Rowing, 71, 74
Rubaiyat, 320
Rubella, *see* German measles
Rubeola, immunization, 738, 739
Rubin test, *215*, 216, **694**
Running, 71, 74
Rupture, **694**
Rupture of membranes (bag of waters), 181

Saccharin, 49, **694**
Sacroiliac, **694**
Sacrum, *6*
Saddle block anesthesia, 195
Sadism, **695**
Safety precautions, aging and, 463–65
Saf-T-Coil, 144
Sailing, 71, 74
Saline abortion, **695**
Saliva, 14, **695**
Salmonella, **695**
Salpingectomy, **695**
Salpingitis, **695**
Salt, 48–50, 56, 58, **695**
Samaritans, The, 751
Saphenous nerve, *18*
Sarcoma, **696**
Sartorius muscle, *8*
Scabies, 255–56, **696**
Scalp, emotion and, *392*
Scanning machines, **696**
Scapula, *6*
Scars, 305
    cosmetic surgery, 298, 299, 301, 302, 306
Scarsdale Diet, 60
Scheimann, Dr. Eugene, 105
Schizophrenia, 394–95, **697**
    drug induced, 337, 340
School
    athletic programs, 67
    returning to, 436–37, 477
Schulz, Charles, 481
Sciatica, **697**
Sciatic nerve, *18*
Scopolamine, 337, 343–44, **698**
Scrotum, *24, 25*
Scurvy, 44, **698**
Seat belts, use of, 30
Sebaceous glands, **698**
Seconal, 328, 329, **698**
Secondary sex characteristics, 21
Sedatives, 326, 328–30, **698**
    cross-tolerance, as, 328
    depressants, as, 327
    pregnancy and, 350
Self-care, 32–33
Self-help groups, 33–34, 488
Self-respect, 108–9, 117
Semen, 167, **699**

analysis, 207, 209, *214*
Seminal vesicle, *24*
Senescence, **699**
Senility, 448, **699**
Senile macular degeneration, 444
Separation anxiety, 434–35
Serum, blood, **545**
Sewage disposal, 29
Sex Book, A Modern Pictorial Encyclopedia, The, 131
"Sex Can Help You Live Longer," 105
Sex Can Save Your Heart, 105
Sex determination, 167, 169
Sex education, 102, 104, 129, 750
    birth control information, 129–30
Sex Information and Education Council of the United States (SIECUS), 131, 750
Sex-linked abnormalities, **699**
Sex organs, female, *see* individual organs; Reproductive system
Sex organs, male, **700**
Sexual health, 102–31
    adolescence, 103–4
    birth control and, 129–30
    bisexualism, 127–29
    childhood and infancy, 102–3
    fantasies, 126
    love and, 107–8
    masturbation, 124–26
    sexual activity, *see* Sexual relations
    society and, 102–5
    therapy, sexual, 115–19
Sexual intercourse, *see* Sexual relations
Sexual therapy, 115–19, 750
    group therapy, 118
    physical examination, 116
    physical problems, 116–17
    psychological problems, 117–18
    therapists, finding, 118–19
Sexual relations, 105–7, **700**
    aging and, 471–72
    casual, 119, 120
    childbirth, resumption after, 202
    communication in, 113, 115
    disease and, *see* Sexually transmissible diseases
    extramarital, 121–24
    lesbianism, 127–29
    love and, 107–8
    pregnancy and, 167, 180–81
    rape, *see* Rape
    response in, 109–15
    single woman, 119–21
    types of, 108
Sexually transmissible diseases, 245–62
    (*see also* individual diseases)
    anally transmitted, 261–62
    associations concerned with, 750
    attitudes toward, 107, 117

barrier contraceptives and, 150–52
carriers, 246
descriptions, 249–62
diagnostic tests, 185, 248–49, 737
education concerning, 246
incidence, factors in, 246
orally transmitted, 261–62
partners, treatment of, 249
pregnancy, 185, 186, 248, 250
prevention, 247
rape and, 374
reporting, 246
Sheirman, Dr. Gail, 77
Shigellosis, 261–62
Shingles, *see* Herpes zoster
Shock, **700**
Shock treatment, **593**
Shoulder Stand, 82
Sickle cell disease, **701**
associations concerned with, 750
Sickle Cell Disease Foundation of
    Greater New York, 750
Side Bender, 81
SIECUS, 131, 750
Silicone implantation, **702**
Single woman, 408–9
casual sex, 119, 120
celibacy, 121
Sinoauricular node, *5*
Sinuses, **702**
Sinusitis, **702**
Sit-up, 85
Skating, 71
Skeletal system, 4, *6, 7* (color inserts)
Skiing, 71, 75
Skin, *5*, 392, **703**
dermabrasion, 305–6
diseases, *see* individual diseases
pigmentation, oral contraceptives and,
    141
Skin care, 442–44, **704, 750**
Skull, *6*
Slavery, rape and, 365
Sleep, 30, 473–74, **704**
exercise and, 69
Sleeping pills, 30
(*see also* individual drugs; Barbi-
    turates)
alcohol and, 328
availability, 325, 326
Slide test, 172
Slipped disc, **582**
Smallpox, **705, 739**
Smegma, **705**
Smith, Bradley, 131
Smokenders, 751
Smoking, 30, 450, 452, **765**
associations concerned with, 751
breast-feeding and, 179, 352

contraceptive choice and, 136, 140,
    141
discontinuance, 348
heart attacks and, 141
physiological effects, 347–48
pregnancy and, 177, 179, 352
safety precautions, 464
social acceptance, 326
Snoring, **706**
Soap, **706**
Soccer, 71, 75
Social security system, 467
Social workers, qualifications of, 397
Sodium, 45
Sodium chloride, *see* Salt
Sodium warfarin (Coumadin), 743
Softball, benefits of, 75
Soleus muscle, *8*
Sonography, 191, 226
Sontag, Susan, 472
Sopor, 328
Spas, health, 66
Spasm, **706**
Specialist, selection of, 495
Speculum, 222, *223,* **706**
Speech, 751
disorders, **706**
Speech and Hearing Institute, 751
Sperm, 21, 167, 207, **707**
antibodies, 212
artificial insemination, 219–20
Sperm banks, **707**
Spermicides, 135, 150, *151*
Spider hemangiomas, 316
Spinal anesthesia, 195
Spinal cord, 17, *18,* **707**
Spinal tap, **707**
Spine, *6,* 17, **729**
backache and, **538**
slipped disc, **582**
Spironazide (Aldacazide), 742
Spironolactone (Aldactone), 742
Spleen, *12,* **707**
Sports, 66, 71–76
(*see also* individual sports)
age-appropriate, 97–100
calories burned, table of, 71
clothing and equipment, 72, 73, 271
injuries, 73
menstruation and, 75
pregnancy and, 74
selection in personal fitness program,
    76
Spotting, **708**
Spouse abuse, 122, 379–81
Sprain, **708**
Sprinter's Drive, 82
Squash (game), 71
Squat Bender, 78
Squat Thrust, 80

Stabilizers as food additives, 48
Staphylococcus infection, **708**
Starches, digestion of, 14
STD, *see* Sexually transmissible diseases
Stelazine, 328
Sterility, *see* Infertility; Sterilization
Sterilization, 130, 136, 155, 158, **709**
    associations, concerned with, 751
    female, *135*, 155–56
        hysterectomy, *see* Hysterectomy
    involuntary, 158
    male, *135*, 156, *157*, 158
    reversal, 158, 163
Sternocleidomastoid, *8*
Sternum, *6*
Steroids, *see* Corticosteroids
Stethoscope, **709**
Stillbirth, **709**
Stillman, Dr., 61
Stimulants, 322, 327, 334–35, **709**
    (*see also* individual stimulants)
    pregnancy and, 350–51
Stomach, *12*, *13*, 14, *392*, **709**
Strength exercises:
    Abdominal lift, 87
    Arch back, 86
    Back lift, 86
    Back-up, 85
    Broomstick exercises, 90–91
    Dumbbells, with, 92–94
    Flutter legs, 82
    Knee lift, 81
    Leg raiser, 86
    Push-back, 89
    Push-up, 84
    Push-up, knee, 84
    Reach and lift, 87
    Sit-up, 85
    Squat bender, 78
    Squat thrust, 80
    Toe raise, 92
    Weights, with, 94–96
Strain, **709**
Streptococcus infection, **709**
Streptomycin, **710**
Stress, 384–85, **710**
    controlling, 30
    cosmetic surgery and, 295
    exercise and, 69
    infertility and, 207
    love and, 107
    menstrual period and, 227
    overloads, 390
    pregnancy and, 176–77
    transition periods, in, 387–88
Stretch marks, 203, **710**
Stroke, 448–51, **710**
    oral contraceptives and, 138
    smoking and, 141
Stuttering, **711**

Sty, **711**
Sudafed (pseudoephedrine), 743
Sugars, 14, 48, 49, **711**
Suicide, 475, **711**, 751
Sulfa drugs, 249, 253
    allergy to, 249
Sulfisoxazole (Gantrisin), 743
Sulfonamides, **712**
Sunburn, **712**
    aging and, 442
Superficial peroneal nerve, *18*
Superior vena cava, *9*
"Support groups," 400–1
Suppositories, **712**
Surgeon, role of, 502
Surgery, 243, **712**
    (*see also* individual condition or
        procedure)
Surrogate mother, 219–20, **713**
Sutton, Laird, 131
Sweat, *see* Perspiration
Sweeteners, artificial, 49, 180
Swelling, **713**
Swimming, 71, 74
Synapses, 15
Syndrome, **714**
Synovial membrane, *7*
Syphilis, 248, 256–57
    pregnancy and, 185, 186

Taller, Dr. Herman, 60
Talwin (pentazocine), 328, 344, 743
Tampon, **714**
Tanning, 305, 442
Tarnower, Dr., 60
Tars, 347
Tarsals, *6*
Tatum-T, 146
Tay-Sachs disease, **714**, 751
TB, *see* Tuberculosis
Tear glands, *see* Lacrimal ducts
Teenagers
    contraceptive choice, 136
    motherhood by, 129
Teeth
    aging and, 447
    care of, *see* Dental care
Telemetry, **714**
Temperature, *see* Fever
Temperature rhythm family planning,
    153–54
Tendons, 4
Tennis, 71, 75
Tension, 385, 386, **714**
Tenuate (diethylpropion), 743
Terramycin, **714**
Test tube baby, **714**
Testicles, 21, *24*, *25*, **715**
Testosterone, 21
    infertility and, 209, 216

Tetanus, 29, **715**, 738, 739
  drug use and, 324
Tetracycline (Achromycin), 185, **715**
  chancroid, for, 249
  granuloma inguinale, 253
  syphilis, 258
Tetrahydrocannabinol, see Hashish;
  Marijuana
Thalidomide, 179, 350
THC, 337, 341–43
Therapy, sexual, see Sexual therapy
Thermography, **716**
Thiamine (Vitamin B₁), 40–42, **716**
Thorazine (Chlorpromazine), 328, 398,
  559, **716**, 743
Throat disorders, **716**
Thromboembolism, see Blood clots
Thrombosis, **716**
Thymus, *20*, 21
Thyroid, 19, *20*, 48, 70–71, 448
  goiter, 48, **612**
  hyperthyroidism, 19, 212, **633**
  hypothyroidism, 19, 212
  therapy involving, 63, 208, 209, *210*,
    212
Thyroid stimulating hormone (TSH), *20*
Thyroxin, 19, *20*
Tibia, *6*
Tibialis anterior muscle, *8* (color insert)
Tibial nerve, *18*
Tic, **716**
Ticks, **717**
Tigan (trimethobenzamide), 743
Tinnitus, **717**
Tobacco, see Smoking
Toe Raise, 92
Tofranil, 398
Tolbutamide (Orinase), **668**, 743
Tolerance, drug, defined, 319
Tolinase, **717**
Tonsils, **717**
TOPS (Take Off Pounds Safely), 63
Touching, emotional importance of, 106
Toxemia, **717**
Toxic shock syndrome, **718**
Toxoplasmosis, 176, **718**
Trachea, 10, *11*
Trachoma conjunctivitis, 739
Tranquilizers, 30, 320, 326–30, **718**
  pregnancy and, 179, 350
Transcendental meditation, see Medi-
  tation
Transfusion, **718**
Transition periods, stress in, 387–88
Transplant, **719**
Transportation, 468
Transverse presentation, 199, *200*
Trapezius muscle, *8*
Travel, pregnancy and, 180
Treatment, early diagnosis and, 29, 30–31

Tremor, **719**
Trench mouth, see Gums
Triamcinolone (Aristocort, Kenalog),
  742, 743
Triceps, *8*
Trichomonas vaginalis, 232, **720**
Trichomoniasis, 258
Tricuspid valve, *8*
Trigeminal neuralgia, **720**
Triglycerides, **720**
Trimethobenzamide (Tigan), 743
Trisomy, 21, *190*
Trisomy X, *190*
Trunk Rotator, 89
TSH, see Thyroid stimulating hormone
Tubal ligation, *135*, 155–56, **720**
  reversal possibility, 156
Tubal pregnancy, see Ectopic pregnancy
Tuberculosis (BCG), **720**, 739
Tularemia, immunization, 739
Tumors, **721**
  radiation therapy, 243
  types, 230, 234
Turner's syndrome, *190*
Twilight sleep, 195
Twins, 169
Tylenol (acetaminophen), **721**, 743
Typhoid fever, **721**, 739
Typhus, **722**, 739

Ulcers, 29, **722**
Ulna, *6*
Ulnar artery, *9*
Ulnar nerve, *18*
Ultrasound, 191
Umbilical cord, 169, *170*, 192, **723**
Undulant fever, **723**
Unitarian Church, 478
United Cerebral Palsy Associations,
  Inc., 745
United Ostomy Association, 749
University hospital centers, 497–98
University of San Francisco, 477
Uremia, see Kidney disorders
Ureters, 15, *16*, **723**
Urethra, 15, *16*, *24*, 25, **724**
Urethral meatus, see Meatus
Urethritis, 231
Urinary system, 15, *16*, **724**, 748 (color
  insert)
  aging and, 453–54
  disorders, 185, 203
  diuretics and, see Diuretics
Urine, 15, 29, 183, 231, **725**
Urologists, 207, **584**
Uterus, *22*, *23*, 25, *170*, 202, *392*, **725**
  abnormalities, *211*, 212
  conception and, 167, *168*
  fibroids, *211*, 212, 228, 229, 235, 239
  lining, see Endometrium

menstrual cycle and, 26, *27*, 28, 229
perforation, 148
prolapse, 231
removal, *see* Hysterectomy
tumors, 230, 235

Vaccination, 29, 180, **726**
Vacuum extractor, 196
Vagina, *22, 23, 25, 170, 224, 392,* **726**
care of, **727**
delivery through, *197*
examination, 222, *223,* 224
infertility and, *210,* 211, 212
menstrual cycle changes, 28
tumors, 234
Vaginal discharge, 141, 230–33, **727**
Vaginal smear, **727**
Vaginismus, 116
Vaginitis, 232–33, 258–59, **728**
Valium (diazepam), 325–26, 328–29,
398, **728,** 743
fetus, effect on, 179
Varicella (chickenpox), 739
Varicocele, 207, *208,* 209
Varicose veins, 451, **728**
Variola, *see* Smallpox
Vas deferens, 24
Vasectomy, *135, 156, 157,* 158, **729**
Vasopressin, 19
V-Cillin K (penicillin V [K]), 743
VD, *see* Sexually transmissible diseases
Vegetarianism, **729**
Vein, **729**
Venereal disease, *see* Sexually transmis-
sible diseases
Ventricles, *5*
Vertebra, *6,* 17, **730**
Vertigo, **730**
Vibramycin (doxycycline), 743
Vibrators, 114
Vincent's angina, *see* Gums
Violence, rape as crime of, 262
Virus, **730**
Vision disorders, *see* Eyes
Visiting Nurse Association, 507–8
Vitamin A, 39–41
Vitamin B_1 (thiamine), 40–42, **716**
Vitamin B_2 (riboflavin), 40–43
Vitamin B_3 (niacin), 40, 41, 43
Vitamin B_6 (pyridoxine), 40, 41, 43
Vitamin B_{12} (cobalamin), 40, 41, 43,
44
Vitamin C (ascorbic acid), 40, 41, 44,
48, **535**
Vitamin D, 39–41
Vitamin E, 39–42
Vitamin K, 40–42
Vitamins (generally), 38–44, 48,
56–57, **730**
Vitiligo, **731**

Vocal cords, **731**
Volatile solvents as depressants, 328,
333
Volleyball, 71, 75
Vomiting, **731**
Vulva, 21, 234, **732**

Walking, benefits of, 63, 74
War, rape and, 365
Warm-up period, 76, 77
Warts, 237, 257, 259–60, **732**
Waste removal, 15, 69
urine, *see* Urine
Water, fluoridation of, 29, 48, **603**
Water skiing, 71, 75
Weapon in rape, 366
Weight control, 29, 59–64, 203, **667**
associations concerned with, 751
drug use for reduction, 322, 334
ideal weight table, 52–54
Weight lifting, 75, 94–96
Weight Watchers International, 33, 61,
63, 751
Whooping cough (pertussis), 29, 738,
739
Widowhood, 435, 469–70, 478
Widow-to-Widow program, 478
Wife beating, *see* Spouse abuse
Windpipe, *see* Trachea
Wing Stretch, 88
Withdrawal, drug, 346
Withdrawal method of contraception,
154, **562**
Womb, *see* Uterus
Women, changing roles of, 403–18
adolescence, 103–4
conflicts, 404
expectations, rigidity of, 404–5
family size and, 133
history, 403–4
Women's Crisis Center, Rape, 750
Work
elderly, availability for, 467
mothers, by, 406–7, 413–14, 436–37
Worms, **732**
Wound, **733**
Wrestling, 71
Wrinkles, **734**

Xerography, **734**
X-rays, 225–26, **734**

Yeast infections (monilia), 232, 233,
259–60, **657**
Yellow fever immunization, 29, 739
Yoga, 75, **735**
Yogurt, **735**

Zero Population Growth, Inc., 745,
751

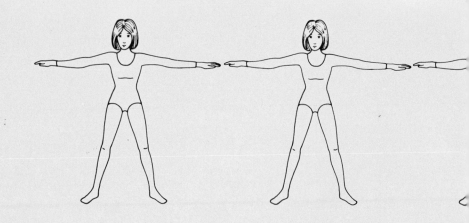

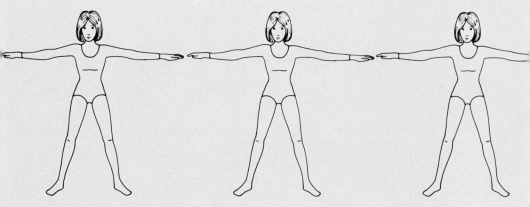

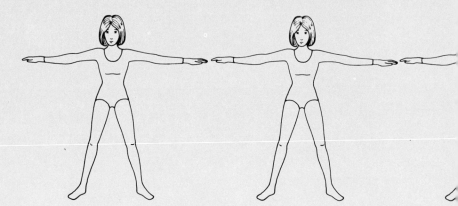

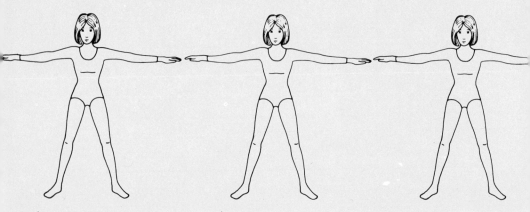